Clinical Cardio-oncology

Clinical Cardio-oncology

JOERG HERRMANN, MD
Department of Cardiovascular Diseases
Mayo Clinic
Rochester, MN, USA

ELSEVIER

ELSEVIER

1600 John F. Kennedy Blvd.
Ste 1800
Philadelphia, PA 19103-2899

Clinical Cardio-oncology
ISBN: 978-0-323-44227-5

Notices

Knowledge and best practice in this field are constantly changing. As new research and experience broaden our understanding, changes in research methods, professional practices, or medical treatment may become necessary.

Practitioners and researchers must always rely on their own experience and knowledge in evaluating and using any information, methods, compounds, or experiments described herein. In using such information or methods they should be mindful of their own safety and the safety of others, including parties for whom they have a professional responsibility.

With respect to any drug or pharmaceutical products identified, readers are advised to check the most current information provided (i) on procedures featured or (ii) by the manufacturer of each product to be administered, to verify the recommended dose or formula, the method and duration of administration, and contraindications. It is the responsibility of practitioners, relying on their own experience and knowledge of their patients, to make diagnoses, to determine dosages and the best treatment for each individual patient, and to take all appropriate safety precautions.

To the fullest extent of the law, neither the Publisher nor the authors, contributors, or editors, assume any liability for any injury and/or damage to persons or property as a matter of products liability, negligence or otherwise, or from any use or operation of any methods, products, instructions, or ideas contained in the material herein.

Library of Congress Cataloging-in-Publication Data

A catalog record for this book is available from the Library of Congress

Content Strategist: Maureen Iannuzzi
Content Development Specialist: Susan Showalter
Design Direction: Renee Duenow

Printed in United States of America

Last digit is the print number: 9 8 7 6 5 4 3 2 1

Contributors

EDITOR

JOERG HERRMANN, MD
Department of Cardiovascular Diseases
Mayo Clinic
Rochester, MN, USA

AUTHORS

MICHAEL JACOB ADAMS, MD, MPH, FACPM
Associate Professor
Department of Public Health Sciences
University of Rochester School of Medicine and Dentistry
Rochester, NY, USA

YEHUDA ADLER, MD, MHA
The Chaim Sheba Medical Center
Tel Hashomer
The Sackler School of Medicine
Tel Aviv University
Tel Aviv, Israel

SHAHNAWAZ M. AMDANI, MBBS, MD
Division of Pediatric Cardiology
Department of Pediatrics
Children's Hospital of Michigan
Detroit, MI, USA

PHILIP A. ARAOZ, MD
Professor of Radiology
College of Medicine
Mayo Clinic
Rochester, MN, USA

OLEXIE ASEYEV, MD, PhD
The Ottawa Hospital Cancer Center
Department of Medicine
University of Ottawa
Ottawa, Ontario, Canada

NEHA BANSAL, MD
Division of Pediatric Cardiology
Department of Pediatrics
Children's Hospital of Michigan
Detroit, MI, USA

ANA BARAC, MD, PhD, FACC
MedStar Heart and Vascular Institute
Georgetown University
Washington, DC, USA

MICHAEL BAUM, MD
Attending Physician
Memorial Hospital
Clinical Member
Memorial Sloan Kettering
Assistant Professor of Clinical Medicine
Weill Cornell Medical College
New York, NY, USA

GINA BIASILLO, MD
Cardioncology Unit
European Institute of Oncology
Milan, Italy

ALLEN BURKE, MD
Professor of Pathology
Section Head, Thoracic Pathology
University of Maryland School of Medicine
Baltimore, MD, USA

ALAN C. CAMERON, BSc (Hons), MB ChB, MRCP
Clinical Research Fellow in Cardiovascular Medicine
Institute of Cardiovascular and Medical Sciences
BHF Glasgow Cardiovascular Research Centre
University of Glasgow
Glasgow, Scotland, UK

DANIELA CARDINALE, MD, PhD, FESC
Director, Cardioncology Unit
European Institute of Oncology
Milan, Italy

JOSEPH R. CARVER, MD
Abramson Family Cancer Research Institute
Abramson Cancer Center of the University of Pennsylvania
Philadelphia, PA, USA

CAROL CHEN, MD
Associate Attending Physician
Memorial Hospital
Associate Clinical Member
Memorial Sloan Kettering
Associate Professor of Clinical Medicine
Weill Cornell Medical College
New York, NY, USA

JENNIFER CROMBIE, MD
Clinical Fellow, Medical Oncology
Dana Farber Cancer Institute
Boston, MA, USA

GIUSEPPE CURIGLIANO, MD, PhD
Division of Development of New Drugs
European Institute of Oncology
Milano, Italy

SUSAN DENT, MD, FRCPC
Division of Medical Oncology
The Ottawa Hospital Cancer Centre
Ottawa, Ontario, Canada

WILLIAM FINCH, MD
Cardiovascular Fellow
Division of Cardiology, Department of Medicine
University of California, Los Angeles
Los Angeles, CA, USA

VIVIAN I. FRANCO, MPH
Division of Pediatric Cardiology
Department of Pediatrics
Children's Hospital of Michigan
Detroit, MI, USA

RYAN K. FUNK, MD
Department of Radiation Oncology
Mayo Clinic
Rochester, MN, USA

DIPTI GUPTA, MD, MPH
Assistant Attending Physician
Memorial Hospital
Assistant Member
Memorial Sloan Kettering
Instructor in Medicine
Weill Cornell Medical College
New York, NY, USA

W. GREGORY HUNDLEY, MD
Section on Cardiovascular Medicine
Professor, Department of Internal Medicine
Wake Forest School of Medicine
Winston-Salem, NC, USA

CEZAR ILIESCU, MD, FACC, FSCAI
Associate Professor
Department of Cardiology
Director, Cardiac Catheterization Laboratory
The University of Texas MD Anderson Cancer Center
Houston, TX, USA

GLORIA ILIESCU, MD
Assistant Professor
Department of General Internal Medicine
The University of Texas MD Anderson Cancer Center
Houston, TX, USA

MASSIMO IMAZIO, MD, FESC
Cardiology Department
Maria Vittoria Hospital
Department of Public Health and Pediatrics
University of Torino
Torino, Italy

MICHELLE JOHNSON, MD, MPH
Attending Physician
Memorial Hospital
Clinical Member
Memorial Sloan Kettering
Assistant Professor of Clinical Medicine
Weill Cornell Medical College
New York, NY, USA

LEE W. JONES, PhD
Attending Physiologist
Memorial Hospital
Member
Memorial Sloan Kettering
New York, NY, USA

ROBIN L. JONES, MD, BSc, MRCP, MB
The Royal Marsden Hospital NHS Foundation Trust
London, England, UK;
The Institute of Cancer Research
London, England, UK;
Seattle Cancer Care Alliance
Seattle, Washington, USA

JENNIFER H. JORDAN, PhD, MS
Section of Cardiovascular Medicine
Assistant Professor, Department of Internal Medicine
Wake Forest School of Medicine
Winston-Salem, NC, USA

GHAZALEH KAZEMI, MD
Assistant Professor
Department of Oncology
McMaster University
Hamilton Health Sciences Juravinski Cancer Centre
Hamilton, Ontario, Canada

BIJOY K. KHANDHERIA, MD, FASE, FAHA, FESC, FACC
Clinical Adjunct Professor of Medicine
University of Wisconsin School of Medicine
Karen Yontz Center for Cardio-Oncology
Aurora Health Care
Milwaukee, WI, USA

NADIA N. ISSA LAACK, MD, MS
Department of Radiation Oncology
Mayo Clinic
Rochester, MN, USA

NINIAN N. LANG, MB, ChB, PhD, MRCP
Consultant Cardiologist and Honorary Senior Lecturer
Institute of Cardiovascular and Medical Sciences
BHF Glasgow Cardiovascular Research Centre
University of Glasgow
Glasgow, Scotland, UK

MICHAEL S. LEE, MD
Associate Clinical Professor of Medicine
Division of Cardiology
Department of Medicine
University of California, Los Angeles
Los Angeles, CA, USA

DANIEL J. LENIHAN, MD
Professor of Cardiovascular Medicine
Vanderbilt University Medical Center
President, International Cardio-Oncology Society-North America (ICOSNA)
Nashville, TN, USA

AMIR LERMAN, MD
Department of Cardiovascular Diseases
Mayo Clinic
Rochester, MN, USA

MARK N. LEVINE, MD, MSc
Professor and Chair
Department of Oncology
McMaster University
Hamilton Health Sciences Juravinski Cancer Centre
Hamilton, Ontario, Canada

OREN LEVINE, MD
Research Fellow
Department of Oncology
McMaster University
Hamilton Health Sciences Juravinski Cancer Centre
Hamilton, Ontario, Canada

STEVEN E. LIPSHULTZ, MD, FAAP, FAHA
Schotanus Family Endowed Chair of Pediatrics
Carman and Ann Adams Endowed Chair in Pediatric Research
Professor, Carman and Ann Adams Department of Pediatrics
Professor of Medicine (Cardiology), Oncology, Obstetrics-Gynecology, Molecular Biology-Genetics, Family Medicine-Public Health Sciences, and Pharmacology
Member, Center for Urban Responses to Environmental Stressors
Professor, Center for Molecular Medicine and Genetics
Wayne State University School of Medicine
President, University Pediatricians and Interim Director
Children's Research Center of Michigan
Pediatrician-in-Chief
Children's Hospital of Michigan
Specialist-in-Chief, Pediatrics
Detroit Medical Center
Scientific Member
Karmanos Cancer Institute
Detroit MI, USA

JENNIFER LIU, MD
Attending Physician
Memorial Hospital
Clinical Member
Memorial Sloan Kettering
Associate Professor of Clinical Medicine
Weill Cornell Medical College
New York, NY, USA

MARZIA LOCATELLI, MD
Division of Development of New Drugs
European Institute of Oncology
Milano, Italy

DAN L. LONGO, MD
Professor of Medicine
Harvard Medical School
Deputy Editor
New England Journal of Medicine
Boston, MA, USA

DOR LOTAN, MD
The Chaim Sheba Medical Center
Tel Hashomer
The Sackler School of Medicine
Tel Aviv University
Tel Aviv, Israel

JOSEPH J. MALESZEWSKI, MD
Associate Professor of Laboratory Medicine & Pathology
Associate Professor of Medicine
Consultant
Divisions of Anatomic Pathology, Cardiovascular Diseases, and Clinical Genomics
Mayo Clinic
Rochester, MN, USA

KONSTANTINOS MARMADGKIOLIS, MD, MBA, FACC, FSCAI
Clinical Assistant Professor of Medicine
University of Missouri
Columbia, MO, USA;
Pepin Heart Institute
Florida Hospital
Tampa, FL, USA

EILEEN McALEER, MD
Assistant Attending Physician
Memorial Hospital
Assistant Clinical Member
Memorial Sloan Kettering
Assistant Professor of Clinical Medicine
Weill Cornell Medical College
New York, NY, USA

ROHIT MOUDGIL, MD, PhD
Department of Cardiology
The University of Texas MD Anderson Cancer Center
Houston, TX, USA

EZEQUIEL MUNOZ, MD
The University of Texas
MD Anderson Cancer Center
Houston, TX, USA

LARA F. NHOLA, MD
Department of Cardiovascular Diseases
Mayo Clinic
Rochester, MN, USA

RUPAL O'QUINN, MD
Penn Heart and Vascular Center
Perelman Center for Advanced Medicine
Philadelphia, PA, USA

MATTHEW S. PIEPER, MD
Instructor
College of Medicine
Mayo Clinic
Rochester, MN, USA

SHAWN C. PUN, MD
Fellow
Cardiology Service
Memorial Hospital
New York, NY, USA

BASEL RAMLAWI, MD
Cardiothoracic Surgery
Valley Health System
Winchester, VA, USA

MICHAEL J. REARDON, MD, FACS, FACC
Department of Cardiovascular Surgery
Houston Methodist DeBakey Heart and Vascular Center
Houston Methodist Hospital
Houston, TX, USA

NANCY ROISTACHER, MD
Attending Physician
Memorial Hospital
Clinical Member
Memorial Sloan Kettering
Assistant Professor of Clinical Medicine
Weill Cornell Medical College
New York, NY, USA

JOHN SASSO, MS
Physiologist
Memorial Hospital
New York, NY, USA

WENDY SCHAFFER, MD, PhD
Associate Attending Physician
Memorial Hospital
Associate Clinical Member
Memorial Sloan Kettering
Assistant Professor of Clinical Medicine
Weill Cornell Medical College
New York, NY, USA

RICHARD M. STEINGART, MD
Chief Attending Physician
Memorial Hospital
Member
Memorial Sloan Kettering
Professor of Medicine
Weill Cornell Medical College
New York, NY, USA

ABIGAIL L. STOCKHAM, MD
Department of Radiation Oncology
Mayo Clinic
Rochester, MN, USA

KEITH M. SWETZ, MD, MA, FACP, FAAHPM, HMDC
Section Chief-Medical Director
Palliative Care at the Birmingham VA Medical Center
Assistant Director
UAB Center for Palliative and Supportive Care
Associate Professor of Medicine
University of Alabama School of Medicine
Birmingham, AL, USA

ZOLTAN SZUCS, MD, PhD
The Royal Marsden Hospital NHS Foundation Trust
London, England, UK

MARIA CHIARA TODARO, MD
University of Messina
Messina, Italy

RHIAN M. TOUYZ, MBBCh, PhD, FRCP, FRSE
BHF Chair in Cardiovascular Medicine
Director, Institute of Cardiovascular and Medical Sciences
BHF Glasgow Cardiovascular Research Centre
University of Glasgow
Glasgow, Scotland, UK

HECTOR R. VILLARRAGA, MD
Department of Cardiovascular Diseases
Mayo Clinic
Rochester, MN, USA

YISHAY WASSERSTRUM, MD
The Chaim Sheba Medical Center
Tel Hashomer
The Sackler School of Medicine
Tel Aviv University
Tel Aviv, Israel

JONATHAN W. WEINSAFT, MD
Associate Attending Physician
Memorial Hospital
Associate Member
Memorial Sloan Kettering
Associate Professor of Medicine
Weill Cornell Medical College
New York, NY, USA

HOWARD WEINSTEIN, MD
Associate Attending Physician
Memorial Hospital
Associate Clinical Member
Memorial Sloan Kettering
Assistant Professor of Clinical Medicine
Weill Cornell Medical College
New York, NY, USA

SARA E. WORDINGHAM, MD
Instructor of Medicine
Mayo Clinic College of Medicine
Mayo Clinic
Phoenix, AZ, USA

ERIC H. YANG, MD
Assistant Clinical Professor of Medicine
Division of Cardiology
Department of Medicine
University of California, Los Angeles
Los Angeles, CA, USA

EDWARD T.H. YEH, MD
Professor and Chairman
Department of Internal Medicine
University of Missouri School of Medicine
Columbia, MO, USA

ANTHONY YU, MD
Assistant Attending Physician
Memorial Hospital
Assistant Member
Memorial Sloan Kettering
Instructor in Medicine
Weill Cornell Medical College
New York, NY, USA

PREFACE

Cardio-oncology: What Do You Know?

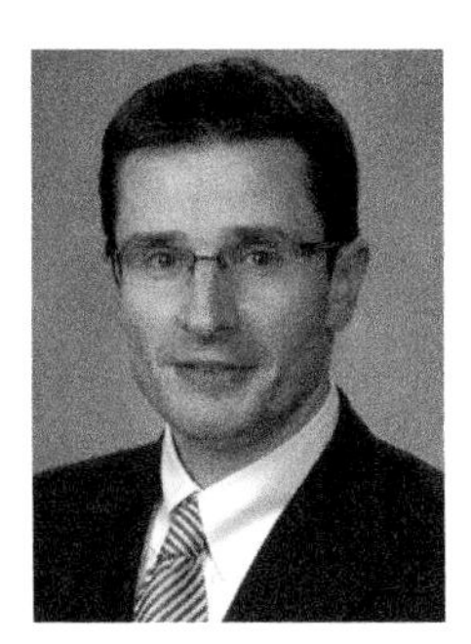

Joerg Herrmann, MD, *Editor*

Cardio-oncology: for some this topic may be rather familiar; for others, it may be the first encounter. Undeniably there is a rapid increase in the number of Cardio-oncology clinics in the United States and globally over the last few years. This is phenomenal in view of the relative paucity of practice guidance in this area. Accordingly, there is a need for a fundamental framework that will sustain this field and its excitement.

This book was developed with the intention to address this need. It provides the reader with the necessary knowledge base of the principles of cancer therapy in the first section, the cardiovascular toxicities that can be caused by cancer therapy in the second section, and the practical integration into the clinic in the third section.

Accordingly, this book should meet the demands of every one engaged in Cardio-oncology, that is, physicians, nurses, nurse practitioners, and pharmacists, and from student to director level.

The content is designed for easy orientation to the relevant needs. For instance, a comprehensive table of the cardiovascular side effects of cancer drugs at the end allows for quick review. For further in-depth study, a specific chapter is available for the main cancer therapy–induced diseases states. Case scenarios are provided to enhance the topic and facilitate translation to personal practice. By reviewing and studying this material and learning on the go, the reader should become very educated and proficient in the practice of Cardio-oncology.

The algorithms, protocols, and tables may be appealing not only as a "guide" to those starting this line of service but also as a "reference" to those who have been in this type of practice for some time. Beyond the more familiar algorithms of surveillance for cardiotoxicity and emerging monitoring algorithms for vascular toxicity, examples of new algorithms include those for general management and care models of patients with cancer before, during, and after their cancer therapy. These aspects may be particularly appealing to those who are intending to start a Cardio-oncology clinic. Further guidance on how to do so is given by pioneers in this particular field.

Moreover, the framework of this book is not only ideal for self-learning and practice building but also for teaching and training programs. Indeed, the content and structure of this book can be directly converted into a formal curriculum in Cardio-oncology, with lectures that follow the three-section template of this book and the individual topics in each section. Unique to this book, experts and pioneers in Cardio-oncology education provide recommendations and suggestions on the elements and start of Cardio-oncology fellowship programs.

To the distinguished expert panel that made this book possible, I am very deeply, personally, and individually indebted. All of them are world-renowned leaders in their fields, and their expertise, commitment, and efforts are truly exemplary, visionary, and extraordinary. Furthermore, I would like to express my deepest gratitude to the publisher and the editorial team for taking on this project and for working relentlessly in order to produce and release this book in just over a year's time.

Collectively, may the work of everyone engaged improve the outcome of those patients who are confronted not only with one but both leading causes of death: cardiovascular diseases and cancer: "Cardio-oncology."

Joerg Herrmann, MD
Department of Cardiovascular Diseases
Mayo Clinic
Rochester, MN, USA

Contents

Section IV
Cardio-oncology in Practice

Clinical Cardio-oncology

Introduction

The care for patients with cancer has advanced tremendously over the past century. Closely related to mustard gas, which was used in the First World War for chemical warfare, nitrogen mustard became the first chemotherapeutic agent to be tested in a clinical lymphoma trial during the Second World War and the first to be introduced as mustine.[1] Thereafter, numerous other agents were discovered and used, inducing remission not only in patients with lymphoma but also in patients with leukemia and even solid cancers.[2] In the 1950s, the concept of cure of cancer emerged, and this became even more a reality in the 1990s, when targeted therapies were introduced. Since then, the cancer-related mortality has declined. On the flip side, a number of agents were found to be associated with cardiac and vascular toxicity (Fig. 1). As a consequence, more than ever, patients with cancer survive with greater chances to experience cardiovascular side effects.

Indeed, since 1990, there has been an increase in cancer survivors to currently almost 15 million in the United States alone and a projection to nearly 20 million by 2020 (Fig. 2). Those who survived their cancer by 5 years or more will constitute the largest group, which is important as the cumulative incidence of chronic health conditions increases with increasing time from cancer diagnosis, including cardiovascular diseases.[3] For instance, childhood cancer survivors face a 15 times higher relative risk of heart failure than their siblings, with anthracyclines and radiation therapy being the strongest risk factors.[3] These risk factors are combined in the treatment of Hodgkin's lymphoma, and the survival course takes three characteristic stages (Fig. 3). In the first phase of nearly 8 years, relapse of the hematologic disease can threaten survival. This is followed by a plateau stage of 8 years, and thereafter, an exponential rise in mortality due to secondary malignancies and cardiovascular disease. In fact, cardiovascular disease is becoming the leading cause of death after 20 years, and cardiovascular mortality is 7 times higher than expected.[4] These dynamics match well with the emergence of clinical heart failure 15 years after anthracycline-based chemotherapy and chest radiation therapy.[5]

Even though the onset is sooner (commonly <10 years), similar dynamics are seen in the adult population, and the consequences are equally severe.[6] It is estimated that currently over 5 million cancer survivors are at a high lifetime risk of cardiomyopathy/heart failure because of exposure to anthracyclines alone. Furthermore, two thirds of the cancer survivors are 65 years or older and with a higher propensity towards comorbidities. A significant proportion of cancer survivors may thus face the burden of morbidity and mortality of cardiovascular diseases in general. Indeed, elderly patients with breast cancer are more likely to die from cardiovascular diseases than cancer over time.[7]

It is important to consider that the 5-year survival rates of heart failure and after the first hospitalization for myocardial infarction are significantly worse than those of Hodgkin's lymphoma, breast cancer, and even colorectal cancer up to their regional disease stage (Fig. 4). Moreover, anthracycline-induced heart failure may carry a prognosis that is worse than that of idiopathic dilated and ischemic cardiomyopathy (Fig. 5). It may be even worse (median survival 2 years) than the prognosis of patients with metastatic breast cancer on dual HER-2–directed therapy (median survival 5 years).[8,9] Cardiotoxicity with HER-2–directed therapy has also received attention; in fact, it received seminal attention in 2001 with a major clinical trial reporting an extremely high and unanticipated incidence of heart failure in patients undergoing HER-2–directed therapy in conjunction with anthracyclines.[10] These observations also provided the final momentum

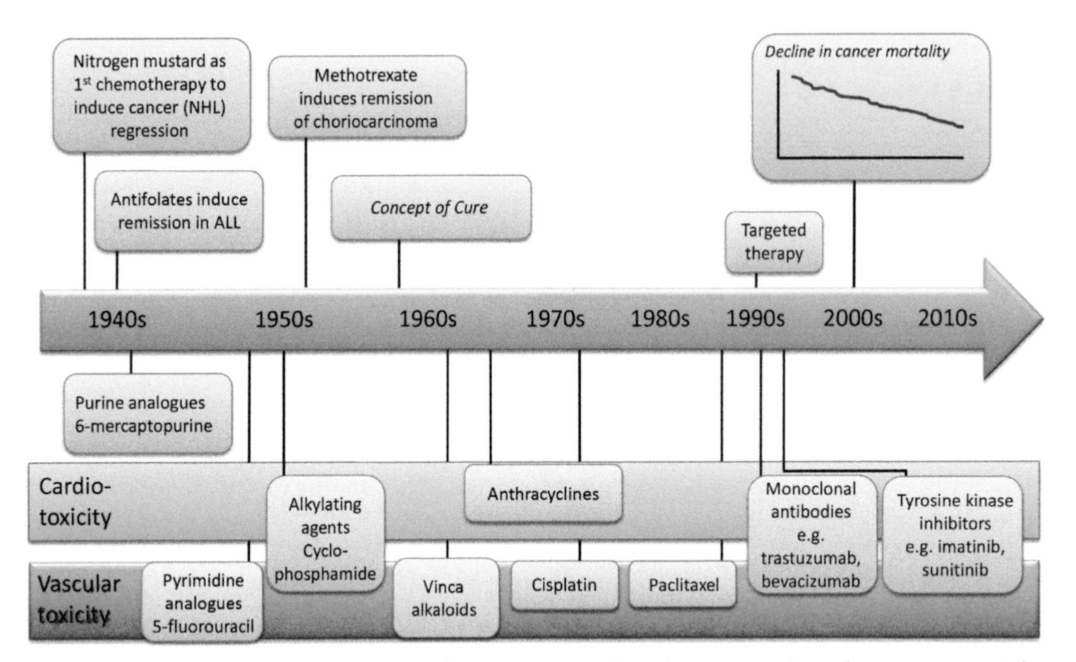

Fig. 1 The history and success of cancer chemotherapy. Agents with cardiotoxicity and vascular toxicity potential are indicated by the alignment with the cardiovascular side-effect bar. ALL, acute lymphoblastic leukemia; NHL, non-Hodgkin's lymphoma.

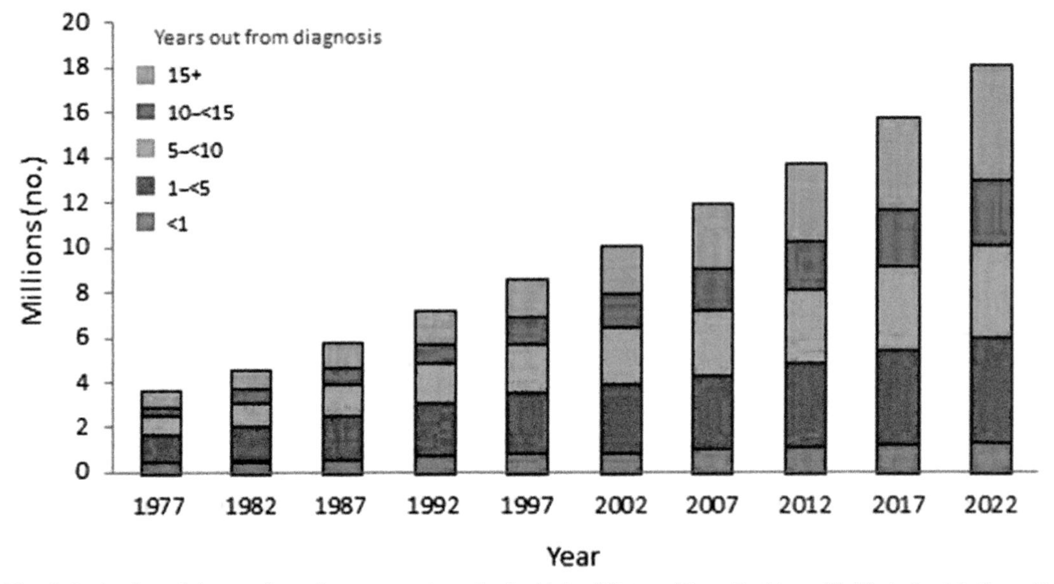

Fig. 2 Projection of the number of cancer survivors in the United States. (*From* De Moor JS, Mariotto AB, Parry C, et al. Cancer survivors in the United States: prevalence across the survivorship trajectory and implications for care. Cancer Epidemiol Biomarkers Prev 2013;22(4):561–70; with permission.)

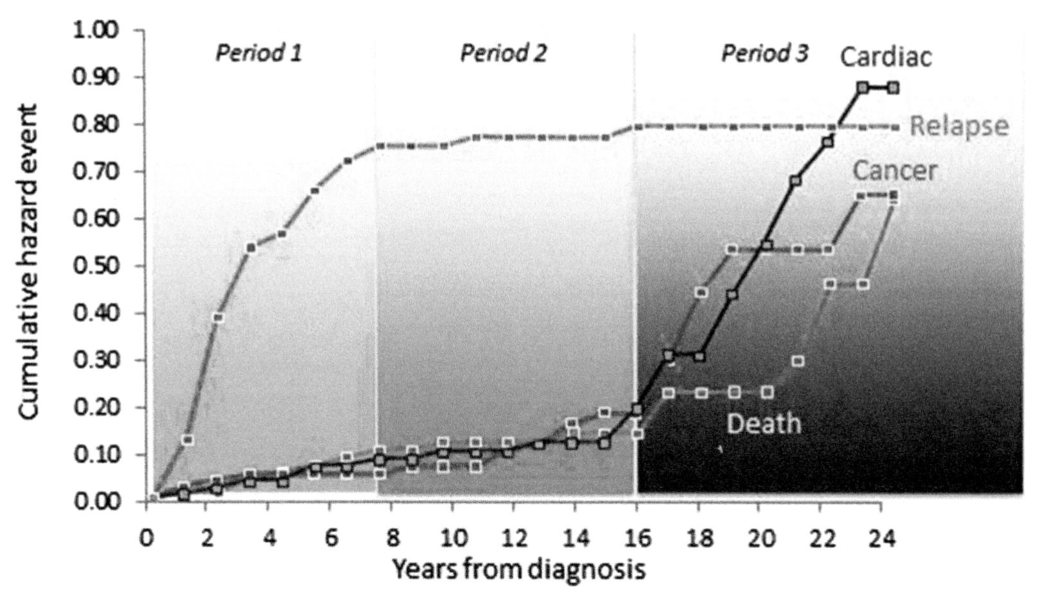

Fig. 3 Number of cancer survivors stratified by years from diagnosis. (*Adapted from* Lee CK, Aeppli D, Nierengarten ME. The need for long-term surveillance for patients treated with curative radiotherapy for Hodgkin's disease: University of Minnesota experience. Int J Radiat Oncol Biol Phys 2000;48:169–79.)

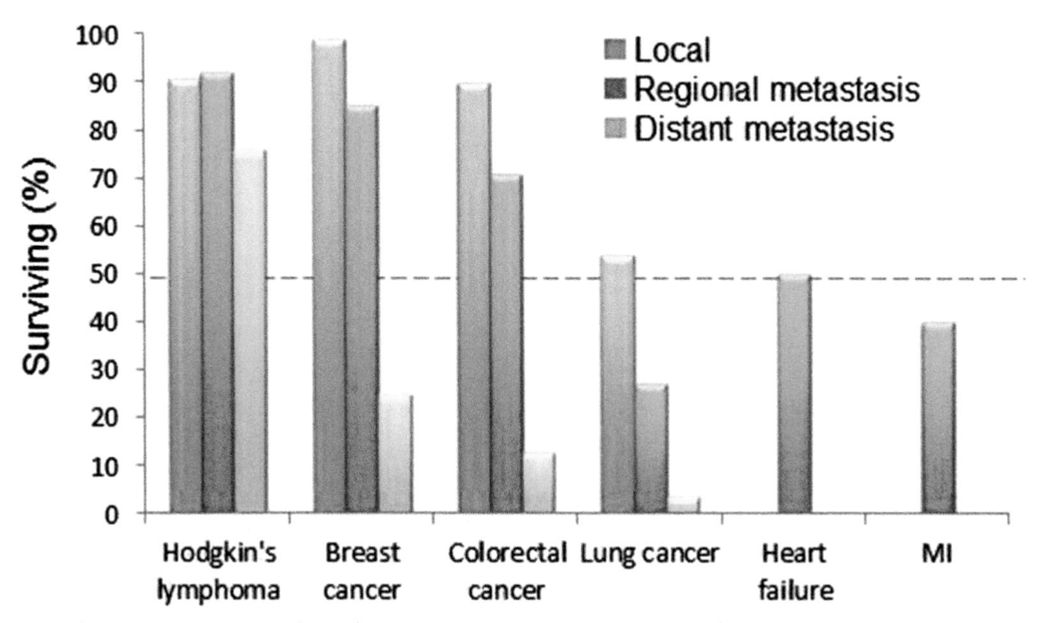

Fig. 4 The 5-year survival rates of specified malignancies, heart failure, and after first hospitalization for acute myocardial infarction (MI). (*From* Howlader N, Noone AM, Krapcho M, et al (eds). SEER Cancer Statistics Review, 1975-2013, National Cancer Institute. Bethesda, MD, http://seer.cancer.gov/csr/1975_2013/, based on November 2015 SEER data submission, posted to the SEER web site, April 2016; Go AS, Mozaffarian D, Roger VL, et al. Heart disease and stroke statistics–2014 update: a report from the American Heart Association. Circulation. 2014;129:e28–292.)

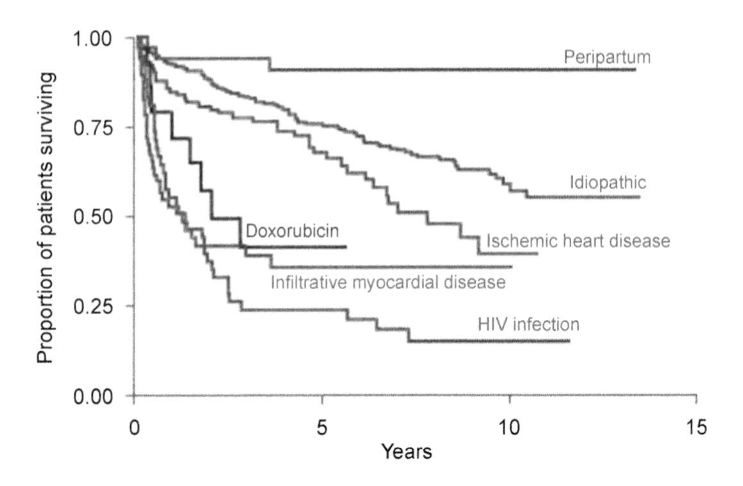

Fig. 5 Cumulative incidence of comorbidities by year from cancer diagnosis. HIV, human immunodeficiency virus. (*Adapted from* Felker GM, Thompson RE, Hare JM, et al. Underlying causes and long-term survival in patients with initially unexplained cardiomyopathy. N Engl J Med 2000;342(15):1077–84.)

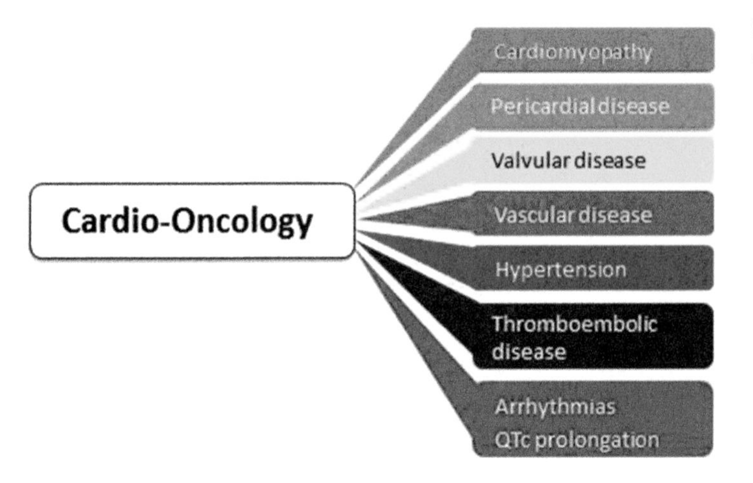

Fig. 6 The spectrum of cardio-oncology.

for a field that has become known as "cardio-oncology."

Sometimes misunderstood as a specialty for "cancer of the heart," cardio-oncology should be considered as the specialty of "cancer and the heart," in fact, the entire spectrum of cardiovascular diseases (Fig. 6). Cardio-oncology may thus be best defined as the specialty that is directed toward the cardiovascular care of patients with cancer. Herein, experts compiled a state-of-the-art collection on these various aspects and a practical companion to Cardio-oncology in clinical practice: "Clinical Cardio-oncology."

Joerg Herrmann, MD
Department of Cardiovascular Diseases
Mayo Clinic
Rochester, MN, USA

REFERENCES

1. DeVita VT Jr, Chu E. A history of cancer chemotherapy. Cancer Res 2008;68(21):8643–53.
2. Chabner BA, Roberts TG Jr. Timeline: Chemotherapy and the war on cancer. Nat Rev Cancer 2005;5(1):65–72.
3. Oeffinger KC, Mertens AC, Sklar CA, et al. Chronic health conditions in adult survivors of childhood cancer. N Engl J Med 2006;355(15):1572–82.
4. Lee CK, Aeppli D, Nierengarten ME. The need for long-term surveillance for patients treated with curative radiotherapy for Hodgkin's disease: University of Minnesota experience. Int J Radiat Oncol Biol Phys 2000;48(1):169–79.
5. Yeh JM, Nohria A, Diller L. Routine echocardiography screening for asymptomatic left ventricular dysfunction in childhood cancer survivors: a model-based estimation of the clinical and economic effects. Ann Intern Med 2014;160(10):661–71.

6. Qin A, Thompson CL, Silverman P. Predictors of late-onset heart failure in breast cancer patients treated with doxorubicin. J Cancer Surviv 2015; 9(2):252–9.
7. Patnaik JL, Byers T, DiGuiseppi C, et al. Cardiovascular disease competes with breast cancer as the leading cause of death for older females diagnosed with breast cancer: a retrospective cohort study. Breast Cancer Res 2011;13(3):R64.
8. Felker GM, Thompson RE, Hare JM, et al. Underlying causes and long-term survival in patients with initially unexplained cardiomyopathy. N Engl J Med 2000;342(15):1077–84.
9. Swain SM, Baselga J, Kim SB, et al. Pertuzumab, trastuzumab, and docetaxel in HER2-positive metastatic breast cancer. N Engl J Med 2015; 372(8):724–34.
10. Slamon DJ, Leyland-Jones B, Shak S, et al. Use of chemotherapy plus a monoclonal antibody against HER2 for metastatic breast cancer that overexpresses HER2. N Engl J Med 2001;344(11): 783–92.

CHAPTER 1

Principles of Cancer Treatment

Jennifer Crombie, MD[a,*], Dan L. Longo, MD[b]

CANCER PRESENTATION

Introduction

Cancer is currently the second leading cause of death in the United States, second only to heart disease, but has already overtaken heart disease as the number one cause of death among those younger than 85 years of age.[1] Although many patients with cancer will ultimately succumb to their disease, advances in current treatment strategies with the use of surgery, radiation therapy, chemotherapy, and biologic agents have resulted in improved survival for patients with cancer. When treating patients with underlying malignancy, it is important to be aware of the complex nature of their disease, possible disease complications, and treatment-related side effects. Given the multisystem nature of disease, care of the patient with cancer must cross multiple disciplines, including cardiology. The need for a multidisciplinary approach is especially relevant as two-thirds of all cancers are diagnosed in those older than 65 years of a age, a population with a high burden of pre-existing cardiovascular disease.[2] Another important aspect is the emotional and psychological dimensions to these diseases. In general, a diagnosis of cancer is perceived far more devastating than a diagnosis of cardiovascular disease, even though the prognosis of the latter can be the same or even worse. On the other hand, when the diagnosis of cardiovascular disease is made in addition to or as a consequence of cancer and its treatment, the devastation is even of greater magnitude.

Cancer Detection

The approach to cancer in the current era is sequentially from the first steps of screening to early diagnosis, staging, and treatment, supportive care, and finally, palliative care (Fig. 1.1). Although not all cancers are curable at presentation, establishing the diagnosis as early as possible often affords the patient the greatest opportunity for cure (Table 1.1).

With the implementation of a variety of screening modalities, cancer can be detected before there are appreciable symptoms. Mammography, colonoscopy, Papanikolaou smears, and low-dose computerized tomography (CT) have allowed for the early detection of breast, colon, cervical, and lung cancer, respectively. Tumor markers, or cancer-specific biomarkers, can also signify the presence of a tumor. Prostate-specific antigen (PSA), for example, is a glycoprotein secreted by epithelial cells within the prostate gland. When elevated in the blood, the PSA can denote prostate cancer. The benefit of early detection of malignancy must be carefully weighed against the harms of overdiagnosis and false positive results when applying these screening modalities in clinical practice.

Although the above-mentioned screening tools can allow for the early detection of tumors, most cancers are detected with the onset of symptoms. It is now understood that tumors result from the abnormal proliferation of either benign or malignant cells. This growth can result in localized swelling and mass effect and can also affect the function of the organ involved, resulting, for example, in hemoptysis from lung cancers, jaundice from tumors obstructing the hepatobiliary tree, bowel obstruction from colon cancers, and neurologic symptoms or seizures from the presence of brain tumors. Hematologic malignancies, such as leukemia, result from abnormal growth of hematopoietic cells within the bone marrow rather than a definable tumor mass. Leukemia often presents with fatigue or dyspnea from

[a] Medical Oncology, Dana Farber Cancer Institute, 50 Brookline Avenue, Boston, MA 02115, USA; [b] New England Journal of Medicine, 10 Shattuck Street, Boston, MA 02115, USA
* Corresponding author.
E-mail address: jlcrombie@partners.org

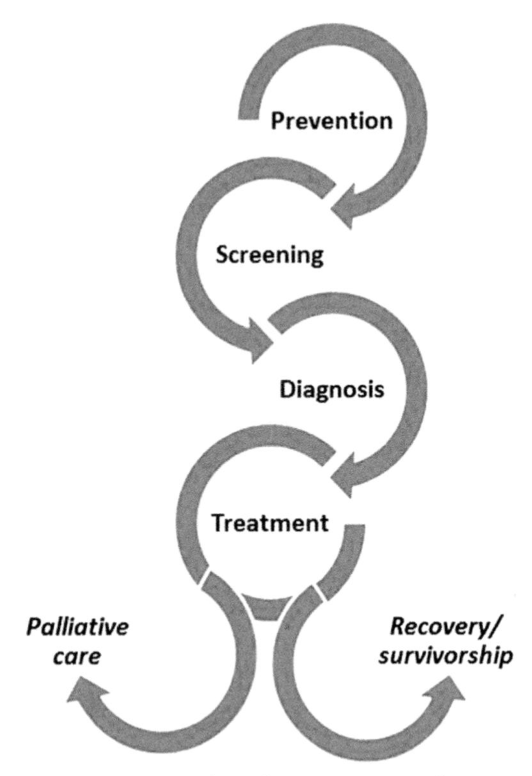

Fig. 1.1 Sequence of care for cancer patients from prevention to survivorship and end of life care.

anemia and bleeding and bruising from thrombocytopenia. The detection of cancer can be made by identifying a mass on physical examination or with the use of imaging modalities, such as plain radiograph, CT, PET, or nuclear MRI. In the case of leukemia, cancer is detected by standard laboratory evaluation, that is, complete blood count with differential (and smear). Endoscopies, which allow for the direct visualization of tumors within gastric, intestinal, colonic and bladder mucosa, also allow for the identification of malignancies of certain organs.

Establishing a Cancer Diagnosis

Although imaging can be used to identify a mass, a pathologic diagnosis is often required to formally make the diagnosis of cancer. Typically, biopsies are performed with the attempt to obtain enough tissue for adequate evaluation in the least invasive way possible. Excisional biopsies are often preferred, because the entire tumor is removed with only a small margin of malignant cells remaining. A core needle biopsy typically contains less tissue, although that can be enough to make a diagnosis. Fine needle biopsy results in a suspension of cells from within the mass. This technique often will allow for the identification of malignant cells, although it may not be adequate to make a formal diagnosis. In rare instances, as in hepatocellular carcinoma, the diagnosis can sometimes be made from MRI alone.[3]

Further analysis of the tumor by light microscopy can demonstrate the proliferation index, degree of atypia, and the presence of microvascular invasion, which provide additional prognostic information. More specifically, the use of immunohistochemistry and protein expression patterns allows for subclassification of a tumor within a cancer type. For example, the presence of Reed-Sternberg cells, a large cell characteristic of Hodgkin lymphoma, can be seen on examination by light microscopy. Further staining of cellular markers, including CD30 and CD15, can confirm their presence and allow for a confirmed diagnosis. Similarly, staining for the presence of estrogen, progesterone, and the human epidermal growth factor receptor 2 (HER2) receptors, can further classify breast cancer and aid in prognostication and therapeutic management.

There are occasions in which metastatic disease is seen, although no clear primary malignancy is identified. The pathologic information from the metastatic lesions, as well as factors such as age, sex, and sites of involvement, should be used in an attempt to define the primary source of malignancy.

CANCER STAGING

Assessing the Extent of the Cancer

Determining the stage of the malignancy is often the most critical for determining prognosis and formulating a treatment strategy because the curability of a tumor is usually inversely related to the tumor burden. For solid tumors originating from a primary site, the TNM staging system, defined by the International Union Against Cancer and the American Joint Committee on Cancer, is classically used to define tumor stage. "T" refers to the size of the tumor and its invasion into local structures. "N" refers to the total number of involved lymph nodes adjacent to the primary tumor. Last, "M" is based on the presence of metastatic or distant disease. Radiographic techniques are typically used to identify areas of possible metastases and complement the physical examination for clinical staging. It is also important to keep staging in mind when choosing a biopsy site at the time of diagnosis. For example, if the patient is found to have a primary colonic mass as well as numerous hepatic lesions, a biopsy of the liver demonstrating colon cancer allows for diagnosis of malignancy and confirmation of metastatic disease. Similarly, staging can also be performed intraoperatively

TABLE 1.1
Curability of cancers with various treatment modalities

Advanced Cancers with Possible Cure with Chemotherapy	Cancers Responsive with Useful Palliation, But Not Cure, by Chemotherapy
Acute lymphoid and acute myeloid leukemia Hodgkin disease Lymphomas—certain types Germ cell neoplasms Embryonal carcinoma Teratocarcinoma Seminoma or dysgerminoma Choriocarcinoma Gestational trophoblastic neoplasia Embryonal rhabdomyosarcoma Peripheral neuroepithelioma Neuroblastoma Small-cell lung cancer Ovarian carcinoma	Bladder carcinoma Chronic myeloid leukemia Hairy cell leukemia Chronic lymphocytic leukemia Lymphoma—certain types Multiple myeloma Gastric carcinoma Cervix carcinoma Endometrial carcinoma Soft tissue sarcoma Head and neck cancer Adrenocortical carcinoma Islet cell neoplasms Breast carcinoma Colorectal carcinoma Renal carcinoma
Advanced Cancers Possibly Cured by Chemotherapy and Radiation	**Cancers Possibly Cured with "High-Dose" Chemotherapy with Stem Cell Support**
Squamous carcinoma (head and neck) Squamous carcinoma (anus) Breast carcinoma Carcinoma of the uterine cervix Non–small-cell lung carcinoma (stage III) Small-cell lung carcinoma	Relapsed leukemias, lymphoid and myeloid Relapsed lymphomas, Hodgkin and non-Hodgkin Chronic myeloid leukemia Multiple myeloma
Cancers Possibly Cured with Chemotherapy as Adjuvant to Surgery	**Tumors Poorly Responsive in Advanced Stages to Chemotherapy**
Breast carcinoma Colorectal carcinoma Osteogenic sarcoma Soft tissue sarcoma	Pancreatic carcinoma Biliary tract neoplasms Thyroid carcinoma Carcinoma of the vulva Non–small-cell lung carcinoma Prostate carcinoma Melanoma (subsets) Hepatocellular carcinoma

with the sampling of surrounding lymph nodes at the time of the primary tumor resection as part of pathologic staging. For example, during a lumpectomy for breast cancer, sentinel lymph node dissection is typically performed to assess for malignancy in the lymph nodes most likely to drain the tumor. Of note, the TMN staging system is only used for patients with solid malignancies. For most malignancies, tumor burden and extent of disease are inversely correlated with curability.

Hematologic malignancies are often disseminated on presentation and therefore have alternative prognostic indicators. In most leukemias, for example, the subtype of disease as well as certain molecular markers determines prognosis. In most lymphomas, stage is determined according to the Ann Arbor classification, which categorizes the location of lymph nodes involved, with either localized disease, disease limited to one side of the diaphragm, disease on both sides of the diaphragm, or disseminated involvement in extralymphatic organs. Other anatomic staging systems include the Dukes classification for colorectal cancer and the International Federation of Gynecologic and Obstetricians classification for gynecologic malignancies.

Assessing the Biological Features of the Cancer

Further understanding of the molecular basis of malignancy has also revealed biologic features specific to certain cancer types. In many cases, these provide further prognostic information. Oncogenes, translocations, antiapoptotic factors, and the presence of genes influencing metastasis may contribute to predictions of how a tumor will behave, respond to therapy, and recur. In many cases, the histology can look identical under the microscope, although the identification of specific biologic features can greatly impact differences in prognosis and even treatment. For example, in diffuse large B-cell lymphomas, the presence of a chromosomal breakpoint affecting the MYC locus in combination with a breakpoint in the gene encoding the antiapoptotic factor Bcl-2 confers a poor prognosis.[4] Patients with these 2 mutations, also known as "double-hit" lymphomas, are typically treated differently than those patients without these mutations.[5] The absence of certain biologic markers can also provide prognostic information. The absence of the estrogen and progesterone receptor, as well as lack of overexpression of HER2 in breast cancer, known as "triple-negative breast cancer," limits the use of targeted therapy and thus has been found to predict an increased risk of disease recurrence.[6]

Assessing the Physiologic Reserve of the Patient

In addition to assessing the extent of disease and biologic features of the tumor, the patient's physiologic reserve is a key determinant of treatment outcome, and this can be significantly influenced by cardiovascular diseases, such as cardiomyopathies and valvular or ischemic heart disease. The patient's physical abilities can predict how likely they are to tolerate the stress of the malignancy as well as the often toxic treatment options. There are a variety of tools that have been designed to quantify the underlying health and baseline performance status of a patient. The Eastern Cooperative Oncology Group (ECOG) performance status uses activity level to assign a score of 0-5 (Table 1.2).[7] A similar system, the Karnofsky Performance Index, uses a scoring system from 20 to 100 to classify a patient's activity level and degree of independence. An ECOG score greater than or equal to 3 or a Karnofsky performance status less than 70 often suggests a poorer prognosis. These scoring systems are also critical to standardizing patients in clinical trials.

TABLE 1.2
Eastern Cooperative Oncology Group performance status

ECOG Score	Description
0	Fully active, able to carry on all predisease performance without restriction
1	Restricted in physically strenuous activity but ambulatory and able to carry out work of light sedentary nature
2	Ambulatory and capable of all self-care but unable to do any work activities. Up and about more than 50% of waking hours
3	Capable of only limited self-care, confined to bed or chair more than 50% of waking hours
4	Completely disabled. Cannot carry on any self-care. Totally confined to bed or chair
5	Dead

CANCER TREATMENT

Setting Treatment Goals—Curative Versus Palliative

Once the diagnosis of cancer is established, a treatment plan can be made, preferably as a multidisciplinary effort, including oncologists, pharmacists, social workers, rehabilitation specialists, primary care physicians, and consulting specialists such as cardio-oncologists. The extent of disease, the patient's performance status, and the patient's wishes are all factors in establishing the most appropriate plan. If possible, the goal is usually for cancer eradication with a curative intent, as for those malignancies listed in Table 1.1. This goal can be achieved with a variety of treatment modalities, although most often by the combination of surgery, chemotherapy, and radiation. If a patient presents with an advanced stage and cure is not possible, the goal is often palliative. In these cases, there is an attempt to use treatment to ameliorate symptoms, preserve quality of life, and increase overall survival. A list of malignancies that is often meaningfully managed with palliative intent is provided in Table 1.1. Patients considered for palliative therapy should have a sound understanding of their diagnosis, prognosis, and treatment limitations and goals, ready access to supportive care, and a suitable performance status (Karnofsky or ECOG; see Table 1.2). Only patients with ECOG performance status 0-2 are generally fit for palliative therapy. With curative intent, even patients with poor performance status may undergo treatment, but face an inferior prognosis compared with those with a good performance status in general. Although the choice of treatment approaches used to be dominated by the practice setting, advances in communication have allowed for access to cross-institutional treatment protocols and every approved clinical research study in North America. Involvement of specialists of different disciplines is particularly important when new drugs are administered to receive guidance on potential toxicity profiles.

Localized Cancer Treatments

Cancer therapy is typically divided into either local or systemic therapy. Local therapy is classically achieved with surgery, radiation therapy, or a combination of the two. The goal with this type of treatment is to remove the tumor cells and treat the surrounding tissue in order to decrease the risk of local recurrence. With surgical excision of a tumor, there must be an adequate margin of normal tissue. The size of the margin is variable and depends on both the type of tumor and its anatomic location. In breast cancer, a patient can undergo either a lumpectomy with subsequent radiation therapy or have a mastectomy in order to remove the tumor and prevent local recurrence. Similarly, in prostate cancer, patients can opt for either resection of the prostate gland through surgical resection or radiation therapy targeted at the prostate. Overall, at least 40% of patients with cancer are cured by surgery, whereas 60% have evidence of metastatic disease, which does not allow for a cure. Under these latter circumstances, tumor removal does not typically improve outcomes, although it can have important palliative benefits, including preservation of organ function, reduction in pain, or improvement in other associated symptoms. For example, if a patient presents with metastatic colon cancer with recurrent intestinal obstructions, resection of the primary mass can dramatically improve quality of life.

RADIATION THERAPY

Systemic Cancer Treatments: Actions and Toxicities

Systemic therapy is fundamental to the treatment of cancer. Although local disease management eliminates the primary lesion, systemic therapy is required to kill micrometastatic disease and prevent metastasis (Fig. 1.2). The need for systemic therapy following local therapy is often dictated by stage and extent of disease at diagnosis. When chemotherapy is given after surgical

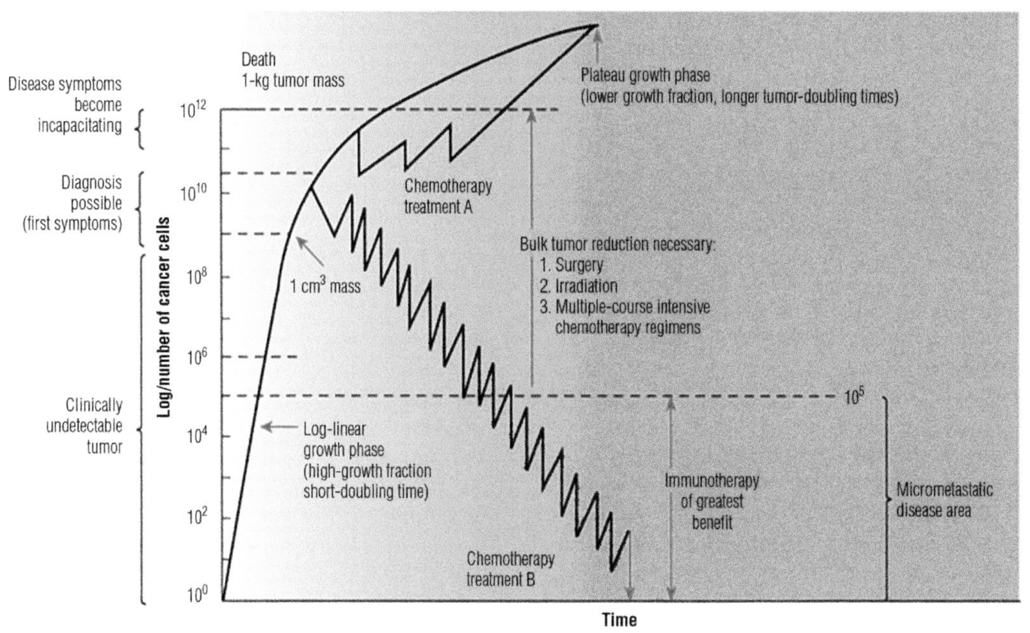

Fig. 1.2 Tumor growth kinetics and the log kill hypothesis of cancer therapy. As outlined, there is a long subclinical period of rapid proliferation. The longer the delay, the higher the overall tumor cell burden. Chemotherapy regimens started late, with infrequent scheduling of treatment courses and low (1 log kill) dosing, prolong survival but do not cure the patient (chemotherapy A, kill rate<growth rate). On the contrary, regimens with more intensive and frequent treatment cycles, adequate (2 log kill) dosing, and an earlier start are geared toward cure (chemotherapy B, kill rate>growth rate). Surgical removal or radiation therapy can reduce the level B-type chemotherapy regimens are starting at, which henceforth can be of shorter duration, geared to eliminate any persistent tumor. (*From* DiPiro JT, Talbert RL, Yee GC, et al. Pharmacotherapy: a pathophysiologic approach. 7th edition. The McGraw-Hill Companies, Inc; with permission.)

resection, it is referred to as *adjuvant* therapy (Box 1.1).

Adjuvant treatment is given to eliminate microscopic residual disease after curative surgery and therefore minimize the risk of reoccurrence and development of distant metastasis, with the aim of improving survival. For solid tumors, the risk of recurrence following resection generally increases with the extent of invasion of the primary tumor and the degree of regional lymph node involvement. In solid tumors, adjuvant therapy ranges from chemotherapy that has shown benefit in advanced disease to more specific application of hormonal, immune, and molecularly targeted therapies. Adjuvant use of these agents is based on increased understanding of tumor biology and signaling pathways. The balance between the therapeutic outcome, acute toxicity, and long-term side effects is an important consideration for adjuvant therapy and should be determined on an individual patient basis. Although most adjuvant therapies are associated with toxicity, the benefits are generally agreed to outweigh the potential risks, given unequivocal improvements in disease-free survival and/or overall survival. The tolerability of more intensive chemotherapy regimens may decrease with increasing intensity of therapy.

A prime example of adjuvant therapy is given in patients with stage I–III breast cancer. The choice of regimen is individualized based on each patient's underlying estimated risk of recurrence, their comorbidities, and likely tolerance of toxicity. The anthracyclines, doxorubicin and epirubicin, were introduced in the 1990s, followed by the addition of taxanes in the early 2000s, which resulted in a reduction of mortality by one-third and the current foundation of adjuvant chemotherapy in early breast cancer. In premenopausal women with estrogen receptor positive (ER+) breast cancer, endocrine treatment with tamoxifen further reduces the risk of recurrence and mortalities.[8] Similar reductions in recurrence rates are seen with the use of aromatase inhibitors in postmenopausal women. In HER-2–positive breast cancers, the addition of trastuzumab to paclitaxel after doxorubicin and cyclophosphamide leads to a substantial and durable improvement in survival as a result of a sustained marked reduction in cancer recurrence.[9]

In non–small-cell lung cancer, adjuvant chemotherapy with cisplatin-based chemotherapy can lead to 100% relative improvement in overall survival, even though the absolute gain is only in the order of 2.5% to 4.1%.

5-Fluorouracil (5-FU) is a component of the standard adjuvant therapy for resected stage III colorectal cancer; its relative contribution in stage II disease remains controversial. National Comprehensive Cancer Network (NCCN) guidelines recommend 6 months of adjuvant chemotherapy with combinations of 5-FU/oxaliplatin–based treatment for stage III disease. Adjuvant chemotherapy with 5-FU–based therapy has a 30% reduction in the risk for recurrence of all stages of colon cancer and a 26% risk of reduction in death. The addition of oxaliplatin and leucovorin to 5-FU further increases the 5-year survival rate by 5%.

Finally, immunity plays a key role in the pathogenesis of melanoma, and induction of immune response is important for disease control in both the adjuvant and advanced disease settings. Adjuvant interferon-α (IFN-α) treatment can be recommended following resection of melanoma at high risk of recurrence (stage IIB–III). IFN-α had significant benefits upon relapse, however with questionable benefits upon survival.

There are instances when systemic treatment is indicated before surgery in order to reduce the size of the tumor and decrease undetectable metastatic disease. This treatment strategy is referred to as *neoadjuvant* therapy. *Neoadjuvant treatment* for potentially operable disease has several potential benefits, including tumor downsizing and improvement in resectability, increased rate of complete macroscopic and

BOX 1.1
Oncology key terms

Adjuvant therapy: Additional cancer treatment given after curative surgery. Adjuvant therapy may include chemotherapy, radiation therapy, hormone therapy, targeted therapy, or biological therapy.

Neoadjuvant therapy: Treatment given as a first step to shrink a tumor before a curative surgery. Examples of neoadjuvant therapy include chemotherapy, radiation therapy, and hormone therapy.

Disease-free survival: The length of time after the primary treatment that the patient survives without any signs or symptoms of that cancer.

Overall survival: The length of time from either the date of diagnosis or the start of treatment that patients are still alive.

Complete response: The disappearance of all signs of cancer in response to treatment.

Partial response: A decrease in the size of a tumor, or in the extent of cancer in the body, in response to treatment.

microscopic clearance of the primary tumor (R0 resection), earlier treatment of micrometastatic disease, as well as the use of the tumor as in vivo marker of response. On the contrary, there is of course the risk of tumor progression, making the tumor inoperable as well as the possibility of clinical deterioration and the increased risk of perioperative complications. Neoadjuvant strategies are best established in the treatment of breast and rectal cancers, where they form current standards of care.

Induction chemotherapy is commonly used in the treatment of acute leukemias, with an aim to achieve optimal remission. *Consolidation chemotherapy* is given once a remission is achieved. The goal of this therapy is to sustain a remission. *Maintenance chemotherapy* is given in lower doses to assist in prolonging a remission. Maintenance chemotherapy is most commonly used in the curative treatment of acute leukemias; however, it is getting more acceptance in the palliative management of solid tumors as well.[3]

Palliative chemotherapy is given specifically to address symptom management without expecting cure. However, as the example of the palliative treatment of advanced/metastatic colorectal cancer shows, life can be significantly prolonged with sequential multiple lines of chemotherapy. Over the last 20 years, the number of effective systemic therapies available to treat patients with metastatic colorectal cancer has increased considerably, with a corresponding improvement in median overall survival from about 6 months to approximately 30 months. These improvements have resulted from the completion of well-designed randomized controlled trials.[3]

Cancer chemotherapy

Systemic cancer treatments take several different approaches (Fig. 1.3), which can be broadly categorized into 4 types. *Conventional "cytotoxic" chemotherapy agents* mainly target DNA structure or segregation of DNA as chromosomes in mitosis (Fig. 1.4A). *Targeted agents* interact with a defined molecular target important in maintaining the malignant state or expressed by the tumor cells (Fig. 1.4B). *Hormonal therapies* capitalize on the biochemical pathways underlying estrogen and androgen function and act as a therapeutic basis for approaching patients with tumors of breast, prostate, uterus, and ovarian origin (Fig. 1.4C). *Biologic therapies* expand on these to regulate growth of tumor cells by inducing differentiation or dormancy or a host immune response to kill tumor cells (Fig. 1.4D). Any of the drugs used for systemic treatment has been designed to kill tumor cells but can also exert toxic effects to the host. The separation of the two has become known as the *therapeutic index*. A large therapeutic index is ideal, leveraging, for instance, on the selective expression of the drug

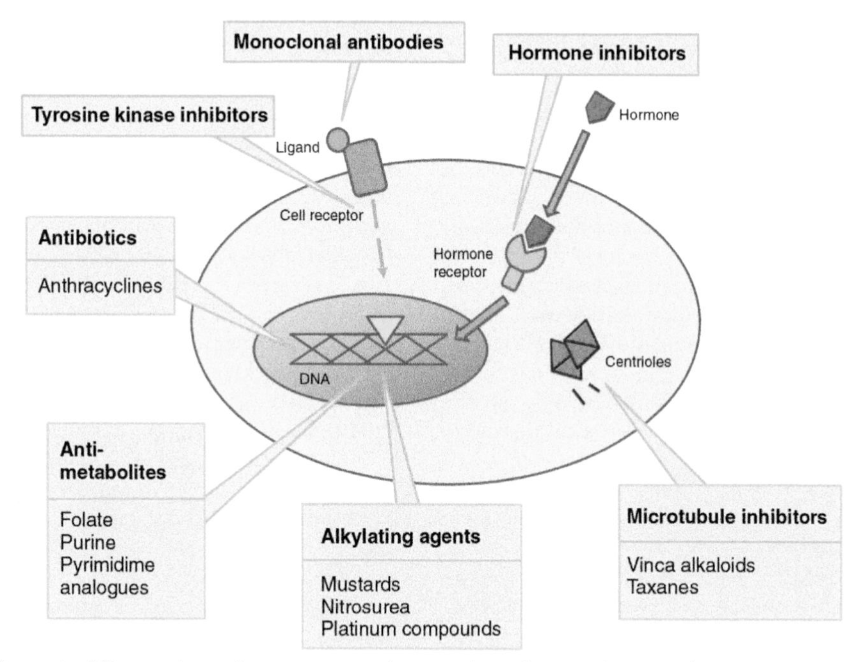

Fig. 1.3 The main different chemotherapies currently in use based on mechanism of action and target within the cancer cell.

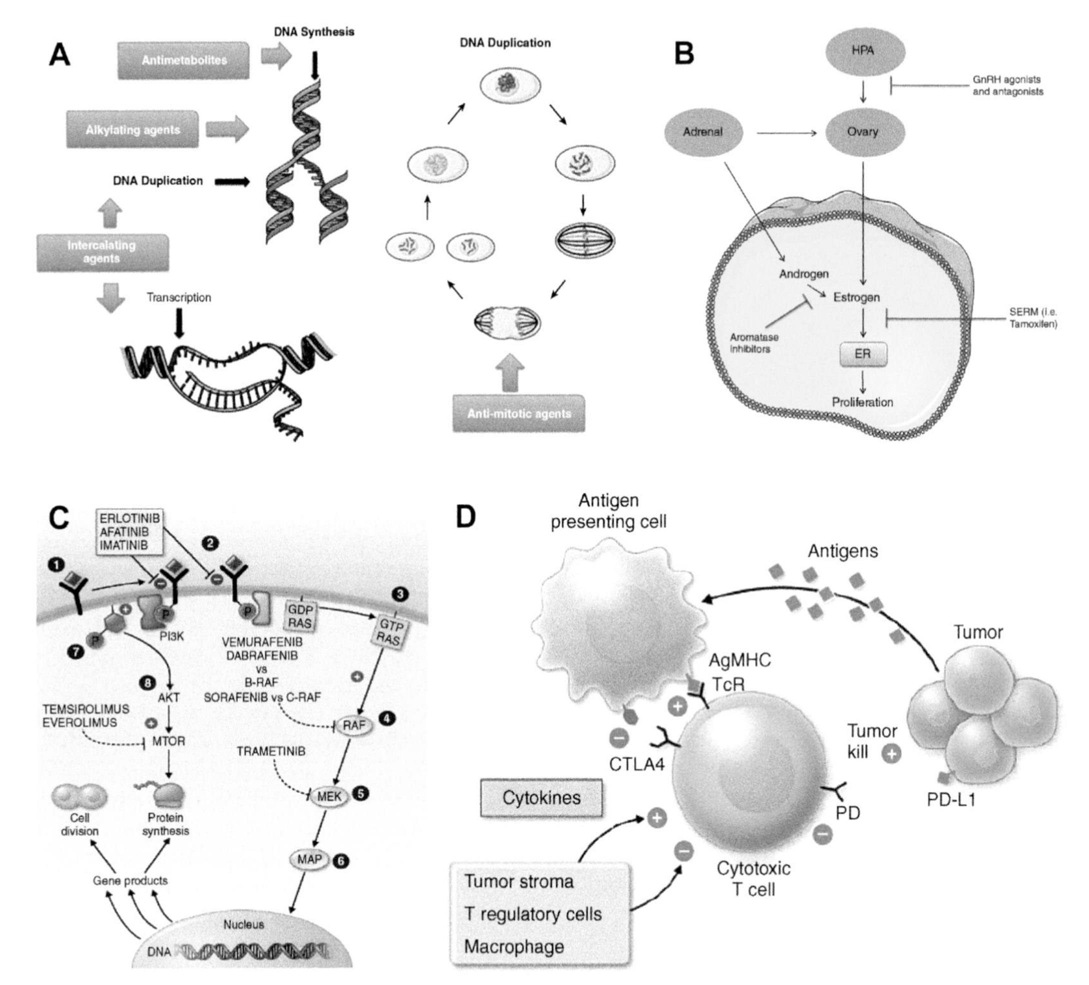

Fig. 1.4 Classes of systemic cancer therapies: (*A*) conventional "cytotoxic" chemotherapy agents, (*B*) hormonal therapies, (*C*) targeted therapies, (*D*) biologic therapies. ER, estrogen receptor; HPA, hypothalamic-pituitary-adrenal axis; SERM, selective estrogen receptor modulator. (*Adapted from* Kasper D, Fauci A, Hauser S, et al, editors. Harrison's principles of internal medicine. 19th edition. New York: McGraw-Hill; 2015. p. 103e-16–22; with permission.)

target in the disease-causing compartment as opposed to the normal compartment. However, current chemotherapeutic agents have relatively narrow therapeutic indices because their targets are present in both normal and tumor tissues. Determination of the therapeutic as well as the toxic response has thus become a critical element in the care of patients who undergo chemotherapy. A decrease by at least 50% in a tumor's bidimensional area is considered a partial therapeutic response, whereas disappearance of all tumor connotes a complete response. On the other hand, the clinical efficacy of therapeutic responses is often measured in overall survival, or an increased time to further progression of disease. Progression of disease is defined by the development of new lesions or an increase in size of existing lesion by at least 25% from baseline or best response state. As a rule of thumb, conventional chemotherapy agents induce partial response rates of at least 20% to 25% with reversible, non–life-threatening side effects. Side effects or toxicities are conventionally graded on a scale of 1 to 5, whereby grade 1 toxicities do not require treatment; grade 2 toxicities may require symptomatic treatment but are not life-threatening; grade 3 toxicities are potentially life-threatening if untreated; grade 4 toxicities are actually life-threatening; and grade 5 toxicities are those that result in the patient's death. Most chemotherapies are administered in "conventional" dose regimens with (predictable) usually reversible acute side effects. Indeed, it is to be emphasized that any new symptoms that develop over the course of cancer treatment should be assumed to be reversible until proven otherwise. "High-dose" chemotherapy regimens aim for a markedly increased therapeutic effect, albeit at the cost of potentially life-threatening complications that require intensive support, for example, stem cell transplantation or pharmacologic "rescue" strategies to repair the effect of the high-dose chemotherapy on normal tissues.

SUPPORTIVE CARE FOR THE PATIENT WITH CANCER

Patients with an underlying malignancy can have a variety of disease- and treatment-related side effects. Management of these symptoms is critical to the quality of life of the patient and his or her ability to proceed with possibly life-saving therapy. Studies have also shown the incorporation of palliative care can improve survival.[10] Underlying medical conditions, including heart disease and renal dysfunction, can also lead to life-threatening complications, further exacerbation of symptoms, and limitation of available therapies. It is important for cardiologists to be aware of these risks and possible management approaches.

In many aspects, the success of the cancer treatment depends on the success of the supportive care these patients receive. Failure to control the symptoms resulting from the malignancy or treatment can lead not only to significant morbidity, but also the inability to proceed with life saving therapy.

Acute side effects from radiation therapy are discussed (see Ryan K. Funk, Abigail L. Stockham, Nadia N. Issa Laack's chapter, "Basics of Radiation Therapy," in this volume). Herein, the most common primarily noncardiotoxic side effects of chemotherapies are presented (Fig. 1.5). Details regarding the classes and use of chemotherapies are provided (see Zoltan Szucs and Robin L. Jones's chapter, "Introduction to systemic antineoplastic treatments for cardiologists," in this volume).

Nausea and Vomiting

The incidence and severity of nausea and vomiting depends on chemotherapy regimen, dose, association with other treatments, and patient risk factors. Chemotherapy-induced nausea and vomiting (CINV) is classified into 3 categories: acute emesis, occurring within 24 hours of initial administration of chemotherapy; delayed emesis, occurring 24 hours to several days after initial administration of chemotherapy; and anticipatory nausea and vomiting, occurring at the perception of special stimuli. CINV risks are patient or chemotherapy dependent. Younger age, female gender, anxiety, a history of nausea and vomiting during earlier chemotherapy, or vomiting during pregnancy or motion sickness increases the risk of CINV, whereas higher age, male gender, and regular consummation of alcohol seem to be protective. Carmustine, cisplatin, cyclophosphamide (at a dose of >1500 mg/m^2), dacarbazine, dactinomycin, and streptozotocin are all highly emetogenic, as emesis occurs in greater than 90% of patients receiving these agents without antiemetic protection. Anthracyclines are of moderate/high emetogenic potential. Although there is some variability in the estimation of the emetogenic risk of chemotherapies by the different scientific societies as the Multinational Association

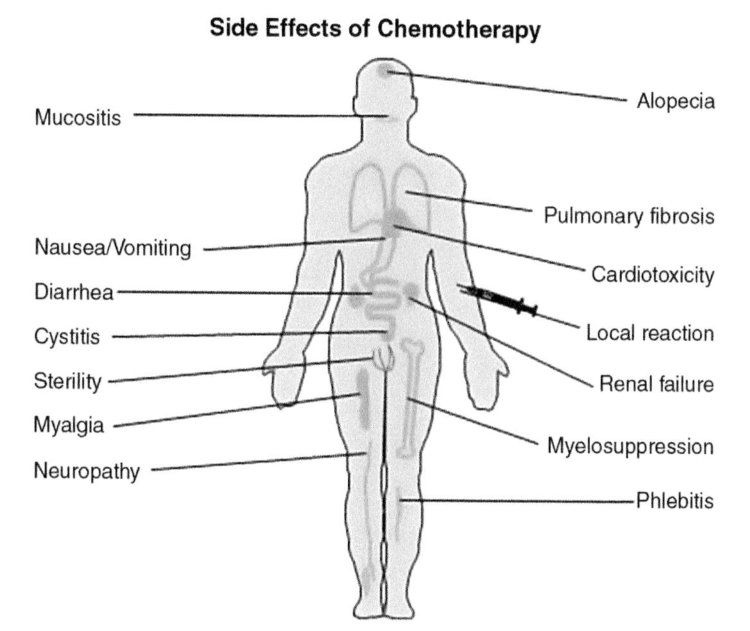

Fig. 1.5 The most common and important side effects of chemotherapy.

of Supportive Care in Cancer, the NCCN, the European Society of Medical Oncology, and the American Society of Clinical Oncology, their basic concept and recommendations are homogenous.

A variety of treatment options exist for prevention and management of nausea, including serotonin antagonists (ie, palonosetron and ondansetron), neurokinin receptor antagonists (ie, aprepitant), and antidopaminergic phenothiazines (ie, compazine). Dexamethasone is also commonly used for prevention of nausea around the time of chemotherapy administration. Serotonin antagonists have been shown to prolong the QTc interval, and thus, this should be monitored in patients receiving high doses of therapy.

Although antiemetics can be highly effective at controlling symptoms, patients may still be able to tolerate limited oral intake, including critical cardiovascular medications. In these cases, it is helpful to convert important oral medications to intravenous or sublingual formulations if possible.

MYELOTOXICITY

Antineoplastic agents almost invariably affect bone marrow function. These effects can be indirect with chemotherapy-induced damage to the bone marrow microenvironment or alterations in hematopoietic regulators. These effects can be indirect with chemotherapy-induced damage to the bone marrow microenvironment or alterations in hematopoietic regulators. Alternatively, chemotherapeutics can interact with bone marrow cells or their progenitors. The dynamics are to a certain degree predictable; for instance, neutrophil counts decline to the lowest level, the so-called nadir, around 10 to 14 days after chemotherapy with complete recovery by day 21 to 28. Some cell-cycle nonspecific agents like busulfan, nitrosoureas, and mitomycin C, however, can induce a prolonged duration of neutropenia. The overall magnitude of neutropenia depends on the intensity of the antineoplastic agent regimen and sequential order of drug administration. Anemia is a common dose-limiting toxicity of platinum-containing agents and docetaxel. Agents with dose-limiting thrombocytopenia include carboplatin and gemcitabine, among others. Anemia may be very relevant for patients with coronary artery disease, because it may increase the risk of myocardial demand-supply mismatch ischemia. It is also relevant for procedures such as cardiac catheterization percutaneous coronary intervention. Thrombocytopenia can pose an additional problem, predisposing to bleeding and challenges to antiplatelet therapies.

The most severe consequence is febrile neutropenia with variable incidence based on type of cancer and antineoplastic regimen. Febrile neutropenia is defined as an absolute neutrophil count of less than 500 cells per cubic millimeter and a temperature of more than 38.5°C. Colony-stimulating factors (CSF) like granulocyte CSF (G-CSF) stimulate the proliferation of neutrophil progenitors, promote their differentiation into mature neutrophils, and enhance their survival. Primary prophylaxis with G-CSF (ie, G-CSF administered immediately after cycle 1 of chemotherapy) can reduce the risk of febrile neutropenia by 50% in patients with solid tumors, without affecting the rates of tumor response, infection-related death, early-treatment–related death, or overall survival. Filgrastim and pegfilgrastim are the principal CSF products in current clinical use.

HYPERSENSITIVITY REACTIONS

The incidence of hypersensitivity is significant for certain anticancer agents, including platinum drugs (cisplatin, carboplatin, oxaliplatin), taxanes (paclitaxel, docetaxel), epipodophyllotoxins (teniposide, etoposide), monoclonal antibodies, procarbazine, and to a lesser extent, 6-mercaptopurine. A major feature of hypersensitivity to platinum drugs, compared with other types of agents, is that allergic reactions can appear after a significant number of infusions with no prior clinical signs. Taxane-related hypersensitivity symptoms generally develop within the first 10 to 15 minutes after infusion, and in 95% of cases, reactions occur during the first or second infusion. Some patients can develop skin reactions several days or up to a week after infusion. The incidence of paclitaxel and docetaxel hypersensitivity varies and can affect up to half of the patients exposed. Premedication with antihistamines, H2 blockers, and corticosteroids are typically not effective in preventing hypersensitivity reactions to platinum agents. Predmedication does, however, decrease the incidence of hypersensitivity to taxanes.[11] Desensitization protocols allow for readministration of either platinum- or taxane-based chemotherapy to some patients without causing severe hypersensitivity reactions.

Peripheral Neuropathy

Chemotherapy-induced peripheral neuropathy (CIPN) is a major dose-limiting side effect of many commonly used chemotherapeutic agents, including platinum drugs, taxanes, epothilones, and vinca alkaloids, but also newer agents such as bortezomib and lenolidamide. Neurotoxic chemotherapeutic agents may cause structural damage to peripheral nerves, resulting in aberrant somatosensory processing of the peripheral and/or central nervous system. Approximately 30% to 40% of patients receiving chemotherapy can be affected by CIPN. The incidence of CIPN is related to dose intensity, cumulative dose, coadministration of other neurotoxic chemotherapy agents, and pre-existing conditions such as diabetes and alcohol abuse. Although symptoms may resolve completely, in some instances CIPN is only partly reversible, and in other cases, it does not appear to be reversible at all. CIPN can be extremely painful and/or disabling, causing significant loss of functional abilities and decreasing quality of life.

Mucositis

Mucositis refers to mucosal damage secondary to cancer therapy potentially affecting any part of the gastrointestinal tract and can be a highly significant, and sometimes dose-limiting, toxicity of cancer therapy. It affects 20% to 40% of patients receiving conventional chemotherapy and 80% of patients receiving high-dose chemotherapy as conditioning for hematopoietic stem cell transplantation. Oral mucositis can become very painful, requiring opioid analgesics, and impairing nutritional intake and quality of life. Gastrointestinal mucositis presents with debilitating symptoms, such as pain, nausea/vomiting, and diarrhea. Antimetabolites and anthracyclines (especially at high doses) and tyrosine kinase inhibitors often predispose to the development of mucositis.

Hand and Foot Syndrome

Palmar plantar erythrodysesthesia, also referred as hand-foot syndrome (HFS), has long emerged as a common, dose-dependent toxicity associated with certain chemotherapeutical agents. HFS is mostly characterized by erythematous skin lesions on hands and feet; however, other unusual presentations have been described, such as unilateral spread, involvement of other cutaneous regions, and in extreme cases, secondary infection. HFS has been increasingly associated not only with some specific cytotoxic agents, such as pegylated liposomal doxorubicin and capecitabine, but also with targeted therapies, such as tyrosine kinase inhibitors (particularly sorafenib, pazopanib, regorafenib, axitinib, and sunitinib), with incidence rates up to 60%.

Nephrotoxicity

Antineoplastic agents, such as bevacizumab and gemcitabine, can injure the renal vasculature and cause thrombotic microangiopathy (TMA). TMA presents clinically as microangiopathic hemolytic anemia, thrombocytopenia, hypertension, and acute kidney injury (AKI) with hematuria and proteinuria, although renal-limited TMA does occur. Nephrotoxicity is the major adverse effect of the first-generation platinum agent cisplatin, although ototoxicity also occurs. Cisplatin injures multiple renal compartments, including blood vessels, glomeruli, and most commonly, the tubules. Although AKI can recover, renal outcomes, such as progressive chronic kidney disease from chronic tubulointerstitial fibrosis and irreversible chronic tubulopathies, may result. In order to minimize its nephrotoxicity, intensive hydration is given preadministration and postadministration of cisplatin. Ifosfamide's major adverse effect can be kidney injury. Nephrotoxic manifestations include tubulopathies such as proximal tubular injury or Fanconi syndrome and nephrogenic diabetes insipidus; in addition, AKI is often reversible, but can be permanent. The difference in adverse effects for ifosfamide (nephrotoxicity) and cyclophosphamide (hemorrhagic cystitis), which are related compounds, is caused by the major toxic metabolite that they produce. Acrolein produced by cyclophosphamide is nonnephrotoxic, whereas chloroacetaldehyde produced by ifosfamide injures kidney tissue. Preventive measures are limited for ifosfamide. Mesna, which is effective for hemorrhagic cystitis, is of limited value for ifosfamide-induced kidney injury. Nephrotoxicity is a known complication of high-dose dihydrofolate reductase inhibitor methotrexate (MTX) therapy (1–12 g/m^2) but rarely occurs with long-term conventional dosing. The incidence is highly variable depending on the patient's risk factors and the appropriate employment of preventive measures, such as intravenous fluids. MTX and its major metabolite, 7-OH methotrexate, are filtered by the glomerulus and secreted into the urinary space by proximal tubules. AKI is primarily the result of acute tubular injury from precipitation of MTX/7-OH methotrexate in distal tubular lumens. Risk factors for MTX nephrotoxicity include intravascular volume depletion with sluggish urinary flow, acid urine pH, and underlying kidney disease (glomerular filtration rate <60 mL/min). Based on these factors, prevention is focused on volume repletion before/during drug infusion, appropriate drug dosing, and alkalinization of the urine (pH >7.1). Treatment includes leucovorin rescue at 24 to 36 hours of MTX therapy to reduce nonmalignant cell injury. Glucarpidase cleaves MTX to noncytotoxic metabolites and is a reserved salvage agent in use when toxic MTX levels occur.

Effusions

Malignancy can lead to fluid accumulation within a variety of locations, including the pleura, pericardium, and peritoneum. Effusions are most commonly seen in patients with lung cancer, breast cancer, and lymphoma. Asymptomatic malignant effusions can often be closely observed, whereas symptomatic accumulations usually require drainage. In the case of cardiac tamponade, percutaneous drainage (ie, pericardiocentesis) and surgical drainage are highly effective at removing fluid and preventing hemodynamic compromise. As reaccumulation is seen in up to 60% of patients with malignant effusions, patients must be closely monitored if they receive a pericardiocentesis alone.[12] Strategies to prevent reaccumulation include continued catheter drainage, sclerosis, and formation of a pericardial window.

Volume Overload

Many chemotherapeutic regimens are given in conjunction with large volumes of hydration, often with the goal of renal and bladder protection. Patients with underlying cardiomyopathy must be monitored closely in order to prevent significant volume overload. Similarly, treatment with chemotherapy and volume expansion can exacerbate underlying atrial fibrillation. Patients may require diuresis or adjustment in their cardiac medications in order to prevent further complications in these settings.

Gonadotoxicity/Infertility

Infertility represents one of the main long-term consequences of combination chemotherapy given for lymphoma, leukemia, and other malignancies in young women. The gonadotoxic effect of various chemotherapeutic agents varies and has been categorized into 3 risk categories: high-risk, medium-risk and low-risk chemotherapeutic agents. High-risk chemotherapeutic agents include several alkylating agents (cyclophosphamide, busulphan, chlorambucil, procarbazine, melphalan, ifosfamide, chlormethamine). Platinum agents (cisplatin, carboplatin), anthracycline antibiotics (doxorubicin), and taxanes (docetaxel and paclitaxel) are considered to be of medium risk. Low-risk agents include vinca plant alkaloids (vincristine and vinblastine), anthracycline antibiotics (bleomycin), and antimetabolites (MTX, 5-FU, 6-mercaptopurine). The reported rate of premature ovarian failure after various diseases and chemotherapeutic protocols differ enormously and depend mainly on the chemotherapeutic protocol used and age range of the woman. Overall, the rate of premature ovarian failure ranges from 10% to almost 100%, although it is usually around 30% to 70% for premenopausal women exposed to gonadotoxic regimens, and 90% to 100% for adult, premenopausal women undergoing hematopoietic stem-cell transplantation, combined with preceding aggressive chemotherapy-conditioning protocols. Several options have been proposed for preserving female fertility, despite gonadotoxic chemotherapy: ovarian transposition, cryopreservation of embryos, unfertilized metaphase II oocytes and ovarian tissue, and administration of gonadotropin-releasing hormone agonistic analogues in an attempt to decrease the gonadotoxic effects of chemotherapy by simulating a prepubertal hormonal milieu. None of these methods has proved to be ideal, and none guarantees future fertility in all survivors.

It is also important to be aware that hormonal shifts following chemotherapy can have a significant impact on cardiovascular health.

Secondary Malignancies

The most worrisome late effect of chemotherapy is the development of secondary malignant neoplasms (SMN). SMN are defined as histologically distinct malignant neoplasms developing at least 2 months after completion of treatment of the primary malignancy; however, most occur years to decades after primary treatment has been completed. Common alkylating agents like cyclophosphamide, ifosfamide, mechlorethamine, melphalan, busulfan, dacarbazine, nitrosoureas, and cisplatin have been shown to be an important risk factor for developing SMN. In particular, exposure to alkylating agents has been associated with increased risk of the development of hematologic malignancies, often referred to as therapy-related acute myelogenous leukemia (t-AML). Treatment with topoisomerase II inhibitors, like anthracyclines, anthracenediones (eg, mitoxantrone), as well as epipodophyllotoxins, such as etoposide and tenoposide, is also associated with an increased risk of SMN. The incidence of t-AMLs from topoisomerase II inhibitors varies in published reports but has been reported as high as 8.3%.

Survivorship Programs

As treatment options for patients with cancer improve, there are an increasing number of people who are living with or being cured of their malignancies. Having undergone cancer treatment can be associated with a variety of both medical and psychological side effects. Oncology patients, therefore, require long-term surveillance, prevention services, and management related to the cancer itself or the toxicities of prior treatment. Over the past decade, there has been an increased focus on developing programs aimed at addressing the needs of this growing population. Survivorship programs are aimed at working with patients to outline potential late effects and develop the most appropriate future care plan. They also typically involve a multidisciplinary approach. Cardiologists, for example, are important for assessing for increased risk of coronary artery disease associated with prior radiation and management of treatment-related cardiomyopathies and arrhythmias. Other specialists, including endocrinologists, nephrologists, gynecologists, nutritionists, and exercise consultants, can also play a role in providing comprehensive care to a cancer survivor. Survivorship programs also include various types of support in the form of classes, group meetings, and individual appointments aimed at addressing the social, mental, and emotional side effects that can affect patients and their families.

REFERENCES

1. Siegel RL, Miller KD, Jemal A. Cancer statistics, 2015. CA Cancer J Clin 2015;65(1):5–29.
2. Al Kindi SG, Oliveira GH. Prevalence of preexisting cardiovascular disease in patients with different types of cancer: the unmet need for onco-cardiology. Mayo Clin Proc 2016;91(1):81–3.
3. Bruix J, Sherman M. American Association for the Study of Liver Diseases. Management of hepatocellular carcinoma: an update. Hepatology 2011;53(3):1020–2.
4. Aukema SM, Siebert R, Schuuring E, et al. Double-hit B-cell lymphomas. Blood 2011;117(8):2319–31.
5. Petrich AM, Gandhi M, Jovanovic B, et al. Impact of induction regimen and stem cell transplantation on outcomes in double-hit lymphoma: a multicenter retrospective analysis. Blood 2014;124(15):2354–61.
6. Anders C, Carey LA. Understanding and treating triple-negative breast cancer. Oncology 2008; 22(11):1233–9 [discussion: 1239–40, 1243].
7. Oken MM, Creech RH, Tormey DC, et al. Toxicity and response criteria of the Eastern Cooperative Oncology Group. Am J Clin Oncol 1982;5(6):649–55.
8. Roca J. The mechanisms of DNA topoisomerases. Trends Biochem Sci 1995;20(4):156–60.
9. Piccart-Gebhart MJ, Procter M, Leyland-Jones B, et al. Trastuzumab after adjuvant chemotherapy in HER2-positive breast cancer. N Engl J Med 2005; 353(16):1659–72.
10. Temel JS, Greer JA, Muzikansky A, et al. Early palliative care for patients with metastatic non-small-cell lung cancer. N Engl J Med 2010;363(8):733–42.
11. Boulanger J, Boursiquot JN, Cournoyer G, et al. Management of hypersensitivity to platinum- and taxane-based chemotherapy: cepo review and clinical recommendations. Curr Oncol 2014;21(4):e630–41.
12. Tsang TS, Seward JB, Barnes ME, et al. Outcomes of primary and secondary treatment of pericardial effusion in patients with malignancy. Mayo Clin Proc 2000;75(3):248–53.

CHAPTER 2

Introduction to Systemic Antineoplastic Treatments for Cardiologists

Zoltan Szucs, MD, PhD[a,*],
Robin L. Jones, MD, BSc, MRCP, MB[a,b]

INTRODUCTION

Medical oncology has expanded and evolved with an unforeseen speed. An initial key step was the discovery of the differences in cell kinetics between normal and malignant cells, which has led to the development of the first classes of cytotoxic agents directed against DNA or proteins involved in DNA replication, translation, and transcription. Additional hallmarks of cancer include replicative immortality, sustained proliferative signaling, evasion of growth suppressors, angiogenesis induction, tissue invasion and metastases, resistance to cell death, deregulated cell metabolism, genomic instability, tumor-promoting inflammation, and ability to evade the immune system.[1] Each of these can provide a target for drug treatment in a wide range of cancers.

The aim of this chapter is to give a concise overview, for nononcologists, of the systemic therapies used in treating patients with cancer. Further resources include the American National Comprehensive Cancer Network guidelines[2] and manufacturers' summaries of product characteristics, which provide detailed information on indication, application, pharmacodynamics and pharmacokinetics, and side-effect profile of individual antineoplastic compounds currently in use.[3]

PRACTICAL APPROACHES TO SYSTEMIC ANTICANCER TREATMENTS

Decision to Treat

The initiation and delivery of systemic anticancer treatments is highly regulated, and constant vigilance is required during both commencement of treatment and follow-up. The decision to treat an individual patient should be initiated by a certified oncologist, often following a multidisciplinary team (MDT) discussion. Ideally, every new patient with cancer should have his or her treatment plan discussed in an MDT discussion, as referenced elsewhere in this volume. A treatment plan should always include the exact diagnosis and TNM stage,[4] the intent of treatment (neoadjuvant, adjuvant, curative, palliative), investigations/tests required before treatment (ie, cardiac, pulmonary, hepatic, or renal assessment), planned length or the treatment, and schedule of efficacy assessment. It cannot be emphasized enough how much comorbidities and performance status weigh in for overall patient outcome. A widely used scale is the Eastern Cooperative Oncology Group (ECOG) Performance Status, which describes along standardized criteria a patient's level of functioning in terms of their ability to care for themselves, daily activity, and physical ability (see Table 1.2).[5] As outlined in a study from the United Kingdom, 1 in 5 patients who died within 30 days of systemic anticancer chemotherapy had an ECOG performance score of 3 or 4, that is, severely debilitated, at the time of the decision for treatment. In a similar number of cases, the decision to treat with the most recent course of systemic chemotherapy was inappropriate in the advisors' view.[6]

All patients should receive upfront comprehensive education regarding the potential side effects of therapy and should have access to a 24-hour support line. They are also to be regularly reviewed before each cycle of treatment, often

[a] The Royal Marsden Hospital NHS Foundation Trust, Fulham Road, London SW3 6JJ, United Kingdom; [b] Seattle Cancer Care Alliance, 825 Eastlake Avenue East, Seattle, WA 98109-1023, USA
* Corresponding author.
E-mail address: z.szucs@nhs.net

even within the cycle as well, to assess early toxicities in order to facilitate preemptive management of side effects. Toxicity recording and grading should be performed according to the National Cancer Institutes' Common Terminology Criteria for Adverse Events (Table 2.1).[7]

Tailoring chemotherapy

The decision whether a drug is used on its own or in combination depends on many factors. For example, in the treatment of *metastatic* breast cancer, combination chemotherapy (doublet, triplet) has not led to an overall survival (OS) benefit; therefore, single-agent chemotherapeutics are offered in a sequential manner (targeted agents, like human epidermal growth factor receptor 2 [HER2] inhibitors, can still be given as chemotherapy adjuncts when appropriate).[2]

In the palliative setting, the choice of chemotherapy schedule often involves balancing quality of life and safe delivery with the potential efficacy of different schedules. For instance, in the

TABLE 2.1
Alkylating agents

Group	Agent	Main Indications	Specific Toxicities
Nitrogen mustards	Chlorambucil	HL, NHL, CLL, WM, sarcomas	BMD, CINV, seizures
	Melphalan	MM, PV, ovarian and breast cancers	BMD, CINV, alopecia
	Estramustine	Prostate cancer	Gynecomastia, libido changes
Oxazaphorines	Cyclophosphamide	CLL, CML, AML, ALL, HL, NHL, MM, Ewing sarcoma, SCLC, neuroblastoma, ovarian and breast cancers	BMD, hemorrhagic cystitis, RTN, SIADH, VOLD, pneumonitis, CINV
	Ifosfamide	Sarcomas, pediatric tumors	BMD, nephrotoxicity, hemorrhagic cystitis, neurotoxicity, RTN, SIADH, VOLD, pneumonitis, CINV
Hydrazines and triazines	Procarbazine	HL	BMD, CINV
	Dacarbazine	Melanoma, HL, sarcomas	BMD, CINV, VOLD
	Temozolomide	GBM	BMD-lymphopenia, opportunistic infections, CINV
Nitrosureas	Carmustine	GBM	BMD, cerebral edema-intracranial hypertension
	Lomustine	Brain tumors	BMD, CINV
	Streptozocin	Neuroendocrine tumors	Diarrhea, CINV
Metal salts	Carboplatin	SCLC, NSCLC, GCT, ovarian cancer	BMD-thrombocytopenia, CINV, CIPN, hypersensitivity-reactions/anaphylaxis
	Cisplatin	GCT, NSCLC, esophageal, ovarian, and bladder cancer	Highly emetogenic, nephrotoxicity and ototoxicity, BMD
	Oxaliplatin	CRC	CIPN, BMD, CINV, RPLS, hypersensitivity-reactions/anaphylaxis

Abbreviations: ALL, acute lymphocytic leukemia; AML, acute myelogenic leukemia; BMD, bone marrow depression; CINV, chemotherapy-induced nausea and vomiting; CIPN, chemotherapy-induced peripheral neuropathy; CLL, chronic lymphocytic leukemia; GBM, glioblastoma multiforme; GCT, germ cell tumors; HL, Hodgkin lymphoma; MM, multiple myeloma; NHL, non-Hodgkin lymphoma; NSCLC, non–small cell lung cancer; PV, polycythemia vera; RPLS, reversible posterior leukoencephalopathy syndrome; RTN, renal tubular necrosis; SCLC, small cell lung cancer; SIADH, syndrome of inappropriate secretion of antidiuretic hormone; VOLD, veno-occlusive liver disease; WM, Waldenstrom macroglobulinemia.

treatment of advanced pancreatic cancer, the highly toxic combination of 5-fluorouracil (5-FU; bolus and protracted infusion), leucovorin, irinotecan, and oxaliplatin has led to significant improvements in 1-year OS rates and is recommended as a first-line option.[2,8] However, patients with advanced pancreatic cancer are often frail, and therefore, in many instances, a less toxic schedule (gemcitabine monotherapy or combinations of thereof) would be selected.

Furthermore, patients themselves often make a choice between equally effective treatment options based on the toxicity profile of the agents involved. In the first-line treatment of metastatic colorectal cancer (CRC), irinotecan and oxaliplatin are equally potent agents. A patient fearing alopecia might opt for oxaliplatin as a first choice; on the contrary, a violinist might choose irinotecan as a first-line option, fearing the cumulative peripheral neuropathy associated with oxaliplatin.

Dose intensity/dose density

The dose of a particular drug or schedule will often undergo adjustments based on the performance status, comorbidities, and the intent of treatment. In the radical (adjuvant, curative) setting, generally the policy would be to maintain dose density/intensity. Chemotherapy dose intensity represents a treatment strategy with a focus geared on maximum unit dose administered per unit time (the dose per course). Standard chemotherapy regimens implement these standard doses of chemotherapeutics every 3 to 4 weeks to allow for normal cells to recover. However, this time interval may also allow smaller, more rapidly growing cancer cells to recover tumor growth. Dose-dense protocols aim to maximize tumor killing by increasing the rate and not the dose of chemotherapy. Accordingly, the same dose of chemotherapy given every 3 weeks, for instance, will be given every 2 weeks instead.

In contrast, in the palliative setting, quality of life is paramount, and effective treatments with significant cumulative toxicities do not necessarily need to be given until disease progression; treatment breaks and reinitiation of the same treatment can also be a safe and effective option. When concurrent radiotherapy is given, specific dose adjustments need to be made to avoid compounded toxicity.

Method of Delivery

Chemotherapy regimens can be administered in different ways, including bolus or continuous infusion. Most treatments are given intravenously, through a temporary angiocatheter. Peripherally inserted central catheters, or PICC lines, are ideal for multiple short infusions or continuous infusions given in a hospital or at home with a portable pump. Tunneled catheters (Groshong, Hickman) with multiple lumens are most often used for extensive chemotherapy regimens such as bone marrow transplant procedures. A more permanent option involves the placement of a Port-a-Cath by an interventional radiologist or by a surgeon and can function for many years. Intraventricular or intrathecal chemotherapy can be given through a lumbar puncture or through an implanted Ommaya reservoir.

Intraperitoneal treatment given through temporary single-use catheters, Tenckhoff catheters, or Port-a-Cath remains controversial; other than for treatment of ovarian cancer, this technique has not gained much popularity and is considered experimental. Intra-arterial chemotherapy has been used most commonly for colon cancer that has spread to the liver. Although the local tumor responses have been better with this therapy, there has been no survival benefit to date; thus, it is not a standard approach in the everyday clinical practice. Intravesical chemotherapy for superficially invasive bladder cancer can significantly reduce local recurrence rates after surgical intervention. Intrapleural delivery of chemotherapeutics has been used for pleurodesis rather than as an antineoplastic measure.

Implantable chemotherapy treatment with carmustine wafers is a unique form of delivering chemotherapy straight into the surgical cavity, for example, after removal of a glioblastoma multiforme. Subcutaneous administration of chemotherapy agents is often challenged by an irritation effect; it has, however, recently been approved as alternative delivery method for biologicals like trastuzumab or bortezomib.[3]

Mechanism of Action of Traditional Antineoplastic Agents

Traditional chemotherapeutics aim to interfere with cell division, and thus, the greater the proliferation or replication rate, the higher the vulnerability of cells to these drugs. Cell division consists of 2 consecutive processes: (1) DNA replication, and (2) segregation of replicated chromosomes into 2 separate cells. The latter is called mitosis (M), the former, the interphase (Fig. 2.1). The interphase includes G1 (or gap 1; a growth phase during which the cell is preparing for DNA synthesis), S (synthesis; the replication of DNA occurs), and G2 phases (gap 2; a growth phase during which the cell prepares for mitosis). The M phase (mitosis; the actual division from 1 cell into 2) includes prophase, metaphase, anaphase, and telophase. Cells in G1 can, before commitment to

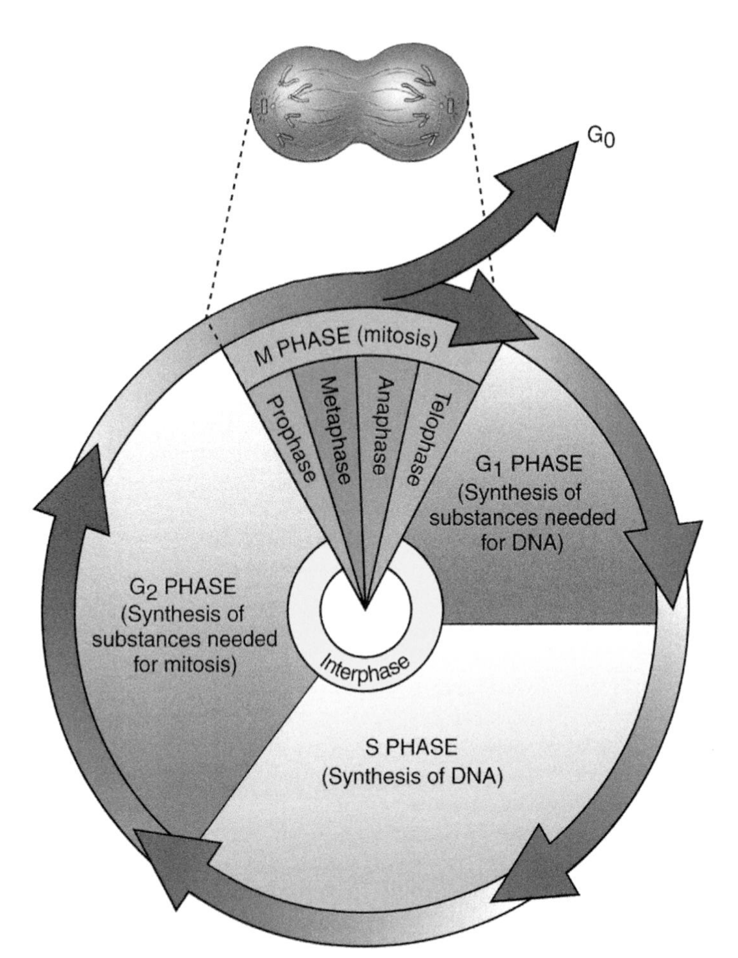

Fig. 2.1 The cell cycle. (*From* Herlihy B, Maebius N. The human body in health and illness. Philadelphia: Saunders; 2000; with permission.)

DNA replication, enter a resting state called G0. Cells in G0 account for most of the nongrowing, nonproliferating cells in the human body. The restriction point (R) is defined as a point of no return in G1, following that the cell is committed to enter the cell cycle. Additional controls or checkpoints exist further in the cell cycle, ensuring an orderly sequence of events in the cell cycle. In response to DNA damage, checkpoints arrest the cell cycle in order to provide time for DNA repair. DNA damage checkpoints are positioned before the cell enters S phase (G1-S checkpoint) or after DNA replication (G2-M checkpoint), and there appears to be DNA damage checkpoints during S and M phases.[9]

Some chemotherapy agents are able to kill cells during any phase of the cycle (cell-cycle nonspecific), whereas others operate only during a specific phase and not in the resting phase (cell-cycle specific) (Fig. 2.2). The action of the different chemotherapies can be further stratified and illustrated along the sequence of DNA synthesis, replication, and transcription.

Alkylating agents

Alkylating agents are considered to be cell-cycle nonspecific chemotherapeutics and include a variety of drugs with different chemical structures and mechlorethamine as the first one to be approved by the US Food and Drug Administration (FDA) in 1949. Although alkylating agents are one of the oldest classes of anticancer agents, their use still lies at the core of the treatment for an extensive range of malignancies (Table 2.2). Alkylating agents are electrophilic and react with nucleophilic moieties of DNA or proteins, resulting in the covalent transfer of an alkyl group. The alkylation of DNA bases impairs essential DNA processes such as DNA replication and/or transcription. Although monofunctional agents generate covalent adducts with the target molecule, bifunctional derivatives (chlorambucil, melphalan) can form cross-links (interstrands or intrastrand) in DNA or between DNA and proteins.

One of the best known alkylating agents is cyclophosphamide, used commonly in the

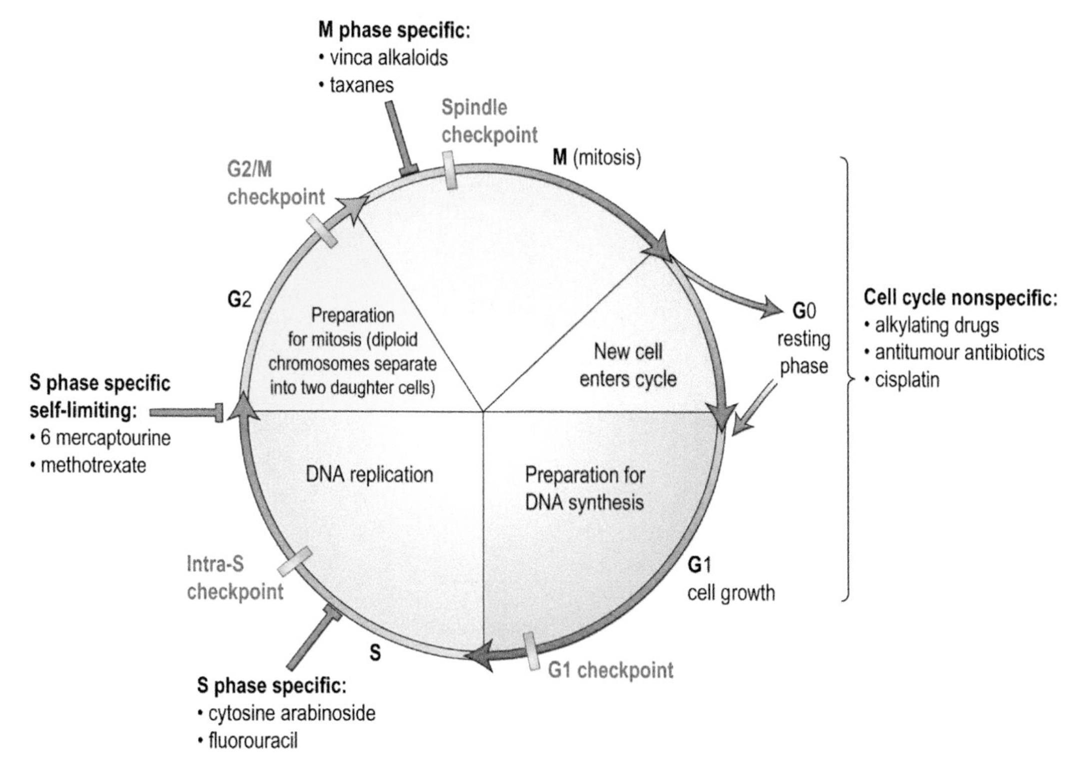

Fig. 2.2 Chemotherapeutics target the replication cycle of cancer cells and can act at a specific point of the cell cycle or less specifically. (*From* Kumar P, Clark M. Malignant disease. In: Kumar & Clark's clinical medicine. Philadelphia: Elsevier; 2012. p. 431–84; with permission.)

treatment of lymphomas and breast cancer. It is a prodrug that requires activation in the liver and may therefore not be appropriately activated in patients with underlying hepatic dysfunction. Furthermore, one of its breakdown products (acrolein) causes cystitis, and thus, it is critical to administer hydration as well as mesna (2-mercaptoethanesulfonate) for bladder protection when the drug is used at high doses. If used in very high doses, as is done before bone marrow transplantation, there can be cardiac toxicity and resulting cardiomyopathy.[10] Ifosphamide is a cyclophosphamide analogue that has demonstrated efficacy in a variety of malignancies, including lymphomas and sarcomas. As with cyclophosphamide, it is important to provide hydration and mesna for prevention of hemorrhagic cystitis. Ifosphamide can also rarely be associated with neurotoxicity and encephalopathy that is generally self-limited and reversible.[10]

Platinum derivatives have emerged in the clinic in the late 1970s with the use of cisplatin and its spectacular results in testicular cancers.[10] It is also used in the systemic treatment of small-cell and non–small-cell lung cancer, and esophageal, ovarian, and bladder cancer. Cisplatin can lead to renal dysfunction, hypomagnesemia, hearing loss, and neurotoxicity as well as vascular toxicity. Carboplatin, which is a similar platinum-based agent, has decreased rates of described toxicities, although associated with more prominent myelosuppression. Carboplatin is typically the preferred platinum agent for ovarian cancer, uterine cancer, and breast cancer. Oxaliplatin is another platinum-based therapy with activity against refractory colon cancers (see Table 2.1).

Other alkylating agents are available, although less commonly used, including nitrogen mustard, chlorambucil, dacarbazine, and temozolamide.

Mitotic inhibitors

Mitosis defines the critical time of the cell cycle during which replicated chromosomes are separated into 2 identical sets of chromosomes, each within their own nucleus. Microtubules are required for the segregation of chromosomes during this process. These ubiquitous fibrillar structures are part of the cytoskeleton within the cytoplasm and are composed of tubulin polymers. Chemotherapeutics that target and interfere with the normal formation and function of microtubules can effectively disrupt cells in the M phase of the cell cycle and ultimately result in cell death. Most of the mitotic inhibitors (Table 2.3) are plant alkaloids or their derivatives (vinca alkaloids from the periwinkle plant, taxanes from the bark of the Pacific yew tree).

TABLE 2.2
Common terminology criteria for adverse events (CTCAE)

CTCAE v4.0 Term	Grade 1	Grade 2	Grade 3	Grade 4	Grade 5
Acute coronary syndrome	—	Symptomatic, progressive angina; cardiac enzymes normal; hemodynamically stable	Symptomatic, unstable angina, and/or acute myocardial infarction, cardiac enzymes abnormal, hemodynamically stable	Symptomatic, unstable angina, and/or acute myocardial infarction, cardiac enzymes abnormal, hemodynamically unstable	Death
Aortic valve disease	Asymptomatic valvular thickening with or without mild valvular regurgitation or stenosis by imaging	Asymptomatic; moderate regurgitation or stenosis by imaging	Symptomatic; severe regurgitation or stenosis by imaging; symptoms controlled with medical intervention	Life-threatening consequences; urgent intervention indicated (eg, valve replacement, valvuloplasty)	Death
Asystole	Periods of asystole; nonurgent medical management indicated	—	—	Life-threatening consequences; urgent intervention indicated	Death
Atrial fibrillation	Asymptomatic, intervention not indicated	Nonurgent medical intervention indicated	Symptomatic and incompletely controlled medically, or controlled with device (eg, pacemaker), or ablation	Life-threatening consequences; urgent intervention indicated	Death
Atrial flutter	Asymptomatic, intervention not indicated	Nonurgent medical intervention indicated	Symptomatic and incompletely controlled medically, or controlled with device (eg, pacemaker), or ablation	Life-threatening consequences; urgent intervention indicated	Death
Atrioventricular block complete	—	Nonurgent intervention indicated	Symptomatic and incompletely controlled medically, or controlled with device (eg, pacemaker)	Life-threatening consequences; urgent intervention indicated	Death
Atrioventricular block first degree	Asymptomatic, intervention not indicated	Nonurgent intervention indicated	—	—	—

Cardiac arrest	—	—	—	Life-threatening consequences; urgent intervention indicated	Death
Chest pain, cardiac	Mild pain	Moderate pain; limiting instrumental activities of daily living (ADL)	Pain at rest; limiting self-care ADL	—	—
Conduction disorder	Mild symptoms; intervention not indicated	Moderate symptoms	Severe symptoms; intervention indicated	Life-threatening consequences; urgent intervention indicated	Death
Constrictive pericarditis	—	—	Symptomatic heart failure or other cardiac symptoms, responsive to intervention	Refractory heart failure or other poorly controlled cardiac symptoms	Death
Heart failure	Asymptomatic with laboratory (eg, BNP [B-natriuretic peptide]) or cardiac imaging abnormalities	Symptoms with mild to moderate activity or exertion	Severe with symptoms at rest or with minimal activity or exertion; intervention indicated	Life-threatening consequences; urgent intervention indicated (eg, continuous intravenous (IV) therapy or mechanical hemodynamic support)	Death
Left ventricular systolic dysfunction	—	—	Symptomatic due to drop in ejection fraction responsive to intervention	Refractory or poorly controlled heart failure due to drop in ejection fraction; intervention, such as ventricular assist device, intravenous vasopressor support, or heart transplant indicated	Death
Mitral valve disease	Asymptomatic valvular thickening with or without mild valvular regurgitation or stenosis by imaging	Asymptomatic; moderate regurgitation or stenosis by imaging	Symptomatic; severe regurgitation or stenosis by imaging; symptoms controlled with medical intervention	Life-threatening consequences; urgent intervention indicated (eg, valve replacement, valvuloplasty)	Death

(continued on next page)

TABLE 2.2
(continued)

CTCAE v4.0 Term	Grade 1	Grade 2	Grade 3	Grade 4	Grade 5
Mobitz (type) II atrioventricular block	Asymptomatic, intervention not indicated	Symptomatic; medical intervention indicated	Symptomatic and incompletely controlled medically, or controlled with device (eg, pacemaker)	Life-threatening consequences; urgent intervention indicated	Death
Mobitz type I	Asymptomatic, intervention not indicated	Symptomatic; medical intervention indicated	Symptomatic and incompletely controlled medically, or controlled with device (eg, pacemaker)	Life-threatening consequences; urgent intervention indicated	Death
Myocardial infarction	—	Asymptomatic and cardiac enzymes minimally abnormal and no evidence of ischemic electrocardiogram (ECG) changes	Severe symptoms; cardiac enzymes abnormal; hemodynamically stable; ECG changes consistent with infarction	Life-threatening consequences; hemodynamically unstable	Death
Myocarditis	Asymptomatic with laboratory (eg, BNP) or cardiac imaging abnormalities	Symptoms with mild to moderate activity or exertion	Severe with symptoms at rest or with minimal activity or exertion; intervention indicated	Life-threatening consequences; urgent intervention indicated (eg, continuous IV therapy or mechanical hemodynamic support)	Death
Palpitations	Mild symptoms; intervention not indicated	Intervention indicated	—	—	—
Paroxysmal atrial tachycardia	Asymptomatic, intervention not indicated	Symptomatic; medical management indicated	IV medication indicated	Life-threatening consequences; incompletely controlled medically; cardioversion indicated	Death
Pericardial effusion	—	Asymptomatic effusion size small to moderate	Effusion with physiologic consequences	Life-threatening consequences; urgent intervention indicated	Death

Pericardial tamponade	—	—	—	Life-threatening consequences; urgent intervention indicated	Death
Pericarditis	Asymptomatic, ECG, or physical findings (eg, rub) consistent with pericarditis	Symptomatic pericarditis (eg, chest pain)	Pericarditis with physiologic consequences (eg, pericardial constriction)	Life-threatening consequences; urgent intervention indicated	Death
Pulmonary valve disease	Asymptomatic valvular thickening with or without mild valvular regurgitation or stenosis by imaging	Asymptomatic; moderate regurgitation or stenosis by imaging	Symptomatic; severe regurgitation or stenosis by imaging; symptoms controlled with medical intervention	Life-threatening consequences; urgent intervention indicated (eg, valve replacement, valvuloplasty)	Death
Restrictive cardiomyopathy	—	—	Symptomatic heart failure or other cardiac symptoms, responsive to intervention	Refractory heart failure or other poorly controlled cardiac symptoms	Death
Right ventricular dysfunction	Asymptomatic with laboratory (eg, BNP) or cardiac imaging abnormalities	Symptoms with mild to moderate activity or exertion	Severe symptoms, associated with hypoxemia, right heart failure; oxygen indicated	Life-threatening consequences; urgent intervention indicated (eg, ventricular assist device); heart transplant indicated	Death
Sick sinus syndrome	Asymptomatic, intervention not indicated	Nonurgent intervention indicated	Severe, medically significant; medical intervention indicated	Life-threatening consequences; urgent intervention indicated	Death
Sinus bradycardia	Asymptomatic, intervention not indicated	Symptomatic, medical intervention indicated	Severe, medically significant, medical intervention indicated	Life-threatening consequences; urgent intervention indicated	Death
Sinus tachycardia	Asymptomatic, intervention not indicated	Symptomatic; nonurgent medical intervention indicated	Urgent medical intervention indicated	—	—
Supraventricular tachycardia	Asymptomatic, intervention not indicated	Nonurgent medical intervention indicated	Medical intervention indicated	Life-threatening consequences; urgent intervention indicated	Death

(*continued on next page*)

TABLE 2.2
(continued)

CTCAE v4.0 Term	Grade 1	Grade 2	Grade 3	Grade 4	Grade 5
Tricuspid valve disease	Asymptomatic valvular thickening with or without mild valvular regurgitation or stenosis	Asymptomatic; moderate regurgitation or stenosis by imaging	Symptomatic; severe regurgitation or stenosis; symptoms controlled with medical intervention	Life-threatening consequences; urgent intervention indicated (eg, valve replacement, valvuloplasty)	Death
Ventricular arrhythmia	Asymptomatic, intervention not indicated	Nonurgent medical intervention indicated	Medical intervention indicated	Life-threatening consequences; hemodynamic compromise; urgent intervention indicated	Death
Ventricular fibrillation	—	—	—	Life-threatening consequences; hemodynamic compromise; urgent intervention indicated	Death
Ventricular tachycardia	—	Nonurgent medical intervention indicated	Medical intervention indicated	Life-threatening consequences; hemodynamic compromise; urgent intervention indicated	Death
Wolff-Parkinson-White syndrome	Asymptomatic, intervention not indicated	Nonurgent medical intervention indicated	Symptomatic and incompletely controlled medically or controlled with procedure	Life-threatening consequences; urgent intervention indicated	Death
Cardiac disorders, other, specify	Asymptomatic or mild symptoms; clinical or diagnostic observations only; intervention not indicated	Moderate; minimal, local, or noninvasive intervention indicated; limiting age-appropriate instrumental ADL	Severe or medically significant but not immediately life-threatening; hospitalization or prolongation of existing hospitalization indicated; disabling; limiting self-care ADL	Life-threatening consequences; urgent intervention indicated	Death

Capillary leak syndrome	—	Symptomatic; medical intervention indicated	Severe symptoms; intervention indicated	Life-threatening consequences; urgent intervention indicated	Death
Flushing	Asymptomatic; clinical or diagnostic observations only; intervention not indicated	Moderate symptoms; medical intervention indicated; limiting instrumental ADL	Symptomatic, associated with hypotension and/or tachycardia; limiting self-care ADL	—	—
Hematoma	Mild symptoms; intervention not indicated	Minimally invasive evacuation or aspiration indicated	Transfusion, radiologic, endoscopic, or elective operative intervention indicated	Life-threatening consequences; urgent intervention indicated	Death
Hot flashes	Mild symptoms; intervention not indicated	Moderate symptoms; limiting instrumental ADL	Severe symptoms; limiting self-care ADL	—	—
Hypertension	Prehypertension (systolic blood pressure [BP] 120–139 mm Hg or diastolic BP 80–89 mm Hg)	Stage 1 hypertension (systolic BP 140–159 mm Hg or diastolic BP 90–99 mm Hg); medical intervention indicated; recurrent or persistent (≥24 h); symptomatic increase by >20 mm Hg (diastolic) or to >140/90 mm Hg if previously within normal limits; monotherapy indicated Pediatric: recurrent or persistent (≥24 h) BP > ULN; monotherapy indicated	Stage 2 hypertension (systolic BP ≥ 160 mm Hg or diastolic BP ≥ 100 mm Hg); medical intervention indicated; more than one drug or more intensive therapy than previously used indicated Pediatric: Same as adult	Life-threatening consequences (eg, malignant hypertension, transient or permanent neurologic deficit, hypertensive crisis); urgent intervention indicated Pediatric: same as adult	Death
Hypotension	Asymptomatic, intervention not indicated	Nonurgent medical intervention indicated	Medical intervention or hospitalization indicated	Life-threatening and urgent intervention indicated	Death

(continued on next page)

TABLE 2.2 (*continued*)

CTCAE v4.0 Term	Grade 1	Grade 2	Grade 3	Grade 4	Grade 5
Lymph leakage	—	Symptomatic; medical intervention indicated	Severe symptoms; radiologic, endoscopic, or elective operative intervention indicated	Life-threatening consequences; urgent intervention indicated	Death
Lymphedema	Trace thickening or faint discoloration	Marked discoloration; leathery skin texture; papillary formation; limiting instrumental ADL	Severe symptoms; limiting self-care ADL	—	—
Lymphocele	Asymptomatic; clinical or diagnostic observations only; intervention not indicated	Symptomatic; medical intervention indicated	Severe symptoms; radiologic, endoscopic, or elective operative intervention indicated	—	—
Peripheral ischemia	—	Brief (<24 h) episode of ischemia managed nonsurgically and without permanent deficit	Recurring or prolonged ($\geq$24 h) and/or invasive intervention indicated	Life-threatening consequences; evidence of end organ damage; urgent operative intervention indicated	Death
Phlebitis	—	Present	—	—	—
Superficial thrombophlebitis	—	Present	—	—	—
Superior vena cava syndrome	Asymptomatic; incidental finding of superior vena cava thrombosis	Symptomatic; medical intervention indicated (eg, anticoagulation, radiation, or chemotherapy)	Severe symptoms; multimodality intervention indicated (eg, anticoagulation, chemotherapy, radiation, stenting)	Life-threatening consequences; urgent multimodality intervention indicated (eg, lysis, thrombectomy, surgery)	Death

Thromboembolic event	Venous thrombosis (eg, superficial thrombosis)	Venous thrombosis (eg, uncomplicated deep vein thrombosis), medical intervention indicated	Thrombosis (eg, uncomplicated pulmonary embolism [venous], nonembolic cardiac mural [arterial] thrombus), medical intervention indicated	Life-threatening (eg, pulmonary embolism, cerebrovascular event, arterial insufficiency); hemodynamic or neurologic instability; urgent intervention indicated	Death
Vasculitis	Asymptomatic, intervention not indicated	Moderate symptoms, medical intervention indicated	Severe symptoms, medical intervention indicated (eg, steroids)	Life-threatening; evidence of peripheral or visceral ischemia; urgent intervention indicated	Death
Visceral arterial ischemia	—	Brief (<24 h) episode of ischemia managed medically and without permanent deficit	Prolonged (≥24 h) or recurring symptoms and/or invasive intervention indicated	Life-threatening consequences; evidence of end-organ damage; urgent operative intervention indicated	Death
Vascular disorders, other, specify	Asymptomatic or mild symptoms; clinical or diagnostic observations only; intervention not indicated	Moderate; minimal, local, or noninvasive intervention indicated; limiting age-appropriate instrumental ADL	Severe or medically significant but not immediately life-threatening; hospitalization or prolongation of existing hospitalization indicated; disabling; limiting self-care ADL	Life-threatening consequences; urgent intervention indicated	Death

Data from http://evs.nci.nih.gov/ftp1/CTCAE/CTCAE_4.03_2010-06-14_QuickReference_5x7.pdf.

TABLE 2.3
Mitotic inhibitors

Group	Agent	Main Indications	Specific Toxicities
Vinca alkaloids	Vincristine	CLL, CML, AML, ALL, HL, NHL, MM, sarcomas, breast cancer	CIPN, BMD, constipation
	Vinblastine	HL, NHL, breast cancer	BMD, CINV
	Vinorelbine	NSCLC, breast cancer	BMD, CIPN, CINV
Taxanes	Paclitaxel	NSCLC, sarcomas, Ovarian and breast cancer	Hypersensitivity reaction/ anaphylaxis, CIPN, BMD
	Nab-paclitaxel	NSCLC, breast and pancreatic cancer	CIPN, BMD
	Docetaxel	NSCLC, breast, prostate and gastric cancer	BMD, alopecia, hypersensitivity reaction/ anaphylaxis, fluid retention, CIPN
Epothilones	Ixabepilone	Breast cancer	BMD, CIPN
Halichondrin	Eribulin	Breast cancer	BMD, CIPN

Abbreviations: ALL, acute lymphocytic leukemia; AML, acute myelogenic leukemia; BMD, bone marrow depression; CINV, chemotherapy-induced nausea and vomiting; CIPN, chemotherapy-induced peripheral neuropathy; CLL, chronic lymphocytic leukemia; HL, Hodgkin lymphoma; MM, multiple myeloma; NHL, non-Hodgkin lymphoma; NSCLC, non–small-cell lung cancer.

Microtubule destabilizers consist predominantly of drugs that act at the Vinca alkaloid and colchicine-binding sites. Vinca alkaloids, such as vincristine, vinblastine, and vinorelbine, used for the treatment of malignancies, such as lymphoma and acute lymphoblastic leukemia, interact with the central portion of the tubulin subunit and thus prevent polymerization into microtubules. Common side effects include distal neuropathy, constipation, and alopecia.

Microtubule stabilizers like paclitaxel and docetaxel bind to tubulin, stabilize the microtubule, and inhibit its disassembly, leading ultimately to cell death by apoptosis. They are used in the treatment of a variety of solid tumors, including those of ovarian, breast, prostate, pancreatic, and lung origin.

Hypersensitivity reactions (particularly related to its vehicle polyoxyethylated castor oil, cremaphor) can occur with paclitaxel, and thus, premedication with glucocorticoids and antihistamines is commonly used. Advances in the formulation, such as the albumin-bound, vehicle-free nab-paclitaxel, have led to lower risk of these reactions at higher intracellular concentrations and antitumor activity in preclinical models. Other side effects include myelosuppression and peripheral neuropathy and are also observed with docetaxel, which can also cause fluid retention and worsening effusions as well as rash and stomatitis.

Epothilones, like ixabepilone, are macrolide antibiotics and represent a novel class of antimicrotubule agents, which by binding near the taxane-binding site cause microtubular stabilization and cellular arrest.[11,12] Eribulin mesylate is a nontaxane, completely synthetic microtubule inhibitor approved as third-line treatment of metastatic breast cancer refractory to anthracyclines and taxanes. Eribulin is a synthetic analogue of halichondrin B. Unlike other antimicrotubule drugs, such as vinblastine and paclitaxel, which suppress the shortening and growth phases of microtubule dynamic instability, eribulin works through an end-poisoning mechanism, resulting in the inhibition of microtubule growth but not of shortening. Tubulin is also sequestered into nonfunctional aggregates, resulting in irreversible G2- to M-phase arrest and apoptosis.[13]

Antitumor antibiotics and topoisomerase inhibitors

Antitumor antibiotics are natural products of *Streptomyces* species. These drugs act during multiple phases of the cell cycle and are considered cell-cycle nonspecific (Table 2.4). Several different mechanisms have been proposed for their cytostatic and cytotoxic actions. These mechanisms include intercalation into DNA leading to inhibition of macromolecular biosynthesis, free radical formation with consequent induction of DNA damage or lipid peroxidation, DNA binding and alkylation, DNA cross-linking, interference with DNA unwinding or DNA strand separation and helicase activity, direct membrane effects,

TABLE 2.4
Antitumor antibiotics

Group	Agent	Main Indications	Specific Toxicities
Anthracyclines	Doxorubicin	AML, ALL, NHL, HL, MM, sarcomas, SCLC, breast, gastric and bladder cancer	CINV, BMD, alopecia, cardiotoxicity
	Liposomal doxorubicin	MM, sarcomas, breast and ovarian cancer	PPE, BMD, alopecia, cardiotoxicity
	Epirubicin	AML, ALL, breast cancer	CINV, BMD, alopecia, cardiotoxicity
	Daunorubicin	AML, ALL	CINV, BMD, cardiotoxicity
	Mitoxantrone	NHL, ALL, breast cancer	CINV, BMD, cardiotoxicity
	Idarubicin	AML, breast cancer	CINV, BMD, cardiotoxicity
Chromomycins	Dactinomycin	Sarcomas, gestational trophoblastic tumor	CINV, BMD
Miscellaneous	Mitomycin	Bladder, breast and anal cancer	CINV, BMD
	Bleomycin	GCT, malignant effusion	Pneumonitis, lung fibrosis

Abbreviations: ALL, acute lymphocytic leukemia; AML, acute myelogenic leukemia; BMD, bone marrow depression; CINV, chemotherapy-induced nausea and vomiting; CIPN, chemotherapy-induced peripheral neuropathy; CLL, chronic lymphocytic leukemia; GCT, germ cell tumors; HCL, hairy cell leukemia; HL, Hodgkin lymphoma; MM, multiple myeloma; NHL, non-Hodgkin lymphoma; PPE, palmar-plantar erythrodysesthesia; SCLC, small-cell lung cancer.

and the initiation of DNA damage via the inhibition of topoisomerase II (TOP I).

Topoisomerases are enzymes that facilitate the unwinding DNA that is required for normal replication or transcription.[14,15] TOP I inhibition leads to single-stranded breaks in DNA, whereas topoisomerase II (TOP II) inhibition causes double-stranded breaks. The TOP1 inhibitor camptothecin (CPT), first isolated from the Chinese tree *Camptotheca acuminate*, was clinically used for cancer treatment long before it was identified as a TOP1 inhibitor. Because of side effects, CPT is no longer used clinically, and more effective and safer derivates like topotecan and irinotecan have replaced it.[14] Irinotecan is used primarily for the treatment of colon cancer, and topotecan has activity in gynecologic malignancies. Both medications can cause myelosuppression. Irinotecan is also known to cause a secretory diarrhea.

TOP II inhibitors (see Table 2.3; Table 2.5) include etoposide, which is used for the treatment of small-cell lung cancer, certain types of lymphomas, and testicular cancer. The most commonly observed side effects are myelosuppression, alopecia, and nausea. If administered rapidly, it can also lead to a transient reduction in blood pressure.

The best-known antitumor antibiotic TOP II inhibitors are the anthracyclines, doxorubicin and daunorubicin, from which idarubicin and epirubicin are derived.[15] Doxorubicin is a critical chemotherapeutic in the treatment of a variety of cancers, including leukemia, lymphoma, breast cancer, and sarcoma. Common side effects include

TABLE 2.5
Topoisomerase inhibitors

Group	Agent	Main Indications	Specific Toxicities
Podophyllo-toxins	Etoposide	Sarcomas, SCLC, GCT	BMD, CINV, alopecia, pneumonitis
	Tenisopide	ALL	BMD, CINV, alopecia
Camptothecan analogues	Irinotecan	CRC, sarcomas	Alopecia, acute cholinergic syndrome, BMD, CINV
	Topotecan	Ovarian cancer	BMD, CINV

Abbreviations: ALL, acute lymphocytic leukemia; BMD, bone marrow depression; CINV, chemotherapy-induced nausea and vomiting; SCLC, small-cell lung cancer.

alopecia, nausea, mucositis, and myelosuppression. Furthermore, treatment with doxorubicin can lead to acute and chronic cardiotoxicity as discussed elsewhere in this volume.

Actinomycin D is a natural antibiotic that inhibits the transcription of genes by interacting with a GC-rich duplex, a single-stranded or hairpin form of DNA, and then interfering with the action of RNA polymerase.[16]

Mitomycin-C is an antitumor antibiotic that is activated in the tissues to an alkylating agent, which disrupts DNA in cancer cells by forming a complex with DNA and also acts by inhibiting division of cancer cells by interfering with the biosynthesis of DNA.[17]

Bleomycin is a basic, water-soluble glycopeptide with cytotoxic activity isolated from a strain of *Streptomyces verticillus*.[18] It acts by forming complexes with Fe^{2+} while binding to DNA. Oxidation of Fe^{2+} subsequently leads to the formation of free radicals, which result in DNA damage.[18] It is used for the treatment of germ cell tumors and lymphoma. Common side effects include fever, facial flushing, and Raynaud phenomenon. Although less common, the most concerning side effect is pulmonary fibrosis. Lung fibrosis is dose dependent and is more commonly seen with cumulative doses that are greater than 300 units. Typically, pulmonary function testing with assessment of the carbon monoxide diffusing capacity is obtained before initiation of therapy and with the onset of any symptoms.

Antimetabolites

Antimetabolites act by mimicking purines and pyrimidines that are required for DNA synthesis or by interfering with native synthesis. They most commonly affect cells in the S phase of the cell cycle (cell-cycle specific) when DNA replication is occurring (Table 2.6).

Methotrexate was rationally designed nearly 60 years ago to potently block dihydrofolate reductase (DHFR) as an antimetabolite, thereby achieving temporary remissions in childhood acute leukemias. DHFR regenerates the reduced form of folate, a requirement for the biosynthesis of purines and thymidylate, which when missing leads to ineffective DNA synthesis and replication. When given in high doses, methotrexate is able to diffuse directly into cells, leading to significant toxicity. Therapy is also toxic to nonmalignant cells, although leucovorin is able to bypass DHFR and rescue these cells. The strategy of high-dose therapy followed by leucovorin rescue is commonly used for the treatment of osteosarcoma and hematologic malignancies, especially

TABLE 2.6
Antimetabolites

Group	Agent	Main Indications	Specific Toxicities
Folic acid antagonists	Methotrexate	AML, ALL, NHL, sarcomas, breast, bladder, GCT	Mucositis, CINV, nephrotoxicity, pneumonitis
	Pemetrexed	Mesothelioma, NSCLC	CIPN, BMD, CINV
Pyrimidine analogues	5-FU	CRC, breast cancer	CINV, mucositis, BMD, cardiotoxicity
	Capecitabine	CRC, breast cancer	PPE, diarrhea, N/V, mucositis, BMD, cardiotoxicity
	Gemcitabine	NSCLC, breast, pancreas, bladder and ovarian cancer	BMD-thrombocytopenia, CINV, LFT changes
	Cytarabine	ALL, AML	BMD-thrombocytopenia, rash, mucositis
Purine analogues	6-Mercaptopurine	ALL, AML	BMD, CINV
	6-Thioguanine	ALL, AML	BMD, CINV
	Cladribine	HCL, CLL	BMD, CINV neurotoxicity
	Fludarabine	CLL	BMD, CINV
	Pentostatin	HCL	BMD, CINV

Abbreviations: ALL, acute lymphocytic leukemia; AML, acute myelogenic leukemia; BMD, bone marrow depression; CINV, chemotherapy-induced nausea and vomiting; CIPN, chemotherapy-induced peripheral neuropathy; GCT, germ cell tumors; HL, Hodgkin lymphoma; MM, multiple myeloma; NHL, non-Hodgkin lymphoma; NSCLC, non–small cell lung cancer; PPE, palmar-plantar erythrodysesthesia.

when there is involvement of the central nervous system. Like all antimetabolites, methotrexate can cause myelosuppression and mucositis. It can also lead to renal dysfunction, which can be decreased with the use of urine alkalinization. Transaminitis can also be seen. The new generation antifolate pemetrexed is an antimetabolite with activity against certain lung cancers and mesothelioma. It is thought to affect many targets, including thymidylate synthase, DHFR, and glycinamide ribonucleotide formyltransferase, which ultimately leads to decreased production of purines and pyrimidines. Folic acid and vitamin B12 injections are given in conjunction with chemotherapy to reduce side effects.

Deoxynucleoside analogues are antimetabolites that compete with natural deoxynucleosides used for DNA synthesis, bases, and ribonucleosides. Deoxynucleoside analogues can be divided into purine analogues (eg, fludarabine, cladribine), pyrimidine analogues (eg, cytarabine, gemcitabine), and the fluoropyrimidines (eg, 5-FU, capecitabine). 5-FU is widely used for treatment of various solid tumors. It is readily incorporated into rapidly dividing malignant cells, especially those found within the gut, and is one of the key chemotherapeutic agents used in the treatment of many gastrointestinal malignancies. It has multiple mechanisms of action; its metabolite mediates inhibition of thymidylate synthase, and 5-FU can also be incorporated into RNA and DNA. 5-FU is clinically administered with leucovorin to increase its antitumor activity. Capecitabine is a prodrug of 5-FU that is selectively activated in tumors overexpressing the activating enzyme thymidine phosporylase.[19]

Additional antimetabolites include the cytosine arabinoside (Ara-C), 6-thioguanine, 6-mercaptopurine, and fludarabine. These chemotherapeutic agents, which are used in the treatment of a variety of hematologic malignancies, are incorporated into DNA with resulting S-phase toxicity. Gemcitabine is also a cytosine derivative that is incorporated into DNA, thus rendering the DNA more susceptible to breakage. Unlike Ara-C, gemcitabine has been found to have activity against many solid tumors and is less likely to cause myelosuppression.

TARGETED CANCER THERAPIES

Remarkable scientific advances over the past decade have led to the development of agents for the treatment of cancer targeting enzymes (especially kinases) abnormally activated by mutation or translocation (Fig. 2.3). In some instances, this has led to the inhibition of pathognomonic pathways, as, for example, in chronic myeloid leukemia (CML).

BCR-ABL Inhibitors

A translocation between chromosome 9 and 22 is causally responsive for CML as it leads to the *BCR-ABL* fusion gene, which encodes for a constitutively active tyrosine kinase that activates downstream signaling and unregulated cell division. Imatinib, which is a targeted agent against the ATP binding site of the mutated tyrosine kinase, blocks signaling and induces cell death. Side effects are typically moderate in severity and include hepatoxicity, fluid retention, and diarrhea. Congestive heart failure is also a recognized, although it is a less common adverse effect. Nilotinib, dasatinib, and bosutinib are similar inhibitors, although more potent and possibly effective in patients resistant to imatinib. Ponatinib is another tyrosine kinase inhibitor that is typically active against patients with a T315I mutant

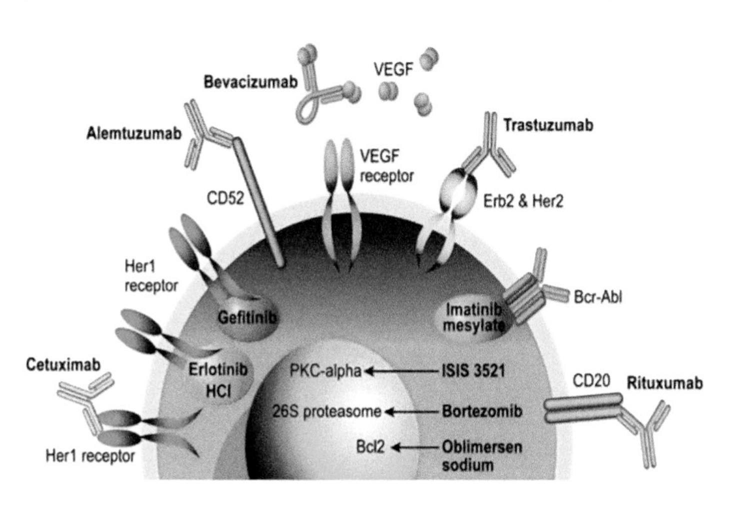

Fig. 2.3 Molecular targeted therapies for HCC and their target signalling pathways. (*From* Llovet JM, Villanueva A, Lachenmayer A, et al. Advances in targeted therapies for hepatocellular carcinoma in the genomic era. Nat Rev Clin Oncol 2015;12(7):408–24; with permission.)

BCR-ABL. This mutation is a common source of drug resistance to imatinib. Ponatinib has similar side effects, although it is also associated with an increased risk of thromboembolic events.

Vascular Endothelial Growth Factor Receptor Inhibitors

The angiogenic switch, a process that signifies the transition from an avascular stage to a vascularized stage through the initiation of angiogenesis, is essential for tumors to grow beyond 1 to 2 mm^3.[1]

The realization of the need of cancers for sufficient blood supply has stimulated the development of various angiogenesis inhibitors (Table 2.7).[20] The vascular endothelial growth factor (VEGF) signaling pathway is one of the most, if not the most, important molecular mediator for tumor angiogenesis. Key members of the VEGF family of angiogenic factors are VEGF-A, VEGF-B, and placental growth factor (PlGF) that can act as potent mitogenic, chemotactic, and vascular permeability factors for endothelial cells. VEGF-A acts via 2 receptor tyrosine kinases, vascular endothelial growth factor receptor-1 (VEGFR-1) and VEGFR-2, present on the surface of endothelial cells. PlGF and VEGF-B bind only to VEGFR-1, which is also present on the surface of leukocytes. Excessive activation of these receptors by VEGF-A can result in pathologic neovascularization and excessive vascular permeability. PlGF is also linked to pathologic neovascularization and recruitment of inflammatory cells into tumors. Drugs designed to inhibit the VEGF receptor kinase have proven efficacy, for instance, in metastatic renal cell carcinoma with 4 drugs being FDA approved: sorafenib, sunitinib, pazopanib, and axitinib. These drugs have also shown single-agent activity in advanced hepatocellular carcinoma and advanced pancreatic neuroendocrine tumors (PNET). Bevacizumab, a humanized monoclonal antibody (mAb) that binds specifically to VEGF-A, has shown efficacy in several indications in the metastatic setting (colorectal, breast cancer). Aflibercept is a fusion protein that binds to 3 VEGF family ligands: VEGF-A, VEGF-B, and PlGF, and proved to be another effective antiangiogenic agent in the treatment of CRC. By targeting VEGF-B and PlGF, which are also implicated in angiogenesis and/or the survival of newly formed vessels, aflibercept may have additional antiangiogenic effects beyond targeting VEGF-A alone.[21]

Epidermal Growth Factor Receptor Inhibitors

The human epidermal growth factor receptor (EGFR) family consists of 4 members that belong to the ErbB lineage of proteins (ErbB1–4). These

TABLE 2.7
Antiangiogenics

Agent	Target	Indication	Specific Toxicity
Bevacizumab	VEGF	CRC, NSCLC, RCC, breast and ovarian cancer	Hypertension, hemorrhage, arterial thromboembolism, gastrointestinal perforations
Aflibercept	VEGF-A; VEGF-B; PlGF	CRC	BMD, hypertension, PPE
Sunitinib	PDGFRα and PDGFRβ, VEGFR1, VEGFR2, VEGFR3, KIT, FLT3, CSF-1R, RET	GIST, RCC, PNET	Hypertension, PPE, skin rash, proteinuria, cardiotoxicity, BMD
Sorafenib	CRAF, BRAF, V600E BRAF, c-KIT, and FLT-3, VEGFR-2, VEGFR-3, and PDGFR-ß	HCC, RCC, thyroid cancer	Hypertension, PPE, skin rash, proteinuria, cardiotoxicity, BMD
Pazopanib	VEGFR-1, -2, and -3, PDGFR-α and -β, c-KIT	RCC, sarcoma	Hypertension, PPE, skin rash, proteinuria, cardiotoxicity, BMD
Axitinib	VEGFR-1, VEGFR-2, and VEGFR-3	RCC	Hypertension, PPE, skin rash, proteinuria, cardiotoxicity, BMD
Regorafenib	VEGFR1, -2, -3, KIT, RET, RAF-1, BRAF, $BRAF^{V600E}$, PDGFR, FGFR	GIST, CRC	Hypertension, PPE, skin rash, proteinuria, cardiotoxicity, BMD

Abbreviations: BMD, bone marrow depression; CSF-1R, colony stimulating factor receptor; FLT3, Fms-like tyrosine kinase-3; GIST, gastrointestinal stromal tumor; HCC, hepatocellular carcinoma; KIT, stem cell factor receptor; PDGFRα and PDGFRβ, platelet-derived growth factor receptors; PPE, palmar-plantar erythrodysesthesia; RCC, renal cell carcinoma; RET, glial cell-line derived neurotrophic factor receptor; VEGFR1, VEGFR2, and VEGFR3, vascular endothelial growth factor receptors.

receptors consist of an extracellular domain, a transmembrane segment, and an intracellular portion with a protein kinase domain. Growth factor binding to EGFR induces a large conformational change in the extracellular domain and leads to dimerization and autophosphorylation of the intracellular receptor tyrosine kinase and subsequent activation of complex downstream signaling, which includes the phosphatidylinositol 3-kinase/Akt pathway, the Ras/Raf/MEK/ERK1/2 pathway, and the phospholipase C pathway (Fig. 2.4). EGFR/ErbB1 is aberrantly activated by various mechanisms, like receptor overexpression, mutation, ligand-dependent receptor dimerization, and ligand-independent activation, and is associated with the development of a variety of tumors. Similar to VEGF receptor inhibitors, 2 major approaches have been developed and demonstrated benefits in clinical trials for targeting EGFR: mAbs and tyrosine kinase inhibitors (Table 2.8).

Several malignancies are associated with the mutation or increased expression of members of the ErbB family, including lung, breast, stomach, colorectal, head and neck, and pancreatic carcinomas, and glioblastoma. Gefitinib, erlotinib, and afatinib are orally effective protein-kinase–targeted quinazoline derivatives that are used in the treatment of ERBB1-mutant lung cancer. Lapatinib is an orally effective quinazoline derivative used in the treatment of ErbB2-overexpressing breast cancer. Trastuzumab and pertuzumab are mAbs that target the extracellular domain and are used for the treatment of ErbB2-positive breast cancer. Cetuximab and panitumumab are mAbs that target ErbB1 and are used in the treatment of CRC.[22]

BRAF Inhibitors

Activating *BRAF* mutations, leading to constitutive activation of the mitogen-activated protein kinase (MAPK) signaling pathway, are common in a variety of human cancers. More specifically, activation of the MAPK pathway is a hallmark of melanoma. Mutations in pathway members or promoters (including *NRAS*, *BRAF*, and *NF1*, and less commonly *KRAS*, *MEK1/2*) occur in most melanomas. The identification of the activating *BRAF* V600 mutations in 40% to 50% of melanomas leads to the development of selective

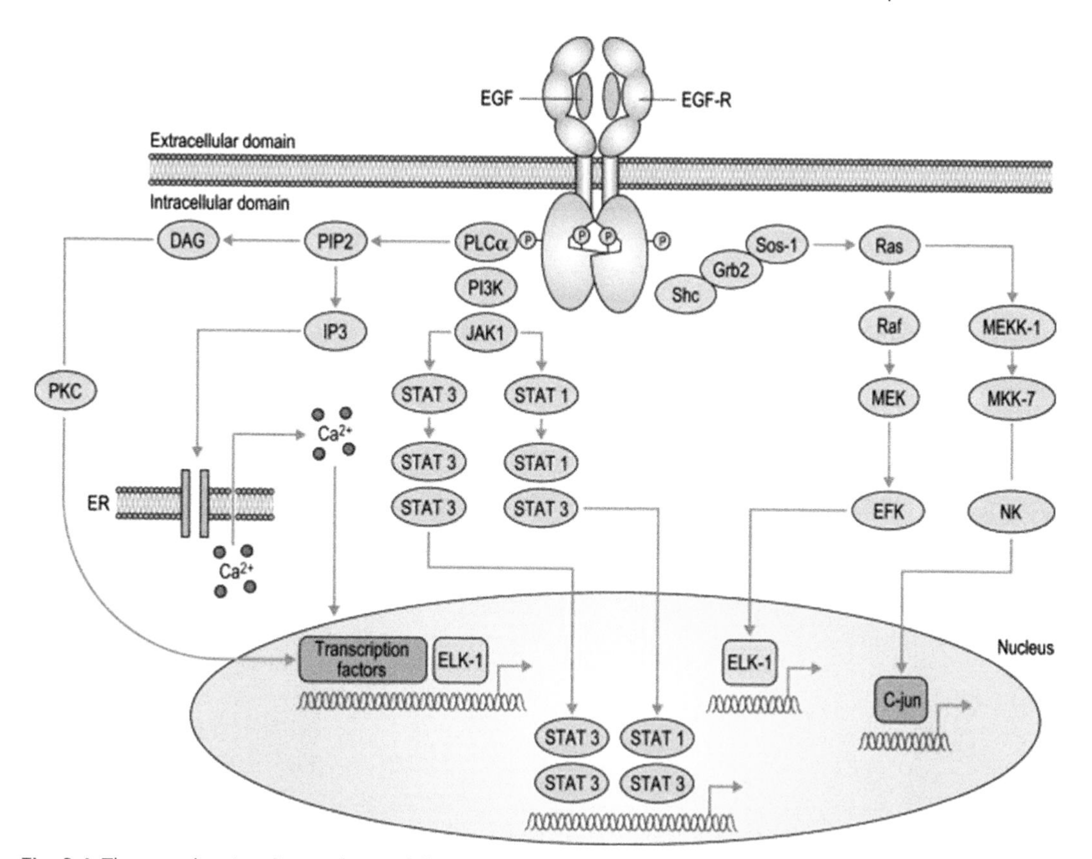

Fig. 2.4 The complex signaling pathways following activation of EGFR. (*From* Hatcher HM. Appendix: a glossary of common targets with examples. In: Ajithkumar TV, Hatcher H, editors. Specialist training in oncology. Philadelphia: Mosby; 2011. p. 370–4; with permission.)

TABLE 2.8
Endothelial growth factor receptor targeting agents

Agent	Target	Indication	Specific Toxicity
Afatinib	ErbB1	NSCLC	Skin rash, mucositis, PPE
Erlotinib	ErbB1	NSCLC, pancreatic cancer	Skin rash, mucositis, PPE
Gefitinib	ErbB1	NSCLC	Skin rash, mucositis, PPE
Lapatinib	ErbB1/2	Breast cancer	Skin rash, mucositis, PPE
Cetuximab	ErbB1	CRC, head and neck SCC	Skin rash, mucositis, PPE,
Panitumumab	ErbB1	CRC	Skin rash, mucositis, PPE
Trastuzumab	ErbB2	Breast and gastric/ gastroesophageal cancer	Hypersenitivity reaction, cardiotoxicity
Pertuzumab	ErbB2	Breast cancer	Hypersenitivity reaction, cardiotoxicity

Abbreviations: NSCLC, non–small-cell lung cancer; PPE, palmar-plantar erythrodysesthesia; SCC, squamous cell carcinoma.

BRAF inhibitors like vemurafenib and dabrafenib. These agents have shown dramatic responses in the treatment of metastatic melanoma. Unfortunately, acquired resistance quickly develops to the BRAF inhibitors, within the first 1 to 2 years of therapy. Unlike in many other cancers, resistance in *BRAF*-mutant melanoma is not the result of second-site mutations in the target gene rather than acquired alterations in the MAPK pathway or parallel signaling networks. BRAF inhibitor–MEK inhibitor combinations of dabrafenib and trametinib targeting distinct MAPK pathway components not only circumvent or delay resistance but also lead to fewer side effects, such as development of secondary squamous tumors.[23]

Other Targeted Agents

The list of targeted agents in development and already in use in the treatment of a wide range of malignancies is expanding day by day. Without aiming for completeness and going into details about their exact mechanism of action, the most frequently used additional targeted agents are listed in Table 2.9.

ANTIBODY DRUG CONJUGATES

mAbs, like trastuzumab, bevacizumab, and cetuximab, have been a success story in the treatment of several malignancies. A critical feature of mAbs is their high specificity and their ability to bind

TABLE 2.9
"Other" targeted agents

Agent	Target	Indication	Specific Toxicity
Bortezomib	26s proteasome	MM	N/V, rash, peripheral neuropathy
Crizotinib	ALK	NSCLC with ALK gene rearrangement	Gastrointestinal and hepatotoxicity
Dasatinib	BCR-ABL (Philadelphia chromosome)	CML, ALL with PCR-proven BCR-ABL transcript	Diarrhea, rash, QT interval prolongation
Everolimus	mTOR	PNET, breast cancer	Mucositis, rash, transaminitis, pneumonitis, BMD
Temsirolimus	mTOR	RCC	Mucositis, rash, transaminitis, pneumonitis, BMD
Imatinib	BCR-ABL (Philadelphia chromosome); c-KIT	CML, ALL, GIST, MDS, DFSP	Rash, edema, BMD, cardiotoxicity, PPE

Abbreviations: ALK, anaplastic lymphoma kinase; ALL, acute lymphocytic leukemia; AML, acute myelogenic leukemia; BCR, ABL-breakpoint cluster region-Abelson; BMD, bone marrow depression; DFSP, dermatofibrosarcoma protuberans; GIST, gastrointestinal stromal tumor; KIT, stem cell factor receptor; MDS, myelodysplastic syndrome; MM, multiple myeloma; mTOR, mammalian target of rapamycin; NSCLC, non–small-cell lung cancer; PPE, palmar-plantar erythrodysesthesia; RCC, renal cell carcinoma.

target antigens, marking them for removal by methods such as complement-dependent cytotoxicity or antibody-dependent cell-mediated cytotoxicity. Traditional chemotherapeutics (alkylating agents, anthracyclines, mitotic inhibitors) have a small therapeutic index (maximum tolerated dose/minimum efficacious dose) resulting in a narrow therapeutic window. Conjugation of mAbs to cytotoxic drugs can expand the utility, potency, and effectiveness of each component. The promise of antibody drug conjugates (ADCs) is that they could selectively deliver toxic compounds to diseased tissue. Brentuximab vedotin licensed for the treatment of anaplastic large cell lymphoma and Hodgkin lymphoma chemically couples an anti-CD30 chimeric antibody with the highly potent antimitotic agent, monomethyl auristatin through a protease cleavable linker. Ado-trastuzumab emtansine targets human epidermal growth factor receptor 2 (HER2)-positive breast cancer and combines an anti-HER2 antibody (trastuzumab) with the cytotoxic agent maytansine (DM1) via a stable linker. Upon ADC binding, the entire antigen-ADC complex is internalized through receptor-mediated endocytosis. Once inside the cell, ADCs are degraded, and free cytotoxic drug is released into the cell, resulting in cell death.[24]

IMMUNE CHECKPOINT THERAPIES

The immune system can act as a powerful defense against tumor cells. It can be envisioned as a cancer-immunity cycle, divided into 7 major steps, starting with the release of antigens from the cancer cell and ending with the killing of cancer cells (Fig. 2.5).[25]

Each step of the cancer-immunity cycle requires the coordination of numerous factors, both stimulatory and inhibitory in nature to allow for appropriate and controlled immunity. Malignant cells, however, have found ways to break the cycle to allow for continued proliferation. For example, cancer cells express programmed death-ligand 1 (PD-L1), which binds to the programmed cell death protein 1 receptor (PD-1) on T cells and B cells. This interaction acts as an immune rheostat and silences the immune response. Another strategy used by cancer cells to circumvent the immune response is the

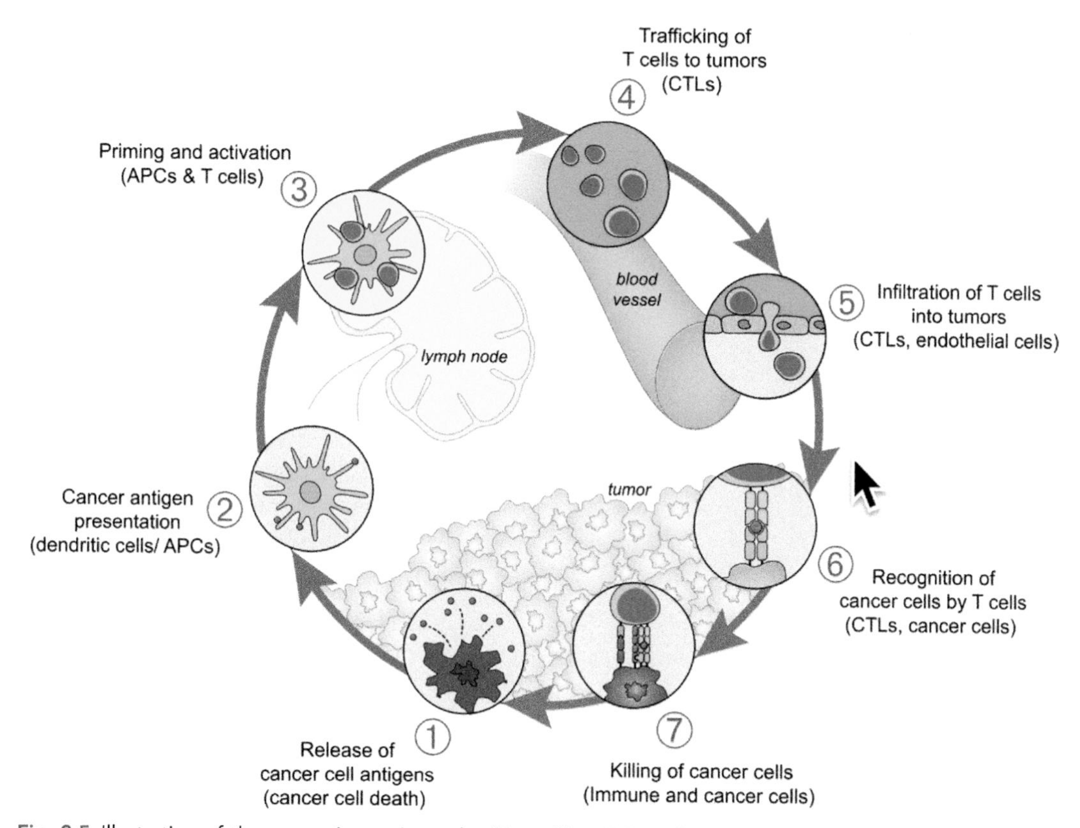

Fig. 2.5 Illustration of the cancer-immunity cycle. (*From* Chen DS, Mellman I. Oncology meets immunology: the cancer-immunity cycle. Immunity 2013;39(1):1–10; with permission.)

expression of cytotoxic T-lymphocyte–associated protein 4 (CTLA4), an immune checkpoint protein that can inhibit the development of an active immune response by acting primarily at the level of T-cell development and proliferation. Ipilimumab is an mAb against CTLA-4 and even when used as monotherapy resulted in more than 20% long-term survival in the treatment of advanced melanoma. Pembrolizumab and nivolumab are antibodies against the programmed cell death 1 (PD-1) receptor, found to be effective in the treatment of melanoma, renal cell carcinoma, and certain types of lung cancer. Antibodies against PD-L1 receptors have similar activity (Fig. 2.6). The stunning successes in treating cancers with anti-CTLA-4 and anti-PD-1 "immune checkpoint therapies" have spawned newfound optimism that targeting of additional immune pathways and optimization of drug regimens will be effective in numerous cancers and in larger proportions of patients.[26] Common side effects of these therapies are fluid retention, edema, and effusions. Nevertheless, the main concern is induction of autoimmune diseases, for example, vasculitis.[26]

Allogeneic bone marrow transplantation is another classic example of the strength of the immune system against malignant cells. T cells from the donor recognize tumor cells as foreign and mediate a "graft-versus-tumor" effect. In the setting of disease relapse after stem cell transplant, reduction in immunosuppression or a donor lymphocyte infusion can result in disease control.

Autologous T cells can also be used to enhance the immune response against a tumor. T cells can be removed from a patient and modified in order to express receptors specific to cancer cells. When reintroduced into patients, the cells are able to recognize and kill cancer cells.

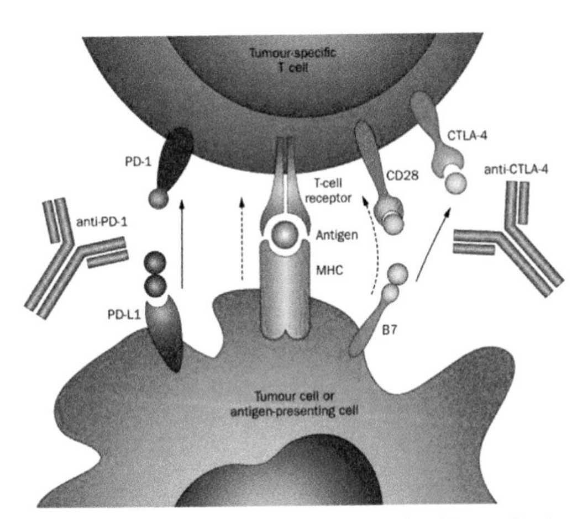

Fig. 2.6 Immune checkpoint blockade. (*From* Drake CG, Lipson EJ, Brahmer JR. Breathing new life into immunotherapy: review of melanoma, lung and kidney cancer. Nat Rev Clin Oncol 2014;11(1):24–37; with permission.)

Tumor vaccines are also under development. Specifically purified antigen-presenting cells have been exposed to tumor antigens and delivered as a vaccine. This technique is used as a treatment option of patients with castration-resistant prostate cancer. A patient's dendritic cells are first isolated with the use of leukapheresis. They are then incubated with the antigen prostatic acid phosphatase as well as granulocyte-macrophage colony stimulating factor, which facilitates cell maturation. These cells are subsequently returned to the patient with a goal of inducing an immune response against the antigen.

Cytokines

Various cytokines have been found to have antineoplastic properties. Interferon (IFN) induces gene expression, inhibits protein synthesis, and affects intracellular signaling. IFN has activity in CML, although it has essentially been replaced by the use of tyrosine kinase inhibitors. It can also induce partial responses in hairy cell leukemia and follicular lymphoma, although it has a limited role given the availability of alternative therapy. Last, IFN is currently the approved adjuvant treatment for melanoma, although the role of checkpoint inhibitors in this setting is currently under investigation. These medications are challenging to tolerate given a host of toxicities. Specifically, treatment can cause fever, flulike symptoms, fatigue, malaise, myelosuppression, and depression. Interleukin-2, also known as T-cell growth factor, which acts indirectly against cancer by stimulating T cells, has had a limited role with a low level of response in the treatment of melanoma and renal cell carcinoma. With the advent of checkpoint blockage with PD-1, PDL-1, and CTLA-4 antibodies, the role for cytokine therapy is becoming more limited.

Hormone Receptor Inhibitors

Targeted therapy against hormone receptors has been identified as a powerful tool in the treatment of breast and prostate cancer. In breast cancer, for example, approximately two-thirds of patients with invasive breast cancer have hormone receptor–bearing tumors. The use of targeted therapies against these receptors can lead to the inhibition of cell proliferation and cell-cycle arrest. Tamoxifen is a selective estrogen receptor modulator, which serves as an antagonist of the estrogen receptor in breast tissue, but also as an agonist in endometrial and vascular tissue. Tamoxifen is often used as adjuvant therapy for women with estrogen receptor–positive disease, especially if premenopausal, resulting in reduction in disease recurrence and mortality. Side effects of tamoxifen include a small increased risk of thrombosis and endometrial carcinoma, especially with prolonged use. Aromatase inhibitors can also lead to hormonal suppression in patients with breast cancer. They work by either irreversibly or reversibly inhibiting aromatase, an enzyme that catalyzes the formation of estrogen within tissues. Exemestane, anastrozole, and letrozole are aromatase inhibitors and are preferable over tamoxifen in postmenopausal patients. A major side effect of aromatase inhibitors is reduction in bone density.

Prostate cancer is also treated with hormone suppression, classically through androgen deprivation. Androgen deprivation is used in conjunction with radiation therapy for patients with high-risk disease and for patients with evidence of metastasis. Hormonal suppression can be achieved with the use of luteinizing hormone–releasing hormone agonists (LHRH), such as leuprolide and goserelin. These agents continuously stimulate the LHRH receptor, resulting in normal loss of pulsatile activation. This leads to the decreased LH production by the anterior pituitary and diminished downstream testosterone production at the level of the testicle. If the cancer cell becomes refractory to suppression, androgen receptor blockers such as bicalutamide or enzalutamide or drugs that block enzymes that lead to production of testosterone within tissue, such as abiraterone, can be used. Side effects of androgen blockade include fatigue, hot flashes, weight gain, and decreased libido.

Differentiating Agents

Acute promyelocytic leukemia (APL) results from the translocation 15;17, which leads to the production of a promyelocytic leukemia-retinoic acid receptor fusion protein. All transretinoic acid (ATRA) is a special class of drug used for the treatment of this malignancy. The binding of ATRA to the fusion protein causes differentiation of malignant promyelocytes into mature granulocytes. It is used for the treatment of APL in combination with arsenic trioxide and possibly chemotherapy, depending on the disease risk. Side effects of ATRA include headache and gastrointestinal upset. There is also the possibility of differentiation syndrome, which is a systemic and respiratory illness characterized by fever, dyspnea, and weight gain that can develop as a consequence of the maturing tumor cells eliciting a cytokine response and sludging in the lungs.

Proteasome Inhibitors

The proteasome is a multi-subunit assembly of proteases that selectively degrades proteins, including transcription factors that regulate the cell cycle. Bortezomib is a proteasome inhibitor that is one of the key components of therapy for patients with multiple myeloma.[11] It also has activity in certain types of lymphoma. Side effects include neuropathy, orthostatic hypotension, and thrombocytopenia. Carfilzomib is another proteasome inhibitor with activity in refractory multiple myeloma.[13] It does not cause significant neuropathy, although it can cause cytopenias as well as a cytokine release response.

Chromatin Modifiers

Gene transcription is also regulated by a variety of factors, including orientation of histones on DNA and DNA methylation status. The proper orientation of histones, proteins that allow for condensation of DNA, determines the transcriptional readiness of a gene. When acetylated, histones allow for the access of transcription factors for gene expression. Histone deacetylase inhibitors have been found to be an effective treatment approach in cutaneous T-cell lymphoma. Vorinostat and romidepsin are inhibitors that are currently approved.

Tumors can similarly methylate DNA in order to silence genes. DNA methyltransferase inhibitors lead to the demethylation of DNA and expression of various genes. 5-Aza-cytidine and 2′-deoxy-5-azacitabine (ie, decitabine) are examples of methyltransferase inhibitors. These drugs have activity in myelodysplastic syndrome and certain types of leukemia.

THE FUTURE OF SYSTEMIC ANTICANCER TREATMENT

Most cancers can be characterized by collections of mutated and aberrantly regulated genes that collaborate to promote tumor growth. Intricate feedback cycles, immune responses, and pharmacokinetics add further complexity to the malignant phenotype. Antineoplastic treatment itself often triggers further mutations as an escape mechanism. These facts suggest that cancer must be managed by treatment regimens comprising a cocktail of drugs that are changed to challenge the evolving disease. The emerging new generation of Precision Oncology uses broad-spectrum pan-omic (such as genomic, transcriptomic, proteomic, metabolomic, and so forth) analyses and sophisticated network-based statistical reverse engineering methods to hypothesize the putative driver networks for a given patient's tumor. Once these are computed, they are combined with important contextual features (such as the patient's treatment history, status, and preferences as well as knowledge of available drugs and drug interactions) to hypothesize a treatment plan that attacks these tumor drivers with cocktails of narrowly targeted therapies. Pan-omic data from tissue samples (tumors and surrounding healthy tissue) are analyzed to produce a list of hypothetical, aberrant driver networks. Drug candidates that target specific molecular pathways are selected and validated in models if possible; for example, in vitro (in tumor-derived cell lines) or in vivo (in mouse models). If the decision is made to move forward with that treatment, the patient is treated and monitored using rapid measures, such as imaging and serum biomarkers. Failure to respond, or disease recurrence, might lead one to choose a different drug or combination based on a fresh analysis. These new approaches will however impose further economic, social, and structural impediments, such as obtaining access to, and reimbursement for, investigational drugs.[27]

REFERENCES

1. Hanahan D, Weinberg RA. Hallmarks of cancer: the next generation [review]. Cell 2011;144(5):646–74.
2. National Comprehensive Cancer Network®. NCCN Clinical Practice Guidelines in Oncology. Available at: http://www.nccn.org/professionals/physician_gls/f_guidelines.asp#site.
3. Electronic Medicines Compendium. Available at: https://www.medicines.org.uk/emc.
4. American Joint Committee on Cancer. Available at: https://www.cancerstaging.org.
5. Oken MM, Creech RH, Tormey DC, et al. Toxicity and response criteria of the Eastern Cooperative Oncology Group. Am J Clin Oncol 1982;5(6):649–55.
6. The national confidential enquiry into patient outcome and death. Available at: http://www.ncepod.org.uk/2008report3/Downloads/SACT_report.pdf.
7. National Cancer Institutes' Common terminology criteria for adverse events. Available at: http://evs.nci.nih.gov/ftp1/CTCAE/CTCAE_4.03_2010-06-14_QuickReference_5x7.pdf.
8. Conroy T, Desseigne F, Ychou M, et al, Groupe Tumeurs Digestives of Unicancer, PRODIGE Intergroup. FOLFIRINOX versus gemcitabine for metastatic pancreatic cancer. N Engl J Med 2011;364(19):1817–25.
9. Vermeulen K, Van Bockstaele DR, Berneman ZN. The cell cycle: a review of regulation, deregulation and therapeutic targets in cancer [review]. Cell Prolif 2003;36(3):131–49.
10. Puyo S, Montaudon D, Pourquier P. From old alkylating agents to new minor groove binders [review]. Crit Rev Oncol Hematol 2014;89(1):43–61.
11. Morris PG, Fornier MN. Microtubule active agents: beyond the taxane frontier. Clin Cancer Res 2008;14(22):7167–72.
12. Moudi M, Go R, Yien CY. Vinca alkaloids. Int J Prev Med 2013;4(11):1231–5.
13. Jain S, Vahdat LT. Eribulin mesylate. Clin Cancer Res 2011;17(21):6615–22.
14. Xu Y, Her C. Inhibition of topoisomerase (DNA) I (TOP1): DNA damage repair and anticancer therapy. Biomolecules 2015;5(3):1652–70.
15. Gewirtz DA. A critical evaluation of the mechanisms of action proposed for the antitumor effects of the anthracycline antibiotics adriamycin and daunorubicin [review]. Biochem Pharmacol 1999;57(7):727–41.
16. Kang HJ, Park HJ. Novel molecular mechanism for actinomycin D activity as an oncogenic promoter G-quadruplex binder. Biochemistry 2009;48(31):7392–8.
17. Paz MM, Zhang X, Lu J, et al. A new mechanism of action for the anticancer drug mitomycin C: mechanism-based inhibition of thioredoxin reductase. Chem Res Toxicol 2012;25(7):1502–11.
18. Froudarakis M, Hatzimichael E, Kyriazopoulou L, et al. Revisiting bleomycin from pathophysiology to safe clinical use. Crit Rev Oncol Hematol 2013;87(1):90–100.
19. Sigmond J, Peters GJ. Pyrimidine and purine analogues, effects on cell cycle regulation and the role of cell cycle inhibitors to enhance their cytotoxicity [review]. Nucleosides Nucleotides Nucleic Acids 2005;24(10–12):1997–2022.
20. Rao N, Lee YF, Ge R. Novel endogenous angiogenesis inhibitors and their therapeutic potential. Acta Pharmacol Sin 2015;36(10):1177–90.
21. Vasudev NS, Reynolds AR. Anti-angiogenic therapy for cancer: current progress, unresolved questions and future directions. Angiogenesis 2014;17(3):471–94.
22. Roskoski R Jr. The ErbB/HER family of protein-tyrosine kinases and cancer. Pharmacol Res 2014;79:34–74.
23. Johnson DB, Sosman JA. Therapeutic advances and treatment options in metastatic melanoma. JAMA Oncol 2015;1(3):380–6.
24. Panowksi S, Bhakta S, Raab H, et al. Site-specific antibody drug conjugates for cancer therapy [review]. MAbs 2014;6(1):34–45.
25. Chen DS, Mellman I. Oncology meets immunology: the cancer-immunity cycle. Immunity 2013;39(1):1–10.
26. Littman DR. Releasing the brakes on cancer immunotherapy. Cell 2015;162(6):1186–90.
27. Shrager J, Tenenbaum JM. Rapid learning for precision oncology. Nat Rev Clin Oncol 2014;11(2):109–18.

CHAPTER 3

Basics of Radiation Therapy

Ryan K. Funk, MD*, Abigail L. Stockham, MD,
Nadia N. Issa Laack, MD, MS

INTRODUCTION

William Roentgen received the first Nobel Prize in physics for his discovery of radiographs in 1895. It was quickly recognized that radiographs had the potential to cause damage to living tissues, and within 1 year, radiographs were used in the treatment of breast cancer. Early radiation treatments were groundbreaking in their time, but the techniques were crude by modern standards. For example, early dose measurements were based on daily changes in skin color. This crude measure of dose to the skin correlates roughly with dose to underlying tumors, but the dose to produce skin erythema varies between patients. Furthermore, early radiation treatment modalities delivered relatively high surface doses (ie, skin dose) compared with dose to deeper areas, where most tumors are found. In addition, radiobiology, the study of the biologic effects of radiation on living tissues, was in its infancy, and early predictions regarding normal and tumor response to radiation were unreliable. The intervening century has resulted in discoveries by physicians and radiobiologists that have improved the understanding of radiobiology. Technological advances, facilitated by radiation physicists, engineers, and physicians, have resulted in techniques that allow for greater precision in radiation dose calculation and treatment delivery. This chapter reviews the basic underpinnings of radiation therapy and practical aspects of modern radiotherapy. Potential side effects from radiotherapy are explored in depth in a separate chapter.

BASIC PHYSICS

A basic understanding of the physical properties governing radiation therapy aids in a clinician's appreciation of the characteristics of radiation that lead to therapeutic and deleterious effects of radiation. This section describes types of radiation, radiation sources of radiation, and how radiation is deposited in tissue.

TYPES OF RADIATION

Radiation is defined as the emission and propagation of energy through space or matter. For the purposes of therapy, radiation can be divided into electromagnetic (EM) radiation and particle radiation. EM and particle radiation can be generated using accelerators (eg, linear accelerators [linacs], cyclotrons, or synchrotrons) or by radioactive materials undergoing decay.

Electromagnetic Radiation

EM radiation is a form of energy propagation where photons with both particle and wavelike properties travel at the speed of light.[1] EM waves carry energy and transfer their energy upon interaction with matter. The energy associated with EM radiation is proportional to frequency and inversely proportional to wavelength. Thus, EM waves with shorter wavelengths have more energy. Examples of EM radiation (from lowest to highest energy) include radio waves, microwaves, infrared, visible light, UV, and radiographs (Fig. 3.1). EM radiation can be further divided into ionizing and nonionizing radiation. EM radiation at or below the UV spectrum is nonionizing, whereas radiographs are ionizing. Ionizing EM has enough energy to remove tightly bound electrons from an atom or molecule. The release of bound electrons leads to the generation of ions and free radicals. Within living cells, ions and free radicals interact with cellular machinery and cause DNA damage, which can ultimately lead to cell death. Radiotherapy uses ionizing radiation in order to cause damage to tumor cells. The photons used for therapeutic radiation generally have wavelengths of 10^{-11} to 10^{-13} m (see Fig. 3.1).[1]

Department of Radiation Oncology, Mayo Clinic, 200 First Street Southwest, Rochester, MN 55905, USA
* Corresponding author.
E-mail address: Funk.Ryan@mayo.edu

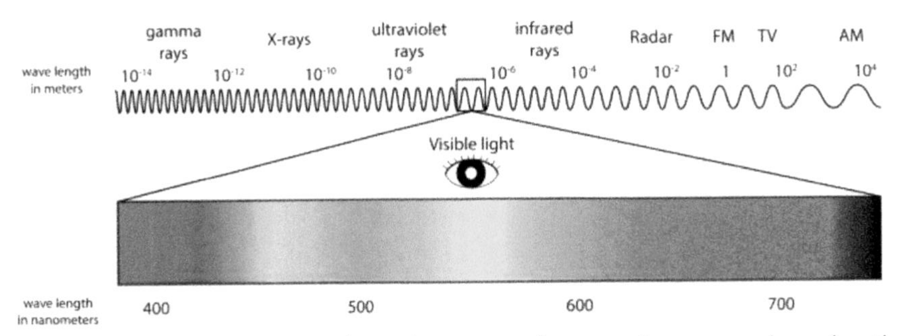

Fig. 3.1 The EM spectrum. The energy per photon increases as frequency increases and wavelength decreases. High-frequency, short-wavelength (eg, high energy) radiation is used for radiotherapy. (*From* Franck P, Henderson PW, Rothaus KO. Basics of lasers: history, physics, and clinical applications. Clin Plast Surg 2016;43(3):505–13; with permission.)

Particle Radiation

Particle radiation refers to energy carried by fast-moving electrons, protons, neutrons, or other atomic nuclei (ie, carbon). Beams of these particles are generated using linear accelerators (electrons) or cyclotrons/synchrotrons (protons, neutrons) and then directed at the target. As the particles interact with matter, they deposit energy in a pattern specific to the particle and the composition of the target medium.

SOURCES OF RADIATION

Radioactive Decay

Radioactive decay is another important source of therapeutic radiation. Radioactivity is a phenomenon whereby radiation (in the form of EM radiation, particle radiation, or both) is generated by the transition of an unstable, high-energy atomic nucleus to a more stable, lower-energy state.[1] The rate of decay can be communicated in terms of the half-life, which is defined as the time it takes for half of the radioactive particles to undergo decay. The half-life for each specific isotope is constant. Radioactive isotopes may emit several types of radiation, but, for therapeutic purposes, the most relevant are α particles (helium nuclei), β particles (electrons), and γ rays (photons). Radioactive decay continues to provide the source of radiation for most brachytherapy treatments and for units using cobalt-60 as a source (Gamma Knife machines [Elekta AB, Stockholm, Sweden] and older external beam radiotherapy machines) (Fig. 3.2). Because they constantly decay, radioactive sources must be periodically replaced.

Radiograph Tubes

Radiograph tubes (Fig. 3.3) are used to generate diagnostic radiographs and low-energy therapeutic radiographs. A radiograph tube has an anode and a cathode. A voltage applied across the tube releases electrons from the cathode. These electrons are directed at the cathode and the interaction between the electrons and the cathode generates radiographs. The maximum energy of the resulting photons is equal to the voltage applied across the radiograph tube. Radiograph tubes are able to generate kilovoltage beams but not higher-energy megavoltage beams.

Accelerators

Megavoltage photon and electron beams and particle beams are generated by various accelerators including linear accelerators (for electrons and photons), cyclotrons (heavy particles), and synchrotrons (heavy particles). A full discussion of how these machines work is beyond the scope of this chapter but a detailed description can be found in Khan, chapter 26.[1] As linear accelerators are the most commonly used accelerators for radiotherapy, a brief description of their function is provided.

Linear accelerators (Fig. 3.4) use EM fields to accelerate a beam of electrons. The accelerated electrons can be used directly for treatment or can be used to generate radiographs that are then used for treatment. Most modern radiotherapy units can treat using either electrons or radiographs. Electrons gain energy as they accelerate. Once the beam is accelerated to the treatment energy, electromagnets then direct the electron beam into the treatment head of the machine and toward the patient. At this point, the beam is only about a millimeter in cross section. Because therapeutic areas, or targets, are much larger than the size of the small beam, steps are taken in the treatment head to spread the beam out to cover a larger area (generally up to

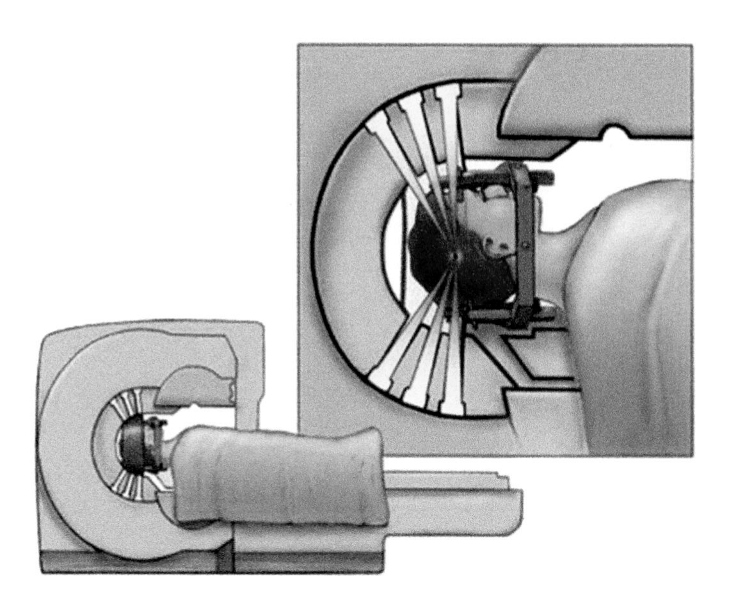

Fig. 3.2 Gamma Knife radiosurgery unit. A Gamma Knife radiosurgery unit is used to deliver high doses of radiation to small areas in the brain (see SBRT discussion in this chapter). Radioactive decay of cobalt-60 provides the radiation for this type of treatment. Radiation from the cobalt sources is shielded, or blocked, when the device is not delivering treatment. The shielding moves to open small channels for the delivery of multiple small radiation beams that are focused on a small area. The small area of high dose is focused on the tumor (or other treated abnormality). The surrounding brain tissue receives much less dose. Cobalt has a half-life of 5.27 years. Without replacement of the cobalt sources, the dose delivered per unit time will drop by half, and the treatment time needed to deliver a specific dose will double every 5.27 years. (Copyright © Mayo Foundation for Medical Education and Research. All rights reserved.)

40 cm × 40 cm in modern radiotherapy units).[2] If the patient is to be treated with photons, a metal target is placed in the beam path (Fig. 3.5A). Electrons strike the target and, secondary to physical characteristics of radiation, result in generation of radiographs. These radiographs pass through a flattening filter to ensure relatively homogenous dose to the center of the field compared with objects further from the center. For treatment with electrons, the radiograph target is removed

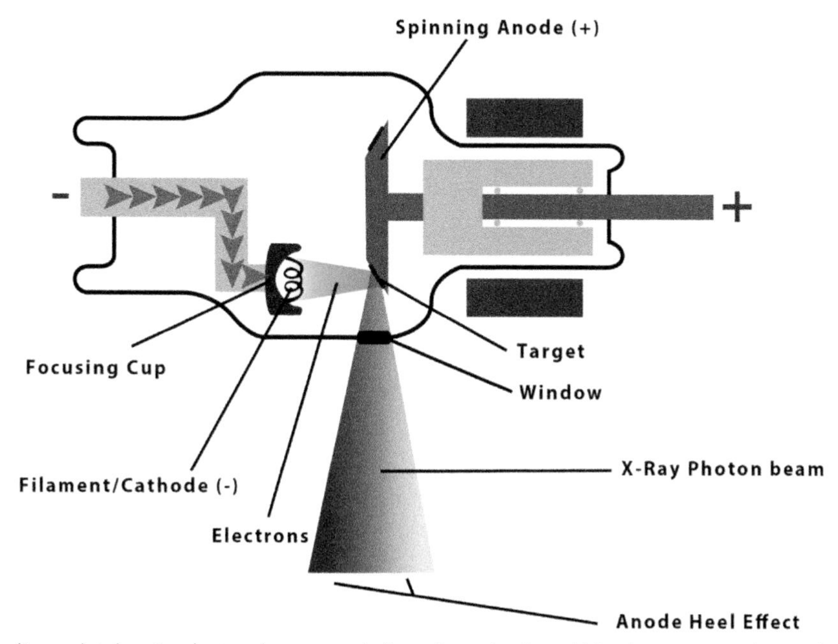

Fig. 3.3 Radiograph tube. An electron beam travels from the cathode and hits the target on the anode resulting in the generation of radiographs. In this figure, a spinning anode is used to dissipate heat. (*Courtesy of* Dr Matt Skalski, Los Angeles, CA.)

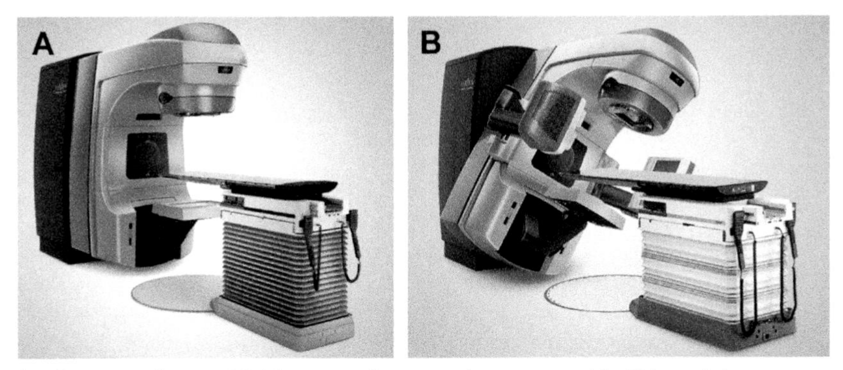

Fig. 3.4 Modern linear accelerator. (*A*) A linear accelerator and treatment table. This model can generate megavoltage images for patient position verification using radiographs from the treatment head. The detector for megavoltage imaging is the retractable panel positioned under the head of the treatment table. (*B*) The gantry can rotate 360° to provide treatment from any angle. This model has the ability to generate kilovoltage images for patient position verification. The kilovoltage radiograph tube and detector are set at 90° to the treatment beam. Kilovoltage imaging allows for higher contrast images compared with magavoltage images. Please refer to the section on IGRT in this chapter for further details. (*Courtesy of* Varian Medical Systems, Palo Alto, CA; with permission.)

from the beam path and the electron beam is spread out using a beam spoiler (Fig. 3.5B). After the flattening filter or scattering foil, the beam is collimated using metal blocks to generate a beam of the appropriate size and shape for treatment. Further discussion of treatment field shaping can be found later in the Intensity-Modulated Radiation Therapy section.

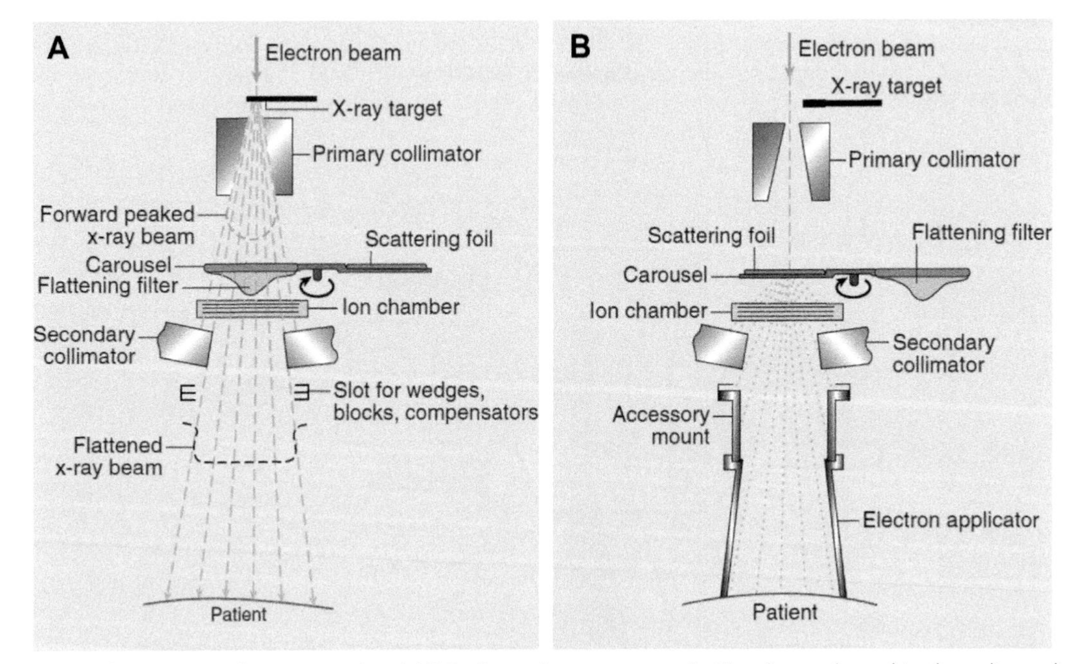

Fig. 3.5 Components of a treatment head. (*A*) Radiograph treatment mode. The electron beam hits the radiograph target and generates radiographs. The primary collimator shapes the beam to the desired size. The flattening filter improves dose homogeneity. The ion chamber measures dose. The secondary collimator shapes the beam further. Further modifications to the beam profile can be made by adding wedges or blocks (discussed in the Specific Modalities section of this chapter). (*B*) Treatment head components for electron treatment. The scattering foil converts the narrow electron beam into a broad beam. The ion chamber measures dose. Collimation, or beam shaping, is achieved with the secondary collimator and the electron applicator. (*From* Zeman EM, Schreiber EC, Tepper JE. Basics of Radiation Therapy. In: Niederhuber JE, Armitage JO, Doroshow JH, et al, editors. Abeloff's Clinical Oncology. Fifth edition; 2014. p. 396; with permission.)

RADIATION INTERACTIONS IN THE BODY

Radiation-induced Cellular Damage

Radiation is thought to act primarily at cellular and molecular levels. Ionizing radiation traverses the entirety of a cell and has the potential to interact with all of the cellular contents. However, the consequences of radiation on cellular functions appear to be mediated primarily by radiation-induced DNA damage. Direct damage occurs as the result of interaction between the incident radiation and the DNA molecule to cause single- or double-strand breaks. Indirect damage occurs when ionizing radiation interacts with water molecules to generate hydroxyl ions. These ions, in turn, interact with DNA to cause strand breaks. Large particles (protons, α particles) primarily cause direct damage, whereas photons and electrons primarily act via indirect damage.[3]

Dose Deposition

The amount of DNA damage caused by a particular beam is proportional to the dose; therefore, an understanding of how dose is distributed in the body is important. Depth dose curves are used to graphically represent energy deposition as radiation hits the surface of an object and then travels through that object (ie, the patient). The specific pattern of dose deposition depends on the type of radiation, the initial energy of the beam, and the composition of the interposing matter. In general, higher energy beams are more deeply penetrating, which means that these beams are often used for treating deep-seated tumors. The following sections describe dose deposition for commonly used radiation beams.

Orthovoltage Photon Beams

Orthovoltage and megavoltage refer to the energy of the photons or particles used in a treatment beam. Orthovoltage photon beams have peak energies in the range of 10 to 400 kV potential (kVp) with most modern commercial units operating in the 50- to 150-kVp range.[4] The surface dose for orthovoltage photons is nearly 100% of maximum with very rapid dose falloff (Fig. 3.6). For example, the relative dose of a 50-kVp radiograph beam at 2-, 10-, and 20-mm

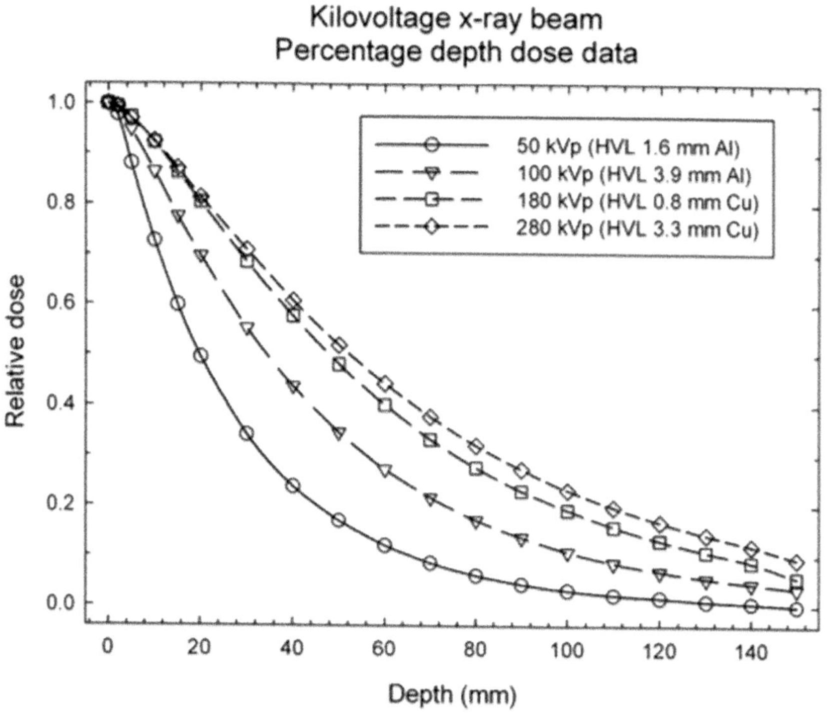

Fig. 3.6 Percentage depth dose curves for kilovoltage radiograph beams with energies of 50 to 280 kVp. The dose at the surface is nearly 100% for beam energies in the kilovoltage range. Half value layer (HVL) refers to the thickness of a material to attenuate half of the beam energy. Al, Aluminum; Cu, Copper. (*From* Hill R, Healy B, Holloway L, et al. Advances in kilovoltage x-ray beam dosimetry. Phys Med Biol 2014;59(6):R185. http://dx.doi.org/10.1088/0031-9155/59/6/R183. © Institute of Physics and Engineering in Medicine. Reproduced by permission of IOP Publishing. All rights reserved.)

depth is approximately 98%, 73%, and 49% of maximum, respectively. The relative dose for a 280-kVp radiograph beam at 2-, 10-, and 20-mm depth is approximately 99%, 93%, and 82%, respectively, and drops to 50% by 5-cm depth.[4] Before the invention of higher-energy treatment machines, orthovoltage machines were used to treat even deep-seated tumors. In the modern era, however, orthovoltage beams are used almost exclusively to treat skin cancers.[5]

Megavoltage Photon Beams

Megavoltage photons (typically with energies of 4–20 MV) are more penetrating than orthovoltage photon beams and reach their maximum doses at varying depths depending on the energy[6] (Fig. 3.7). Megavoltage photons deliver a lower relative dose to the surface than electrons or low-energy photons and are thus commonly referred to as "skin-sparing." Modern teletherapy machines (ie, linacs) operate in the megavoltage range.

Megavoltage Electron Beams

Electrons used for radiotherapy typically have energies of 6 to 25 MeV. They reach their maximum dose at 1 to 3 cm within the target and have a relatively rapid dose falloff thereafter[6] (see Fig. 3.7). Because of their rapid falloff, electrons can be used to treat relatively superficial targets (such as internal mammary lymph nodes) with relative sparing of the deeper tissues compared with megavoltage photons.

Proton Beams

The depth of maximum dose deposition for protons depends on the initial energy of the proton beam. The depth dose curve for a monoenergetic proton beam has an initial plateau that sharply increases at the end of the proton range and then falls off rapidly. The sharp increase in dose deposition is referred to as the Bragg peak. The width of the Bragg peak from a monoenergetic beam is too narrow to cover most clinical targets so multiple beams of decreasing energy are used to provide a wider area of high dose. The summation of these beams is referred to as a spread-out Bragg peak[7] (SOBP; Fig. 3.8). The width of the SOBP is designed to cover the proximal and distal ends of the target.

RADIATION TREATMENT PLANNING AND DELIVERY

Radiation treatment relies heavily on technologies that allow for accurate planning and delivery of the desired dose. This section reviews various common planning and treatment methods used by the radiation oncologist.

Types of Radiation Treatment Delivery

Various terms used in describing radiation therapy delivery are summarized in Table 3.1. Teletherapy, or external beam radiation (EBRT), refers to the delivery of radiation from a source external to the patient. EBRT is the most common form of radiation therapy delivery. Photons, electrons, protons, and neutrons can be used for EBRT. Most modern EBRT machines are isocentric. Isocentric machines rotate around a point, called the isocenter, and the center of the radiation beam is at the isocenter (Fig. 3.9). An isocentric setup allows for precise calculations when determining the relationship between patient position and treatment machine position.

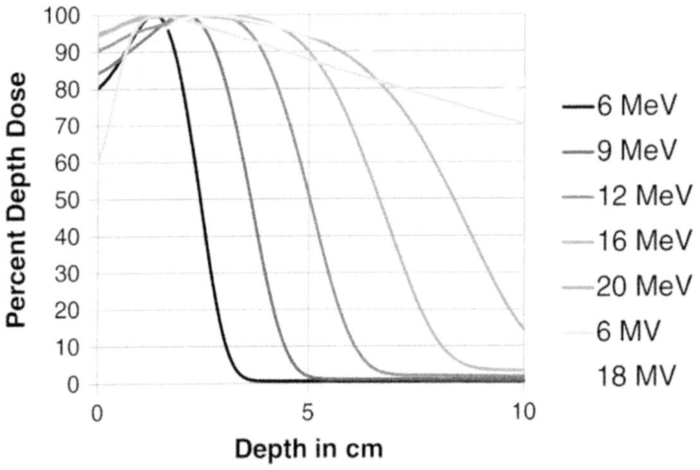

Fig. 3.7 Percentage depth-dose curves for megavoltage radiograph and mega-electron voltage beams. Photon beams (6 MV and 18 MV) deliver less dose at the surface (depth 0 cm) compared with electron beams. Electron beam penetration increases with increasing energy from 6 MeV to 20 MeV, but these beams drop off much more rapidly than MV photon beams. Penetration of radiograph beams also increase as the energy increases from 6 MeV to 18 MV. Note the change in x-axis scale compared with the corresponding orthovoltage figure. (*From* Brengues M, Liu D, Korn R, et al. Method for validating radiobiological samples using a linear accelerator. EPJ Tech Instrum 2014;1(1):4; with permission.)

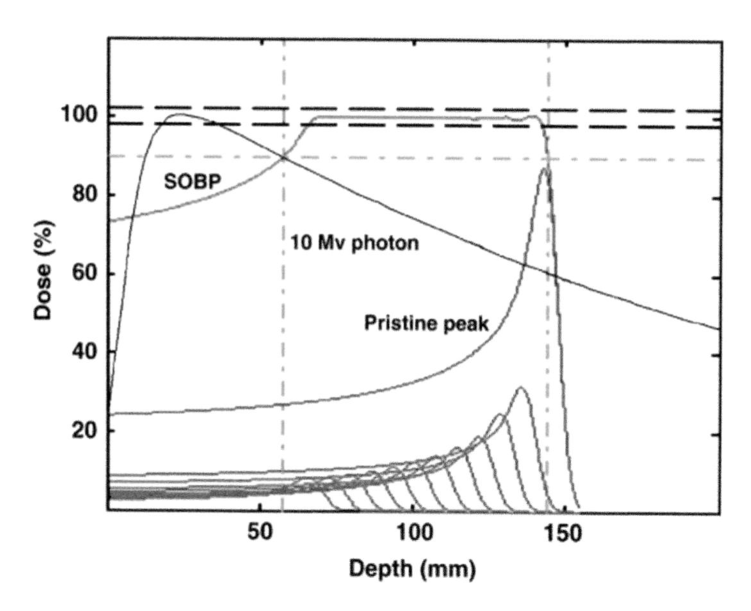

Fig. 3.8 Depth-dose curves for proton beams. Depth-dose curves for a SOBP (*red*), the constituent pristine proton beams of decreasing energy (*blue*), and a 10-MV photon beam (*black*). The SOBP is a summation of the dose from the constituent pristine proton beams. The SOBP in this example could treat a target area spanning approximately 5- to 15-cm depth. The surface dose (depth 0 mm) is higher for SOBP than for the 10-MV photon beam or the individual constituent beams. (*From* Levin WP, Kooy H, Loeffler JS, DeLaney TF. Proton beam therapy. Br J Cancer 2005;93(8):850; with permission.)

Beams from the treatment machine are collimated, or shaped, to match the shape of the target volume. Early radiotherapy machines had relatively rudimentary collimators, or collimation was achieved by creating custom high-density cut-out blocks that were either attached to the treatment machine or placed on the patient. Modern treatment machines have multiple collimators that can move during treatment to better shape the dose. Further specifics of EBRT delivery are discussed later in the chapter.

Brachytherapy refers to delivery of radiation from sources placed inside or very near the patient. The primary advantage of brachytherapy is that radiation exposure from a point source decreases proportional to the inverse square law. That is, exposure is proportional to $1/r^2$ at a distance r from the source. Thus, high doses can be delivered to the tumor with nearby organs receiving much lower dose. For example, if dose is prescribed to 1 cm from a single source, then the dose at 2 cm will be 25% of the prescribed dose. For more complex brachytherapy treatments using multiple sources, the dose falloff is not as steep as for a single source, but the falloff typically surpasses what can be achieved with external treatments.

RADIATION TREATMENT PARAMETERS

Dose

Early radiation oncologists used the skin on their arms to estimate dose. The dose required to produce a pink, sunburnlike reaction was called the "erythema dose" and was considered an appropriate daily dose. Modern dose is measured under standard conditions, and then these standard measurements are used to inform dose calculations in patients. The absorbed dose (commonly referred to as simply "dose") is measured in units of gray. A dose of 1 Gy is defined as the absorption of 1 J of energy per kilogram of matter. Historically, dose was reported in units of rads (radiation absorbed dose). One rad is equivalent to 1 cGy (one-hundredth of a gray, cGy).

RELATIVE BIOLOGICAL EFFECTIVENESS

Different types of radiation have different biologic effects. As a consequence, equivalent absorbed doses of different types of radiation may have different biologic effects. Relative biologic effectiveness (RBE) is defined as the ratio of doses of standard (D_s) and test (D_r) radiation to provide equivalent biologic effect (RBE = D_s/D_r). The selected biologic effect may be cell killing, mutation, or another biologic endpoint. Historically, the standard radiation was 250-kVp radiographs, although sometimes the RBE comparison is made with cobalt-60 γ rays.[1] Relative to 250-kVp radiographs, the RBE of protons (RBE = 1.1) and neutrons (RBE = 1–2) is higher, whereas the RBE of megavoltage photons (RBE = 0.85) is lower.[8] Doses for proton therapies are often reported in units of "cobalt Gray equivalent" (CGE) in order to make the comparison between proton and megavoltage photon plans simpler.[9]

Dose Prescription

Before the development of volumetric radiation planning, targets were delineated on

TABLE 3.1
Terms describing methods of radiation therapy

Modality	Brief Description	Examples
Brachytherapy	The placement of sealed radioactive sources into or immediately adjacent to tumors.	
LDR	The use of low-activity sources for brachytherapy. The implant may be permanent or temporary. Patients are hospitalized for the duration of temporary implants (usually 24–96 h).	Permanent: Prostate seed implant Temporary: Cervical cancer (historical in United States as most centers now use HDR)
HDR	The use of high-activity sources for brachytherapy. A device called an afterloader is used to advance the radioactive source into the patient to deliver dose. After the specified dose is delivered, the afterloader retracts the radioactive source. The treatment takes minutes to deliver.	Cervical cancer (most centers in United States) Accelerated partial breast irradiation (APBI) using balloon-based or multichannel based brachytherapy
Intracavitary	Isotopes are placed into a natural or artificial body cavity.	APBI using balloon- or multichannel-based brachytherapy
Interstitial	Isotopes are embedded directly in the tumor.	Prostate seed implant
Teletherapy (EBRT)	Treatment using an external source of radiation.	
Conventional fractionation	Delivery of daily doses of ~1.8–2 Gy. The total dose is typically delivered over 4–8 wk.	Conventionally fractionated lung, breast, or esophageal cancer treatment
IGRT	The use of imaging in the treatment room to verify patient position.	
Hypofractionation	Delivery of doses >2 Gy per day. May be delivered on consecutive days, every other day or weekly.	Hypofractionated whole breast radiotherapy
Hyperfractionation	The total dose is divided into smaller doses and treatments are given more than once per day.	Early-stage small-cell lung cancer
SBRT	The use of high doses per fraction (usually 6–24 Gy per fraction). SBRT uses advanced immobilization, image-guidance, and treatment planning to minimize dose to nearby normal tissues.	Early-stage (node negative) non–small-cell lung cancer
SRS	SBRT directed at the central nervous system. May be delivered as a single fraction or multiple fractions.	Limited brain metastases

2-dimensional films (2D), and the dose was often prescribed to the isocenter. Modern EBRT plans are typically designed using 3-dimensional (3D) imaging, and dose is prescribed to the planning treatment volume (PTV) as described below.

Fractionation

Most EBRT treatments require that total dose be divided into fractions that are delivered daily. Normal cells typically have greater capacity for radiation damage repair compared with tumor cells.

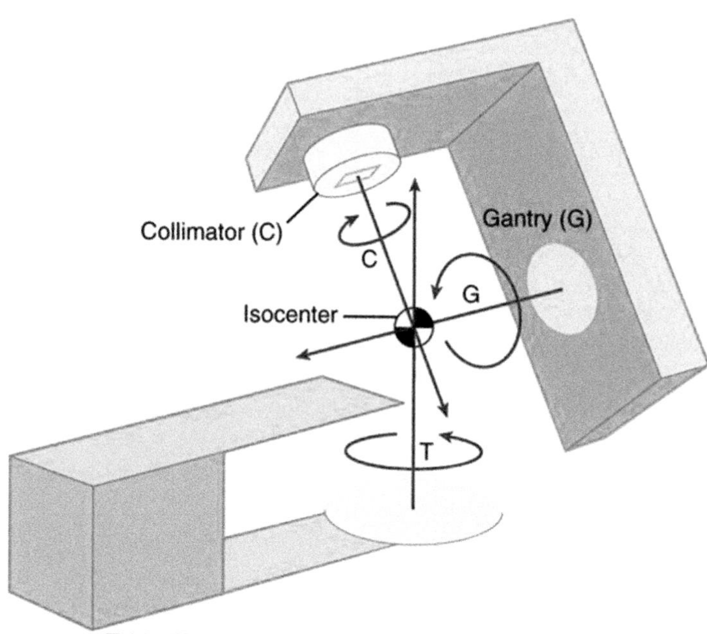

Fig. 3.9 Isocenter of a gantry-based radiotherapy machine. The gantry, collimator, and table all rotate around a single point, called the isocenter. The center of treatment beam is at isocenter. The use of an isocenter allows for reliable and reproducible movement of treatment machine with respect to the patient. (*From* Bourland JD. Radiation oncology physics. In: Gunderson LL, Tepper JS, editors. Clinical radiation oncology. 3rd edition. Philadelphia: Saunders; 2012. p. 98; with permission.)

Fractionation, or delivery of radiotherapy over several different sessions, allows normal tissues to recover between fractions to a greater degree than tumor cells. In general, fraction size (quantity of radiation delivered in a single treatment) correlates with late toxicity, whereas acute toxicity is more dependent on total dose. However, smaller fraction size also lowers the therapeutic effect on the tumor. Conventional fractionation typically refers to daily doses of 180 to 200 cGy, although pediatric and lymphoma patients may be treated with lower daily doses (~150 cGy). These doses were selected to try to balance tumor killing and normal tissue sparing. Subsequent studies have since shown that hypofractionation with daily doses of greater than 250 cGy per day are effective and without increased toxicity in certain clinical scenarios. Stereotactic body radiotherapy (SBRT) (also called stereotactic ablative body radiation, SABR) treats small, critically located targets through high-dose-per-fraction treatments using advanced immobilization and treatment planning techniques to allow large quantities of radiation to reach the tumors. A very steep dose-gradient outside the target results in a much lower dose to surrounding normal tissues. Palliative regimens are often hypofractionated, delivering large quantities of radiation over a small number of treatments, because late effects are unlikely to develop within the patient's lifetime.

Extensive effort has been dedicated to identifying and quantifying normal tissue tolerance to radiation. A more complete discussion of side effects will be addressed in a separate chapter. In brief, tumor and normal tissue response to therapy and the likelihood of acute and late side effects depend on the total dose, the dose per fraction, and the time elapsed for treatment. The development of side effects is also dependent on patient-specific factors, such as prior insults to the irradiated tissue (eg, surgery or radiation), modifiable behavioral factors such as smoking, and nonmodifiable factors such as underlying genetics. The dose-and–fractionation schedule prescribed by the radiation oncologist attempts to maximize the therapeutic ratio (Fig. 3.10), that is, the ratio between the likelihood of controlling the cancer and the likelihood of causing side effects.

PRACTICAL ASPECTS OF RADIATION THERAPY PLANNING AND DELIVERY

Simulation

Most patients will undergo a radiation planning session, called a simulation, days or weeks before initiating radiation therapy. The purpose of the simulation is multifold. First, it allows the radiation oncologist to generate a reproducible setup so that the patient is in the same position each day for treatment. Immobilization devices, often made of thermoplastics, vacuum-evacuated bags, or quick-setting foam, are used to ensure reproducibility. Uncertainty in patient position

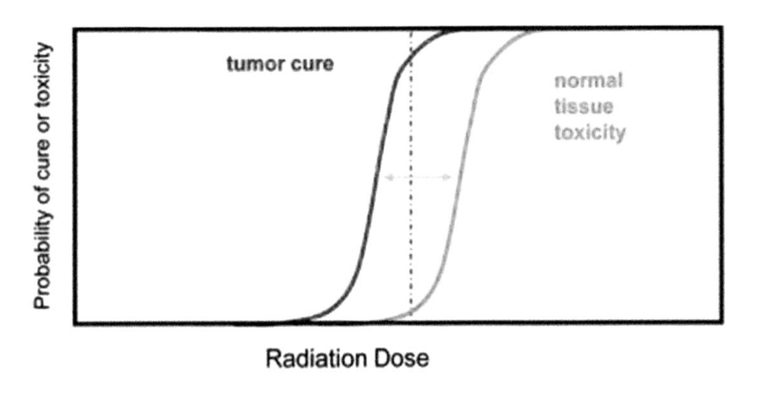

Fig. 3.10 Therapeutic ratio. The probability of tumor control (*red*) and normal tissue toxicity (*blue*) can be plotted as a function of radiation dose. The radiation oncologist seeks to deliver a plan that delivers a high likelihood of cure while minimizing the probability of normal tissue toxicity. In this example, the selected radiation dose (*dashed line*) provides a high probability of tumor control and low probability of normal tissue toxicity. Increasing the dose would increase the probability of tumor control at the expense of higher toxicity. Note that the curve shown is idealized and may not represent the clinical reality. (*From* Citrin DE, Mitchell JB. Altering the response to radiation: sensitizers and protectors. Semin Oncol 2014;41(6):848–59; with permission.)

leads to uncertainty in the delivered dose, and the simulation is one effort to minimize this uncertainty. The simulation also allows imaging of the area to be treated. These images are used to identify the target volumes and normal tissues and for planning and dose calculations. Modern radiotherapy planning systems use tissue-specific information from the computed tomographic (CT) scan to accurately calculate dose. Calculating dose without the tissue-specific information provided by CT can lead to differences between the calculated dose and the actual dose delivered of up to 5% or more.

Target Volume Delineation

An integral part of modern radiation therapy treatment planning is the identification of target (Fig. 3.11) and normal tissue volumes (Fig. 3.12). Most modern treatment-planning systems use CT imaging for target volume delineation, treatment planning, and dose calculation. Previously, target volumes were delineated on 2D images, and calculations were based on patient anatomy as measured at the time of simulation. MRI and ultrasound can also be used for treatment planning purposes, but dose calculations are generally carried out using a CT dataset.

Several factors influence the final volume to be treated. These factors include the size and location/tissue affected by the primary tumor and any visibly involved lymph nodes, the pattern of disease progression for a particular disease type, tissue movement (eg, breathing motion, bladder/stomach distension), anticipated random errors in daily patient setup, and known uncertainties in radiation beam targeting.

The gross tumor volume (GTV) refers to visible tumor on imaging studies. The GTV may be absent if prior therapy (surgery or chemotherapy) has eradicated gross disease. The clinical target volume (CTV) identifies a target volume that accounts for microscopic disease spread. The shape and size of the CTV depend on the clinical features of a particular disease entity but are often concerned with addressing adjacent draining nodal basins. The planning target volume (PTV) is usually a geometric expansion of the CTV to account for uncertainties in daily patient setup, organ and tumor motion, and radiation beam targeting. The size of the PTV expansion depends on anticipated setup uncertainties and the use of image guidance. Predictable organ motion in certain parts of the body can be imaged dynamically in order to assess tumor motion. For example, a 4-dimensional CT (3 dimensions of space and the fourth dimension of time) may be obtained during planning for targets in or near the lungs so as to assess movement during breathing. This dataset provides information on the position of the tumor and normal tissues during different phases of the respiratory cycle. These data can be used to expand the CTV to an internal target volume, which is then expanded to the PTV. If different areas of the patient are to be treated to different doses, then PTVs (and corresponding CTVs) for each dose level will be delineated.

Normal Tissues

Normal tissues are also contoured on the simulation CT (see Fig. 3.12). In the thorax, the most commonly delineated, or contoured, normal tissues include the heart, lungs, spinal cord, and esophagus. If the patient is undergoing SBRT, the proximal bronchial tree, great vessels, and chest wall may also be contoured. Contouring normal structures allows the treatment software

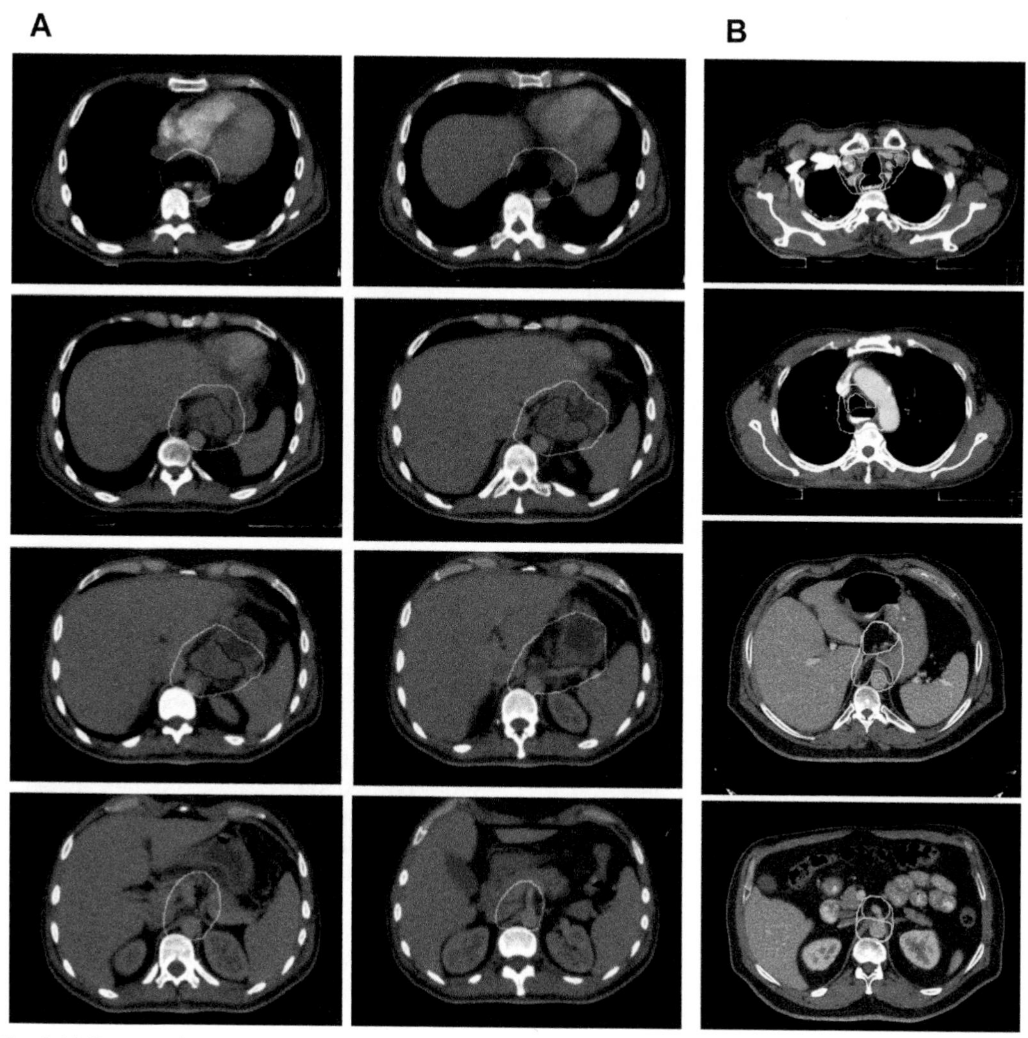

Fig. 3.11 Target volume delineation. Representative gross tumor volume (GTV) and clinical tumor volume (CTV) contours for esophageal cancer (*A*) GTV (*red*) and CTV (*yellow*) for a distal esophageal cancer. The CTV encompases potential microscopic submucosal and lymphatic spread. (*B*) Examples of contours encompassing specific nodal regions. The CTV (*yellow*) encompasses at-risk nodal volumes (*blue* and *purple*) at each level. The volumes included vary based on the location of the primary tumor and any grossly involved nodes. The CTV will be expanded to account for setup and treatment delivery uncertainty to create the planning treatment volume. The CTV-to-PTV expansion is typically between 5-10 mm in all directions depending on the equipment being used. (*From* Wu AJ, Bosch WR, Chang DT, et al. Expert consensus contouring guidelines for intensity modulated radiation therapy in esophageal and gastroesophageal junction cancer. Int J Radiat Oncol Biol Phys 2015;92(4):914–6; with permission.)

to calculate the dose any target or normal tissue of interest receives. Radiation planning and delivery techniques can then be used to maximize target coverage while respecting normal tissue tolerances.

Treatment Planning

Once target volumes and normal tissues are identified, the radiation oncologist prepares a prescription document that identifies the desired dose and fractionation schedule. The document states the desired coverage to the treatment volumes (eg, 95% of the PTV will receive 95% of the prescription dose) and contains any normal tissue constraints that the plan should meet. Radiation dosimetrists use treatment planning software to design a treatment plan that meets the goals specified in the prescription document. The software or the dosimetrist selects beam arrangements that are likely to result in target coverage while minimizing normal tissue dose. Iterative adjustments are made until an acceptable dose distribution is obtained. The final plan finds a balance between optimal target coverage and normal tissue sparing to maximize the likelihood of tumor control and minimize the likelihood of side effects.

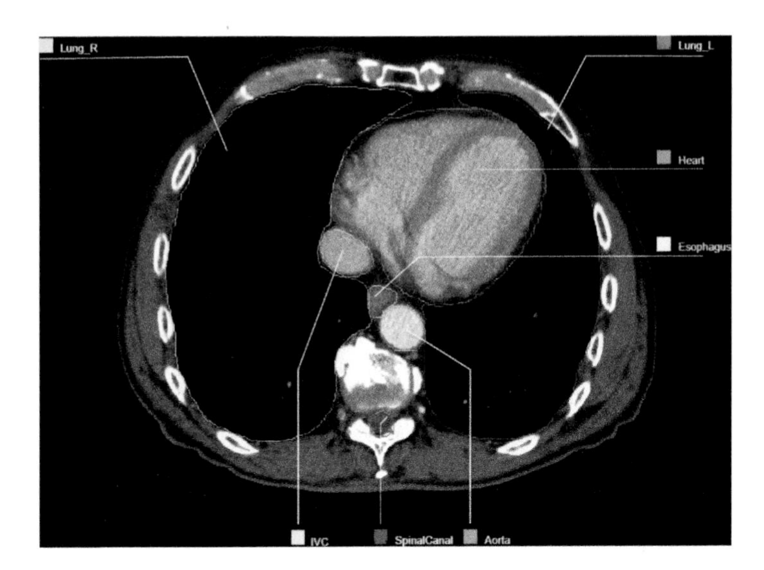

Fig. 3.12 Normal tissue contours. Normal tissue contours allow the planning system to calculate dose to the specified tissues. IVC, inferior vena cava. (*Courtesy of* Radiation Therapy Oncology Group, Philadelphia, PA; with permission.)

Creating an optimal plan requires knowledge of how dose (quantity and volume) affects various tissues. Some organs are highly sensitive to the actual maximum dose, such as the spinal cord. Other organs, such as the lungs, are more sensitive to the volume of tissue irradiated. Balancing the need to deliver effective radiation therapy doses to the treatment target and known acceptable radiation limits (referred to as constraints) results in the challenge of a dosimetrist (or treatment planner) and a physician in balancing the benefits of minimizing heart dose perhaps at the expense of higher lung dose and vice versa. The treating radiation oncologist asks for coverage that is likely to balance risks to each of these organs and minimize overall risk. Physicians review the plan to confirm that it is clinically appropriate and ask for adjustments to the plan as needed. Medical physicists then perform quality assurance measures to confirm that the actual delivered dose distribution will match the calculated dose distribution.

Treatment Delivery

Treatments are delivered with the patient in the same position as at the simulation. As noted above, there are uncertainties regarding organ motion, patient setup, and radiation beam delivery that are accounted for by the PTV margin. The PTV margin takes into account the method of localization to be used to verify correct position at the time of treatment. In the modern era, many patients undergo daily imaging using radiographs, a CT scan, or mounted cameras that evaluate the external surface contour of the patient at the time of treatment. These methods compare positional data from the simulation to the treatment position data. After correct positioning and verification, treatment begins. During treatment, the patient is encouraged to remain as motionless as possible. There is typically no detectable sensation as the radiation is delivered.

SPECIFIC MODALITIES

Photon Radiotherapy

Photons are by far the most used modality for EBRT. Advances in treatment technique now allow for very conformal delivery of radiation. Because many cardiac sequelae may occur decades after treatment, also discussed are outdated methods of treatment delivery.

Although primitive by modern standards, megavoltage machines of 1 MV were available as early as the 1930s. Cobalt machines (1.3 MV) and megavoltage linear accelerators (4–18 MV) became available in the 1950s. Initially, treatment field design was based on the physical examination and clinical judgment. As machines increased in sophistication, 2D radiographic images were used to define treatment volumes. Knowledge of bony anatomy with respect to soft tissue counterparts was used to identify appropriate target volumes. Dose calculations were initially done by hand based on measurements taken under control conditions. Radiation beams could be delivered from multiple angles to maximize dose to the target, but without 3D data (provided by a CT scan), the dose calculations were inexact. Limited dose shaping could be accomplished by placing high-density material of various shapes in the beam path. Specific configurations (for example, a wedge) were available that would provide a calculable change to the dose profile under standard conditions.

Three-Dimensional Conformal Radiotherapy

3D conformal radiation therapy (3D-CRT) gained popularity in the 1990s as improvements in computing and imaging allowed for dose calculations on 3D image sets (see https://www.astro.org/rtevolution/player.html). After delineation of target volumes and normal tissues on the CT simulation images, multiple radiation beams are arranged to maximize target coverage while avoiding normal tissues (Fig. 3.13, left panel). Wedges can be used (as in 2D treatment) to conform the shape of the distal edge of the beam to provide more uniform target coverage. In addition, multileaf collimators (MLCs) in the treatment machine can be used to closely conform the edges of the beam to the shape of the target or to avoid critical normal tissues. MLCs are banks of closely spaced, mobile "leaves" made of high-density, high-atomic number material. Because of the high atomic number, when an individual leaf moves into the beam path, it attenuates, or blocks dose in that area. The individual MLCs can be positioned independently to generate a custom shape that blocks dose to areas outside of the intended target volume. Once the beams are arranged, dose is calculated and the dosimetrist makes adjustments as needed to obtain the desired dose distribution. This method of planning (as with 2D planning) is called forward planning because the beams are arranged first and then the dose distribution is calculated.

Intensity-Modulated Radiation Therapy

IMRT is an advanced method of treatment planning and delivery. In contrast to 3D-CRT, IMRT uses inverse planning, meaning that target and normal tissue constraints describing the desired dose distribution are transferred to the planning software, which then uses algorithms to generate beam arrangements that best meet the objectives specified. IMRT algorithms generate beams that are dynamically modulated during treatment delivery using moving MLCs. The dynamic modulation of the beam allows for much tighter conformality around the target volume and better sparing of nearby normal tissues (see Fig. 3.13,

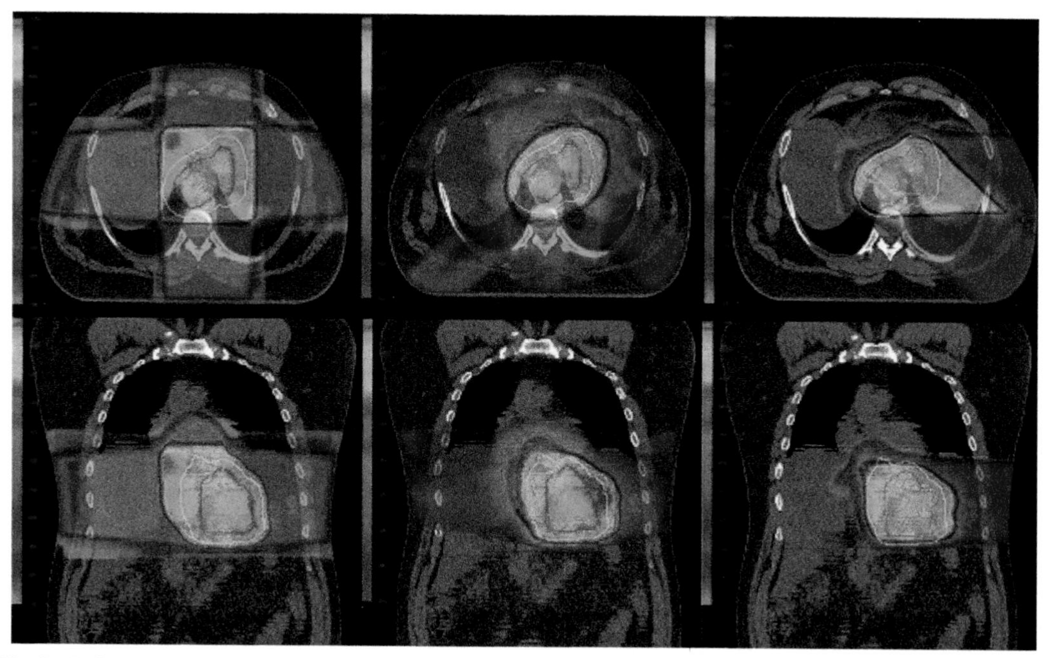

Fig. 3.13 Comparative radiotherapy plans. Axial (*top*) and coronal (*bottom*) images of 3D CRT (*left*), intensity modulated radiotherapy (IMRT, *middle*), and proton radiotherapy (*right*) plans for a patient with esophageal cancer. The target PTV is shown with a yellow line, and the CTV is shown with a purple line. Dose is shown in color wash (see the color key along the left side of each image; high dose is at the top of the key and low dose is at the bottom of the key). The IMRT and proton plans conform more tightly to the PTV than the 3D CRT plan. The IMRT plan has much more low-dose spread than the proton plan. (*From* Ling TC, Slater JM, Nookala P, et al. Analysis of intensity-modulated radiation therapy (IMRT), proton and 3D conformal radiotherapy (3D-CRT) for reducing perioperative cardiopulmonary complications in esophageal cancer patients. Cancers (Basel) 2014;6(4):2356–68.)

middle panel). A potential downside to IMRT is that it spreads low dose into a greater volume of normal tissue when compared with 3D-CRT. Thus, normal tissues directly adjacent to the target volume are often spared from high doses at the expense of spreading more low-dose radiation to normal tissues that are not directly adjacent to the target volume.

Stereotactic Body Radiotherapy

SBRT refers to delivering large doses of highly conformal radiation in few fractions. If the target is in the head, the term, "stereotactic radiosurgery (SRS)" is often used. The high doses used in stereotactic treatments necessitate techniques that minimize delivery uncertainties and maximize dose falloff outside the target volume. Techniques to minimize delivery uncertainty include the use of advanced immobilization devises such as a skull-anchored head-frame in Gamma Knife or custom whole-body vacuum bags for linac-based treatments. In addition, advanced imaging may be used to verify the position of the patient at the time of treatment (see IGRT in the next section). Because of the large fraction size, a steep dose gradient between the target volume and nearby normal tissue is needed to minimize normal tissue exposure (and the attendant side effects). The physics of radiation therapy are such that dose falloff is not as rapid for larger volumes compared with small volumes. Current tumor size limits are approximately 4 cm in the brain[10] and 5 cm in the lung.[11]

Image-Guided Radiotherapy

Image-guided radiotherapy (IGRT) does not refer to a particular treatment modality; rather, it refers to the use of in-room imaging at the time of treatment to minimize positioning errors. Highly conformal techniques such as IMRT and SBRT require high levels of setup reproducibility to ensure that the planned dose is delivered to the specified area. Recent decades have seen several advances in IGRT technology.[12] Planar IGRT techniques compare 2D radiographs obtained with the patient in treatment position with digitally reconstructed radiographs from the simulation imaging. Overlaying the radiograph from simulation with the radiograph from treatment allows for accurate matching to bony anatomy. Volumetric IGRT techniques provide 3D imaging that can be compared with the simulation imaging to verify position. Volumetric IGRT imaging allows for soft tissue matching as well as bony matching. Examples of volumetric IGRT include cone-beam CT, CT on rails, and megavoltage CT imaging.[12]

Electron Radiotherapy

Electrons are typically used to treat superficial targets because dose from electrons falls off rapidly as the beam penetrates deeper into tissue. A common use of electron radiotherapy in the thorax is in patients with breast cancer receiving regional nodal irradiation. An election field can be used for coverage of internal mammary lymph nodes in conjunction with a photon plan to cover the axillary and supraclavicular nodes and the remaining chest wall or breast. Electrons scatter laterally more than photons so care must be taken when designing adjacent photon and proton treatment fields so as to minimize hot spots where the fields abut.

Protons

Proton radiotherapy is available at a limited number of institutions. Construction and treatment-related costs are generally higher than for photon-based treatments, but significant advances have been made to make it viable for more centers to begin offering proton therapy. As noted above, treatment with protons and heavy ions takes advantage of the Bragg peak. A monoenergetic proton beam enters a patient and delivers a low entrance dose of radiation. Near the end of the proton range, the dose deposited increases until it peaks at the Bragg peak. Tissue distal to the Bragg peak receives minimal dose (see Fig. 3.13). Several beams of differing energies are used to create a SOBP so as to cover the entire tumor (see Fig. 3.8). The SOBP allows for homogenous target coverage, but it often increases entrance dose compared with photons. Because of the sharp dose gradient at the end of range, proton therapy treatments tend to be more sensitive to small changes in patient position or anatomy than a corresponding photon plan.

Proton delivery systems can be broadly divided into either passive scatter systems or spot-scanning systems. Passive scatter systems generate a beam that is then passed through materials that scatter the beam to create a broad beam that can be used to treat larger fields. Custom compensators are then used to shape the proton beam to conform to the lateral and distal edges of the target volume. Spot-scanning systems use electromagnets to direct narrow proton beams to specific, precalculated coordinates (spots). The dose is calculated by summing the dose from all of the discrete beamlets. In addition to conforming to the lateral and distal edges of the target volume, spot-scanning allows for conforming to the proximal surface of the target volume. Because of improved conformality, most new proton systems are using spot-scanning technology, whereas older systems generally used passive-scatter techniques.

As noted above, the RBE for protons is generally taken to be 1.1, meaning that the biologic effect of proton radiation is about 10% higher than photons for the same amount of deposited energy. Thus, proton dose is typically reported in cobalt gray equivalents. In other words 60 CGE from a proton plan is thought to be biologically equivalent to 60 Gy from a photon treatment. Currently, most treatment systems assume a uniform RBE for proton dose deposition throughout the treatment field. Recent evidence suggests that the RBE may higher in the Bragg peak region of the treatment beam. Thus, the effective dose to the distal edge of the treatment field could be higher than reported. An example where this may be clinically meaningful to the cardio-oncologist is neoadjuvant proton therapy for distal esophageal cancer. Most proton treatment plans use posterior beams that deliver dose to the esophagus with a small margin into the posterior surface of the abutting heart tissue. This margin is necessary to avoid underdosing the tumor. Because the proton beam does not pass through the entire heart and lungs as photons would, proton plans deliver much less dose to the heart and lungs than a traditional photon plan. However, because the distal edge of the proton beam is in the heart, it is possible that the effective dose to that small portion of the heart is higher than would be calculated using a uniform RBE of 1.1. Active investigations should provide further information that may allow for a better understanding of this phenomenon.

Heavy Ions

Therapeutic heavy ion particle accelerators are much less common than therapeutic proton accelerators. As of June 2015, there were 49 operational proton facilities worldwide with an additional 29 under construction. There were 8 carbon ion facilities with an additional 4 under construction, and none of these were in the United States.[13] Carbon and other heavy ions have a Bragg peak similar to that of protons, but the peak is steeper and the beam scatters less in the lateral directions along the beam path. These physical properties allow for greater dose conformality. In addition, heavy ions deposit energy in a way that causes more double-stranded DNA breaks than other modalities of radiation delivery. This property is thought to be advantageous particularly when treating radioresistant tumor histologies that are less responsive to photon-based radiotherapy.

Brachytherapy

Brachytherapy refers to temporary or permanent placement of radioactive sources into the body. Interstitial brachytherapy uses needles to introduce radioactive sources into solid tumors or organs. Intracavitary brachytherapy uses an applicator to introduce radioactive sources into natural (eg, vagina) or surgical (eg, lumpectomy) body cavities.

Brachytherapy can be further classified as low-dose rate (LDR) or high-dose rate (HDR). In LDR brachytherapy, radioactive sources of relatively low activity are placed by the radiation oncologist into the patient. Some LDR applications are temporary, and the patient remains hospitalized for a few days until the applicator is removed. Other applications, for example, prostate seed implants, are permanent. Isotopes used for permanent implants typically have low energy, decay within months, and typically deliver negligible dose to bystanders.

HDR brachytherapy uses a high-intensity radioactive source on the end of a wire, which is contained in a computerized, shielded afterloader. Once the applicator and/or needles are positioned correctly and connected to guide-tubes, staff leaves the room. A program remotely directs the afterloader to extend the wire to position the HDR source at specified locations. The wire remains extended until the specified dose is delivered, and then the wire (with the source) retracts into the afterloader.

Brachytherapy is often selected in areas with easy access for the placement of catheters or applicators (Fig. 3.14). Brachytherapy plans are capable of delivering highly conformal treatments because the dose drops off quickly as a function of distance from the radiation source. Structures immediately to the surface of the radiation source are expected to receive as much as 400% of the prescribed dose. Because of difficulties in accessing the mediastinum and improvements in other technologies, there has been a decrease in mediastinal brachytherapy, but future studies may lead to a resurgence of this modality. Specific applications of brachytherapy of interest to the cardio-oncologist include intravascular brachytherapy to prevent coronary in-stent restenosis,[14] intravascular brachytherapy to prevent restenosis in peripheral artery occlusive disease after balloon dilatation,[15] lung brachytherapy to prevent local recurrence,[16] and esophageal brachytherapy.[17]

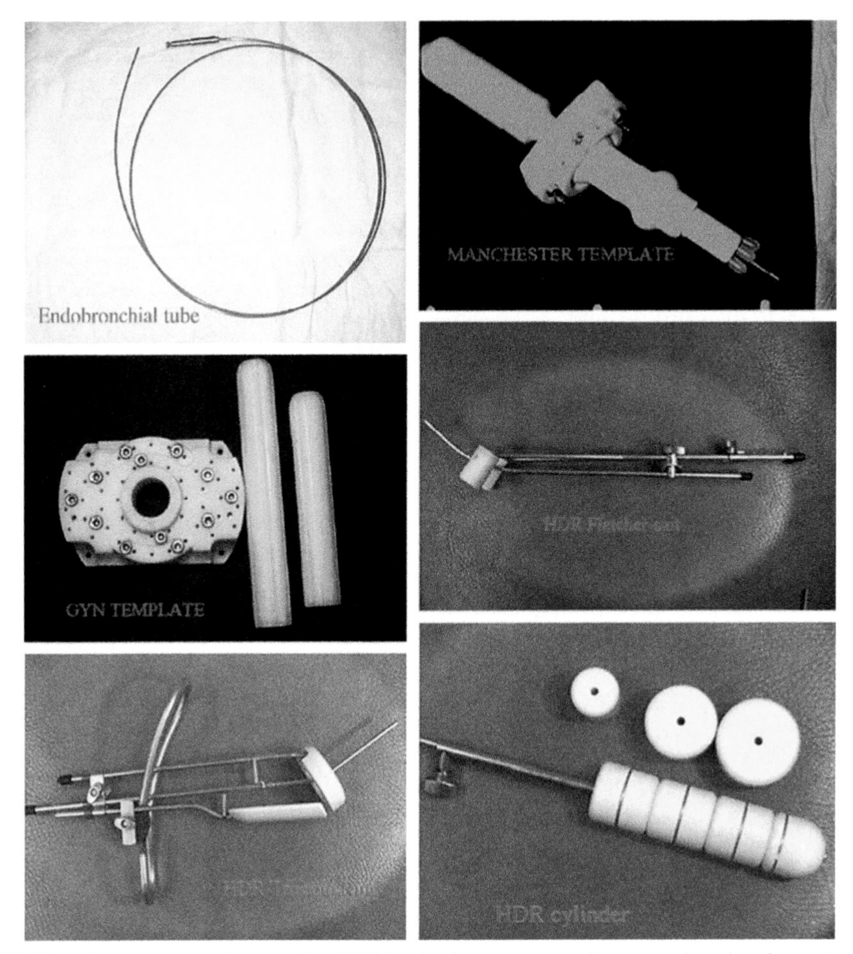

Fig. 3.14 HDR brachytherapy applicators. For HDR brachytherapy, an applicator is placed in the patient. The specific applicator chosen depends on the site to be treated and the anatomy of the patient/tumor. Once proper positioning is verified (typically with imaging), software is used to design a treatment plan. The applicators are connected to the afterloader via catheters. The afterloader has a radioactive source on the end of a wire. The radioactive source is shielded when it is inside the afterloader so that dose to the surrounding area is minimal. The wire is advanced remotely by the computer system through the catheter(s) and into the applicator. Dose is determined by the activity of the source and the time it stays at a precalculated position. Once the desired dose is delivered, the wire retracts into the afterloader, and the applicator is removed from the patient. GYN, gynecologic. (*From* Wilkinson DA. High dose rate (HDR) brachytherapy quality assurance: a practical guide. Biomed Imaging Interv J 2006;2(2):e34.)

SPECIFIC DISEASE SITES

As noted above, sequela from radiation may manifest years or even decades after exposure. Late complications are particularly relevant for patients who are treated at younger ages with high likelihood of cure. In the thorax, patients with breast cancer or Hodgkin lymphoma (HL) are at particular risk for late side effects. Radiation plays an important role in contributing to the high cure rates seen in both of these diseases. However, the relative youth of many of these patients and the high probability for survival signify a longer interval during which the patients might experience the deleterious effects of radiation. In addition, many of the chemotherapeutic agents used for these diseases are associated with cardiac and lung toxicity in addition to the risk posed by radiation. Some of the specifics regarding radiation in the management of these 2 diseases are discussed to better inform the cardio-oncologist as to the potential late risks.

Breast Cancer

Radiation therapy in the management of breast cancer is typically given in the postoperative setting. The volume of tissue irradiated and the prescribed dose of radiation vary based on the type of surgery performed and the findings at the time of surgery. Surgery may address the primary cancer with either a lumpectomy or a mastectomy (with or without reconstruction). Since the development of sentinel lymph node biopsy (SLNB), nodal disease is typically addressed with SLNB with a completion axillary lymph node dissection for select patients at high risk for further node involvement. Patients with a large primary tumor or initially involved lymph nodes may receive neoadjuvant chemotherapy. Appropriate radiotherapy recommendations in the setting of prior chemotherapy are the subject of active investigation.

The target volume varies based on the stage, surgery, and risk factors for recurrence. Current guidelines recommend contouring target and normal tissues, but for many years, treatment fields were generated using clinical landmarks without formal contouring.[18] Postlumpectomy whole breast radiotherapy is the standard of care for patients with early-stage, node-negative disease. Survival and disease control outcomes for patients with early-stage, node-negative disease are similar between patients who undergo mastectomy alone or lumpectomy followed by adjuvant radiation to the remaining ipsilateral breast tissue.[19] Younger patients with risk factors for local recurrence may have a higher dose (a boost) given to the lumpectomy cavity.[20] For very early stage disease, appropriately selected patients may receive partial breast irradiation,[21] that is, irradiation of breast tissue adjacent to the lumpectomy cavity without targeting the remaining breast tissue. Patients with node-positive disease, tumors greater than 5 cm, skin involvement, or pectoral fascia invasion will often receive postmastectomy radiation therapy directed to the chest wall and draining lymph nodes (Fig. 3.15). If a lumpectomy is performed in a patient with nodal disease, the nodal volumes above are often targeted in addition to the ipsilateral breast tissue. Conventionally fractionated breast radiotherapy is typically delivered in 25 to 30 daily fractions (5–6 weeks) to a dose of 50 to 60 Gy. Hypofractionated regimens with equivalent cancer control and toxicity but requiring only 3 weeks for delivery have recently gained wide acceptance for whole breast radiotherapy. Pending studies will determine whether hypofractionation is appropriate when treating nodal volumes.

As with other sites, patients undergo immobilization and simulation before treatment. Patients may be treated in the prone or supine position with various devices used to position the breast such that normal tissues can be reproducibly distanced from the treatment volume. Regardless of patient positioning, most treatment plans use opposing tangential fields to cover the breast or chest wall (Fig. 3.16). These beams can be designed to also provide dose to the internal mammary and low axillary nodal levels if indicated. The high axillary and supraclavicular nodal regions are typically targeted using 1 or 2 separate beams. Alternative photon and/or electron beam arrangements have been studied and may be beneficial in certain clinical situations. Ultimately, the beam arrangement is chosen to maximize target coverage while minimizing organ-at-risk dose.

Heart, particularly for left-sided breast cancers, and lung are the primary organs at risk considered during treatment planning for breast cancer. A better understanding of late toxicity has led to efforts to minimize dose to heart and lung. Management strategies that reduce heart dose include deep inspiration breath-hold (Fig. 3.17), respiratory gating (the treatment machine delivers dose only when sensors on the patient detect that the lungs are filled above a certain threshold), prone positioning, partial breast irradiation for select patients, and the use of IMRT or proton therapy. In general, cardiac sparing is more difficult to achieve for patients with left-sided tumors or who have indications for nodal irradiation.

Hodgkin Lymphoma

Treatment for HL has undergone significant advances in recent decades. A brief historical overview is provided because many patients are still alive following treatment that was given decades ago. Treatment of HL was first described in 1902. Initial responses to radiation therapy were impressive, but recurrences outside the treated field were common, and the disease was thought to be incurable. In the 1950s, Vera Peters[22] described long-term 5-, 10-, and 15-year survival in patients treated with radiation to the involved nodal volumes plus adjacent nodal volumes, so-called extended-field radiotherapy. For several decades, extended-field radiotherapy became the standard of care, but late toxicity after radiation led researchers to seek alternate treatment methods. New chemotherapeutic agents became available in the 1950s and 1960s, and in 1970, the National Cancer Institute published evidence that multiagent chemotherapy could also provide long-term cures.[23] Subsequent studies evolved to use both chemotherapy and radiation in an effort to maximize the benefit of each modality and minimize toxicity. In the context of good response to chemotherapy, significant evidence

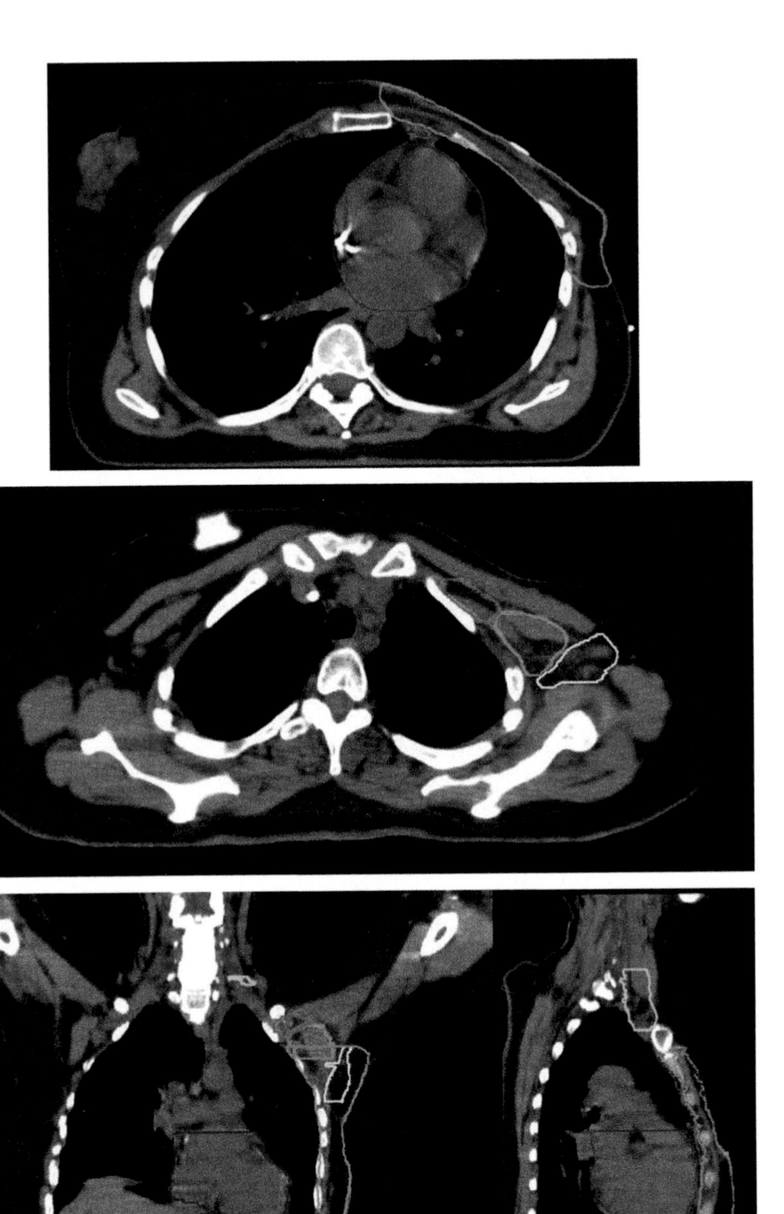

Fig. 3.15 Nodal contours for breast radiotherapy. Contours for the heart (*red*), chest wall (*purple*), levels 1 (*yellow*), 2 (*pink*), and 3 (*blue*) of the axilla, internal mammary (*green*), and supraclavicular (*cyan*) nodal volumes. The chest wall would be a target in this patient with pT3 pN2. (*Courtesy of* Radiation Therapy Oncology Group, Philadelphia, PA; with permission.)

now exists to support treating patients to lower-radiation doses[24–27] and to smaller radiation volumes.[28] Much of the data regarding late cardiac effects after radiotherapy come from patients treated with large radiation fields to higher doses than is currently used. For patients treated during that era, the incidence of HL recurrence plateaus after 5 years. However, the cumulative incidence of second malignancies and cardiovascular events increases and overtakes the incidence of HL recurrence by 15 to 25 years after therapy.[29]

In the early era of combined modality therapy for HL, mediastinal disease was treated with mantle field radiotherapy (Fig. 3.18). Mantle fields were designed to cover the initial nodal sites of disease with extension of the field to adjacent nodal volumes (hence the term extended field radiotherapy; EFRT). Bilateral neck, axilla, hilar,

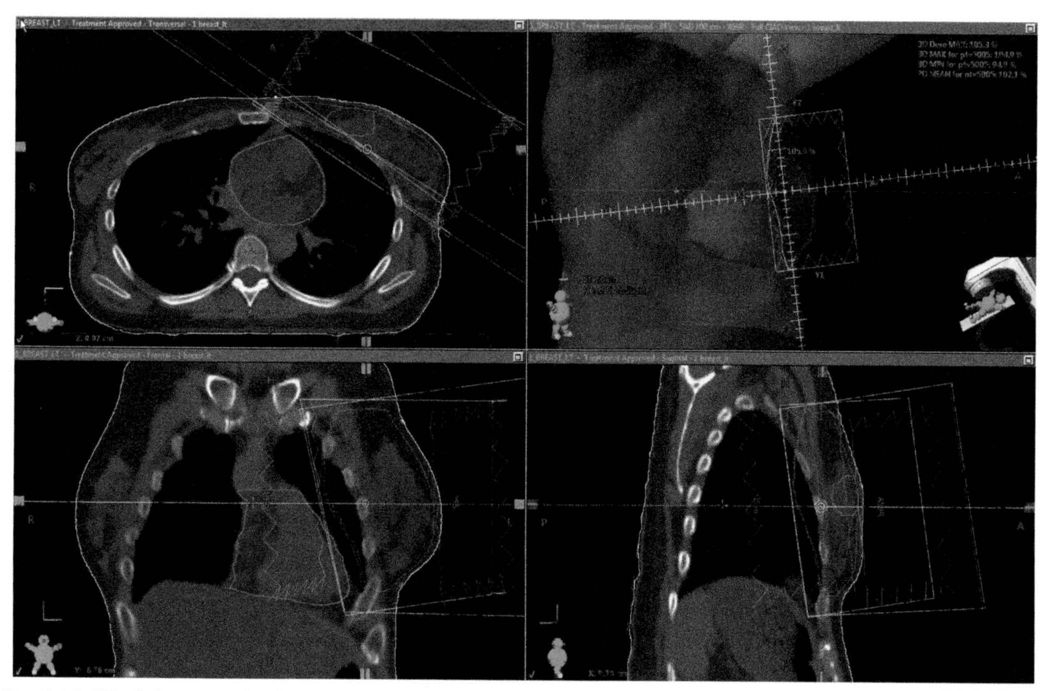

Fig. 3.16 Whole breast radiotherapy. This 43-year-old patient was diagnosed with T1 N0, ER+, PR+, Her2-negative breast. She elected for breast conservation and received adjuvant whole breast radiation therapy with a 10-Gy boost to the lumpectomy cavity. Selected contours (whole breast PTV [*blue*], lumpectomy cavity PTV [*orange*], and heart [*red*]) and the whole breast tangent beams are shown on axial (*upper left*), coronal (*lower left*), and sagittal (*lower right*) CT slices. A beams' eye projection of the medial tangent field is shown in the upper right. Opposing tangent beams are designed to cover the breast tissue while minimizing dose to the heart and lungs. A 1- to 2-cm sliver of lung is included in the beam to provide adequate coverage to the PTV. Examination of the beams' eye projection shows the 3D relationship between the heart and the target volumes.

and mediastinal nodes were included in a standard mantle field. Subsequent advances showed that smaller radiation fields were acceptable in the setting of improved chemotherapy. The first iteration of radiation volume reduction was from EFRT (eg, mantle) to involved field radiotherapy (IFRT). IFRT treatment volumes included the entire involved field (eg, the entire mediastinum in the setting of initial mediastinal disease) without targeting fields that were note initially involved (Fig. 3.19). Smaller volumes, termed involved site radiotherapy (ISRT), are now thought to be

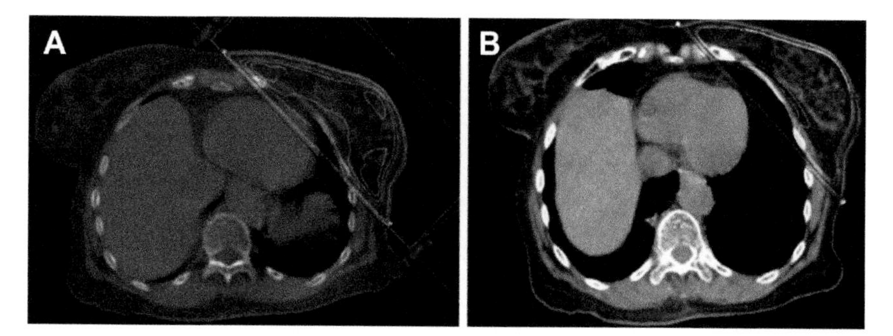

Fig. 3.17 Deep inspiration breath-hold. Radiation treatment plans for a patient with left-sided breast cancer in free-breathing (*A*) and deep inspiration breath-hold (DIBH) (*B*). The images are taken at the same patient level. In free-breathing, the left ventricle and left coronary artery may be in the beam path. In DIBH, the heart moves inferior and away from the left breast, allowing for better sparing of the heart without sacrificing target coverage. (*From* Beck RE, Kim L, Yue NJ, et al. Treatment techniques to reduce cardiac irradiation for breast cancer patients treated with breast-conserving surgery and radiation therapy: a review. Front Oncol 2014;4:327.)

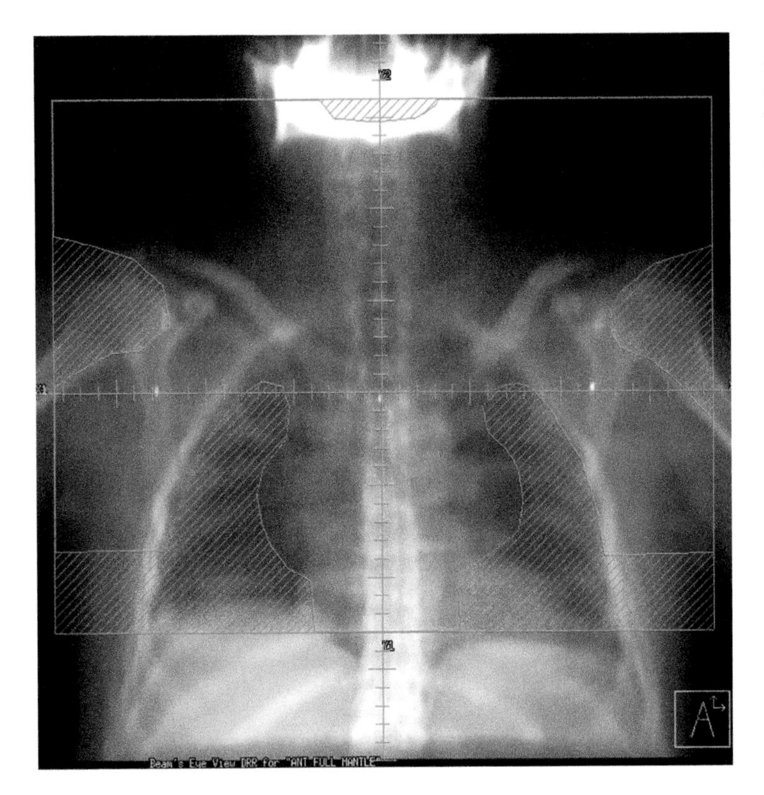

Fig. 3.18 Mantle field radiotherapy. The anterior mantle field showing coverage of the mediastinum and bilateral neck, axilla, and hilar regions. The patient would have been treated with both anterior and posterior mantle fields to provide more uniform dose. (*From* Koh ES, Tran TH, Heydarian M, et al. A comparison of mantle versus involved-field radiotherapy for Hodgkin's lymphoma: reduction in normal tissue dose and second cancer risk. Radiat Oncol 2007;2:13.)

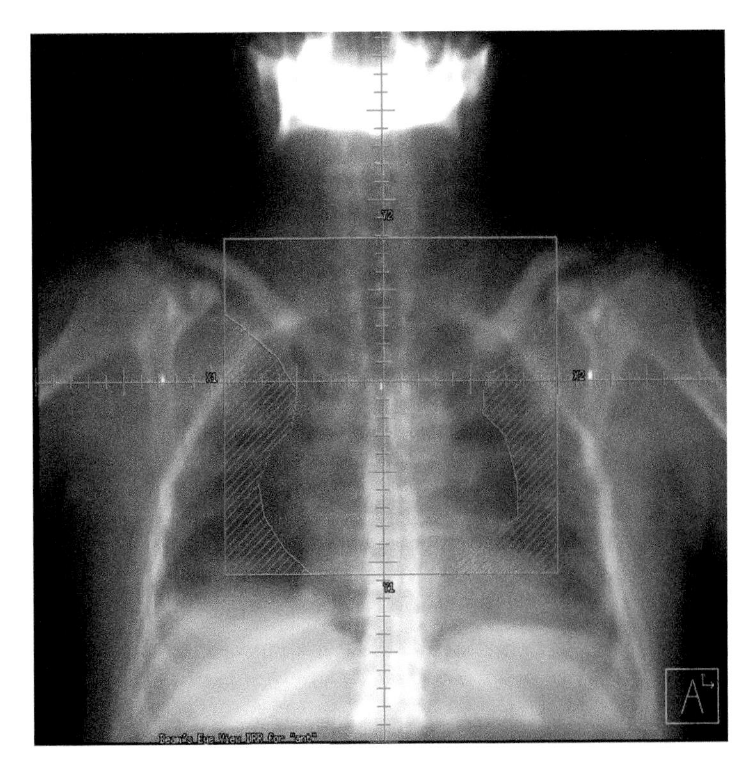

Fig. 3.19 IFRT. Mediastinal IFRT covering the mediastinum. The patient would have been treated with both anterior and posterior mediastinal fields. (*From* Koh ES, Tran TH, Heydarian M, et al. A comparison of mantle versus involved-field radiotherapy for Hodgkin's lymphoma: reduction in normal tissue dose and second cancer risk. Radiat Oncol 2007;2:13.)

acceptable.[30] ISRT volumes cover only the initial disease with a small margin (ie, only the involved mediastinum is treated instead of the entire mediastinum as was covered by IFRT).

As of 2016, adult patients in the United States with early-stage HL are often treated with 2 to 4 cycles of chemotherapy (for example, adriamycin, bleomycin, vinblastine, and dacarbazine) followed by 20- to 30-Gy ISRT. Pediatric patients are often treated with chemotherapy (often a different regimen than that used for adults) followed by 21-Gy ISRT. Indications for radiation therapy after good response to chemotherapy in advanced-stage HL include pediatric patients, partial response to therapy, and initial bulky disease.

SUMMARY

Radiation therapy continues to play an important role in curative and palliative cancer treatment. The cardio-oncologist will encounter patients at many phases in their cancer care from initial workup to decades after treatment. Modern radiotherapy benefits from advances in radiobiology and in treatment delivery that allow modern treatments to better limit dose outside of the intended target tissue while still delivering curative doses to the tumor. The techniques discussed above affect the acute, subacute, and delayed effects of radiotherapy. A working knowledge of current and historic radiotherapy principles, techniques, and effects will help the cardio-oncologist understand, anticipate, and treat various forms of cardiovascular sequela of radiotherapy.

REFERENCES

1. Khan FM. The physics of radiation therapy. 4th edition. Philadelphia: Lippincott Williams & Wilkins; 2010.
2. Zeman EM, Schreiber EC, Tepper JE. Basics of Radiation Therapy. In: Niederhuber JE, Armitage JO, Doroshow JH, et al, editors. Abeloff's Clinical Oncology. Fifth edition; 2014. p. 396–7.
3. Hall EJ, Giaccia AJ. Radiobiology for the radiologist. 7th edition. Philadelphia: Wolters Kluwer Health/Lippincott Williams & Wilkins; 2012.
4. Hill R, Healy B, Holloway L, et al. Advances in kilovoltage x-ray beam dosimetry. Phys Med Biol 2014;59(6):R183–231.
5. Amdur RJ, Kalbaugh KJ, Ewald LM, et al. Radiation therapy for skin cancer near the eye: kilovoltage x-rays versus electrons. Int J Radiat Oncol Biol Phys 1992;23(4):769–79.
6. Brengues M, Liu D, Korn R, et al. Method for validating radiobiological samples using a linear accelerator. EPJ Tech Instrum 2014;1(1).
7. Levin WP, Kooy H, Loeffler JS, et al. Proton beam therapy. Br J Cancer 2005;93(8):849–54.
8. Singh AD, Pelayes DE, Seregard S, et al. Ophthalmic radiation therapy: techniques and applications. Basel, Switzerland: Karger; 2013. p. 24–5.
9. Paganetti H, Niemierko A, Ancukiewicz M, et al. Relative biological effectiveness (RBE) values for proton beam therapy. Int J Radiat Oncol Biol Phys 2002;53(2):407–21.
10. Nieder C, Grosu AL, Gaspar LE. Stereotactic radiosurgery (SRS) for brain metastases: a systematic review. Radiat Oncol 2014;9:155.
11. Videtic GM, Chang JY, Chetty IJ, et al. ACR Appropriateness Criteria(R) early-stage non-small-cell lung cancer. Am J Clin Oncol 2014;37(2):201–7.
12. Verellen D, De Ridder M, Storme G. A (short) history of image-guided radiotherapy. Radiother Oncol 2008;86(1):4–13.
13. Kramer D. Carbon-ion cancer therapy shows promise. Physics Today 2015;68(6):24–5.
14. Oliver LN, Buttner PG, Hobson H, et al. A meta-analysis of randomised controlled trials assessing drug-eluting stents and vascular brachytherapy in the treatment of coronary artery in-stent restenosis. Int J Cardiol 2008;126(2):216–23.
15. Gorenoi V, Dintsios CM, Schonermark MP, et al. Intravascular brachytherapy for peripheral vascular disease. GMS Health Technol Assess 2008;4:Doc08.
16. Jones GC, Kehrer JD, Kahn J, et al. Primary treatment options for high-risk/medically inoperable early stage NSCLC patients. Clin Lung Cancer 2015;16(6):413–30.
17. Gaspar LE, Winter K, Kocha WI, et al. A phase I/II study of external beam radiation, brachytherapy, and concurrent chemotherapy for patients with localized carcinoma of the esophagus (Radiation Therapy Oncology Group Study 9207): final report. Cancer 2000;88(5):988–95.
18. van der Laan HP, Dolsma WV, Maduro JH, et al. Dosimetric consequences of the shift towards computed tomography guided target definition and planning for breast conserving radiotherapy. Radiat Oncol 2008;3:6.
19. Fisher B, Anderson S, Bryant J, et al. Twenty-year follow-up of a randomized trial comparing total mastectomy, lumpectomy, and lumpectomy plus irradiation for the treatment of invasive breast cancer. N Engl J Med 2002;347(16):1233–41.
20. Bartelink H, Horiot JC, Poortmans PM, et al. Impact of a higher radiation dose on local control and survival in breast-conserving therapy of early breast cancer: 10-year results of the randomized boost versus no boost EORTC 22881-10882 trial. J Clin Oncol 2007;25(22):3259–65.

21. Smith BD, Arthur DW, Buchholz TA, et al. Accelerated partial breast irradiation consensus statement from the American Society for Radiation Oncology (ASTRO). Int J Radiat Oncol Biol Phys 2009;74(4): 987–1001.
22. Peters MV. A study of survivals in Hodgkin's disease treated radiologically. Am J Roentgenol Radium Ther 1950;63:299–311.
23. Devita VT Jr, Serpick AA, Carbone PP. Combination chemotherapy in the treatment of advanced Hodgkin's disease. Ann Intern Med 1970;73(6): 881–95.
24. Duhmke E, Franklin J, Pfreundschuh M, et al. Low-dose radiation is sufficient for the noninvolved extended-field treatment in favorable early-stage Hodgkin's disease: long-term results of a randomized trial of radiotherapy alone. J Clin Oncol 2001; 19(11):2905–14.
25. Ferme C, Eghbali H, Meerwaldt JH, et al. Chemotherapy plus involved-field radiation in early-stage Hodgkin's disease. N Engl J Med 2007;357(19): 1916–27.
26. Eich HT, Diehl V, Gorgen H, et al. Intensified chemotherapy and dose-reduced involved-field radiotherapy in patients with early unfavorable Hodgkin's lymphoma: final analysis of the German Hodgkin Study Group HD11 trial. J Clin Oncol 2010;28(27):4199–206.
27. Engert A, Plutschow A, Eich HT, et al. Reduced treatment intensity in patients with early-stage Hodgkin's lymphoma. N Engl J Med 2010;363(7): 640–52.
28. Noordijk EM, Carde P, Mandard AM, et al. Preliminary results of the EORTC-GPMC controlled clinical trial H7 in early-stage Hodgkin's disease. EORTC Lymphoma Cooperative Group. Groupe Pierre-et-Marie-Curie. Ann Oncol 1994;5(Suppl 2):107–12.
29. Castellino SM, Geiger AM, Mertens AC, et al. Morbidity and mortality in long-term survivors of Hodgkin lymphoma: a report from the Childhood Cancer Survivor Study. Blood 2011;117(6): 1806–16.
30. Specht L, Yahalom J, Illidge T, et al. Modern radiation therapy for Hodgkin lymphoma: field and dose guidelines from the international lymphoma radiation oncology group (ILROG). Int J Radiat Oncol Biol Phys 2014;89(4):854–62.

CHAPTER 4

Cardiac Tumors

Overview and Pathology

Joseph J. Maleszewski, MD[a,*], Allen Burke, MD[b]

OVERVIEW

Cardiac tumors are a broad group of entities that encompass both neoplastic and nonneoplastic lesions. Nonneoplastic tumors include thrombi, infections, cysts, varices, degenerative processes (calcification), heterotopias, and occasionally, extracardiac processes that by imaging appear to involve the heart/pericardium (eg, hiatal hernia, esophageal diverticulum).

Among the neoplastic lesions, benign and malignant tumors can be distinguished as well as primary (arising within the heart) and metastatic (arising outside of the heart, but traveling to it) processes.[1] Metastatic lesions are, by very definition, malignant in nature and are far more commonly encountered than primary tumors. Fewer than 10% of primary cardiac neoplasms are malignant. Cardiac neoplasms occur across the human lifespan, but certain entities (eg, rhabdomyoma) are encountered almost exclusively in children, whereas others (eg, myxoma, sarcoma) are usually seen in adults. The recommended classification system is the one endorsed by the World Health Organization (Table 4.1).

The classification of some lesions, such as the papillary fibroelastoma, is yet unclear despite the fact that this is thought to be one of the most common adult cardiac tumors, and why precisely they arise is poorly understood. Although most think them to be reactive growths, neoplastic and hamartomatous causes have been posited.

Although most primary cardiac neoplasms are not malignant, benign histology does not necessarily equate to a benign clinical course, owing to the precarious location in which many of these tumors arise. Lesion size and location also impact the clinical behavior. Small, histologically benign lesions can still cause devastating consequences through thromboembolic events or arrhythmogenesis. Large, histologically benign lesions can obstruct blood flow and result in heart failure.

Definitive characterization of cardiac tumors usually requires sampling, either by way of excision or by biopsy sampling. Such sampling is often quite challenging because of location. Nevertheless, some tumors (particularly those arising in the right heart) are amenable to endomyocardial sampling by wave of a bioptome. Malignant lesions that involve the pericardium may be diagnosed by way of cytologic analysis of pericardial fluid.

NONNEOPLASTIC TUMORS

Mural Thrombi

Mural thrombi are admixtures of variable quantities of erythrocytes, fibrin, and platelets that may form masses that are adherent to the endocardium or sometimes free floating within the cardiac chambers (Fig. 4.1).

Most mural thrombi are associated with underlying heart disease in which the normal cardiac hemodynamics are altered. Atrial thrombosis is more common than ventricular thrombosis. Cardiac amyloidosis, valvular heart disease (mitral stenosis, in particular), and atrial fibrillation have strong associations with atrial thrombosis. Ischemic heart disease can be associated with ventricular mural thrombosis. The presence of intracardiac devices is also a risk factor for thrombus formation. Mural thrombi may also occur sporadically in the absence of heart disease or coagulopathy; also clotting disorders should be ruled out clinically.

Mural thrombi are often asymptomatic, but they may cause cyanosis, dyspnea, and heart failure. They may form spherical masses ("ball thrombi"), especially when they occur in

[a] 200 First Street Southwest, Rochester, MN 55902, USA; [b] University of Maryland Medical Center, UMMS, 21 S.Greene Street, Baltimore, MD 21201, USA
* Corresponding author.
E-mail address: Maleszewski.Joseph@mayo.edu

TABLE 4.1
World Health Organization histologic classification of tumors of the heart

Benign tumors and tumorlike lesions	
Rhabdomyoma	8900/0
Histiocytoid cardiomyopathy	
Hamartoma of mature cardiac myocytes	
Adult cellular rhabdomyoma	8904/0
Cardiac myxoma	8840/0
Papillary fibroelastoma	
Hemangioma	9120/0
Cardiac fibroma	8810/0
IMT	8825/1
Lipoma	8850/0
Cystic tumor of the AV node	
Malignant tumors	
Angiosarcoma	9120/3
Epithelioid hemangioendothelioma	9133/3
Malignant pleomorphic fibrous histiocytoma/undifferentiated pleomorphic sarcoma	8830/3
Fibrosarcoma and myxoid fibrosarcomas	8840/3
Rhabdomyosarcoma	8900/3
Leiomyosarcoma	8890/3
Synovial sarcoma	9040/3
Liposarcoma	8854/3
Cardiac lymphomas	
Metastatic tumors	
Pericardial tumors	
Solitary fibrous tumor	8815/1
Malignant mesothelioma	9050/3
Germ cell tumors	
Metastatic pericardial tumors	

Morphology code of the International Classification of Diseases for Oncology (ICD-0)[1] and the Systematized Nomenclature of Medicine (http://snomed.org). Behavior is coded /0, for benign tumors /3, for malignant tumors, and /1, for borderline or uncertain behavior.

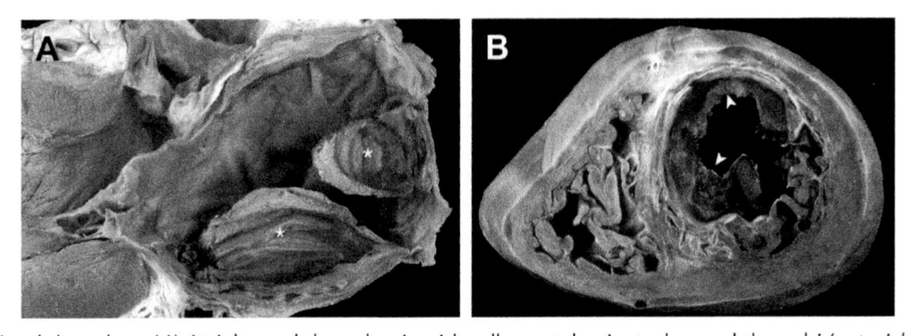

Fig. 4.1 Mural thrombus. (*A*) Atrial mural thrombosis with adherent, laminated, mural thrombi (*asterisks*) involving the inferior and posterior aspects of the left atrium. (*B*) Ventricular mural thrombosis (*arrowheads*) in the setting of a transmural myocardial infarction of the left anterior descending coronary artery territory.

the left atrium, which can then obstruct the valvular orifice. Transesophageal echocardiography is an excellent modality for detection of atrial thrombi, as is cardiac MRI (cMRI) and computed tomography. Nevertheless, it can be difficult to distinguish them from other cardiac tumors, such as atrial myxomas. Location within the atrial appendage (as opposed to the atrial septum) and the presence of underlying heart disease both tend to favor a diagnosis of thrombus.

Cardiac calcifying amorphous tumors are thought to represent calcified and degenerated mural thrombi.[2,3] Such may occur in any cardiac chamber, most commonly the right atrium, and are associated with coagulopathic states, including antiphospholipid syndrome and factor V Leiden. The presence of renal failure may accelerate calcification. They tend to be irregular calcified nodules of chalky material (Fig. 4.2). Histologically, these lesions consist of nodular calcification in a background of amorphous eosinophilic material that likely represents degenerating blood and fibrin.

Mitral Annular Calcification

Mitral annular calcification (MAC) is the degenerative deposition of calcium and lipid along the fibrous annulus (Fig. 4.3). It occurs much more commonly along the posterior portion of the annulus and can occasionally be exuberant and cause a mass-lesion within the heart. MAC may undergo central softening, wherein the calcified material becomes a gritty "toothpastelike" substance. As the annulus undergoes normal flexion and movement throughout the cardiac cycle, the calcified rind of MAC may fissure, causing the gritty material to extrude onto the surface of the valve or into the cardiac chamber. This material may also produce a mass lesion that may organize and further calcify or potentially lead to a thromboembolic event.

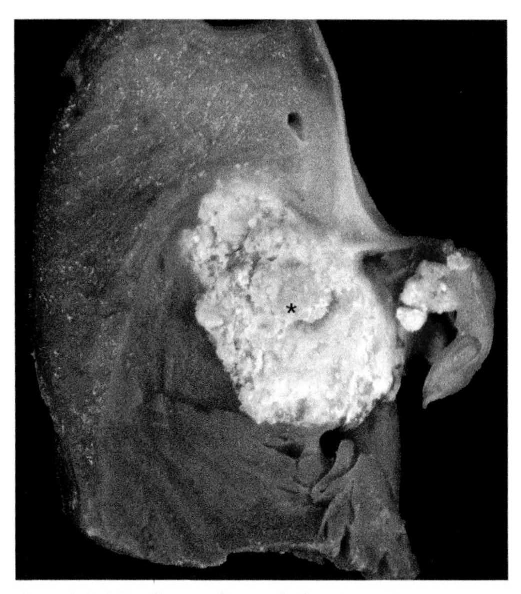

Fig. 4.3 Mitral annular calcification. Degenerative calcification of the fibrous mitral annulus can present as a mass lesion (*asterisk*), usually along the posterior portion of the mitral annulus.

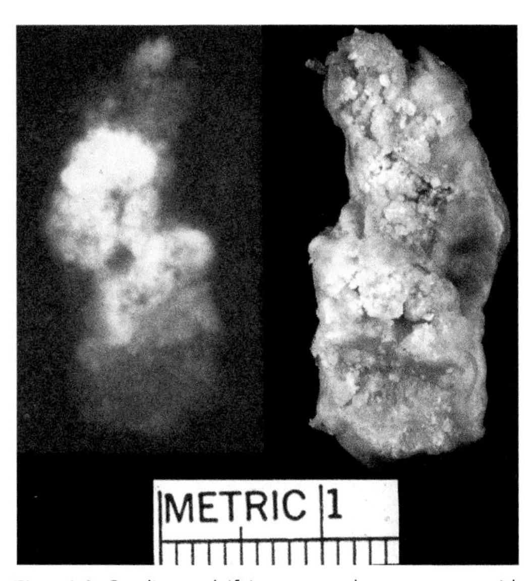

Fig. 4.2 Cardiac calcifying amorphous tumor with irregular, chalky white tissue that is densely calcified. Such calcification is best illustrated by the radiography show on the left of the image.

MAC is a relatively common finding in women over the age of 60 years. The presence of myxomatous mitral valve disease or a left ventricular pressure load (eg, chronic aortic stenosis, systemic hypertension, hypertrophic cardiomyopathy) may also hasten the development of MAC.

Cardiac False Tendons

False tendons are fibrotic or fibromuscular bands that span 2 nonvalvular endocardial surfaces within or across a cardiac chamber (Fig. 4.4). They can be found in either the atria or the ventricles and have a wide-ranging prevalence that, in some studies, has been reported as high as 50%. In the left atrium, they are associated with patent foramen ovale, Chiari network, and supraventricular arrhythmias.[4] Imaging studies have generally focused on the left ventricle, where false tendons have been associated with benign murmurs, premature ventricular contractions, and idiopathic ventricular tachycardia.[5]

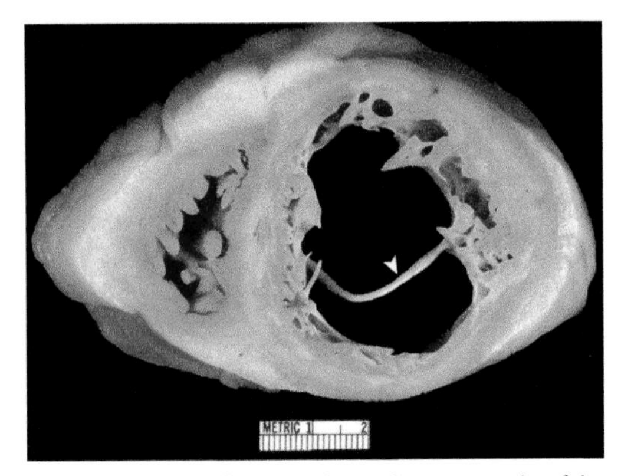

Fig. 4.4 Cardiac false tendon. This ventricular false tendon (*arrowhead*) spans the septum and free wall of the left ventricle.

Grossly, the most common left ventricular location is from the left-sided posteromedial papillary muscle to the ventricular septum (66%), followed by lesions that span the anterolateral and posteromedial papillary muscles (12%).[5] Histologically, false tendons contain fibrous tissue and variable amounts of myocardium, elastic tissue, and blood vessel. Surgical excision may be warranted, particularly if the location precludes deployment of an intracardiac device.

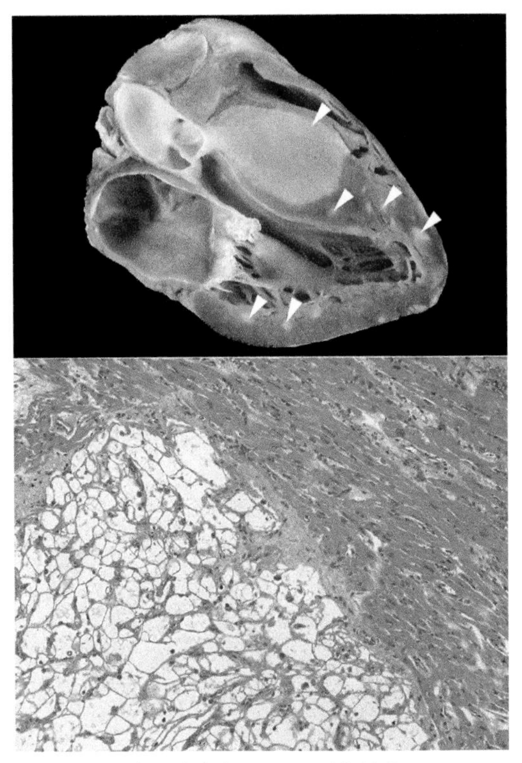

Fig. 4.5 Cardiac rhabdomyomas. Multiple tumors are seen here in the setting of tuberous sclerosis (*arrowheads*). The large lesion caused significant obstruction of both the right and the left outflow tracts. Histologically, the tumors are composed of vacuolated myocytes that form a sharp border with the adjacent, normal, myocardium.

PEDIATRIC AND CONGENITAL TUMORS

Cardiac Rhabdomyoma

Rhabdomyoma is the most common cardiac tumor of infancy and childhood, accounting for 50% to 75% of pediatric cardiac tumors. They are thought to be hamartomatous lesions that arise from cardiac myocytes. Cardiac rhabdomyomas comprise 90% of heart tumors diagnosed prenatally.[6]

Cardiac rhabdomyomas are congenital lesions with a tendency to spontaneously regress and are therefore rarely seen in children older than age 10. Although cardiac rhabdomyomas are often not surgically resected, they are still the most frequently excised tumors in children.[7,8]

About 80% of children with cardiac rhabdomyoma have clinical, radiologic, or family history of tuberous sclerosis complex (TSC).[9] Conversely, almost half of all children with TSC have cardiac rhabdomyoma. It is common to have multiple synchronous lesions, especially when associated with TSC. Sporadic rhabdomyoma is more likely to be single, cause outflow tract obstruction, and result in surgical treatment.[10,11]

Grossly, cardiac rhabdomyomas are circumscribed, homogeneous, pale tan masses that occur most frequently in the ventricles (Fig. 4.5). They may be very large and obstruct the normal flow of blood within the heart. Histologically, they are composed of a uniform population of cardiac myocyte-derived cells with abundant intracellular glycogen and disordered myofilaments. The increased glycogen causes vacuoles that separate strands of cytoplasm into so-called spider cells, which are a useful diagnostic finding.

Because of their propensity to spontaneously regress, conservative management is common in asymptomatic children. Pharmaceuticals that inhibit the mTOR signaling pathway (eg, everolimus) have been shown to hasten regression in some cases.[12]

Cardiac Fibroma

Cardiac fibroma is a benign congenital tumor that occurs within the ventricular myocardium. It has sometimes been reported with different names, such as *fibromatosis*, *fibrous hamartoma*, and *fibroelastic hamartoma*.[13] They most commonly arise in the ventricular septum followed by the left ventricular free wall, right ventricular free wall, right atrium, and the left atrium.[13,14]

Cardiac fibroma is the second most common tumor of childhood. Almost 90% of cardiac fibromas occur in children, one-third of whom are less than 1 year of age.[13] Fewer than 10% of cases are diagnosed antenatally or in the neonatal period. Presenting symptoms include heart failure, cyanosis, arrhythmias, and syncope. The tumor is an incidental finding in one-third of patients. Sudden death may be the initial presentation.[15]

Cardiac fibroma may be a manifestation of Gorlin syndrome, which is caused by mutations in *PTCH1*. Homozygous and heterozygous losses of the *PTCH1* gene have been found in sporadic cardiac fibromas.[16]

Grossly, cardiac fibromas are rounded masses that, upon sectioning, have a white and whorled appearance (Fig. 4.6). The degree of cellularity often decreases with age of the patient, whereas the amount of collagen increases. Calcification is a common finding in fibromas from patients of all ages, and, in addition to their solitary nature, helps distinguish these tumors from rhabdomyomas. Identification of microcalcifications, by imaging, within an intramural tumor is a strong indicator of a cardiac fibroma.

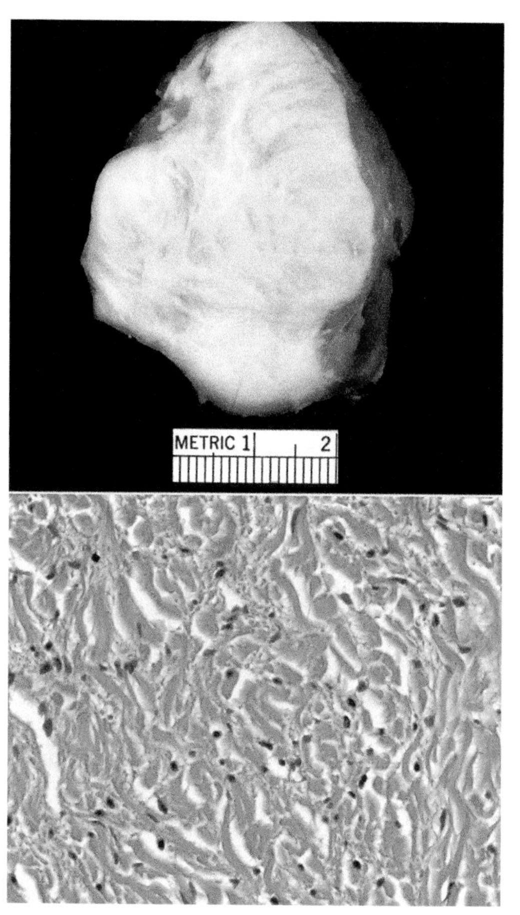

Fig. 4.6 Cardiac fibroma. This whorled, white, grossly well-circumscribed lesion was surgically resected from the left ventricular free wall. Histologically, the tumor consists primarily of collagen with scattered fibroblasts.

Surgical excision is the mainstay of therapy, particularly in those that are symptomatic. However, many are incidental findings, and spontaneous regression has been reported (although much less commonly than with cardiac rhabdomyoma).[17]

Histiocytoid Cardiomyopathy

Histiocytoid cardiomyopathy is a multicentric congenital hamartomatous lesion of cardiac myocytes. Most cases of histiocytoid cardiomyopathy are sporadic, but familial cases have been reported in association with mutation of the *NDUFB11* gene.[18]

There is a female predominance of 4:1. The age range at presentation is birth to 4 years, with a mean age of onset at 10 to 13 months. The most common presenting features are arrhythmias, followed by sudden death and seizures.[19–22]

Grossly, the heart can appear normal. More commonly, there are endocardial nodules, typically at the base of the heart near the valves, which are raised and yellowish with an average size of 2 mm. Lesions can occur anywhere in the heart, including the endocardium, epicardium, atrioventricular (AV) node, and valves.[22]

The cells of histiocytoid cardiomyopathy are somewhat larger than normal myocytes, but smaller than those of rhabdomyoma. They are pale, rounded to oval, often surrounded by thin collagen fibers, and stain faintly with periodic acid-Schiff. In contrast to rhabdomyoma, large vacuoles and cytoplasmic streaming are absent. Associated endocardial fibroelastosis may also be present, and an association with left ventricular noncompaction has been reported.[23]

Treatment is typically targeted at the refractory arrhythmias, either by pharmacotherapy or ablation. Successful therapies with surgical excision and cardiac transplantation have also been reported.

Cardiac Inflammatory Myofibroblastic Tumor

Cardiac inflammatory myofibroblastic tumor (IMT) is a mesenchymal neoplasm of uncertain malignant potential. Synonyms, over the years, have included *inflammatory pseudotumor* and *myofibroblastic inflammatory tumor*.

In the heart, there have been scattered reports of "inflammatory pseudotumors" that are probably a heterogeneous group of both neoplastic and nonneoplastic conditions. Nevertheless, in order to maintain uniformity with other mesenchymal lesions, the term IMT should be restricted to a histologically uniform set of endocardial lesions. Tumors that occur in association with immunoglobulin 4–related sclerosing disease, Behçet disease, hypogammaglobulinemia, and pulmonary inflammatory pseudotumor, or infection should be designated as their respective primary disease.[24–27]

IMT is a low-grade mesenchymal neoplasm with smooth muscle and fibrocytic (myofibroblastic) differentiation and chronic inflammation.

The mean patient age at presentation is 16 years, with a median age of 5.5 years. The endocardial location and surface fibrin result in a propensity for embolization to the brain or lower extremities. Prolapse into the coronary arteries can result in ischemia, myocardial infarction, and sudden death.[11,28]

Sites of involvement include the endocardium of the mitral valve, right atrium, right ventricle, tricuspid valve, pulmonary valve, aortic valve, left atrium, and left ventricle.[28–33]

Grossly, they are polypoid lesions, reflected in the histologic appearance, which is similar to IMTs of soft tissue. These features include variable myxoid background, spindled cells with abundant cytoplasm ("tissue culture" cells), absent or minimal mitotic activity, a chronic inflammatory background of lymphocytes, plasma cells, and macrophages, and variable fibrosis.[28]

In general, these lesions respond very well to surgical excision, with excellent survival. There are only very rare reports of tumor-associated death.

Heterotopic Tissue

Tissue heterotopias refer to congenital entrapments or rests of tissue that can present as mass lesions within the heart. Bronchogenic cysts and cystic tumors of the AV node are the most commonly encountered.

Cystic tumor of the AV node is thought to represent an ultimobranchial heterotopia that occurs near the membranous septum in the area of the AV node and penetrates the bundle of His. It usually results in congenital heart block and may precipitate sudden death. Rarely, cystic AV nodal tumors can be incidental. They are usually grossly unapparent, but may be characterized by multiple small cysts seen within the AV septum. Histologically, AV nodal tumors are collections of small cystic structures composed of cuboidal cells.

Bronchogenic and enteric cysts may occasionally occur within the pericardium, and exceptionally within the myocardium. There is a 2:1 female predilection. They are usually incidental findings, but surgical excision is usually curative in those that are symptomatic.

LESIONS OF UNCERTAIN CAUSE

Papillary Fibroelastoma

Papillary fibroelastoma is a benign, papillary, endocardial growth that consists of endothelium overlying avascular fibroelastic fronds. Although in the past some have referred to these lesions as "cardiac papillomas," this is strongly discouraged to avoid confusion with human papilloma virus–associated lesions that have no relation to the papillary fibroelastoma.

Papillary fibroelastoma is the most common surgically excised cardiac tumor.[34] Advances in imaging resolution have certainly fostered the recognition of how common these lesions truly are. The mean age at presentation is 64 years.[34] Although their exact nature is unclear, there is a clear association with endocardial injury and/or hemodynamic trauma.

Although usually incidental, some papillary fibroelastomas may produce significant symptoms. Although usually less than 1 cm, larger lesions have been reported.[35] Chest pain, syncope, transient ischemic attacks, and stroke have all been reported presentations. Sudden cardiac death has also been documented.[36]

These growths may occur on any endocardium-lined surface, but they most commonly arise on the cardiac valves (left>right). By imaging, they tend to exhibit a very characteristic shimmering appearance, which correlates with their many fronds. These fronds that arise from a common stalk and arborize are highly characteristic gross findings that may be unapparent unless the lesion is in solution (Fig. 4.7).

Unlike papillary fibroelastoma, Lambl excrescences tend to have a simpler (single frond) architecture and occur exclusively on the closing surface of cardiac valves.

Owing to the possibility of thromboembolic events and serious sequelae, many investigators contend that these lesions should be excised (particularly when left-sided). Surgical excision, in experienced hands, has been shown to have excellent results and can often spare the underlying valve.

Lipomatous Hypertrophy of the Atrial Septum

Considered by some to represent a form of heterotopic or entrapped tissue, lipomatous hypertrophy of the atrial septum (LHAS) is characterized by a nonencapsulated fatty thickening of the atrial septum. Nevertheless, a single case of LHAS harboring a neoplastic gene rearrangement has

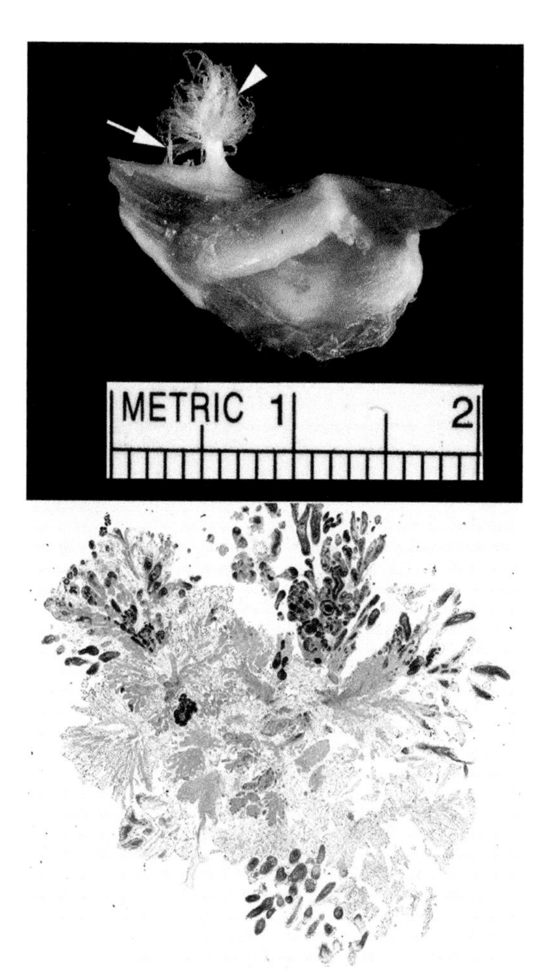

Fig. 4.7 Papillary fibroelastoma. This endocardial tumor (*arrowhead*) has multiple branching fronds arising from a common stalk on the free edge of the aortic valve cusp. Contrast this lesion with the simpler, nonbranching, Lambl excrescence to the left of it (*arrow*). Histologically, the fronds are avascular and consist of collagen (*pink*) and elastin (*black*).

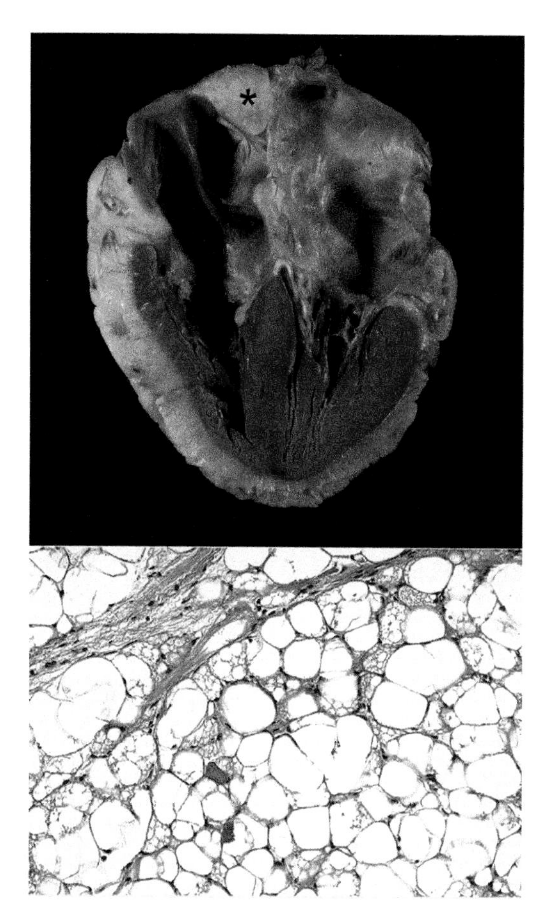

Fig. 4.8 LHAS. The posterior portion of the limbus of the fossa ovalis is markedly thickened by yellow fat (*asterisk*). Histologically, the lesion contains an admixture of mature (*white*) fat, immature (*brown*; vacuolated) fat, and atrial myocytes.

been identified, bringing into question the precise cause of this entity.[37]

The mean age of presentation of LHAS is approximately 69 years. There is an association with body mass index, with about a third of patients being obese. Although usually asymptomatic, LHAS can present with arrhythmia or heart failure, the latter owing to obstruction of venous return to the right atrium via compression of the vena cava. cMRI is an excellent imaging modality, because the fatty attenuation and location are characteristic.

LHAS usually involves the posterior limbus of the fossa ovalis, usually with sparing of the valve portion (Fig. 4.8). In general, this thickening is usually in excess of 1.5 to 2.0 cm. If both anterior and posterior portions of the limbus are involved, the septum may have a dumbbell morphology. Histologically, the lesion is composed of mature fat, brown (immature) fat, and entrapped atrial myocytes.

Surgical resection can be helpful in symptomatic cases, but is not necessary in most with this condition.

BENIGN PRIMARY CARDIAC NEOPLASMS

Cardiac Myxoma

Cardiac myxoma is the most common primary adult cardiac neoplasm, with the exception of the papillary fibroelastoma (which may not be truly neoplastic). Cardiac myxomas can occur in any age group, but are most common between the fourth and seventh decades of life.[38] There is, in some series, a female predilection of 2:1 that appears to lessen after the age of 65 years. As with most cardiac tumors, presentation is dependent on location, size, shape, mobility, and rate of growth. Tumors may be asymptomatic, result in embolic phenomena if irregular and friable, or cause obstruction. The inflammatory infiltrate can result in systemic symptoms related to interleukin-6 production. In young children, cardiac myxomas may, indeed, represent other processes, such as IMTs.

Some myxomas (<10%) arise in association with the Carney complex (myxoma syndrome), an autosomal-dominant condition that can result from mutation in the *PRKAR1A* gene.[39] The Carney complex includes previously described LAMB (lentigines, atrial myxomas, mucocutaneous myxomas, and blue nevi) and NAME (nevi, atrial myxoma, myxoid neurofibroma, and ephelides) syndromes. In addition to cardiac myxomas, the syndrome is associated with extracardiac myxomas, endocrinopathy, and spotty skin pigmentation. Cardiac myxomas occurring in the context of the Carney complex are more likely to occur in atypical (non-left atrium) locations; be multiple; and occur earlier in life.

Cardiac myxomas usually arise from the left side of the atrial septum. Grossly, they may be sessile and broad-based, or pedunculated on a stalk that can allow mobility of the tumor within the atrium or through a valvular orifice (typically mitral) (Fig. 4.9). They can be smooth walled or villiform, with the latter having a higher potential to be associated with thromboembolic events (from either adherent surface thrombus or tumor embolization).

Histologically, cardiac myxomas are heterogeneous, due to intratumoral hemorrhage, calcification, and other degenerative changes. The "myxoma cell" is oval or spindled and often forms vasoformative rings. There is, in nondegenerative areas, a myxoid background rich in proteoglycans, lymphocytes, macrophages, and dendritic cells, which typically express factor 13A. Degenerative changes include ossification, and mineralization of elastic tissue can occur. Occasionally, glandular elements identified within the tumor can cause diagnostic confusion with a metastatic process.

The prognosis for a cardiac myxoma is generally good with a very low risk of recurrence, which is almost always associated with incomplete tumor resection in nonsyndromic cases. It is important to identify those cases arising in the setting of Carney complex, and therefore, a careful family and medical history should be obtained in each instance. Routine immunohistochemical staining for PRKAR1A can also be helpful in screening for such.[39]

Hamartoma of Mature Cardiac Myocytes

Hamartoma of mature cardiac myocytes is a benign overgrowth of differentiated, mature, disorganized cardiac myocytes. It is very rare and has been noted in both pediatric and adult populations.

Most are thought to be asymptomatic, and most are identified at autopsy. However, there

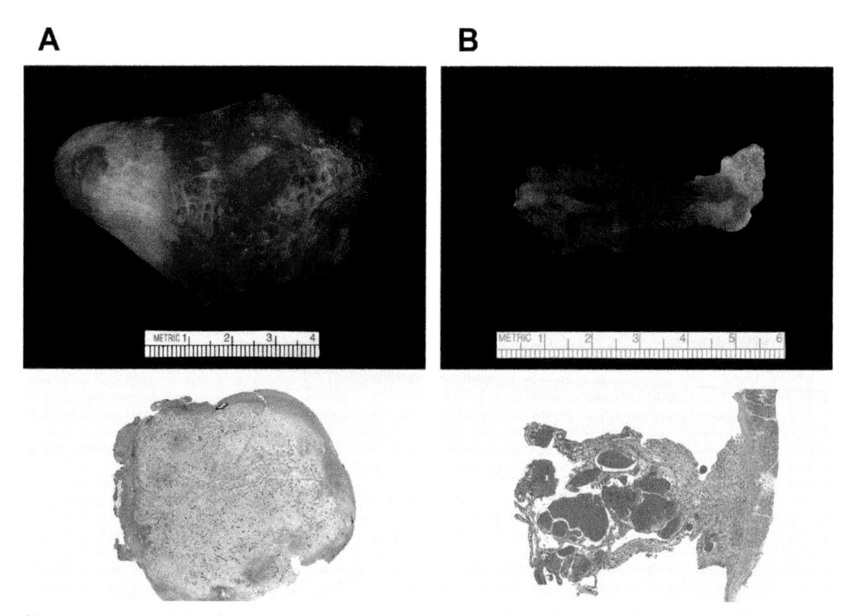

Fig. 4.9 Cardiac myxoma. (*A*) Cardiac myxomas may have a smooth surface or (*B*) a more villiform architecture. The latter are more likely to be associated with thromboembolic phenomena. Histologically, the tumor is characterized by myxoma cells proliferating within an abundant myxoid stroma. Variable intratumor hemorrhage is seen.

have been reports associated with arrhythmia, chest pain, and sudden death.[40] They are usually found within the ventricular wall and manifest as a poorly defined area of pale tissue (Fig. 4.10). Histologically, they are composed of large and disorganized myofibers, within a fibrotic backdrop. There is some histologic overlap between hamartoma of mature cardiac myocytes and hypertrophic cardiomyopathy, although the latter typically does not present as a mass lesion.

Hemangioma

Cardiac hemangiomas are a heterogeneous group of tumors that include congenital neoplasms with a tendency to regress, and malformations occurring in adults that are of uncertain histogenesis, a subset of which are probably neoplastic.

Cardiac hemangiomas are rare, accounting for less than 5% of benign tumors of the heart in adults and 10% of heart tumors in children.[8,11] Most patients are asymptomatic, although they may cause dyspnea, palpitations, arrhythmias, conduction disturbances, and pericardial effusion. The right atrium is the most common location; however, they have been identified in all 4 chambers.[41–44]

Grossly, tumors are usually infiltrative, hemorrhagic lesions without clear borders (Fig. 4.11).

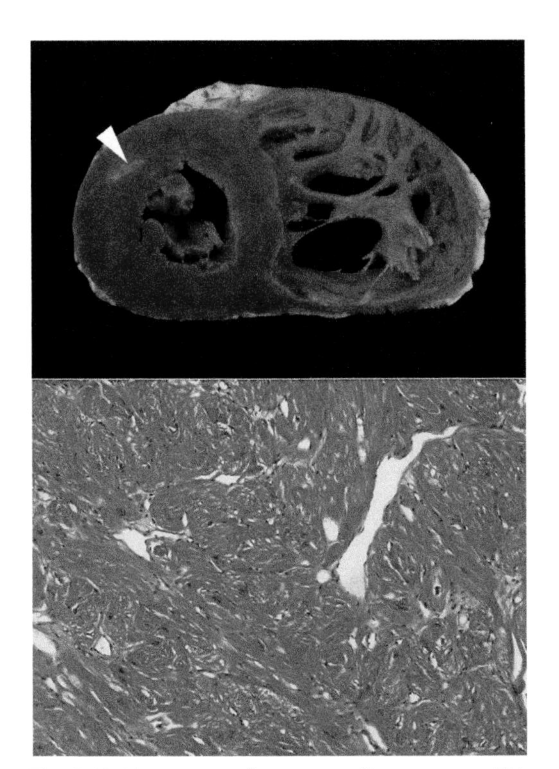

Fig. 4.10 Hamartoma of mature cardiac myocytes. This lesion usually manifests as a pale, myocardial lesion (*arrowhead*) grossly. Histologically, the lesion consists of enlarged, disorganized myocytes.

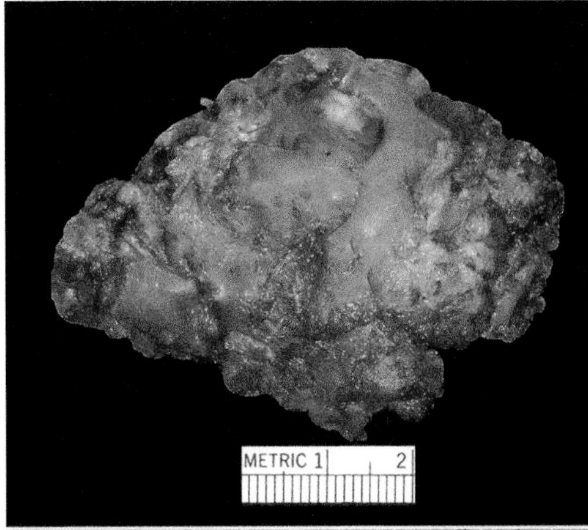

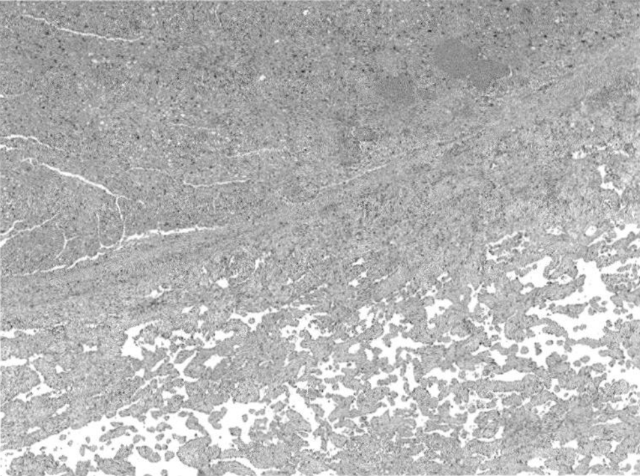

Fig. 4.11 Cardiac hemangioma. The red-brown appearance of this lesion is a clue to its vascular nature. Histologically, the vascular nature of the lesion is evident, consisting of collections of blood vessels.

Occasionally, they are endocardially based polypoid or pedunculated tumors.[45] Histologically, most cardiac hemangiomas are of the cavernous or capillary type.[41–43,45] There is often infiltration of the endocardial recesses of the right atrium with superimposed thrombosis. Occasionally, the histologic appearance can mimic an intramuscular hemangioma of soft tissue, with variable amounts of fat and fibrous tissue.[46]

As is the case with other cardiac tumors, surgery is the mainstay of therapy for symptomatic lesions.

Lipoma

Cardiac lipomas are benign mesenchymal neoplasms of mature adipocytes. They are very rare and can affect any age with no sex predilection. There are rare reports of associations with Cowden syndrome and tuberous sclerosis.

They are usually located on the epicardial surface, but intramural and endocardial tumors have also been described. They are usually yellow, smooth, and well-circumscribed and are composed entirely of fat (Fig. 4.12). Resection is usually curative.

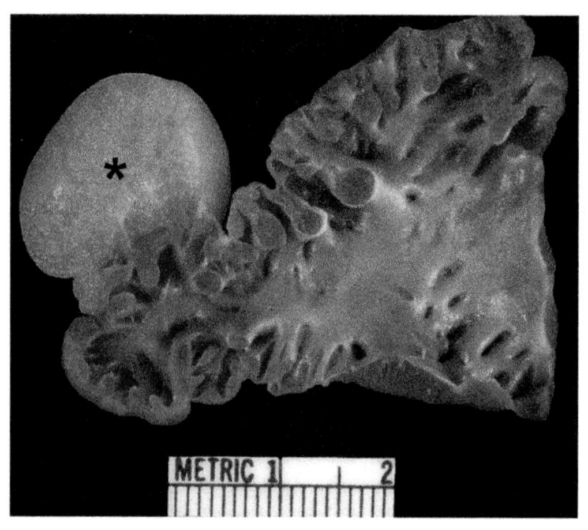

Fig. 4.12 Cardiac lipoma. A well-circumscribed, yellow mass (*asterisk*) is seen arising from the epicardial surface of the left atrial appendage.

MALIGNANT PRIMARY CARDIAC NEOPLASMS

Staging

Because of their rarity, there are no accepted methods of staging of cardiac sarcomas, as there is no American Joint Committee on Cancer/TNM staging system yet agreed on. Grading of cardiac sarcomas is also not standardized, although adaptation of existing systems for soft tissue tumors is common. In general, the prognosis of most cardiac sarcomas is grim, regardless of the grade or stage.

Undifferentiated Pleomorphic Sarcoma

Undifferentiated pleomorphic sarcomas are high-grade neoplasms without apparent differentiation. This group of tumors includes what was formerly referred to as *undifferentiated sarcoma* and *malignant fibrous histiocytoma.*

These lesions, along with cardiac angiosarcoma, are far and away the most commonly encountered primary cardiac malignancies. Undifferentiated pleomorphic sarcomas usually present in the fifth or sixth decades of life without an obvious sex predilection.

Two-thirds of tumors are left atrial and typically cause symptoms related to obstruction or heart failure. Symptoms from pulmonary or cerebral metastasis may also be the first manifestation. Because of their left atrial location, they may initially be mistaken for myxomas, but they tend to exhibit a more infiltrative growth pattern and involve the atrial wall directly. Extension into the pulmonary veins or the ventricles is common (Fig. 4.13).

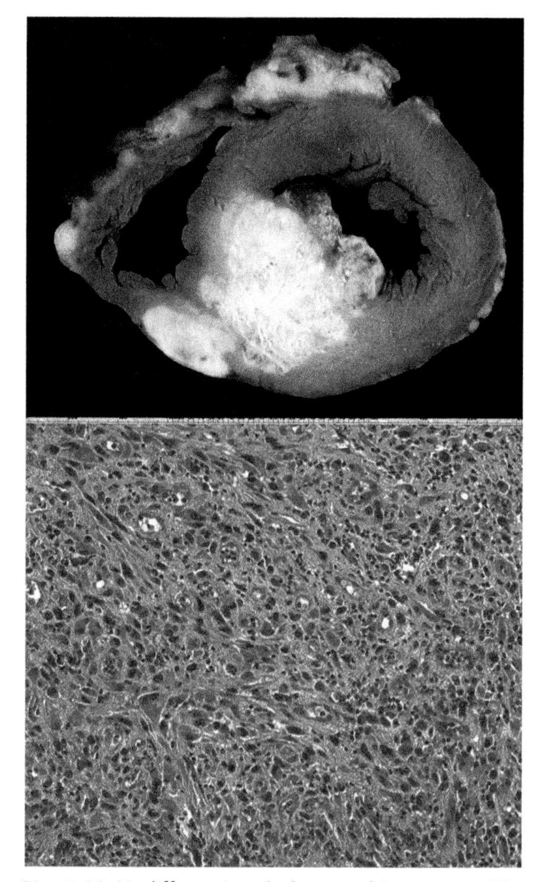

Fig. 4.13 Undifferentiated pleomorphic sarcoma. The pale tumor can be seen infiltrating the biventricular inferior myocardium. Histologically, the lesion consists of highly atypical, pleomorphic cells.

Histologically, the lesions are variable but often consist of high-grade, pleomorphic cells within a myxoid or collagenized stroma. Mitotic activity and necrosis are usually conspicuous.

There most important predictive factor is completeness of resection, in those cases that are amenable to such. Most patients succumb to complications of the disease within 18 months of diagnosis. Surgical debulking can, in some instances, improve symptoms.

Angiosarcoma

Cardiac angiosarcomas are primary sarcomas of the heart that exhibit endothelial differentiation. They are the most common primary cardiac malignancy that exhibits a differentiation along a specific cell lineage.

There is a relatively wide age range at presentation, spanning from childhood to 80+ years, but the peak incidence is in the fourth to fifth decades of life. A slight male predilection has also been reported.

Cardiac angiosarcomas most commonly arise within the right atrium, in the region of the AV groove. The pericardium is commonly involved and may incite a hemorrhagic pericardial effusion that can lead to tamponade as an initial presentation.[47] Other common presenting symptoms include chest pain, dyspnea, heart failure, and arrhythmia. On imaging, cardiac angiosarcomas will often appear as a heterogeneous, nodular mass. cMRI sequences are sensitive for hemorrhage and may show areas of nodularity on T1-weighted imaging. Administration of contrast agents can reveal the vascular nature of these lesions ("blood-sponge" sign).

Grossly, these lesions appear as infiltrative, hemorrhagic tumors with solid and cystic areas (Fig. 4.14). Histologically, the primitive spindle or epithelioid cells form primitive vascular structures that usually show frank infiltration into the adjacent myocardium. Cardiac epithelioid hemangioendothelioma is a distinctive histopathologic entity that is much rarer than cardiac angiosarcoma, but similar in poor prognosis.

Because of their right atrial location, these tumors are often amenable to biopsy via endomyocardial bioptome. The prognosis is usually poor, with a median survival of approximately a year.

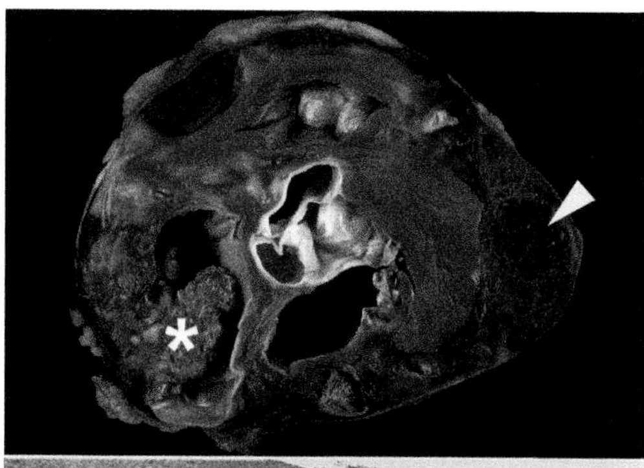
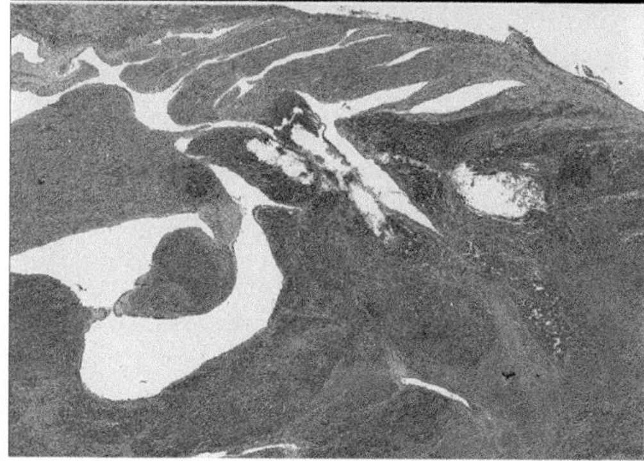

Fig. 4.14 Cardiac angiosarcoma. The tumor (*asterisk*) is arising from the right AV groove and is associated with a hemorrhagic pericardial effusion (*arrowhead*). Histologically, this lesion is characterized by malignant, often pleomorphic cells, with vascular differentiation that invades into adjacent cardiac structures.

Leiomyosarcoma

Cardiac leiomyosarcoma is a sarcoma showing smooth muscle cell differentiation. As with other sarcomas, primary cardiac leiomyosarcomas should be distinguished from metastatic tumors, especially when right-sided. In addition, intravascular leiomyomatosis may also involve the heart, but is histologically benign and results from extension from the uterus via the inferior vena cava.

Cardiac leiomyosarcomas usually present around 60 years of age with no distinct sex predilection. They most commonly arise in the left atrium, with involvement of the pulmonary veins. As such, presenting symptoms often include shortness of breath and chest pain.

Grossly, they are virtually indistinguishable from undifferentiated sarcomas, but histologically exhibit smooth muscle differentiation. Mitosis and necrosis are common and help to confirm the malignant nature of these lesions. As with other cardiac sarcomas, completeness of resection is the most important prognostic indicator.

Synovial Sarcoma

Synovial sarcoma is a malignant mesenchymal neoplasm characterized by a specific chromosomal translocation (X;18) that results in a specific fusion gene *SS18-SSX*. It is a very rare cardiac sarcoma with a male predilection (M:F = 3:1).

The mean age at presentation is approximately 35 years, but they have been reported in both the young and the old. Dyspnea is the most common presenting symptom, and the tumors usually involve the pericardium. They are usually smooth and polypoid. Grossly, the tumors usually have a pale yellow-white "fish-flesh" appearance. Histologically, the lesions may be monophasic or biphasic depending on the whether epithelioid cells accompany the neoplastic spindle cell population.

Survival is poor, with many patients dying within 24 months of diagnosis. Chemotherapy with or without radiation may improves survival.

Other Sarcomas

There is a range of other primary sarcomas that can involve the heart and great vessels. Intimal sarcomas are peculiar lesions that tend to exhibit an intimal growth pattern within the great vessels. The pulmonary artery is most commonly affected. Intimal sarcomas have a slightly better prognosis than other cardiac sarcomas and have been noted to exhibit amplification of *MDM2*. This finding, however, is not entirely unique to intimal sarcomas and may be seen in undifferentiated cardiac sarcomas as well as extracardiac liposarcomas.[37,48]

Other rare sarcomas, such as osteosarcoma, malignant peripheral nerve sheath tumors, liposarcomas, malignant solitary fibrous tumors, rhabdomyosarcoma, and myxofibrosarcoma, have also been reported to arise primarily within the heart. Like other primary cardiac sarcomas, the prognosis is usually poor, regardless of histologic subtype.

Cardiac Lymphoma

Primary cardiac lymphoma is a rare, extranodal lymphoma, involving the heart and/or pericardium. They affect men twice as often as women and usually occur in patients older than 60 years of age.

Most primary cardiac lymphomas are of B-cell lineage. Certain types occur in the setting of immune compromise (primary effusion lymphoma and Burkitt lymphoma), whereas others can occur in association with intracardiac devices and cardiac myxomas, such as the Epstein-Barr virus–associated diffuse large B-cell lymphoma associated with chronic inflammation.[49,50]

Cardiac lymphoma usually manifests as hypoechoic lesions that infiltrate the myocardium, seen on echocardiography. Biopsy, with tissue reserved for flow cytometry, is usually requisite for the diagnosis and appropriate therapy.

Although most cardiac lymphomas impart a poor prognosis, anthracycline-based chemotherapy can be effective depending on the subtype. Interestingly, those primary cardiac lymphomas associated with devices do not appear to have the same poor prognosis as other types of primary cardiac lymphoma.

Malignant Mesothelioma

Like its pleural counterpart, pericardial malignant mesothelioma is a malignant neoplasm of mesothelial lineage. It is exquisitely rare with only a handful of reports. Most cases occur in the fifth to seventh decades of life with a slight male predominance.[51]

Unlike pleural and peritoneal mesothelioma, a correlation with asbestosis has not been definitively established, but this is possibly owing to the relative rarity of these lesions. Symptoms are generally related to direct compressive effects of the tumor or an associated effusion. Diffuse pericardial involvement is generally the rule. Cytology is often not of significant utility because demonstration of invasive growth into tissue is requisite for the diagnosis.

METASTATIC CARDIAC NEOPLASMS

Metastatic tumors to the heart are far more common than the primary variety, outnumbering them more than 10 to 1. In fact, it is estimated that 10% of those with advanced stage cancer have cardiac involvement (usually pericardial).[52]

Metastases from nearby primary sites, such as the lung, breast, and esophagus, are the most common. Extracardiac sarcomas and melanoma may also move to involve the heart, and cardiac symptoms may be the presenting feature of occult cases.

Tumors may travel to the heart by hematogenous seeding (eg, sarcomas, melanoma), retrograde lymphatic extension (eg, carcinomas), or contiguous spread (eg, lung carcinoma) (Fig. 4.15 and 4.16). Diffuse, multifocal involvement is common and should raise suspicions for a metastatic process.

Sampling via cytology (pericardial effusion) or endomyocardial biopsy can help to confirm the diagnosis. Involvement of the heart by a metastatic process generally portends a poor prognosis.

SECONDARY EFFECTS OF NEOPLASMS ON THE HEART

Extracardiac neoplasms can have important secondary effects on the heart. For example, multiple myeloma may cause the elaboration of light chains that can aggregate in the cardiac interstitium as amyloid.[53] These deposits of amyloid can dramatically affect the normal hemodynamics of the heart and are a major source of morbidity among those with myeloma.

Carcinoid tumors from the small bowel may, through elaboration of serotonin metabolites, cause valvular heart disease.[54] Valvular heart disease usually occurs in the setting of the so-called *serotonin syndrome* after the tumor has metastasized to the liver (subverting the first-pass effect

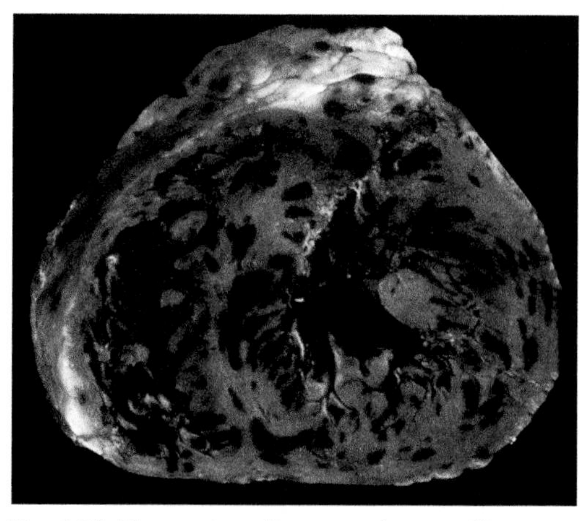

Fig. 4.15 Metastatic malignant melanoma. Numerous tumors can be seen involving the epicardium, myocardium, and endocardium.

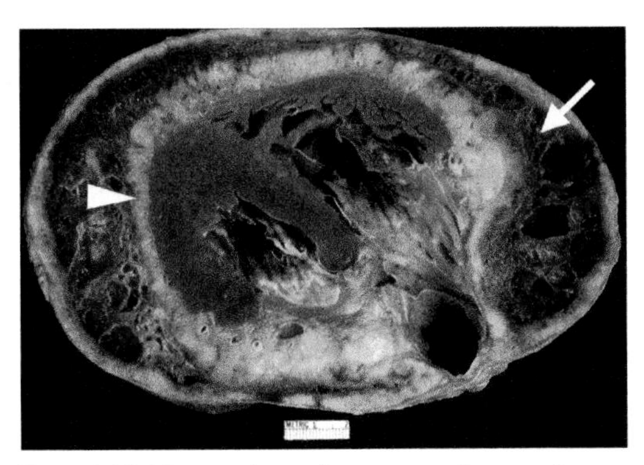

Fig. 4.16 Metastatic pulmonary adenocarcinoma. Diffuse metastatic involvement of the visceral pericardium (epicardium) is seen (*arrowhead*) in association with a hemorrhagic pericardial effusion (*arrow*).

of the portal circulation). Colon cancer also has a curious association with *Streptococcus bovis* endocarditis.[55]

Pheochromocytomas may elaborate catecholamines that can cause impressive cardiac symptoms and chronically lead to catecholamine-cardiotoxicity that may manifest as biventricular dilatation and poor cardiac function.[56]

Aside from the extracardiac neoplasms themselves, treatment of such can also have important effects on the heart. External beam radiation used to treat malignancies of the thorax (breast cancer, mediastinal lymphoma, thymoma) may also damage the myocardium or the cardiac valves and lead to chronic heart disease.[57] Anthracycline-based chemotherapeutics have been long known to be potentially cardiotoxic, but other agents, such as monoclonal antibodies, taxanes, alkylating agents, vinka alkaloids, and fluoropyrimidines, may also have toxic effects on the heart.[58]

REFERENCES

1. Travis WD, Brambilla E, Burke AP, et al. Tumors of the heart and great vessels. In: Silverberg SG, editor. AFIP Atlas of tumor pathology. 4th edition. Silverspring (MD): American Registry of Pathology; 2015. p. 419.
2. Miller DV, Tazelaar HD. Cardiovascular pseudoneoplasms. Arch Pathol Lab Med 2010;134(3):362–8.
3. Reynolds C, Tazelaar HD, Edwards WD. Calcified amorphous tumor of the heart (cardiac CAT). Hum Pathol 1997;28(5):601–6.
4. Yamashita T, Ohkawa S, Imai T, et al. Prevalence and clinical significance of anomalous muscular band in the left atrium. Am J Cardiovasc Pathol 1993;4(4):286–93.
5. Liu Y, Mi N, Zhou Y, et al. Transverse false tendons in the left ventricular cavity are associated with early repolarization. PLoS One 2015;10(5):e0125173.
6. Groves AM, Fagg NL, Cook AC, et al. Cardiac tumours in intrauterine life. Arch Dis Child 1992; 67(10 Spec No):1189–92.
7. Jain D, Maleszewski JJ, Halushka MK. Benign cardiac tumors and tumorlike conditions. Ann Diagn Pathol 2010;14(3):215–30.
8. Padalino MA, Vida VL, Boccuzzo G, et al. Surgery for primary cardiac tumors in children: early and late results in a multicenter European Congenital Heart Surgeons Association study. Circulation 2012; 126(1):22–30.
9. Tworetzky W, McElhinney DB, Margossian R, et al. Association between cardiac tumors and tuberous sclerosis in the fetus and neonate. Am J Cardiol 2003;92(4):487–9.
10. Stiller B, Hetzer R, Meyer R, et al. Primary cardiac tumours: when is surgery necessary? Eur J Cardiothorac Surg 2001;20(5):1002–6.
11. Thomas-de-Montpreville V, Nottin R, Dulmet E, et al. Heart tumors in children and adults: clinicopathological study of 59 patients from a surgical center. Cardiovasc Pathol 2007;16(1):22–8.
12. Tiberio D, Franz DN, Phillips JR. Regression of a cardiac rhabdomyoma in a patient receiving everolimus. Pediatrics 2011;127(5):e1335–7.
13. Torimitsu S, Nemoto T, Wakayama M, et al. Literature survey on epidemiology and pathology of cardiac fibroma. Eur J Med Res 2012;17:5.
14. Burke AP, Rosado-de-Christenson M, Templeton PA, et al. Cardiac fibroma: clinicopathologic correlates and surgical treatment. J Thorac Cardiovasc Surg 1994;108(5):862–70.
15. Cronin B, Lynch MJ, Parsons S. Cardiac fibroma presenting as sudden unexpected death in an adolescent. Forensic Sci Med Pathol 2014;10(4):647–50.
16. Scanlan D, Radio SJ, Nelson M, et al. Loss of the PTCH1 gene locus in cardiac fibroma. Cardiovasc Pathol 2008;17(2):93–7.
17. Filiatrault M, Béland MJ, Neilson KA, et al. Cardiac fibroma presenting with clinically significant arrhythmias in infancy. Pediatr Cardiol 1991;12(2): 118–20.
18. Shehata BM, Cundiff CA, Lee K, et al. Exome sequencing of patients with histiocytoid cardiomyopathy reveals a de novo NDUFB11 mutation that plays a role in the pathogenesis of histiocytoid cardiomyopathy. Am J Med Genet A 2015;167A(9):2114–21.
19. Zangwill SD, Trost BA, Zlotocha J, et al. Orthotopic heart transplantation in a child with histiocytoid cardiomyopathy. J Heart Lung Transplant 2004;23(7): 902–4.
20. Grech V, Ellul B, Montalto SA. Sudden cardiac death in infancy due to histiocytoid cardiomyopathy. Cardiol Young 2000;10(1):49–51.
21. Shehata BM, Patterson K, Thomas JE, et al. Histiocytoid cardiomyopathy: three new cases and a review of the literature. Pediatr Dev Pathol 1998;1(1):56–69.

22. Malhotra V, Ferrans VJ, Virmani R. Infantile histiocytoid cardiomyopathy: three cases and literature review. Am Heart J 1994;128(5):1009–21.
23. Edston E, Perskvist N. Histiocytoid cardiomyopathy and ventricular non-compaction in a case of sudden death in a female infant. Int J Legal Med 2009; 123(1):47–53.
24. Ishizaka N. Letter to the editors: IgG4-related inflammatory pseudotumor in the heart. Methodist Debakey Cardiovasc J 2014;10(1):58.
25. Sunbul M, Cagac O, Birkan Y. A rare case of inflammatory pseudotumor with both involvement of lung and heart. Thorac Cardiovasc Surg 2013; 61(7):646–8.
26. Yao FJ, Liu D, Zhang Y, et al. Inflammatory pseudotumor of the right ventricle in a 35-year-old woman with Behcet's disease: a case report. Echocardiography 2012;29(6):E134–6.
27. Jenkins PC, Dickison AE, Flanagan MF. Cardiac inflammatory pseudotumor: rapid appearance in an infant with congenital heart disease. Pediatr Cardiol 1996;17(6):399–401.
28. Burke A, Li L, Kling E, et al. Cardiac inflammatory myofibroblastic tumor: a "benign" neoplasm that may result in syncope, myocardial infarction, and sudden death. Am J Surg Pathol 2007;31(7): 1115–22.
29. Anvari MS, Soleimani A, Abbasi A, et al. Inflammatory myofibroblastic tumor of the right ventricle causing tricuspid valve regurgitation. Tex Heart Inst J 2009;36(2):164–7.
30. Butany J, Dixit V, Leong SW, et al. Inflammatory myofibroblastic tumor with valvular involvement: a case report and review of the literature. Cardiovasc Pathol 2007;16(6):359–64.
31. de Winkel N, Becker K, Vogt M. Echogenic mass in the right atrium after surgical ventricular septal defect closure: thrombus or tumour? Cardiol Young 2010;20(1):86–8.
32. Gandy KL, Burtelow MA, Reddy VM, et al. Myofibroblastic tumor of the heart: a rare intracardiac tumor. J Thorac Cardiovasc Surg 2005;130(3): 888–9.
33. Jha NK, Trudel M, Eising GP, et al. Inflammatory myofibroblastic tumor of the right atrium. Case Rep Med 2010. [Epub ahead of print].
34. Tamin SS, Maleszewski JJ, Scott CG, et al. Prognostic and bioepidemiologic implications of papillary fibroelastomas. J Am Coll Cardiol 2015;65(22): 2420–9.
35. Fine NM, Foley DA, Breen JF, et al. Multimodality imaging of a giant aortic valve papillary fibroelastoma. Case Rep Med 2013;2013:705101.
36. Takada A, Saito K, Ro A, et al. Papillary fibroelastoma of the aortic valve: a sudden death case of coronary embolism with myocardial infarction. Forensic Sci Int 2000;113(1–3):209–14.
37. Bois MC, Bois JP, Anavekar NS, et al. Benign lipomatous masses of the heart: a comprehensive series of 47 cases with cytogenetic evaluation. Hum Pathol 2014;45(9):1859–65.
38. Jain S, Maleszewski JJ, Stephenson CR, et al. Current diagnosis and management of cardiac myxomas. Expert Rev Cardiovasc Ther 2015;13(4):369–75.
39. Maleszewski JJ, Larsen BT, Kip NS, et al. PRKAR1A in the development of cardiac myxoma: a study of 110 cases including isolated and syndromic tumors. Am J Surg Pathol 2014;38(8):1079–87.
40. Burke AP, Ribe JK, Bajaj AK, et al. Hamartoma of mature cardiac myocytes. Hum Pathol 1998;29(9): 904–9.
41. Chiappini B, Gregorini R, Vecchio L, et al. Cardiac hemangioma of the left atrial appendag: a case report and discussion. J Card Surg 2009;24(5):522–3.
42. Eftychiou C, Antoniades L. Cardiac hemangioma in the left ventricle and brief review of the literature. J Cardiovasc Med (Hagerstown) 2009;10(7):565–7.
43. Yuan SM, Shinfeld A, Kuperstein R, et al. Cavernous hemangioma of the right atrium. Kardiol Pol 2008; 66(9):974–6.
44. Zanati SG, Hueb JC, Cogni AL, et al. Cardiac hemangioma of the right atrium. Eur J Echocardiogr 2008;9(1):52–3.
45. Han Y, Chen X, Wang X, et al. Cardiac capillary hemangioma: a case report and brief review of the literature. J Clin Ultrasound 2014;42(1):53–6.
46. Zhang B, Xu Z, Tang H. Intermuscular hemangioma of the left ventricle. J Card Surg 2012;27(5): 572–5.
47. Kupsky DF, Newman DB, Kumar G, et al. Echocardiographic features of cardiac angiosarcomas: the Mayo Clinic experience (1976-2013). Echocardiography 2016;33(2):186–92.
48. Neuville A, Collin F, Bruneval P, et al. Intimal sarcoma is the most frequent primary cardiac sarcoma: clinicopathologic and molecular retrospective analysis of 100 primary cardiac sarcomas. Am J Surg Pathol 2014;38(4):461–9.
49. Bonnichsen CR, Dearani JA, Maleszewski JJ, et al. Recurrent Ebstein-Barr virus-associated diffuse large B-cell lymphoma in an ascending aorta graft. Circulation 2013;128(13):1481–3.
50. Bagwan IN, Desai S, Wotherspoon A, et al. Unusual presentation of primary cardiac lymphoma. Interact Cardiovasc Thorac Surg 2009;9(1):127–9.
51. Patel J, Sheppard MN. Primary malignant mesothelioma of the pericardium. Cardiovasc Pathol 2011; 20(2):107–9.
52. Abraham KP, Reddy V, Gattuso P. Neoplasms metastatic to the heart: review of 3314 consecutive autopsies. Am J Cardiovasc Pathol 1990;3(3):195–8.
53. Maleszewski JJ. Cardiac amyloidosis: pathology, nomenclature, and typing. Cardiovasc Pathol 2015;24(6):343–50.

54. Simula DV, Edwards WD, Tazelaar HD, et al. Surgical pathology of carcinoid heart disease: a study of 139 valves from 75 patients spanning 20 years. Mayo Clin Proc 2002;77(2):139–47.
55. Corredoira J, Grau I, Garcia-Rodriguez JF, et al. The clinical epidemiology and malignancies associated with Streptococcus bovis biotypes in 506 cases of bloodstream infections. J Infect 2015; 71(3):317–25.
56. De Lazzari M, Cipriani A, Marra MP, et al. Heart failure due to adrenergic myocardial toxicity from a pheochromocytoma. Circ Heart Fail 2015;8(3):646–8.
57. Jaworski C, Mariani JA, Wheeler G, et al. Cardiac complications of thoracic irradiation. J Am Coll Cardiol 2013;61(23):2319–28.
58. Rosa GM, Gigli L, Tagliasacchi MI, et al. Update on cardiotoxicity of anti-cancer treatments. Eur J Clin Invest 2016;46(3):264–84.

CHAPTER 5

Cardiac Tumors
Imaging

Matthew S. Pieper, MD, Philip A. Araoz, MD*

INTRODUCTION

This chapter focuses on the imaging characteristics of benign and malignant primary cardiac neoplasms and metastatic disease. In addition, to provide clarity and prevent incorrect diagnoses of cardiac neoplasms, a section regarding cardiac pseudotumors and normal variants is included. There is considerable overlap in the appearance of cardiac masses, which mandates synthesis of the imaging characteristics, the location of the lesion, and the clinical scenario in order to facilitate a concise and accurate list of differential diagnoses and ultimately reach the correct diagnosis (Figs. 5.1 and 5.2, Case Studies 1–3, available on Expert Consult).

IMAGING MODALITIES

The vast majority of cardiac masses, up to 85% in a large surgical series, are initially imaged with echocardiography.[1] Imaging with echocardiography is due to its widespread availability and feasibility (including bedside examinations and short imaging times) but also the ability for real-time imaging of dynamic cardiac structures, functional evaluation of valves and chambers, and high spatial resolution. Transthoracic echocardiography (TTE) is the more common modality but requires adequate acoustic windows, which can lead to limitations related to patient body habitus. Use of intravenous ultrasound contrast agents can improve the diagnostic utility of echocardiography. Contrast can be used to evaluate the vascularity and perfusion of cardiac masses and can be helpful for differentiating nonvascular thrombi from vascular neoplasms. The use of 3-dimensional echocardiography may be beneficial in select cases, although its routine use is of uncertain benefit.

Transesophageal echocardiography (TEE) avoids the challenges of limited acoustic windows and allows improved visualization of particular cardiac chambers, such as the left atrial appendage with the tradeoff of increased invasiveness. Compared with computed tomography (CT) and MRI, both forms of echocardiography are more operator-dependent and provide limited tissue characterization and very limited evaluation of the mediastinum and extracardiac structures.

CT allows for fast image acquisition, and when optimized for cardiac imaging, provides very high spatial resolution of cardiac structures. Compared with echocardiography, CT provides superior tissue characterization, specifically of fat and calcium, which can allow precise diagnosis in the case of certain cardiac masses. Electrocardiogram (ECG)-gated cardiac CT also allows for functional analysis of cardiac valves and myocardial function as well as multiplanar reconstructions. Acquisitions may also include the entire thorax, which allows for thorough evaluation of associated structures. However, the ability of CT to characterize small and mobile structures is inferior to echocardiography, primarily due to decreased temporal resolution, and tissue characterization remains inferior to MRI.

Cardiac MRI provides the best tissue characterization of all available imaging techniques, including detailed evaluation for edema, iron content, perfusion, and delayed enhancement. It provides functional evaluation of cardiac structures and morphologic evaluation in multiple planes. Like CT, it provides the capability of imaging the entire thorax. However, MRI has the worst spatial resolution of the available imaging modalities, which can limit evaluation of valvular lesions or small masses. In addition, availability and duration of image acquisition are often more problematic with MRI than with other modalities (Table 5.1).

Nuclear imaging provides a role in the diagnosis of specific masses, as outlined in the individual sections. PET with F-18 fluorodeoxyglucose (FDG) is often useful for evaluating tumor spread throughout the body.

Mayo Clinic, 200 First Street Southwest, Rochester, MN 55905, USA
* Corresponding author.
E-mail address: paraoz@mayo.edu

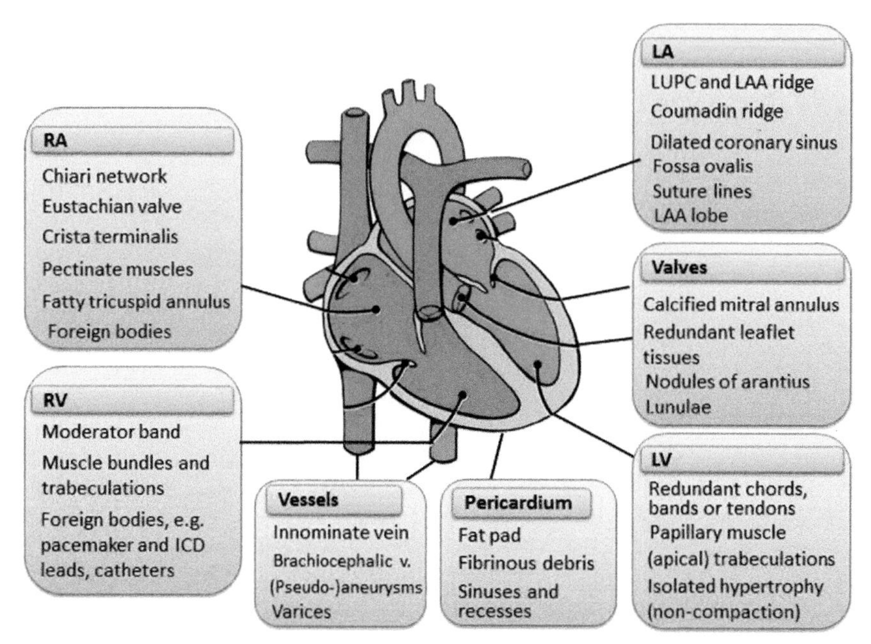

Fig. 5.1 Normal variants/benign conditions with pathologic misinterpretation potential. LA, left atrium; LV, left ventricle; RA, right atrium; RV, right ventricle.

PSEUDOTUMORS

Thrombi

Thrombus is a conglomeration of fibrin and platelets, often containing red and white blood cells, which occurs within a blood vessel or cardiac chamber, adjacent to the endothelium or endocardium. Thrombi occur in areas of slow flow due to stasis or associated with endothelial or endocardial damage. For intracardiac thrombi, this is most frequently seen in the left atrial appendage in patients with atrial fibrillation, in the left ventricle in patients with dilated cardiomyopathy, or in regions of acute or healed scarring in patients with myocardial infarction, with the left ventricular apex as a common location. Right-sided intracardiac thrombi are typically associated with

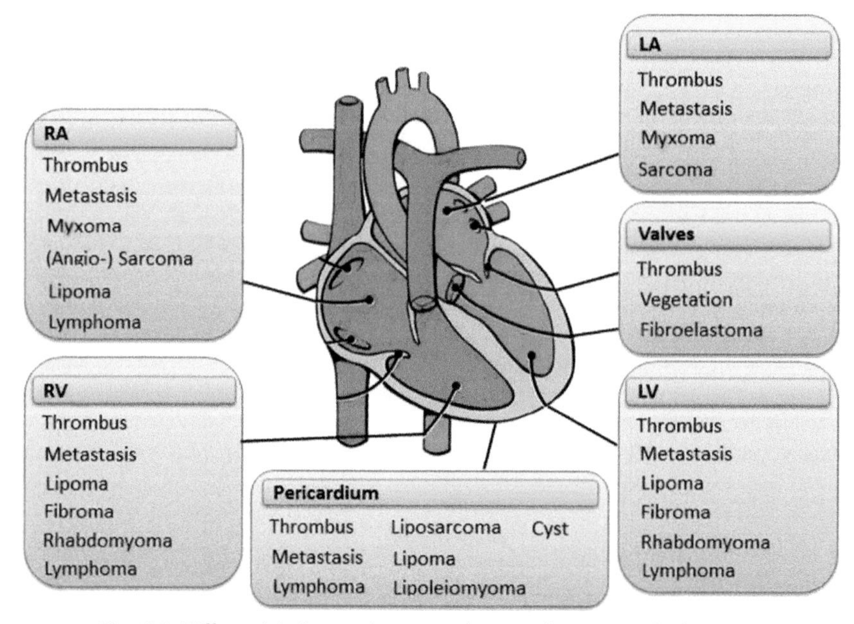

Fig. 5.2 Differential diagnostic approach to cardiac tumors by location.

TABLE 5.1
Imaging modalities of cardiac tumors

Modality	Pros	Cons
Echocardiography	Widely available, highest spatial and temporal resolution, real-time evaluation of dynamic structures	Tissue characterization is limited, most operator-dependent modality, limited evaluation of extracardiac intrathoracic structures
ECG-gated CT	Very fast image acquisition, excellent characterization of fat and calcium, evaluates entire thorax	Tissue characterization is worse than MR, worse temporal resolution than echocardiography, ionizing radiation
Cardiac MRI	Best tissue characterization, allows for structural and functional resolution, can image entire thorax	Worst spatial resolution, long image acquisition time, safety issues with some implanted devices

indwelling catheters or devices. Patients can be asymptomatic or present with systemic emboli.

On gross inspection, cardiac thrombi are firm masses, red to tan in color, and histologically they demonstrate layering thrombus with degenerated red cells and variable amounts of fibrin and platelets.[2] On echocardiography, intracardiac thrombi appear as hyperechoic filling defects without internal blood flow. The left atrial appendage is notoriously difficult to image with TTE, but is well visualized with TEE. By CT, intracardiac thrombi are well-circumscribed, hypodense, nonenhancing masses adjacent to the endocardial surface without signs of invasion into myocardium (Fig. 5.3). Similar features can be detected with MRI, although typically first-pass perfusion and subsequent enhancement (or lack thereof) can be more reliably measured with MRI, which means the diagnosis of thrombus can often be made with more confidence by MRI. Internal tissue characteristics of thrombi by MRI depend on the acuity of the thrombus and are variable. The diagnosis of intracardiac thrombus is often made based on the combination of the imaging appearance and location. In uncertain cases, a trial of anticoagulation followed by repeat imaging can often be used for confirmation.

Prominent Crista Terminalis

The crista terminalis is the demarcation of the embryologic sinus venosus and the muscular right atrium. It is a ridge of fibromuscular tissue within the posterolateral right atrial wall.[3] When prominent, it can be perceived as a mass by imaging (Fig. 5.4). However, knowledge of normal

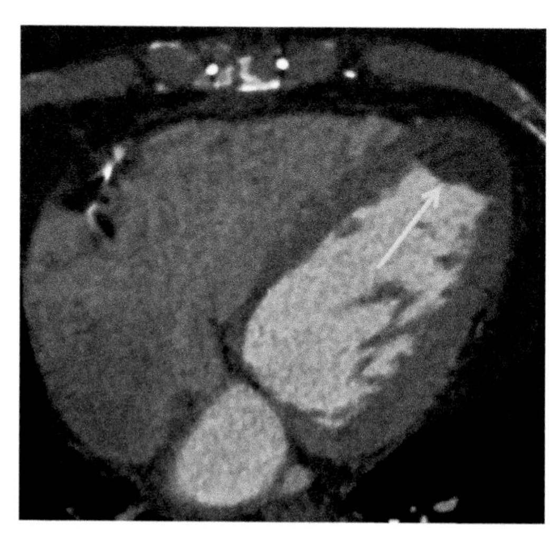

Fig. 5.3 Left ventricular thrombus in a 72-year-old man. Axial image from an ECG-gated CT coronary angiogram demonstrates a filling defect within the left ventricular apex (*arrow*) indicating a left ventricular thrombus.

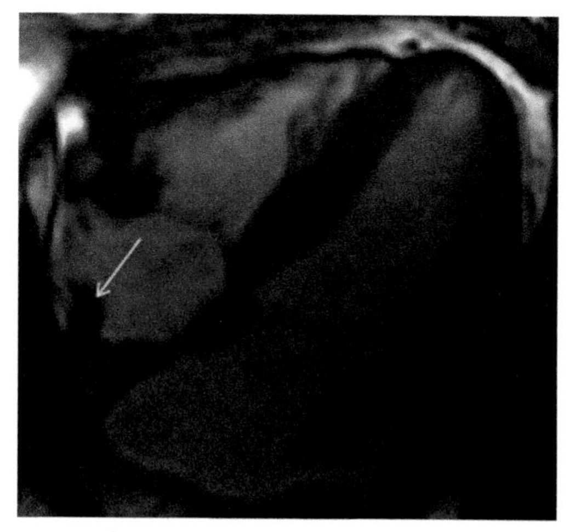

Fig. 5.4 Prominent crista terminalis in a 57-year-old man. Four-chamber Fast Imaging Employing Steady-state Acquisition (FIESTA) image from a cardiac MRI performed to evaluate for primary cardiac amyloidosis demonstrates a prominent crista terminalis (*arrow*).

anatomic variants prevents misdiagnosis. By echocardiography, a prominent crista terminalis appears as a hyperechoic ridge in the posterolateral right atrium.[4] Similarly, on CT and MRI, it follows imaging characteristics of the adjacent right atrial wall on all sequences, including postcontrast.

Lipomatous Hypertrophy of the Interatrial Septum

Lipomatous hypertrophy of the interatrial septum is a benign, nonencapsulated fatty mass, which classically spares the fossa ovalis, resulting in a dumbbell shape with smooth margins. This pseudotumor affects older patients (mean age 70) with greater than 40% being obese (body mass index >30).[5] Microscopically, the mass contains adipocytes and myocytes, which are enlarged and abnormal. The fatty component includes both mature adipocytes and metabolically active brown fat.[2] Imaging characteristics follow fat on all modalities, and the diagnosis can be made based on tissue characteristics and location (Fig. 5.5). Of note, due to the brown fat content, lipomatous hypertrophy of the interatrial septum has been demonstrated to have increased FDG uptake at PET imaging,[6] which makes it particularly important to recognize lipomatous hypertrophy as a benign entity and not malignancy.

Pericardial Hematoma

A hematoma is a collection of blood outside of a blood vessel. Pericardial hematomas have been related to trauma and open heart surgery.[7] Like intracardiac thrombi, they can have varying pathologic appearances based on their acuity. By TTE, pericardial hematomas have the appearance of a hyperechoic extracardiac mass within the pericardial space, which may cause a mass effect on adjacent structures without invasion. Pericardial hematomas will demonstrate varying densities (CT) and signal characteristics (MRI) based on their age and do not show contrast enhancement. A chronic pericardial hematoma may develop peripheral hyperattenuation by CT or T1 prolongation (dark signal) due to calcification.[8]

Pericardial Cyst

Pericardial cysts are congenital bronchogenic cysts that arise from intrapericardial endodermal rests and contain mesodermal and endodermal

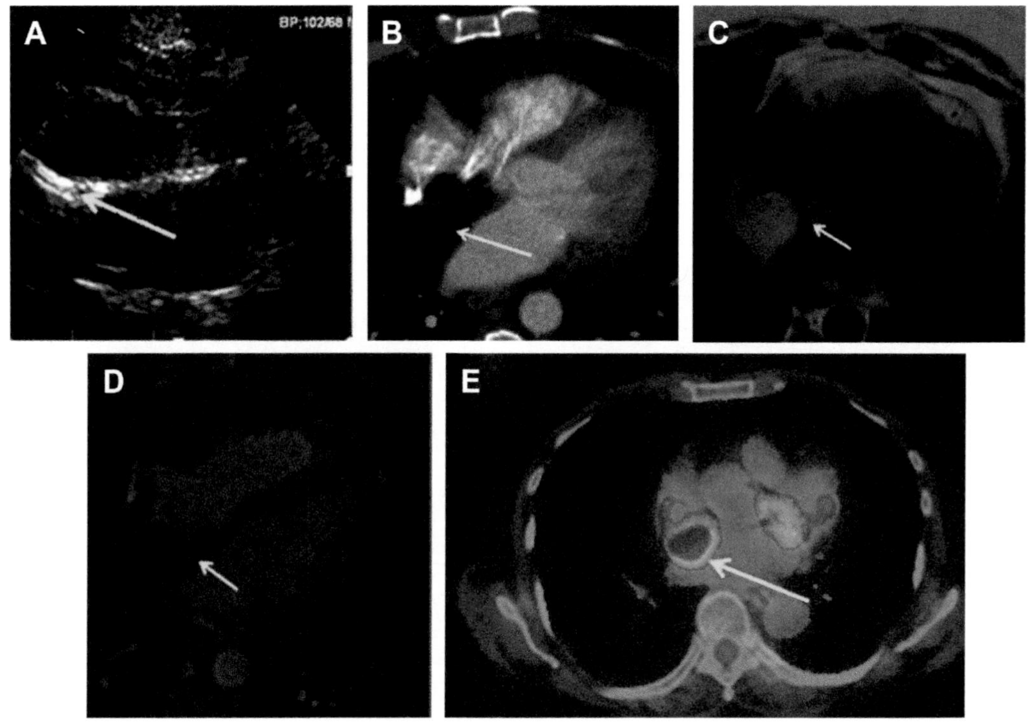

Fig. 5.5 Lipomatous hypertrophy of the interatrial septum in a 54-year-old woman. Parasternal 4-chamber view from a TTE demonstrates increased echogenicity at the interatrial septum (*A*). Axial image (*B*) from a non-ECG-gated CT angiogram demonstrates fatty expansion of the interatrial septum (*arrow*). Axial double-inversion recovery (*C*) and fat-saturated FIESTA (*D*) images demonstrate the fatty mass (*arrow*) and show the sparing of the fossa ovalis. Fusion images from a PET/CT scan (*E*) in a different patient shows radiotracer uptake (arrow) within the fatty tissue within the interatrial septum.

derivatives. They most commonly occur at the right cardiophrenic angle and are typically 1 to 3 cm in diameter.[2] On all imaging modalities, they present as a well-circumscribed, thin-walled cystic mass with fluid characteristics, anechoic by echocardiography, hypoattenuating on CT, and consistent on all MRI sequences (Fig. 5.6). A differential consideration would include a loculated pericardial hematoma; however, the internal contents would not appear consistent with simple fluid.

BENIGN

Myxoma

Myxomas are benign tumors whose cell of origin is a matter of debate, with primitive pluripotent mesenchymal cells proposed due to the presence of epithelial, mesenchymal, endothelial, myofibroblastic, and neuroendocrine proteins by immunohistochemistry.[9] Myxomas typically arise from the atrial septum adjacent to the fossa ovalis (left more common than right) and represent the most common resected intracardiac tumor. The mean age at diagnosis is 53 years with a female preponderance (63%).[2] The clinical presentation can be highly variable, but symptoms related to heart failure, arrhythmia, or embolization are variably present.[10]

In most cases, myxomas are gelatinous to firm masses (mean diameter 4 cm) with focal hemorrhage and/or cavitation and a short, narrow stalk (in 85%).[2,10] A minority of myxomas have a broad-based attachment and are more friable and associated with embolism. Histologically, the diagnosis hinges on the presence of the myxoma, or "lepidic" cell with variable amounts of myxoid matrix present.[2] TTE demonstrates a mobile intracardiac mass (Fig. 5.7), and typically the narrow septal attachment can be identified. The combination of a mobile mass with a narrow stalk attached to the interatrial septum allows confident diagnosis whether seen with echocardiography, CT, or MRI. In those cases, additional tissue characterization is not necessary, in particular because the internal tissue findings are variable. CT can demonstrate variable attenuation as a result of cavitation/hemorrhage or intralesional fat. MRI can add improved tissue characterization with myxoid tissue demonstrating hypointensity on T1-weighted images and hyperintensity on T2-weighted images.

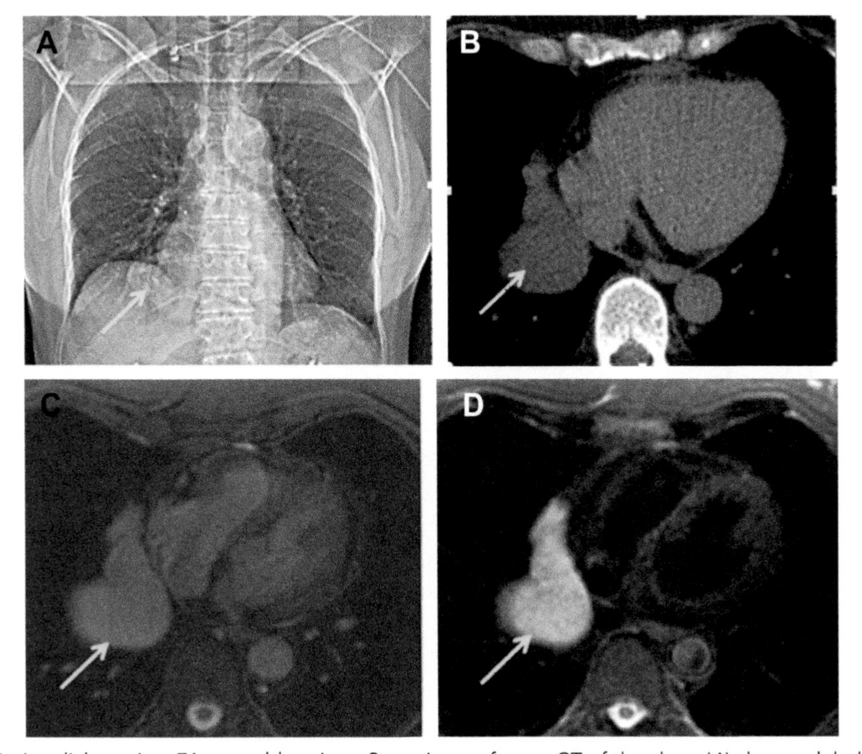

Fig. 5.6 Pericardial cyst in a 71-year-old patient. Scout image from a CT of the chest (*A*) shows a lobulated mass (*arrow*) at the right cardiophrenic angle. Axial noncontrast CT image (*B*) shows a fluid density, smoothly marginated structure at the right cardiophrenic angle (*arrow*). Axial fat-saturated FIESTA (*C*) and triple-inversion recovery (*D*) images confirm that the pericardial cyst (*arrow*) is fluid filled, smoothly marginated, and nonenhancing (not shown).

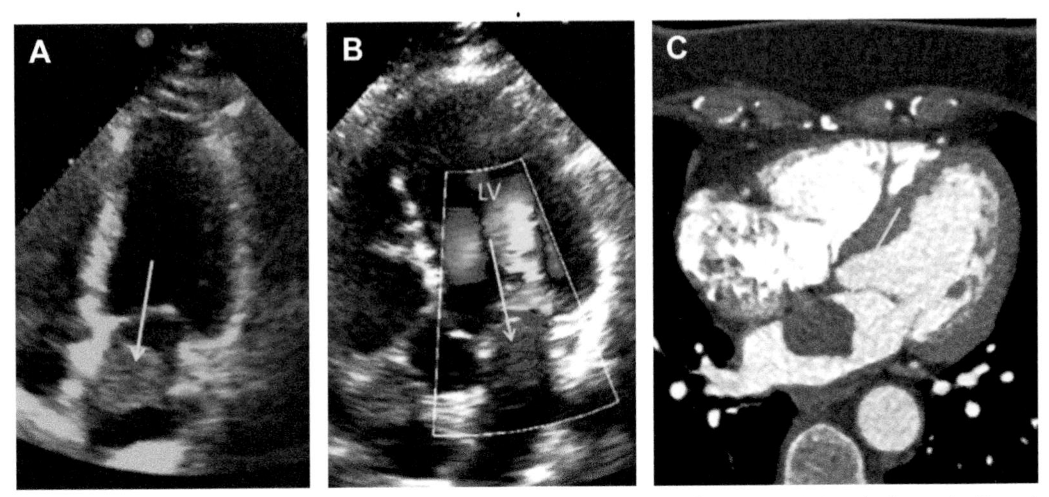

Fig. 5.7 Left atrial myxoma in a 69-year-old woman. Apical 2-chamber view from a TTE (*A*), including color Doppler (*B*) and axial image from an ECG-gated CT angiogram (*C*), demonstrates a 2.5-cm mass within the left atrium (*arrow*) attached to the interatrial septum by a short, wide stalk.

When a narrow stalk is not present or when the mass does not arise from the interatrial septum, the primary differential consideration is a different type of benign neoplasm (in particular, hemangioma) or possibly a malignant neoplasm (either a metastasis or a sarcoma). In these cases, it is often helpful to categorize a lesion as having imaging features suggesting a benign versus aggressive neoplasm, in particular for asymptomatic lesions in the right side of the heart, which possibly could be observed in certain situations. Imaging features that suggest a benign tumor include well-circumscribed borders and mass effect with displacement of adjacent structures without invasion. Aggressive features include irregular margins and invasion of adjacent structures.

In addition, myxomas occurring outside of the atria or in younger patients are more likely to be associated with Carney complex, an inherited autosomal disorder. Identifying this complex is important because the patients are at increased risk for developing neoplasms in other tissues, particularly endocrine tissue, and the myxomas occurring in these patients are more likely to recur than sporadic cardiac myxomas.

Lipoma

Lipomas are rare, benign neoplasms composed of mature adipocytes, representing less than 1% of all intracardiac tumors.[11] They are generally asymptomatic, although there are reported cases of complications related to size, such as left ventricular dysfunction.[12] Pathologically, lipomas are encapsulated masses composed of mature adipocytes with infrequent myocytes. They primarily occur in an epicardial location. Multiple lipomas are associated with tuberous sclerosis and congenital heart defects.[13] Imaging findings of lipomas demonstrate a well-circumscribed mass, which follows fat characteristics in all modalities and sequences (Fig. 5.8).

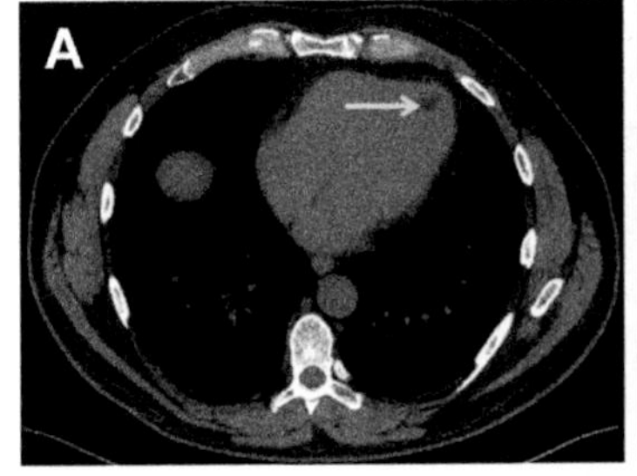

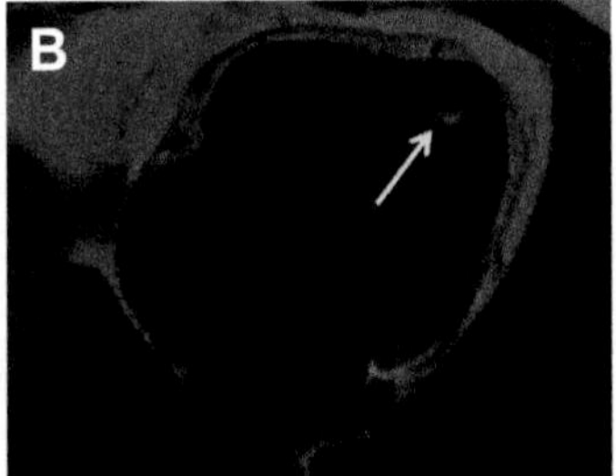

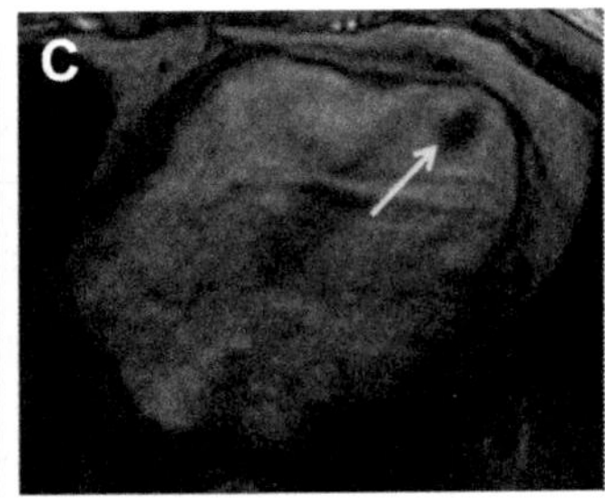

Fig. 5.8 Intramyocardial lipoma in a 57-year-old patient. Axial image from a nongated, noncontrast CT of the chest (*A*) demonstrates a hypodense mass in the left ventricular apex (*arrow*). Axial double-inversion recovery (*B*) and out-of-phase (*C*) images from a cardiac MRI confirm a small, fat intensity mass (*arrow*) within the left ventricular apical myocardium without mass effect or enhancement (not shown). Comparison of the in-phase (not shown) image with the out-of-phase image (*C*) shows signal dropout, confirming fat.

Fibroma

Cardiac fibromas are nonneoplastic tumors composed of fibroblasts that present within cardiac muscle. Fibromas are rare, with fewer than 200 published cases,[14] with the majority diagnosed in childhood.[15] Most affected patients present with symptoms of heart failure or arrhythmia. Fibromas commonly involve the interventricular septum with a mean size of 5.5 cm^2. They are circumscribed, fibrous, white masses that microscopically demonstrate homogenous fibroblasts without atypia and can contain calcification (Fig. 5.9). By echocardiography, fibromas appear as a noncontractile, intramyocardial mass and have occasionally been initially misdiagnosed as hypertrophic cardiomyopathy.[16] They are homogenous by CT and often contain calcification. Their fibrous nature is evident as homogenous T2 hypointensity by MRI, and they typically show little contrast enhancement.

Papillary Fibroelastoma

Papillary fibroelastomas are benign endocardial growths of uncertain cell origin that develop in regions of hemodynamic disturbance or sporadically without a known cause. They have a wide range of age at presentation with a mean age of 52,[17] and the typical symptomatic clinical presentation involves embolic phenomena in left-sided lesions. Average tumors are 1 cm in size, but can be as large as 5 to 7 cm[17] and microscopically contain a matrix of mucopolysaccharides, elastic fibers, and spindle cells.[2] On echocardiogram, a mobile excrescence is seen arising from a cardiac valve (Fig. 5.10). Fibroelastomas are hypodense on CT and demonstrate intermediate T1 signal intensity and intermediate-to-high T2 signal intensity on cardiac MRI without contrast enhancement on either modality. The primary differential diagnosis is endocarditis, and treatment is surgical excision.

Rhabdomyoma

Rhabdomyoma is a hamartomatous growth that occurs in the heart. It occurs most commonly in children and is rarely diagnosed after the age of 10.[18] There is a strong correlation between cardiac rhabdomyomas and tuberous sclerosis complex with nearly 80% of those diagnosed with rhabdomyoma found to have clinical or radiologic diagnosis of tuberous sclerosis.[19] Patients are often diagnosed in utero, but can present with arrhythmia or ventricular outflow tract obstruction (LVOT). Rhabdomyomas are firm, white-tan nodules with a mean size of 3 cm that arise within myocardium, most commonly within the ventricular walls.[2] They appear as homogenously echogenic masses with echocardiography. By MRI, they are well-defined T2 hyperintense masses. The differential diagnosis is limited due to the unique presentation and imaging features.

Hemangioma

A hemangioma is a benign neoplasm of blood vessels. They are most often diagnosed incidentally in the fifth to sixth decades of life, but can be diagnosed in children or even in utero.[2] Symptomatic patients may report palpitations, heart failure, or even angina.[20,21] Hemangiomas are found in all locations within the heart, including the atria, ventricles, and pericardium and range from very small to larger than 8 cm in size.[22] By TTE, hemangiomas are homogenous, hyperechoic masses. Cardiac MRI will demonstrate a mass with increased T2 signal. There is characteristically late contrast enhancement without early

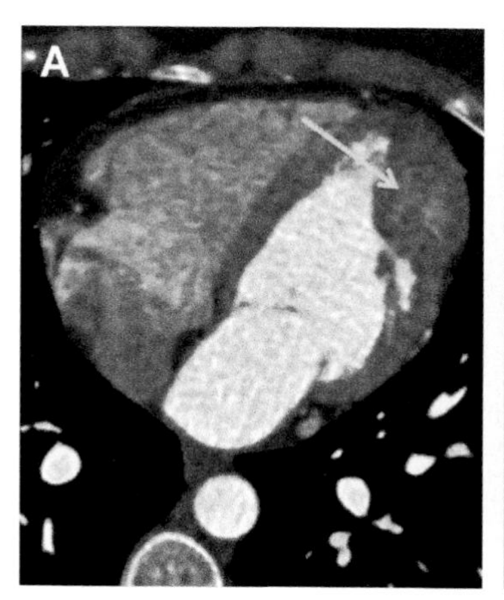

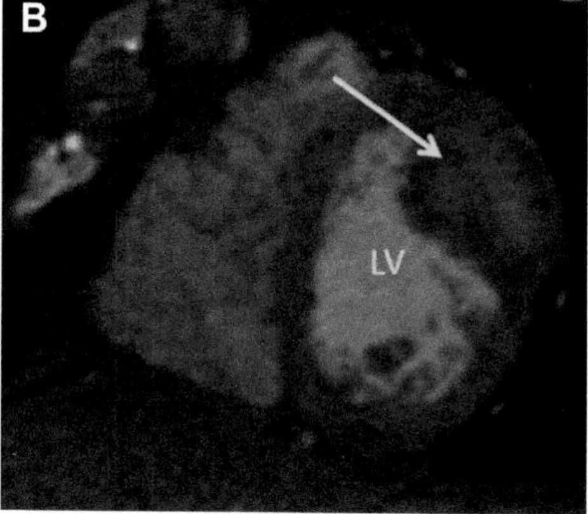

Fig. 5.9 Fibroma in a 34-year-old woman. Axial (*A*) and short-axis reformatted (*B*) images from a multiplanar, ECG-gated coronary CT angiogram demonstrate a heterogenously enhancing mass (*arrow*) in the LV free wall. No calcification was noted on noncontrast examination.

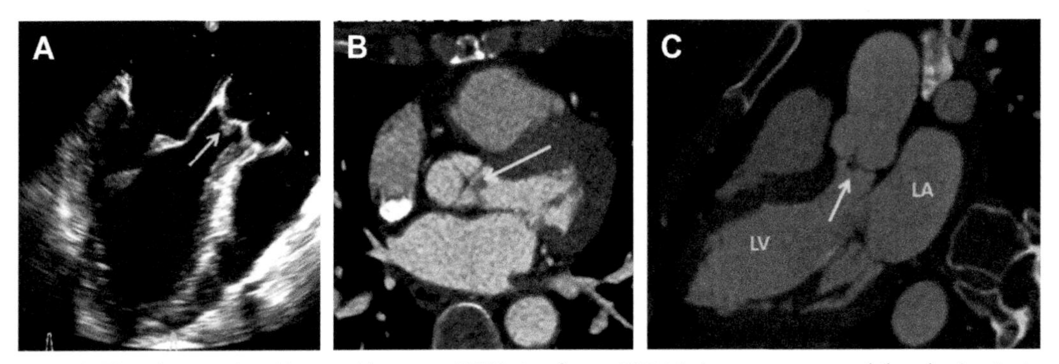

Fig. 5.10 Fibroelastoma in a 61-year-old woman. LVOT view from a TEE (*A*) demonstrates a mobile echodensity (arrow) arising from the left coronary cusp. Axial (*B*) and LVOT (*C*) reformatted images from a multiplanar, ECG-gated CT coronary angiogram demonstrate a 0.6-cm mobile density (*arrow*) arising from the left coronary cusp of the aortic valve. This was a pathology-proven fibroelastoma.

enhancement with both CT and MRI imaging due to slow blood flow within the tumor (Fig. 5.11).

Teratoma

A teratoma is a neoplasm of primordial germ cell origin. These tumors are typically diagnosed in children who present with pericardial effusions, which can be large enough to cause tamponade, due to the pericardial location of the tumor.[23,24] They are classically polycystic masses, which can be up to 15 cm in size.[25,26] They can be diagnosed by ultrasound in utero and appear as a partially cystic mediastinal mass, often with associated pericardial effusion or evidence of hydrops fetalis. With CT and MRI, a heterogenous, partially cystic mass is seen with macroscopic fat, which is low density on CT and hyperintense on T1 and T2 images with loss of signal on fat-saturated sequences.

Paraganglioma

A paraganglioma is a neoplasm arising from paraganglia, neuroendocrine cells widely distributed throughout the body, including within cardiac paraganglia at the roots of the great vessels, within the atria, and along the atrioventricular groove. The mean age at diagnosis is 39 years, and two-thirds occur within the atria, more commonly the left, classically within the atrioventricular groove.[2] Patients often present with hypertension and laboratory evidence of catecholamine overproduction.[27] Subsequently, the tumor is localized to the mediastinum using nuclear medicine imaging with iodine-131 meta-iodobenzylguanidine scan.[28] Paragangliomas appear as large, echogenic masses by TTE. By CT, they typically appear as well-circumscribed, heterogenous, enhancing masses (Fig. 5.12). By MRI, the tumors have markedly increased T2 signal and avidly enhance with contrast, with the exception of regions of central necrosis, which are common and do not enhance.[29] Because of their avid enhancement and possibly large size, paragangliomas may have an appearance similar to primary cardiac angiosarcomas, although

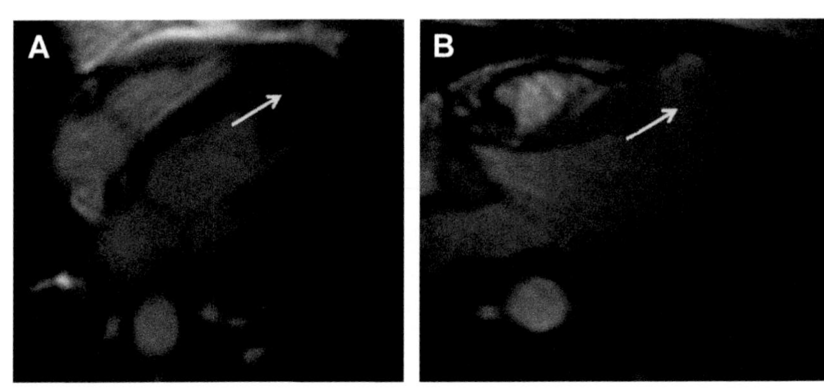

Fig. 5.11 Hemangioma in a 47-year-old woman. Axial precontrast (*A*) and postcontrast (*B*) FIESTA images demonstrate a mass in the left ventricular apex (*arrow*) that protrudes into the left ventricular cavity. The mass is mildly hyperintense to myocardium on precontrast imaging (*A*) and homogenously enhances (*B*), similar to blood pool. This mass was confirmed to be a hemangioma at pathology.

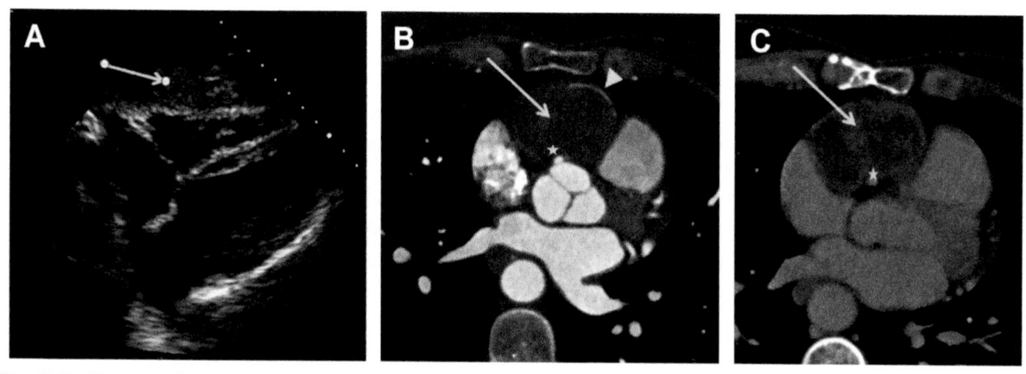

Fig. 5.12 Paraganglioma in a 57-year-old woman. A 4-chamber, parasternal view (*A*) from a TTE shows a hyperechoic mass in the right atrioventricular groove (*arrow*). Axial slices from an ECG-gated CT coronary angiogram in the angiographic (*B*) and delayed (*C*) phases demonstrate a circumscribed mass (*arrow*) in the right atrioventricular groove that displaces the adjacent right coronary artery (*asterisk*) and cause mass effect on the adjacent RA without invasion. The angiographic image demonstrates anterior displacement of a small conus branch (*arrowhead*).

paragangliomas are more often expansile and less likely to invade adjacent structures than angiosarcomas, and paragangliomas have a predilection for either right or left atrioventricular groove or (following the course of paraganglion cells along the coronary arteries), whereas angiosarcomas have a predilection for the right atrium only.

Although paragangliomas are generally categorized as benign, there have been a select few case reports of malignant cardiac paragangliomas,[30,31] and as such, they are sometimes categorized as intermediate.

PRIMARY CARDIAC MALIGNANCIES

Angiosarcoma

Angiosarcoma is a tumor of endothelial cells. It represents the most common differentiated primary cardiac malignancy and 40% of cardiac sarcomas in adults.[2] The tumor occurs most commonly in middle age, with a slight male preponderance. Patients often are symptomatic with fever and weight loss and right-sided heart failure with pericardial effusion with or without tamponade due to the typical location within the right atrium and frequent pericardial invasion.[2] Grossly, angiosarcomas are typically irregular masses that appear dark brown or black due to areas of hemorrhage and necrosis,[32] which can be noted to invade adjacent structures including the pericardium and great vessels. These tumors are often first identified by TTE due to symptoms of dyspnea, which often demonstrates an echogenic mass with an associated pericardial effusion, due to hemorrhage or from growth of the mass into the pericardium. The mass effect and invasion of surrounding structures can often be observed by TTE, but further imaging with CT or MRI is often required.[33] Both CT and MRI demonstrate an infiltrative, irregular mass that appears heterogenous due to hemorrhage and necrosis with avid contrast enhancement in regions of viable tumor (**Fig. 5.13**). Tissue diagnosis can be

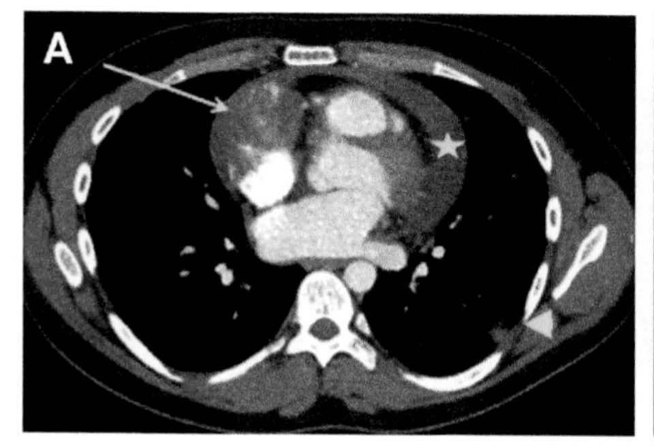

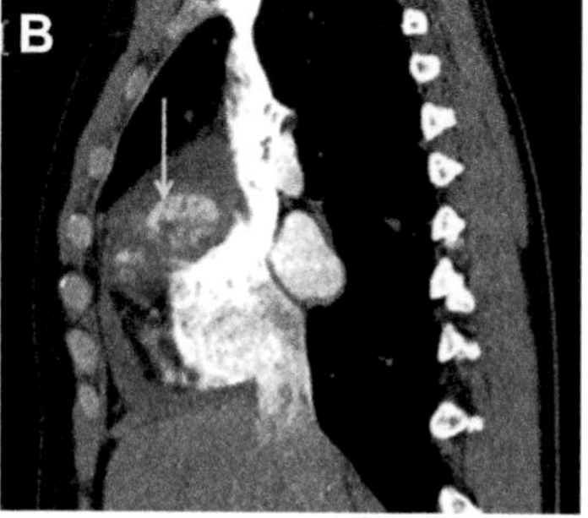

Fig. 5.13 Angiosarcoma in a 23-year-old patient. Axial (*A*) and sagittal (*B*) contrast-enhanced CT images from a non-ECG-gated study demonstrate a heterogeneously enhancing 6-cm pericardial mass (*arrow*) anterior to the right atrium extending into the right atrioventricular groove with an associated high-density circumferential pericardial effusion (*asterisk*) and innumerable pulmonary metastases (*arrowhead*).

made by endomyocardial biopsy,[33] and prognosis is poor.[34,35]

Other Sarcomas

Other primary cardiac sarcomas can occur, including osteosarcoma, rhabdomyosarcoma, and leiomyosarcoma, with the most common being the undifferentiated sarcoma.[32] Undifferentiated sarcomas lack specific histologic differentiation and demonstrate prominent pleomorphism.[32] The most common location for undifferentiated sarcomas, as well as the other differentiated primary cardiac sarcomas (excluding angiosarcomas), is within the left atrium; however, unlike myxomas, these often arise away from the septum and usually have a broad base of attachment.[32] They can invade adjacent structures such as pulmonic veins and have variable appearance on gross pathology, depending on tumor type. They may contain microscopic or macroscopic evidence of their primary tissue type, such as calcification in osteosarcoma. As with pathology, imaging features are variable, but commonly, invasion of the myocardium and/or adjacent structures can be seen on all imaging modalities, which, along with lack of septal involvement, helps to distinguish from myxoma. Like angiosarcoma, prognosis is poor.[13]

Lymphoma

Lymphoma is an abnormal monoclonal proliferation of lymphocytes. Primary cardiac lymphoma is defined as an extranodal occurrence that involves only the heart and pericardium[32] and is rare, representing less than 2% of primary cardiac neoplasms. The tumor often affects immunocompromised middle-aged patients (mean age 63 years old) with men more commonly affected than women.[36] Patients report dyspnea and constitutional symptoms of night sweats, anorexia, and weight loss and may be found to have a pericardial effusion. The most common location of involvement within the heart is the right atrium.[32,37] Gross pathology typically yields multiple firm, white masses as seen in extracardiac lymphoma.[38] By TTE, cardiac lymphoma is

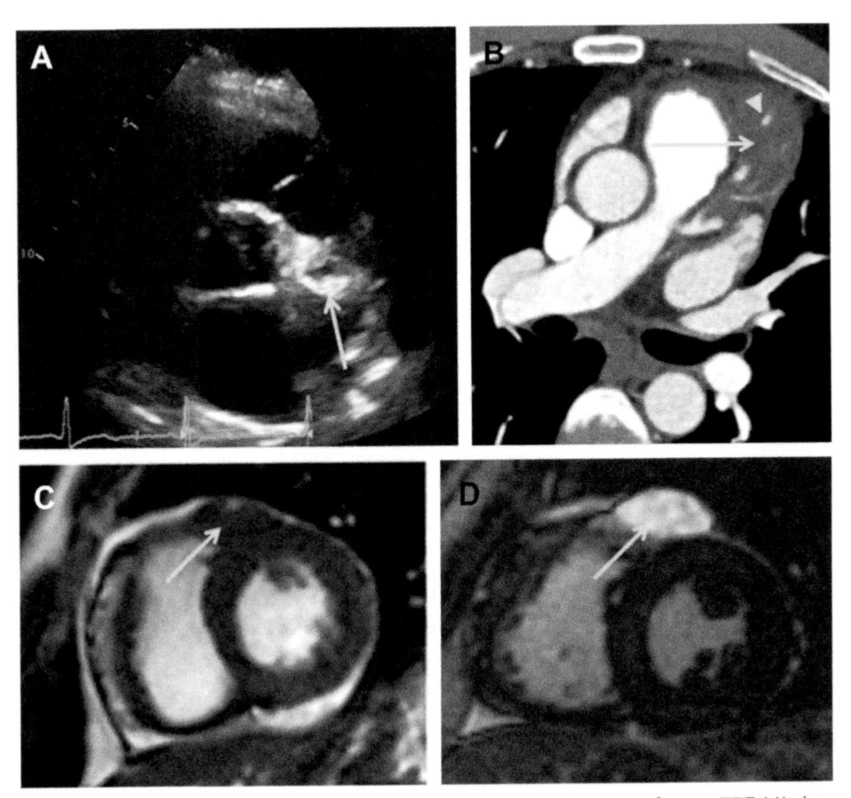

Fig. 5.14 Cardiac lymphoma in a 42-year-old patient. Parasternal short-axis view from a TTE (*A*) demonstrates an echoic mass in the left atrioventricular groove (*arrow*). Axial image from an ECG-gated CT coronary angiogram (*B*) demonstrates a mass (*arrow*) within the atrioventricular groove, which surrounds, but does not narrow, the left anterior descending artery (*arrowhead*). Short-axis FIESTA (*C*) and myocardial delayed enhancement (*D*) images show the mass (*arrow*) within the atrioventricular groove, which is homogenously T1 isointense to myocardium (*C*) with avid, homogenous enhancement (*D*).

appreciated as a hypoechoic, often infiltrative mass within the myocardium. By CT, it is often hypodense and homogenously enhancing. MRI demonstrates a mass that is T1 hypointense and T2 hyperintense[39] with variable contrast enhancement (Fig. 5.14). Because of its predisposition for the right atrium and tendency to infiltration, cardiac lymphoma may have a similar appearance to cardiac angiosarcoma; however, cardiac lymphomas are usually homogenous, without focal regions of necrosis or enhancement and are less likely to have associated pericardial effusions. Diagnosis is important because unlike other primary cardiac malignancies, primary cardiac lymphomas may respond to treatment.[36]

METASTATIC MALIGNANCIES

Metastatic spread of disease to the heart is much more common than primary cardiac malignancies, occurring in 2% of patients in an autopsy series.[40] Metastatic disease reaches the heart by 3 means of spread: hematogenous, lymphatic (pericardial), and direct extension, from an adjacent structure or intravascularly.

Hematogenous

Malignant tumors are composed of neoplastic cells originating from an organ other than the heart. Presentation can be due to symptoms related to the location of the tumor, such as dyspnea if there is outflow tract obstruction or associated pericardial effusion. Some patients are asymptomatic and diagnosed only in the context of staging or screening imaging. The tumors may be a single mass or multiple small masses within the myocardium or pericardium. Renal cell carcinoma and melanoma are examples of tumors that can spread hematogenously to the heart (Fig. 5.15). Imaging characteristics are variable based on the imaging appearance of the primary malignancy. If multiple intracardiac masses are seen, suspicion of malignancy should be high. When a solitary mass is present, a history of malignancy may be the key diagnostic feature in suggesting metastasis.

Lymphatic

Myocardial metastases via lymphatic spread are exceedingly rare because the lymphatics of the heart are efferent, and thus, tumors that reach

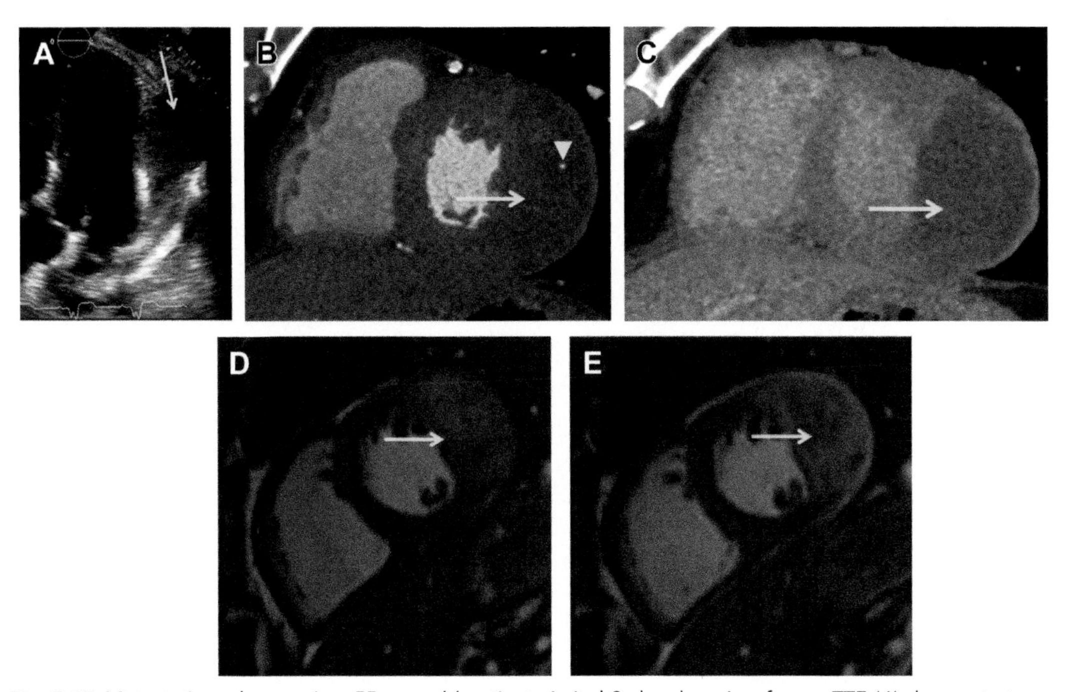

Fig. 5.15 Metastatic melanoma in a 55-year-old patient. Apical 2-chamber view from a TTE (*A*) demonstrates an expansile mass within the left ventricular free wall (*arrow*). Short-axis reformatted views in the angiographic (*B*) and delayed (*C*) phases from an ECG-gated, CT angiogram of the heart demonstrate an expansile mass, hypodense to normal myocardium with minimal enhancement (*arrow*). The angiographic image (*B*) shows an obtuse marginal branch (*arrowhead*) that has been surrounded by the mass. Short-axis steady-state free procession precontrast (*D*) and postcontrast (*E*) images from a multiplanar cardiac MRI show heterogenous increased T1 signal within the mass, which also demonstrates heterogeneous enhancement (*arrow*).

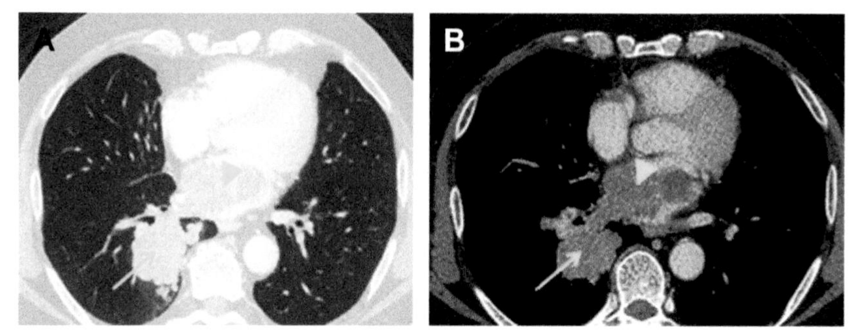

Fig. 5.16 Metastatic rectal cancer in a 67-year-old patient. Axial images from a contrast-enhanced non-ECG gated CT of the chest (*A* and *B*) demonstrate a large metastasis in the right lower lobe (*arrow*), which invades the right inferior pulmonary vein and extends into the left atrium (*arrowhead*).

the heart by lymphatic spread result in pericardial metastases, which are associated with pericardial effusions in up to half of cases.[41] The most common sites of origin of lymphatic metastases are breast and lung carcinoma.[2] These metastases can present as solitary or multiple pericardial masses, which can cause mass effect on adjacent cardiac chambers or great vessels.

Direct Extension

Local invasion of cardiac structures by malignancies of nearby anatomic structures represents a frequent cause of cardiac masses, primarily due to the prevalence of these malignancies. For example, as much as 30% of metastatic cardiac neoplasms have been related to the extension of lung cancer,[32] and esophageal malignancies

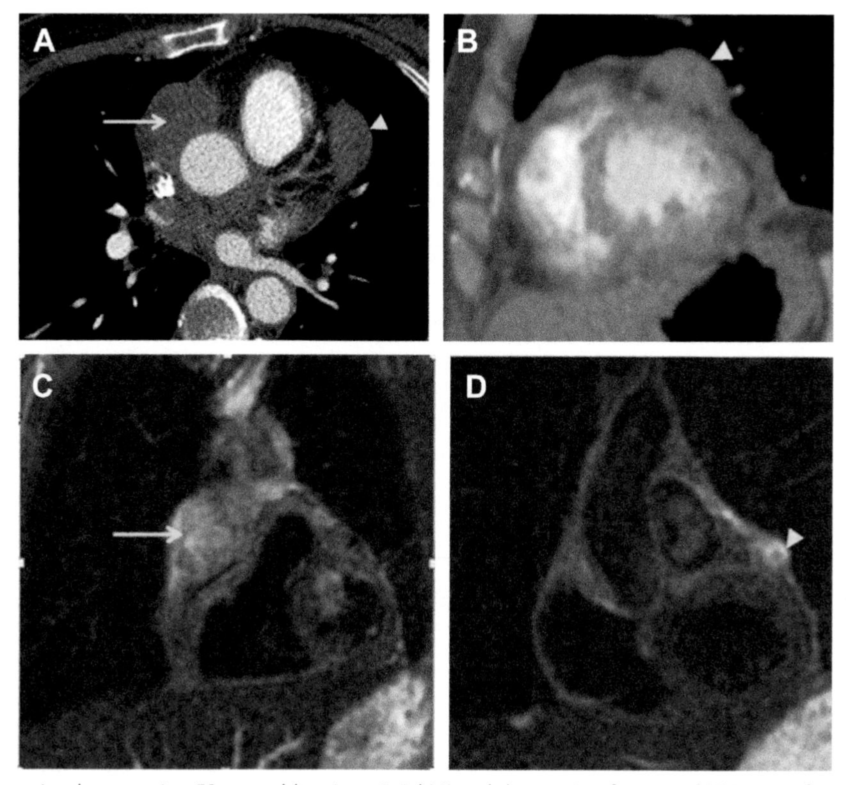

Fig. 5.17 Invasive thymoma in a 50-year-old patient. Axial (*A*) and short-axis reformatted (*B*) images from a contrast-enhanced, non-ECG-gated CT of the chest and coronal triple inversion recovery images (*C* and *D*) from a cardiac MRI demonstrate a primary mediastinal mass (*arrow*) with direct invasion of mediastinal structures and pericardial (lymphatic) metastasis adjacent to the left ventricular free wall (*arrowhead*).

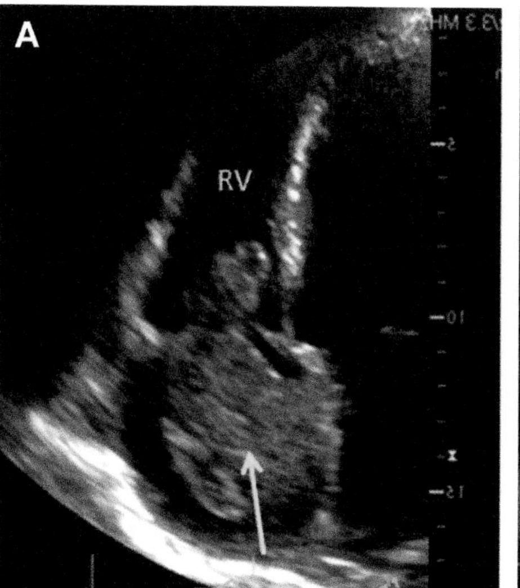

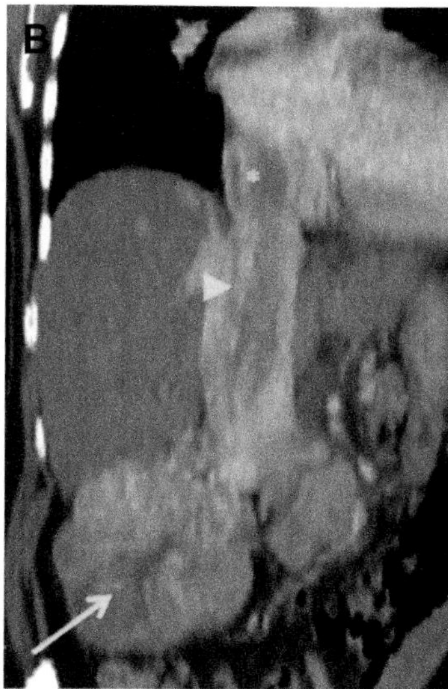

Fig. 5.18 Renal cell carcinoma with intravascular extension in a 69-year-old patient. Apical 2-chamber view from a TTE (*A*) demonstrates dynamic extension of the mass (*arrow*) across the tricuspid valve into the RV. Coronal reformatted image from a contrast-enhanced, non-ECG-gated CT of the chest and abdomen (*B*) demonstrates a large, heterogeneous right renal mass (*arrow*) with extension from the renal vein into the IVC (*arrowhead*) and into the right atrium (*asterisk*).

are also a common consideration. In addition, lung metastases from remote primary tumors can directly invade the pericardium or even cardiac chambers (Fig. 5.16). Other mediastinal tumors, such as thymoma and lymphoma, or other thoracic tumors, such as breast cancer and mesothelioma, can also directly invade cardiac structures (Fig. 5.17).

An additional avenue of direct extension of malignancy to the heart is intravascularly, most commonly via the inferior vena cava (IVC). Renal cell carcinoma classically extends into the renal vein and can ascend the IVC into the right atrium and can even extend into the right ventricle (Fig. 5.18). Additional abdominal neoplasms such as hepatocellular carcinoma and adrenal cortical carcinoma can follow a similar path.

REFERENCES

1. Bakaeen FG, Reardon MJ, Coselli JS, et al. Surgical outcome in 85 patients with primary cardiac tumors. Am J Surg 2003;186(6):641–7.
2. Burke A, Tavora F, Maleszewski JJ, et al, editors. Tumors of the heart and great vessels. Fascicle. 22nd edition. Silver Spring (MD): ARP Press; 2015. p. 140–275. Silverberg S, editor. AFIP Atlas of Tumor Pathology.
3. Loukas M, Tubbs RS, Tongson JM, et al. The clinical anatomy of the crista terminalis, pectinate muscles and the teniae sagittalis. Ann Anat 2008;190(1):81–7.
4. McKay T, Thomas L. Prominent crista terminalis and Eustachian ridge in the right atrium: two dimensional (2D) and three dimensional (3D) imaging. Eur J Echocardiogr 2007;8:288–91.
5. Heyer CM, Kagel T, Lemburg SP, et al. Lipomatous hypertrophy of the interatrial septum*: a prospective study of incidence, imaging findings, and clinical symptoms. Chest 2003;124(6):2068–73.
6. Fan C-M, Fischman AJ, Kwek BH, et al. Lipomatous Hypertrophy of the interatrial septum: increased uptake on FDG PET. Am J Roentgenol 2005; 184(1):339–42.
7. Brown DL, Ivey TD. Giant organized pericardial hematoma producing constrictive pericarditis: a case report and review of the literature. J Trauma Acute Care Surg 1996;41(3):558–60.
8. Wang ZJ, Reddy GP, Gotway MB, et al. CT and MR imaging of pericardial disease. Radiographics 2003; 23(Suppl 1):S167–80.
9. Vaideeswar P, Butany JW. Benign cardiac tumors of the pluripotent mesenchyme. Semin Diagn Pathol 2008;25(1):20–8.
10. Pinede L, Duhaut P, Loire R. Clinical presentation of left atrial cardiac myxoma: a series of 112 consecutive cases. Medicine 2001;80(3):159–72.
11. ElBardissi AW, Dearani JA, Daly RC, et al. Survival after resection of primary cardiac tumors: a 48-year experience. Circulation 2008;118(14 Suppl 1):S7–15.
12. Verkkala K, Kupari M, Maamies T, et al. Primary cardiac tumours–operative treatment of 20 patients. Thorac Cardiovasc Surg 1989;37(6):361–4.

13. Tazelaar HD, Locke TJ, McGregor CGA. Pathology of surgically excised primary cardiac tumors. Mayo Clin Proc 1992;67(10):957–65.
14. Torimitsu S, Nemoto T, Wakayama M, et al. Literature survey on epidemiology and pathology of cardiac fibroma. Eur J Med Res 2012;17(1):5.
15. Burke AP, Rosado-de-Christenson M, Templeton PA, et al. Cardiac fibroma: clinicopathologic correlates and surgical treatment. J Thorac Cardiovasc Surg 1994;108(5):862–70.
16. Veinot JP, O'Murchu B, Tazelaar HD, et al. Cardiac fibroma mimicking apical hypertrophic cardiomyopathy: a case report and differential diagnosis. J Am Soc Echocardiogr 1996;9(1):94–9.
17. Edwards FH, Hale D, Cohen A, et al. Primary cardiac valve tumors. Ann Thorac Surg 1991;52(5):1127–31.
18. Chan HSL, Sonley MJ, Moësmd CAF, et al. Primary and secondary tumors of childhood involving the heart, pericardium, and great vessels a report of 75 cases and review of the literature. Cancer 1985; 56(4):825–36.
19. Tworetzky W, McElhinney DB, Margossian R, et al. Association between cardiac tumors and tuberous sclerosis in the fetus and neonate. Am J Cardiol 2003;92(4):487–9.
20. Han Y, Chen X, Wang X, et al. Cardiac capillary hemangioma: a case report and brief review of the literature. J Clin Ultrasound 2014;42(1):53–6.
21. Koçak H, Özyazıcıoğlu A, Gündoğdu C, et al. Cardiac hemangioma complicated with cerebral and coronary embolization. Heart Vessels 2005;20(6): 296–7.
22. Abad C, Campo E, Estruch R, et al. Cardiac hemangioma with papillary endothelial hyperplasia: report of a resected case and review of the literature. Ann Thorac Surg 1990;49(2):305–8.
23. Mirzaaghayan M, Shabanian R. A huge intrapericardial teratoma in an infant. Pediatr Cardiol 2008; 29(6):1122–3.
24. Singh J, Rana S, Kaur A, et al. Intrapericardial teratoma presenting as recurrent pericardial tamponade: report of a case. Surg Today 2009;39(8):700–4.
25. Rasmussen SL, Hwang WS, Harder J, et al. Intrapericardial teratoma. Ultrasonic and pathological features. J Ultrasound Med 1987;6(3):159–62.
26. Garcia Cors M, Mulet J, Caralps J, et al. Fast-growing pericardial mass as first manifestation of intrapericardial teratoma in a young man. Am J Med 1990;89(6):818–20.
27. Jeevanandam V, Oz MC, Shapiro B, et al. Surgical management of cardiac pheochromocytoma. Resection versus transplantation. Ann Surg 1995; 221(4):415–9.
28. Lin JC, Palafox BA, Jackson HA, et al. Cardiac pheochromocytoma: resection after diagnosis by 111-indium octreotide scan. Ann Thorac Surg 1999;67(2):555–8.
29. Hamilton BH, Francis IR, Gross BH, et al. Intrapericardial paragangliomas (pheochromocytomas): imaging features. AJR Am J Roentgenol 1997; 168(1):109–13.
30. Arai A, Naruse M, Naruse K, et al. Cardiac malignant pheochromocytoma with bone metastases. Intern Med 1998;37(11):940–4.
31. Jirari A, Charpentier A, Popescu S, et al. A malignant primary cardiac pheochromocytoma. Ann Thorac Surg 1999;68(2):565–6.
32. Travis WD, Brambilla E, Muller-Hermelink HK, et al. Pathology and genetics of tumours of the lung, pleura, thymus and heart. 4th edition. IARC; 2004. p. 251–90.
33. Kurian KC, Weisshaar D, Parekh H, et al. Primary cardiac angiosarcoma: case report and review of the literature. Cardiovasc Pathol 2006; 15(2):110–2.
34. Herrmann M, Shankerman R, Edwards W, et al. Primary cardiac angiosarcoma: a clinicopathologic study of six cases. J Thorac Cardiovasc Surg 1992; 103(4):655–64.
35. Murinello A, Mendonça P, Abreu A, et al. Cardiac angiosarcoma. A review. Rev Port Cardiol 2007;26: 577–84.
36. Miguel CE, Bestetti RB. Primary cardiac lymphoma. Int J Cardiol 2011;149(3):358–63.
37. Ceseroli G, Ferreri A, Bucci E, et al. Primary cardiac lymphoma in immunocompetent patients. Diagnostic and therapeutic management. Cancer 1997; 80:1497–506.
38. Araoz PA, Eklund HE, Welch TJ, et al. CT and MR imaging of primary cardiac malignancies. Radiographics 1999;19(6):1421–34.
39. Tada H, Asazuma K-Y, Ohya E, et al. Primary cardiac B-cell lymphoma. Circulation 1998;97(2):220–1.
40. Butany J, Leong SW, Carmichael K, et al. A 30-year analysis of cardiac neoplasms at autopsy. Can J Cardiol 2005;21(8):675–80.
41. García-Riego A, Cuiñas C, Vilanova JJ. Malignant pericardial effusion. Acta Cytol 2001;45(4):561–6.

CHAPTER 6

Cardiac Tumors

Treatment

Basel Ramlawi, MD[a], Michael J. Reardon, MD[b,*]

 **Video content accompanies this chapter.**

Cardiac tumors are divided into primary cardiac tumors arising in the heart and secondary cardiac tumors from metastasis as outlined in prior chapters and pathologic classification systems (Box 6.1).[1,2] Surgical resection is seldom possible or advisable for metastatic tumors, and intervention is usually limited to drainage of malignant pericardial effusions and/or diagnostic biopsies. Regarding primary cardiac tumors, most surgeons will rarely encounter these with the exception of myxomas, the clinical incidence of which is 1 in 500 cardiac surgery patients.[2–6] The purpose of this chapter is to summarize the evaluation and management of patients with cardiac tumors and to provide a reference for additional studies.

When confronted with the diagnosis of a cardiac mass, it is very important to consider patient-specific characteristics (age and clinical context) as well as lesions-specific characteristics (shape, form, and importantly, localization) (Fig. 6.1). Normal variant, thrombus, and vegetation should always be in the differential (Fig. 6.2). Next, one should recall that any true neoplastic process is far more likely to be metastatic than a primary cardiac tumor (Fig. 6.3). If a primary cardiac tumor, a benign process can be assumed in 90% of the cases, with 80% being myxomas and the rest being differentiated by age (see Fig. 6.3; Figs. 6.4 and 6.5). If malignant, primary cardiac tumors are almost always sarcomas (Case Study; see Fig. 6.3).

NONNEOPLASTIC TUMORS

Mural thrombus, although not really a cardiac tumor, may mimic myxoma clinically and pathologically. Most mural thrombi are associated with underlying valvular disease, myocardial infarction, dysfunction, or atrial fibrillation.[7] Mural thrombi also have been noted in hypercoagulable syndromes, particularly antiphospholipid syndrome.[8] With increasing use of long-term central catheters, several right atrial masses have been seen that were difficult to define, and upon removal were mural thrombi. Real-time contrast perfusion imaging may aid in the differentiation against cardiac tumors because thrombi are without perfusion in the vast majority of cases, and if present, only entails mild peripheral slow replenishment (Fig. 6.6). The treatment options for cardiac thrombi include surgical or catheter-based thrombectomy, lytic therapy, and anticoagulation. The choice is based on the size, location, and implication of the thrombus as well as cause and comorbidity spectrum. The need and duration of chronic anticoagulation depends on the underlying substrate as well as the risk for bleeding. For instance, anticoagulation may not be required beyond 4 to 6 weeks after catheter-associated thrombosis, if at all, can be limited to 3 months in cases of unprovoked thrombus, or should be prolonged as in patients with nonbacterial thrombotic endocarditis, which are often those with malignancies, in the absence of any contraindications. Bacterial endocarditis remains an important differential diagnostic consideration and is to be expected within the clinical context. Antibiotic therapy is to be pursued based on societal guidelines in these cases.

Heterotopias and tumors of ectopic tissue include cystic tumors of the atrioventricular (AV) node consisting of multiple benign cysts in the region of the AV node that can cause heart block or sudden death. Most are diagnosed at autopsy, but a biopsy diagnosis of AV nodal tumor has been reported.[9] Germ-cell tumors of the heart

[a] Cardiothoracic Surgery, Valley Health System, Winchester, VA 22601, USA; [b] Department of Cardiovascular Surgery, Houston Methodist DeBakey Heart & Vascular Center, Houston Methodist Hospital, 6550 Fannin, Suite 1401, Houston, TX 77030, USA
* Corresponding author.
E-mail address: mreardon@houstonmethodist.org

BOX 6.1
Types of cardiac tumors by pathology

- Pseudotumors
  - Mural thrombi
- Heterotopias and tumors of ectopic tissue
  - Tumors of the atrioventricular nodal region
  - Teratoma
  - Ectopic thyroid
- Tumors of mesenchymal tissue
  - Hamartoma of endocardial tissue
    - Papillary fibroelastoma
  - Hamartomas of cardiac muscle
    - Rhabdomyoma
    - Histiocytoid cardiomyopathy (Purkinje cell hamartoma)
- Tumors and neoplasms of fat
  - Lipomatous hypertrophy, interarterial septum
  - Lipoma
  - Liposarcoma
- Tumors and neoplasms of fibrous and myofibroblastic tissue
  - Fibroma
  - Inflammatory pseudotumor (inflammatory myofibroblastic tumor)
  - Sarcomas (malignant fibrous histiocytoma, fibrosarcoma, leiomyosarcoma)
- Vascular tumors and neoplasms
  - Hemangioma
  - Epithelioid hemangioendothelioma
  - Angiosarcoma
- Neoplasm of uncertain histogenesis
  - Myxoma
- Neoplasms of neural tissue
  - Granular cell tumor
  - Schwannoma/neurofibroma
- Paraganglioma
- Malignant schwannoma/neurofibrosarcoma (rare)
- Malignant lymphoma
- Malignant mesothelioma
- Metastatic tumors to the heart

usually are teratomas, occurring within the pericardial sac, but yolk sac tumors have been described in infants and children.[10] Ectopic thyroid tissue may occur within the myocardium and is referred to as *struma cordis*. Right ventricular outflow track obstruction may be present, but most patients are asymptomatic.

Most of the remaining tumors arise in the mesenchymal, fat, fibrous, neural, or vascular cells of the heart, with myxoma representing a tumor of undetermined histogenesis. Primary cardiac lymphoma, mesothelioma, and metastatic tumors to the heart represent the remaining pathologic categories that comprise the greater part of this chapter.

BENIGN PRIMARY CARDIAC NEOPLASMS

Myxoma

Myxomas comprise 50% of all benign cardiac tumors in adults and 15% of such tumors in children. Occurrence during infancy is rare (Tables 6.1 and 6.2). A vast majority of myxomas occur sporadically and tend to be more common in women.[4] The peak incidence is between the third and sixth decades of life, and 94% of tumors are solitary.[11] Approximately 75% occur in the left atrium (LA),[12] and 10% to 20% occur in the right atrium. The remaining proportion is equally distributed between the ventricles.[2] The DNA genotype of sporadic myxomas is normal in 80% of patients.[13] Myxomas are unlikely to be associated with other abnormal conditions and have a low recurrence rate.[4,12]

About 5% of myxoma patients show a familial pattern of tumor development based on autosomal-dominant inheritance.[14–16] These patients and 20% of those with sporadic myxoma have an abnormal DNA genotype chromosomal pattern.[13] In contrast to the "typical" sporadic myxoma profile, familial patients are more likely to be younger, equally likely to be male or female, and more often (22%) have multicentric tumors originating from either the atrium or the ventricle.[17–21] Although familial myxomas have the same histology, they have a higher recurrence rate after surgical resection (21%–67%).[12,22] Approximately 20% of familial patients have associated conditions such as adrenocortical nodule hyperplasia, Sertoli cell tumors of the testes, pituitary tumors, multiple myxoid breast fibroadenomas, cutaneous myomas, and facial or labial pigmented spots.[11,22] These conditions often are described as *complex myxomas* within the group of familial myxoma.[13] A familial syndrome with autosomal X-linked inheritance characterized by primary pigmented nodular adrenocortical disease with hypercortisolism, cutaneous pigmentous lentigines, and cardiac myxoma is referred to as *Carney complex*.[11,22]

Pathology

Both biatrial and multicentric myxomas are more common in familial disease. Biatrial tumors

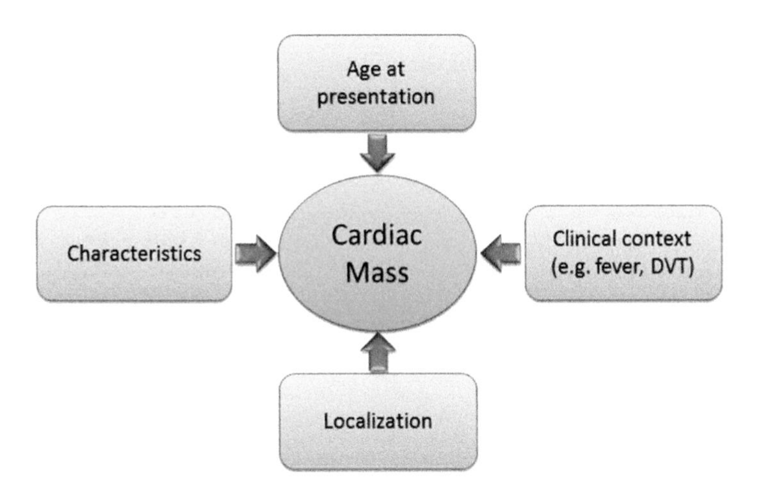

Fig. 6.1 The most important factors to consider in the differential diagnostic approach to a cardiac mass. DVT, deep venous thrombosis.

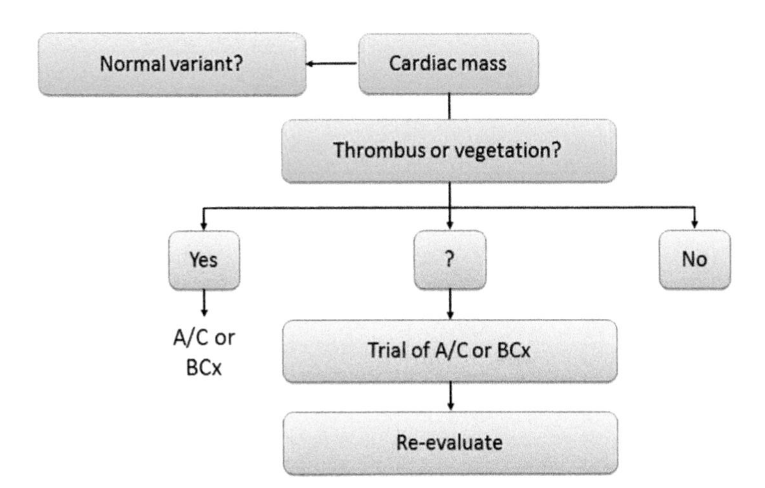

Fig. 6.2 Initial evaluation of cardiac masses focusing on the clinical context. A/C, anticoagulation; BCx, blood culture. (*Adapted from* Bruce CJ. Cardiac tumours: diagnosis and management. Heart 2011;97(2): 152; with permission.)

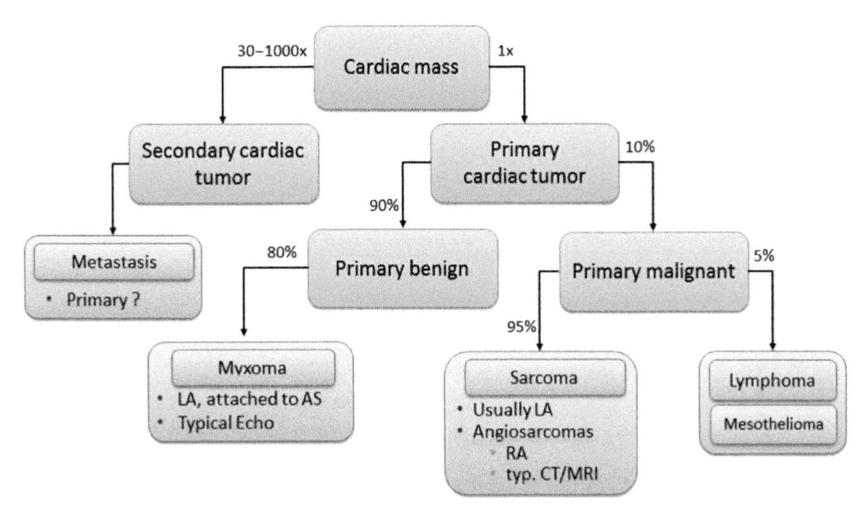

Fig. 6.3 Evaluation of cardiac masses focusing on the histologic context. AS, aortic stenosis; LA, left atrium; RA, right atrium. (*Adapted from* Bruce CJ. Cardiac tumours: diagnosis and management. Heart 2011;97(2):151–60; with permission.)

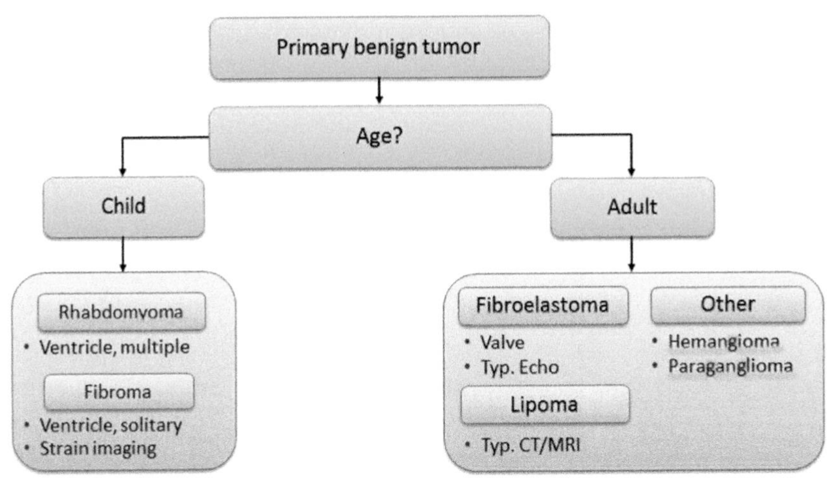

Fig. 6.4 Evaluation of primary benign cardiac tumors focusing on age. (*Adapted from* Bruce CJ. Cardiac tumours: diagnosis and management. Heart 2011;97(2):154; with permission.)

probably arise from bidirectional growth of a tumor originating within the atrial septum.[23] Atrial myxomas generally arise from the interatrial septum at the border of the fossa ovalis but can originate anywhere within the atrium, including the appendage.[4] In addition, isolated reports confirm that myxomas can arise from the cardiac valves, pulmonary artery (PA) and vein, and vena cava.[15,16] Right atrial myxomas are more likely to have broad-based attachments than left atrial tumors; they also are more likely to be calcified[19] and thus visible on chest radiographs. Ventricular myxomas occur more often in women and children and may be multicentric.[2,24,25] Right ventricular tumors typically arise from the free wall, and left ventricular tumors tend to originate in the proximity of the posterior papillary muscle.

Grossly, about two-thirds of myxomas are round or oval tumors with a smooth or lobulated surface. Most are polypoid, compact, pedunculated, mobile, and not likely to fragment spontaneously.[2,4] The less common villous or papillary myxomas are gelatinous and fragile and prone to fragmentation and embolization, occurring about one-third of the time.[26,27] However, myxomas are frequently covered with thrombus.[2] The average size is about 5 cm in diameter, but growth to 15 cm in diameter and larger has been reported.[4] Myxomatous tumors appear to grow rapidly, but growth rates vary, and occasionally, tumor growth arrests spontaneously.[4] Weights range from 8 to 175 g, with a mean between 50 and 60 g.[5]

The base of the tumor contains a large artery and veins that connect with the subendocardium but do not typically extend deep beyond the subendocardium, which is important for coronary angiography when used.[22] Myxomas tend to grow into the overlying cardiac cavity rather

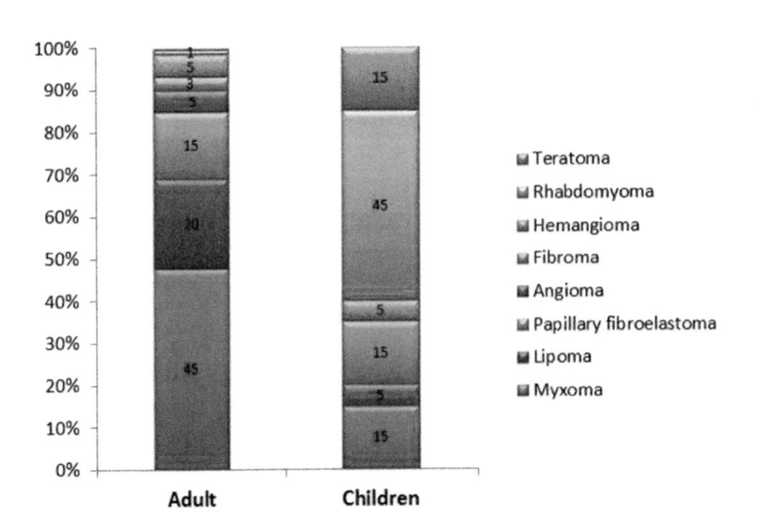

Fig. 6.5 Distribution of benign cardiac tumors in adults and children. (*Data from* Allard MF, Taylor GP, Wilson JE, et al. Primary cardiac tumours. In: Goldhauber S, Braunwald E, editors. Atlas of heart diseases. Philadelphia: Current Medicine; 1995:15.1–15.22.)

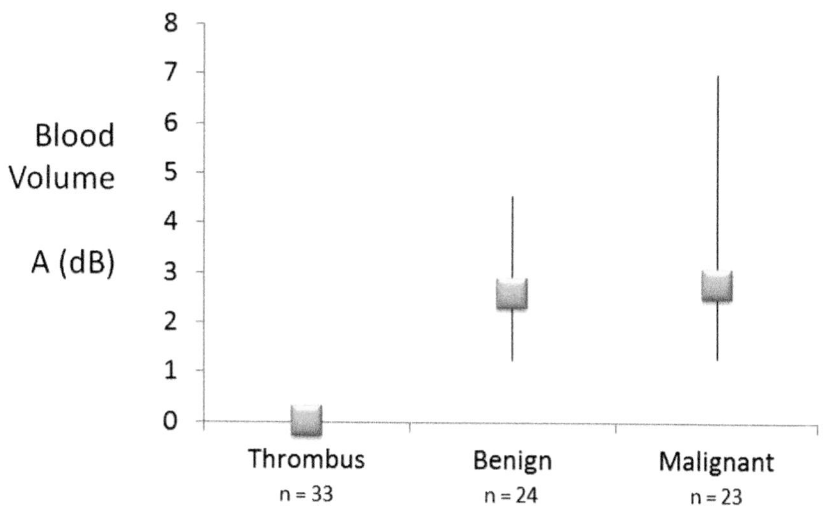

Fig. 6.6 Blood volume by real-time echo perfusion imaging in thrombi versus benign and malignant cardiac tumors (P<.001). (*Data from* Uenishi EK, Caldas MA, Tsutsui JM, et al. Evaluation of cardiac masses by real-time perfusion imaging echocardiography. Cardiovasc Ultrasound 2015;13:23.)

than into the surrounding myocardium. They arise from the endocardium and are considered derivative of the subendocardial multipotential mesenchymal cell.[28–30] This origin accounts for the occasional presence of hematopoietic tissue and bone in these tumors. Interestingly, myxomas have developed after cardiac trauma, including repair of atrial septal defects and transseptal puncture for percutaneous dilatation of the mitral valve.

TABLE 6.1
Benign cardiac neoplasms in adults

Tumor	No.	Percentage
Myxoma	118	49
Lipoma	45	19
Papillary fibroelastoma	42	17
Hemangioma	11	5
AV node mesothelioma	9	4
Fibroma	5	2
Teratoma	3	1
Granular cell tumor	3	1
Neurofibroma	2	<1
Lymphangioma	2	<1
Rhabdomyoma	1	<1
Total	241	100

Data from McAllister HA Jr, Fenoglio JJ Jr. Tumors of the cardiovascular system. In: Atlas of tumor pathology. Washington, DC: Armed Forces Institute of Pathology; 1978.

Clinical Presentation

The classic clinical presentation of a myxoma is intracardiac obstruction with congestive heart failure (67%); signs of embolization (29%); systemic or constitutional symptoms of fever (19%); weight loss or fatigue (17%); and immunologic manifestations of myalgia, weakness, and arthralgia (5%). Cardiac rhythm disturbances and infection occur less frequently.

Constitutional symptoms

Nearly all patients with myxoma admit to a variety of constitutional symptoms. These complaints may be accompanied by a leukocytosis, elevated erythrocyte levels and sedimentation rate, hemolytic anemia, thrombocytopenia, and elevated C-reactive protein. Immunoelectrophoresis may reveal abnormal immunoglobulin levels with increased circulating immunoglobulin G.[31] The recent discovery of elevated levels of interleukin-6 in patients with myxoma has been linked to a variety of associated conditions, including lymphadenopathy, tumor metastasis, ventricular hypertrophy, and development of constitutional symptoms.[24,32,33] Other less frequent complaints include Raynaud phenomenon, arthralgias, myalgias, erythematous rash, and clubbing of the digits.[4,34]

Possible causes of such varied complaints and symptoms include tumor embolization with secondary myalgias and arthralgias and elevated immunoglobulin response.[35] Circulating antibody–tumor antigen complexes with complement activation also may play a role.[36] Such symptom

TABLE 6.2
Benign cardiac neoplasms in children

Tumor	0–1 y Olds Number	0–1 y Olds Percentage	1–15 y Olds Number	1–15 y Olds Percentage
Rhabdomyoma	28	62	35	45.0
Teratoma	9	21	11	14.0
Fibroma	6	13	12	15.5
Hemangioma	1	2	4	5.0
AV node mesothelioma	1	2	3	4.0
Myxoma	—	—	12	15.5
Neurofibroma	—	—	1	1.0
Total	45	100	78	100

Data from McAllister HA Jr, Fenoglio JJ Jr. Tumors of the cardiovascular system. In: Atlas of tumor pathology. Washington, DC: Armed Forces Institute of Pathology; 1978.

complexes tend to resolve following surgical resection of the tumor.[37]

Obstruction

Obliteration of cardiac chambers is the most common cause of acute presenting symptoms. The nature of these symptoms is determined by the anatomic location and extent. For instance, myxomas in the LA tend to produce positional dyspnea and other signs and symptoms of heart failure associated with elevated left atrial and pulmonary venous pressures. Clinically, mitral stenosis often is suspected and leads to echocardiography and diagnosis of myxoma. Syncopal episodes occur in some patients and are thought to result from temporary occlusion of the mitral orifice.[19,38] Right atrial myxomas can produce a clinical picture of right-sided heart failure with signs and symptoms of venous hypertension, including hepatomegaly, ascites, and dependent edema, and can cause tricuspid valve stenosis by partially obstructing the orifice.[19,38] If a patent foramen ovale is present, right-to-left atrial shunting may occur with central cyanosis, and paradoxic embolization has been reported.[39] Large ventricular myxomas may mimic ventricular outflow obstruction. The left ventricular myxoma may produce the equivalent of subaortic or aortic valvular stenosis,[39,40] whereas right ventricular myxomas can simulate right ventricular outflow track or pulmonic valve obstruction.

Embolization

Systemic embolization is the second most common mode of myxomatous presentation, occurring in 30% to 40% of patients.[2,4,19] Because most myxomas are left-sided, approximately 50% of embolic episodes affect the central nervous system, owing to both intracranial and extracranial vascular obstruction. The neurologic deficits following embolization can be transient but are often permanent.[41] Specific central nervous system consequences include intracranial aneurysms, seizures, hemiparesis, and brain necrosis.[42–44] Retinal artery embolization with visual loss has occurred in some patients.[45]

Embolic myxomatous material has been found blocking iliac and femoral arteries.[46,47] Other sites of tumor embolization include abdominal viscera and the renal and coronary arteries.[48] Histologic examination of surgically removed peripheral myxoma that has embolized provides the diagnosis of an otherwise unsuspected tumor.[19] Renal artery specimens from a nephrectomy have shown viable enlarging embolic myxoma after excision of the primary tumor. Right-sided myxomatous emboli mainly obstruct PAs and cause pulmonary hypertension and even death from acute obstruction.[4,39]

Infection

Infection arising in a myxoma is a rare complication and produces a clinical picture of infectious endocarditis.[49,50] Infection increases the likelihood of systemic embolization,[4] and an infected myxoma warrants urgent surgical resection.

Diagnosis

Clinical examination

Findings at the time of clinical assessment of a patient with cardiac myxoma vary according to the size, location, and mobility of the tumor. Left atrial myxomas may produce auscultatory or clinical findings similar to mitral disease. The well-described "tumor plop" can be confused with a third heart sound,[51] occurring just after the opening snap of the mitral valve created from contact between the tumor and endocardial wall.[51] Left atrial myxomas that cause partial obstruction of left ventricular filling may result in elevated pulmonary vascular pressures with augmentation of the pulmonary component of the second heart sound.[52]

Right atrial myxomas may produce similar auscultatory findings as left atrial myxomas with the exception that they are best heard along the lower right sternal border rather than at the cardiac apex. In addition, right atrial hypertension may produce a large *a* wave in the jugular venous pulse and, when severe, may mimic superior vena caval syndrome.

Chest radiograph

The findings on chest roentgenogram may include generalized cardiomegaly, individual cardiac chamber enlargement, and pulmonary venous congestion. More specific rare findings are density within the cardiac silhouette caused by calcification within the tumor occurring more often with right-sided myxomas.[4]

Electrocardiogram

Nonspecific abnormalities, such as chamber enlargement, cardiomegaly, bundle-branch blocks, and axis deviation, can be found.[53] Fewer than 20% of patients have atrial fibrillation.[24] Evaluation of nonspecific electrocardiographic abnormalities occasionally leads to an incidental diagnosis of myxoma, and most electrocardiograms are not helpful in establishing a diagnosis.

Echocardiography

Cross-sectional echocardiography is the most useful test used for the diagnosis and evaluation of myxoma. The sensitivity of 2-dimensional echocardiography for myxoma is 100%, and this imaging technique largely has supplanted angiocardiography.[54] However, coronary angiography usually is performed in myxoma patients more than 40 years of age to rule out significant coronary disease. Transesophageal echocardiography (TEE) provides the best information concerning tumor size, location, mobility, and attachment.[55]

TEEs detect tumors as small as 1 to 3 mm in diameter.[56] Most surgeons obtain a TEE in the operating room before the operation. The authors particularly evaluate the posterior left atrial wall, atrial septum, and right atrium, which often are not well displayed on transthoracic examination, to exclude the possibility of biatrial multiple tumors. In addition, postoperative TEE ensures a normal echocardiogram before leaving the operating room.

Computed tomography and MRI

Although myxomas have been identified using computed tomography (CT),[54,57] this modality is most useful in malignant tumors of the heart because of its ability to demonstrate myocardial invasion and tumor involvement of adjacent structures.[53] Similarly, MRI has been used in the diagnosis of myxomas and may yield a clear picture of tumor size, shape, and surface characteristics.[53–57] MRI is particularly useful in detecting intracardiac and pericardial extension, invasion of malignant secondary tumors, and the evaluation of ventricular masses that occasionally turn out to be myxoma. Both CT and MRI detect tumors as small as 0.5 to 1.0 cm and provide information regarding the composition of the tumor.[4] Neither CT nor MRI is needed for atrial myxomas if an adequate echocardiogram is available. The exception is the occasional right atrial myxoma that extends into one or both caval or tricuspid orifices. CT or MRI should be reserved for the situation in which the diagnosis or characterization of the tumor is unclear after complete echocardiographic evaluation.

Surgical Management

Surgical resection is the only effective therapeutic option for patients with cardiac myxoma and should not be delayed because death from obstruction to flow within the heart or embolization may occur in as many as 8% of patients awaiting operation.[58] A median sternotomy approach with ascending aortic and bicaval cannulation usually is used. Manipulation of the heart before initiation of cardiopulmonary bypass is minimized in deference to the known friability and embolic tendency of myxomas. In the event of known preoperative cerebral embolization without hemorrhage, the tumor should be resected approximately 7 days after the event to prevent further embolization and yet allow time for stabilization of the brain for cardiopulmonary bypass. For *left atrial myxomas*, the venae cavae are cannulated through the right atrial wall, with the inferior cannula placed close and laterally to the inferior vena cava (IVC)–right atrial junction. Caval snares are always used to allow opening of the right atrium, if necessary. If extensive exposure of the LA is needed or a malignant left atrial tumor is suspected, the authors mobilize and directly cannulate the SVC, which allows it to be transected if necessary for additional exposure. Body temperature is allowed to drift down, but there is no attempt to induce systemic hypothermia unless the need for reduced perfusion flow is anticipated. Modern cardioplegic techniques yield a quiet operative field and protect the myocardium from ischemic injury during aortic cross-clamping. Cardiopulmonary bypass is started, and the aorta is clamped before manipulation of the heart.

Exposure of left atrial myxomas is maximized by using several principles from mitral valve repair surgery. The surgeon desires the right side of the heart to rotate up and the left side of the heart to rotate down. Therefore, stay sutures are placed low on the pericardium on the right side, and no pericardial stay sutures are placed on the left before placing the chest retractor. This traction rotates the heart for optimal exposure of both the right atrium and, particularly, the LA. For left atrial tumors, the SVC is mobilized extensively, as is the IVC–right atrial junction, allowing increased mobility and exposing the left atrial cavity. Left atrial myxomas can be approached by an incision through the anterior wall of the LA anterior to the right pulmonary veins. This incision can be extended behind both cavae for greater exposure. Exposure and removal of large tumors attached to the interatrial septum may be aided by a second incision parallel to the first in the right atrium. This biatrial incision allows easy removal of tumor attached to the fossa ovalis with a full-thickness R0 (margin-negative) excision at the site of attachment and easy patch closure of the atrial septum if necessary.

Right atrial myxomas

Right atrial myxomas pose special venous cannulation problems, and intraoperative echocardiography may be beneficial. Both venae cavae may be cannulated directly. When low- or high-lying tumor pedicles preclude safe transatrial cannulation, cannulation of the jugular or femoral vein can provide venous drainage of the upper or lower body. In general, one always can cannulate the SVC distal enough from the right atrium to allow adequate tumor resection, but occasionally femoral venous cannula drainage has been necessary. If the tumor is large or attached near both caval orifices, peripheral cannulation of both jugular and femoral veins may be used to initiate cardiopulmonary bypass and deep hypothermia. After the aorta is cross-clamped and the heart is arrested with antegrade cardioplegia, the right atrium may be opened widely for resection of the tumor and reconstruction of the atrium during a period of circulatory arrest if this is needed for a dry field. Resection of large or critically placed right atrial myxomas often requires careful preoperative planning, intraoperative TEE, and special extracorporeal perfusion techniques to ensure complete removal of the tumor, protection of right atrial structures, and reconstruction of the atrium. Because myxomas rarely extend deep in the endocardium, it is not necessary to resect deeply around the conduction tissue. The tricuspid valve and the right atrium, as well as the LA and ventricle, should be inspected carefully for multicentric tumors in patients with right atrial myxoma. Regardless of the surgical approach, the ideal resection encompasses the tumor and a portion of the cardiac wall or interatrial septum to which it is attached. The authors' policy is to perform a full-thickness resection whenever possible. However, partial-thickness resection of the area of tumor attachment has been performed when anatomically necessary without a noted increase in recurrence rate.[59,60]

Ventricular myxomas

Ventricular myxomas usually are approached through the AV valve[61] or by detaching the anterior portion of the AV valve for exposure and resection and reattachment after resection. Occasional small tumors in either outflow tract can be removed through the outflow valve.[61] If necessary, the tumor is excised through a direct incision into the ventricle, but this is unusual and the least preferred approach. It is not necessary to remove the full thickness of the ventricular wall because no recurrences have been reported with partial-thickness excisions. As with right atrial myxoma, the presence of ventricular myxoma prompts inspection for other tumors because of the high incidence of multiple tumors.

Every care should be taken to remove the tumor without fragmentation. Following tumor removal from the field, the area should be liberally irrigated, suctioned, and inspected for loose fragments. There are rare instances of distant metastases from myxoma many years after tumor resection, and these reports raise the issue of potential intraoperative dissemination of tumor.[62] Cardiotomy suction can be used during the operation, but wall suction should strictly be used during the brief time that the tumor is exposed. The low malignant potential of the vast majority of myxomas and the rarity of metastasis support the authors' current policy of retaining rather than discarding blood, and they believe that most cases of metastatic implantation of myxoma represent a preoperative embolic event.

Minimally invasive approaches to surgical removal

Minimally invasive approaches are being applied with increasing frequency in all areas of cardiac surgery, and cardiac tumors are no exception. Experience is confined to benign tumors and is quite limited. Approaches have included right parasternal or partial sternotomy exposure with standard cardioplegic techniques,[63] right submammary incision with femoral-femoral bypass and nonclamped ventricular fibrillation,[64] and the right submammary port access method with antegrade cardioplegia and ascending aortic balloon occlusion.[65] Thoracoscopic techniques have been used to aid in visualization and removal of ventricular fibroelastomas.[66,67] Myxoma removal is possible via thoracoscopy.[68] Results in this limited number of selected patients have been good, but more experience and longer follow-up are needed before this can be recommended as a standard approach.

Minimally invasive cardiac surgical (MICS) approaches are possible for myxomas and fibroelastomas in appropriate anatomic locations in the right and left atria or AV valves. A right chest (nonsternal) approach is used to gain access to the atria or the ventricles through the mitral or tricuspid valves. Fibroelastomas are also amenable to excision through an MICS approach to the aortic valve and left ventricular outflow tract (LVOT).

MICS approaches are generally performed through a limited right lateral third or fourth intercostal space (ICS) incision (5-8 cm) for exposure of the right and left atria. Exposure of the aortic valve and LVOT is achieved via an upper mini-sternotomy toward the third ICS or anterior thoracotomy with disarticulation of the third rib at the sternum.

In mini-sternotomy approaches, the patient is positioned supine with arms at the side and full exposure to the femoral and axillary spaces. In right lateral approaches, the patient is positioned supine with a bump placed vertically to elevate the right hemithorax, exposing the lateral ribs as well as the axillary and femoral spaces.

Safe and complete cardiopulmonary bypass (CPB) is essential to achieve optimal clinical outcomes. Complete tumor resection, adequate venous drainage, aortic clamping, and complete deairing are essential for a successful result. In left-sided tumors, CPB can be safely performed via femoral vessel Selinger access (percutaneously or cut-down) and multistage venous drainage. In patients wherein right-sided cardiac access is necessary, a separate superior vena cava (SVC) cannula can be inserted and snared separately via the right mini-thoracotomy. Optimal venous drainage is essential for adequate visualization and right ventricular myocardial protection. Arterial cannulation can be performed femorally, directly into the ascending aorta or via the axillary artery.

Myocardial protection in MICS procedures, similar to MICS valve surgery, is dependent on delivery of cardioplegia. Antegrade cardioplegia is usually administered directly into the ascending aorta. Retrograde cardioplegia is performed via direct catheterization of the coronary sinus (CS) through the right atrium. Alternatively, a percutaneous CS catheter can be inserted via a neck approach before surgery. Aortic clamping is optimally performed via standard Chitwood clamp inserted through an axillary stab. Endovascular balloon aortic occlusion may also be performed if the aortotomy is not required. Venting of the left ventricle (LV) may be performed through direct cannulation of the LA/LV via right superior pulmonary vein or percutaneously through PA drainage.

Excellent preoperative imaging (optimally through cardiac magnetic resonance) is necessary to delineate tumor anatomy and involvement before MICS procedures and surgical planning. If performed adequately, MICS tumor resection is a viable and safe option for complete removal of tumors. With these approaches, patients may benefit from decreased transfusions, length of stay, and pain medication requirement.

Results

Removal of atrial myxomas carries an operative mortality of 5% or less. Operative mortality is related to advanced age or disability and comorbid conditions. Excision of ventricular myxomas can carry a higher risk (approximately 10%). The authors' experience over the last 15 years with 85 myxomas shows no operative or hospital mortality.

Recurrence of nonfamilial sporadic myxoma is approximately 1% to 4%.[4,59,60] Many large series report no recurrent tumors.[59,68–71] The 20% of patients with sporadic myxoma and abnormal DNA have a recurrence rate estimated at between 12% and 40%.[4] The recurrence rate is highest in patients with familial complex myxomas, all of whom exhibit DNA mutation, and this is estimated to be about 22%.[4] Overall, recurrences are more common in younger patients. The disease-free interval averages about 4 years and can be as brief as 6 months.[60] Most recurrent myxomas occur within the heart, in the same or different cardiac chambers, and may be multiple.[19,72] Extracardiac recurrence after resection of tumor, presumably from embolization and subsequent tumor growth and local invasion, has been observed.[72,73] The biology of the tumor, dictated by gene expression rather than histology, may be the only reliable factor predicting recurrence. DNA testing of all patients with cardiac myxoma may prove to be the best predictor of the likelihood of recurrence.[74]

Myxomas generally classified as "malignant" are often found on subsequent review to be sarcomas with myxoid degeneration.[75] However, this issue also remains unsettled because of reports of metastatic growth of embolic myxoma fragments in the brain, arteries, soft tissue, and bones.[41,73,76–82] Symptomatic lesions of possible metastatic myxoma should be excised if feasible.[41,76]

The extent to which patients should be subjected to long-term echocardiographic surveillance after myxoma resection is not standardized. It would seem prudent to closely follow patients who are treated initially for multicentric tumors, those whose tumors are removed from unusual locations in the heart, all tumors thought to have been incompletely resected, and all tumors found to have an abnormal DNA genotype. Patients undergoing resection of tumors thought to be myxomas but with malignant characteristics at pathologic examination should have long-term, careful follow-up.

Other Benign Cardiac Tumors

As shown in Table 6.1, myxomas comprise approximately 41% of benign cardiac tumors, with 3 other tumors (ie, lipoma, papillary fibroelastoma, and rhabdomyoma) together contributing a similar proportion. Several rarely encountered tumors account for the remainder.

Lipoma

Lipomas are well-encapsulated tumors consisting of mature fat cells that may occur anywhere in the pericardium, subendocardium, subepicardium, and intra-atrial septum.[2] They may occur at any age and have no sex predilection. Lipomas are slow growing and may attain considerable size before producing obstructive or arrhythmic symptoms. Many are asymptomatic and are discovered incidentally on routine chest roentgenogram, echocardiogram, or at surgery or autopsy.[83,84] Subepicardial and parietal lipomas tend to compress the heart and may be associated with pericardial effusion. Subendocardial tumors may produce chamber obstruction. The right atrium and LV are the sites affected most often. Lipomas lying within the myocardium or septum can produce arrhythmias or conduction abnormalities. Large tumors that produce severe symptoms should be resected. Smaller, asymptomatic tumors encountered unexpectedly during cardiac operation should be removed if excision can be performed without adding risk to the primary procedure. These tumors are not known to recur contrary to other cardiac tumor types (Fig. 6.7).

Lipomatous Hypertrophy of the Interatrial Septum

Nonencapsulated hypertrophy of the fat within the atrial septum is known as *lipomatous hypertrophy*.[2] This abnormality is more common than cardiac lipoma and usually is encountered in elderly, obese, or female patients as an incidental finding during a variety of cardiac imaging procedures.[69] Various arrhythmias and conduction disturbances have been attributed to its presence.[70,85] The main difficulty is differentiating this from a cardiac neoplasm on echocardiography.[86] After the demonstration of a mass by echocardiography, the typical T1- and T2-signal

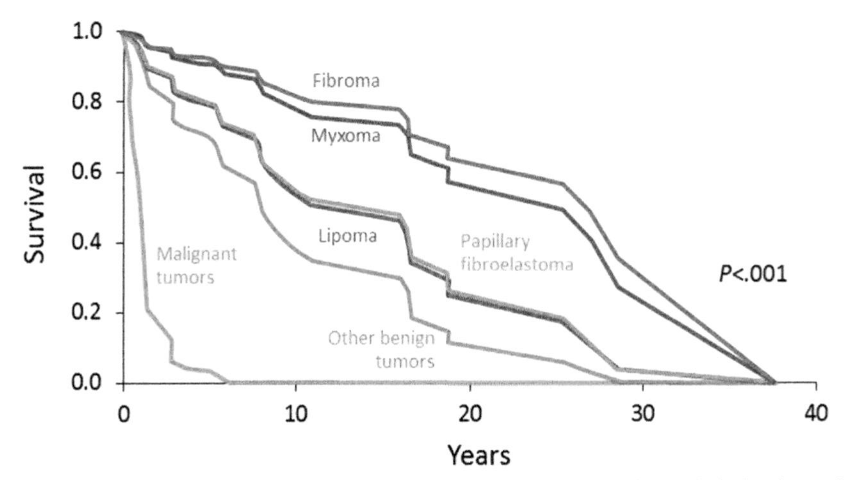

Fig. 6.7 Patient survival after surgical resection based on cardiac tumor type (number included in the analysis = 323). (*From* Elbardissi AW, Dearani JA, Daly RC, et al. Survival after resection of primary cardiac tumors: a 48-year experience. Circulation 2008;118(Suppl 14):S10; with permission.)

intensity of fat on MRI usually can establish a diagnosis.[87,88] Arrhythmias and heart block are considered by some as indications for resection, but data are lacking as to the long-term benefits from resection.[89]

Papillary Fibroelastoma of the Heart Valves

Papillary fibroelastomas are tumors that arise characteristically from the cardiac valves or adjacent endocardium.[90] Cytomegalovirus has been recovered in these tumors, suggesting the possibility of viral induction of the tumor and chronic viral endocarditis.[91] Morphologically these tumors resemble sea anemones with frondlike projections. The AV and semilunar valves are affected with equal frequency. It is now known that these are capable of producing obstruction of flow, particularly coronary ostial flow, and may embolize to the brain and produce stroke.[91–100] They are usually asymptomatic until a critical event occurs. A differential approach has been proposed by some based on location, size, and mobility (see Fig. 6.6). However, one may argue that papillary fibroelastomas of the cardiac valve should be resected whenever diagnosed, and valve repair rather than replacement should follow the resection of these benign tumors whenever technically feasible. Intriguingly, despite resection, patients may still have a lower than expected survival for reasons unknown, which is true for patients with benign cardiac tumors other than myxoma and fibroma (Fig. 6.8).

Rhabdomyoma

Rhabdomyoma is the most frequently occurring cardiac tumor in children. It usually presents during the first few days after birth. It is thought to be a myocardial hamartoma rather than a true neoplasm.[101] Although rhabdomyoma appears sporadically, it is associated strongly with tuberous sclerosis, a hereditary disorder characterized by hamartomas in various organs, epilepsy, mental deficiency, and sebaceous adenomas. Fifty percent of patients with tuberous sclerosis have rhabdomyoma, but more than 50% of patients with rhabdomyoma have or will develop tuberous sclerosis.[102] More than 90% of rhabdomyomas are multiple and occur with approximately equal frequency in both ventricles.[103] The atrium is involved in fewer than 30% of patients. Pathologically, these tumors are firm, gray, and nodular and tend to project into the ventricular cavity. Micrographs show myocytes of twice the normal size filled with glycogen, containing hyperchromatic nuclei and eosinophilic-staining cytoplasmic granules.[2,104] Scattered bundles of myofibrils can be seen within cells by electron microscopy.[103]

Clinical findings may mimic valvular or subvalvular stenosis. Arrhythmias, particularly ventricular tachycardia and sudden death, may be a presenting symptom.[104] Atrial tumors may produce atrial arrhythmias.[104] The diagnosis is made by echocardiography. Rarely, no intramyocardial tumor is found in a patient with ventricular arrhythmias, and the site of rhabdomyoma is located by electrophysiologic study.[104]

Early operation is recommended in patients who do not have tuberous sclerosis before 1 year of age.[71] The tumor usually is removed easily in early infancy, and some can be enucleated.[71] Unfortunately, symptomatic tumors often are both multiple and extensive, particularly in patients with tuberous sclerosis, who, unfortunately, have a dismal long-term outlook. In such circumstances, surgery offers little benefit.

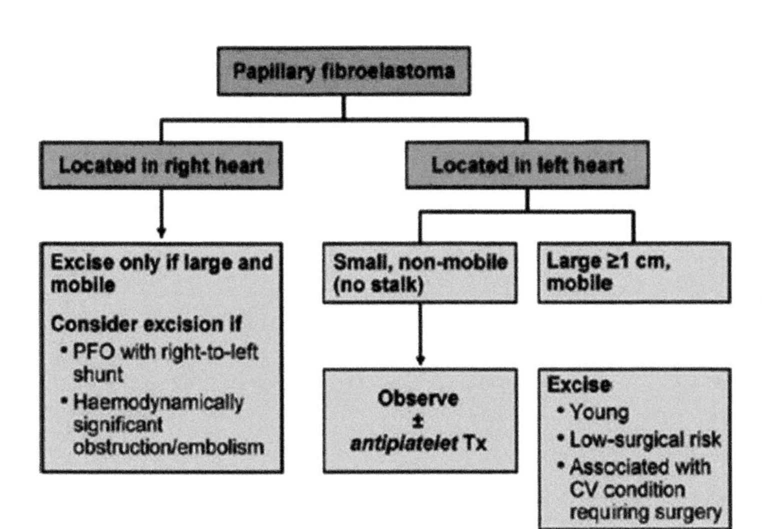

Fig. 6.8 Proposed management algorithm for papillary fibroelastoma based on echocardiographic findings. CV, cardiovascular; PFO, patent foramen ovale; Tx, treatment. (*From* Bruce CJ. Cardiac tumours: diagnosis and management. Heart 2011;97(2):151–60; with permission.)

Fibroma

Fibromas are the second most common benign cardiac tumor, with more than 83% occurring in children. These tumors are solitary, occur exclusively within the ventricle and the ventricular septum, and affect the sexes equally. Fewer than 100 tumors have been reported, and most are diagnosed by the age of 2 years. These tumors are not associated with other disease, nor are they inherited. Fibromas are nonencapsulated, firm, nodular, gray-white tumors that can become bulky. They are composed of elongated fibroblasts in broad spiral bands and whirls mixed with collagen and elastin fibers. Calcium deposits or bone may occur within the tumor and occasionally are seen on roentgenography.

Most fibromas produce symptoms through chamber obstruction, interference with contraction, or arrhythmias. Depending on size and location, such a tumor may interfere with valve function, obstruct flow paths, or cause sudden death from conduction disturbances in up to 25% of patients.[99] Intracardiac calcification on chest roentgenograms suggests the diagnosis, which is confirmed by echocardiogram.

Surgical excision is successful in some patients, particularly if the tumor is localized, does not involve vital structures, and can be enucleated.[71,105–107] However, it is not always possible to remove the tumor completely, and partial removal is only palliative, although some patients have survived many years.[71,106] Operative mortality may be high in infants. Most cases are in adolescents and adults.[105,106,108] Successful, complete excision is curative.[105,106] Children with extensive fibromas have been treated with cardiac transplantation.[107,109]

Mesothelioma of the Atrioventricular Node

Mesothelioma of the AV node, also termed *polycystic tumor, Purkinje tumor,* or *conduction tumor,* is a relatively small, multicystic tumor that arises in proximity to the AV node and may extend upward into the interventricular septum and downward along the bundle of His.[2] Mesothelioma is associated with heart block, ventricular fibrillation,[110] and sudden death. Cardiac pacing alone does not prevent subsequent ventricular fibrillation. Surgical excision has been reported.[9]

Pheochromocytoma

Cardiac pheochromocytomas arise from chromaffin cells of the sympathetic nervous system and produce excess amounts of catecholamines, particularly norepinephrine. Approximately 90% of pheochromocytomas are in the adrenal glands. Fewer than 2% arise in the chest. Only 32 cardiac pheochromocytomas had been reported by 1991.[111] The tumor predominantly affects young and middle-aged adults with an equal distribution between the sexes. Approximately 60% occur in the roof of the LA. The remainder involves the interatrial septum or anterior surface of the heart. The tumor is reddish brown, soft, and lobular and consists of nests of chromatin cells.

Patients often present with symptoms of uncontrolled hypertension or are found to have elevated urinary catecholamines. The tumor is usually located by scintigraphy using (I^{131}) meta-iodo-benzylguanidine[112] and CT or MRI.[112] Cardiac catheterization with differential blood chamber sampling sometimes is necessary in addition to coronary angiography.[111] After the tumor is located, it should be removed using cardiopulmonary bypass with cardioplegic arrest. Patients require preanesthetic α- and β-blockade and careful intraoperative and immediate postoperative monitoring. Most tumors are extremely vascular, and uncontrollable operative hemorrhage has occurred.[112] Resection may require removal of the atrial and/or ventricular wall or a segment of a major coronary artery.[113] Explantation of the heart to allow resection of a large left atrial pheochromocytoma has been attempted.[114] Transplantation has been performed for unresectable tumor and complete excision produces cure.[106,107,109]

Paraganglioma

Paragangliomas are endocrine tumors that can secrete catecholamines. As a result, their presentation is often similar to that of pheochromocytomas. When found within the thoracic cavity, they are located most often in the posterior mediastinum. Paragangliomas typically present with atypical chest pain.[115,116] On echocardiography, they are often large and highly vascular tumors.[117] On cardiac catheterization, they may be intimately associated with the coronary arteries. If they involve the LA, the technique of cardiac autotransplantation may be used to completely resect them.[118,119]

Hemangioma

Hemangiomas of the heart are rare tumors (24 clinical cases reported), affect all ages, and may occur anywhere within the heart.[120,121] These tumors are vascular tumors composed of capillaries or cavernous vascular channels. Patients usually develop dyspnea, occasional arrhythmias, or signs of right-sided heart failure.[122] Diagnosis is difficult, and echocardiography or cardiac catheterization can establish a diagnosis of cardiac tumor by showing an intracavity filling defect.[113] CT and axial T2 weighted MRI should show a high signal mass owing to vascularity. Coronary angiography typically shows a tumor blush and maps the blood supply to the tumor. During resection, meticulous ligation of feeding vessels is required to prevent postoperative residual arteriovenous fistulas or intracavity communications. Partial resections have produced long-term benefits.[120] Tumors rarely resolve spontaneously.[123]

Teratoma

Cardiac teratoma is a rare tumor that typically presents in infants and young children.[124] About 80% of the tumors are benign.[125] These tumors are discovered by echocardiography after a variety of symptoms lead to cardiac or mediastinal evaluation. There is little experience with surgical removal, which should be possible.

Castleman Tumor

Castleman disease is a poorly understood lymphoproliferative disorder. The disease was first described by Castleman and colleagues in 1956.[126] It typically presents as a solitary lesion in the mediastinum. The most common histologic type is hyaline vascular, which accounts for approximately 90% of cases and often behaves in a benign fashion. The more aggressive subgroups are the plasma and mixed-cell types, which have a more malignant behavior.[127] Patients may have a localized or multicentric disease with lymph node involvement, typically in the mediastinum. These tumors typically present as well-circumscribed masses. There have been reports of Castleman disease with myocardial and coronary artery invasion or development of a coronary pseudoaneurysm.[128] In these more aggressive cases, cardiac-assist devices have been used as a bridge to recovery.[128] CT imaging of the lesions reveals atypical or targetlike enhancement that corresponds to various degrees of degeneration, necrosis, and fibrosis. Technetium-99m tetrofosmin and [I^{123}] β-methyliodophenyl pentadecanoic acid (BMIPP) imaging may aid in the diagnosis. On BMIPP, these tumors show reduced uptake compared with the surrounding normal myocardium.[129] Complete surgical resection is considered curative.[130]

PRIMARY MALIGNANT TUMORS

Primary cardiac malignancy is very uncommon, with only 21 surgically treated cases noted in a 25-year surgical experience from 1964 to 1969, combining the experience of 2 large institutions, the Texas Heart Institute and the MD Anderson Cancer Center in Houston.[131] Additional current reports from the Texas Medical Center include a series from the Methodist Debakey Heart and Vascular Center and MD Anderson Cancer Center of 27 patients selected from 1990 to 2006.[131] Approximately 25% of primary cardiac tumors are malignant, and of these, about 75% are sarcomas. McAllister's survey of cardiac tumors found the most common to be angiosarcomas (31%), rhabdomyosarcomas (21%), malignant mesotheliomas (15%), and fibrosarcomas (11%).[2]

Rather than histologic classification of cardiac sarcoma, the authors propose a classification system based on anatomic location. Histology does not greatly affect treatment or prognosis as much as anatomic location.[131,132] The revised classification system divides primary cardiac sarcomas into right heart sarcomas, left heart sarcomas, and PA sarcomas, and these are the categories that will be used in the later discussion.

Right heart sarcomas tend to metastasize early, present as bulky masses, and are characteristically infiltrative.[132] Right heart sarcomas often occupy much of the right atrium, growing largely in an outward pattern, and often avoid heart failure until the latest stage of presentation. This presentation often allows time for neoadjuvant chemotherapy in an attempt to shrink the tumor and sterilize the infiltrating edges to increase chances of obtaining a resection with microscopically negative margins.

Left heart sarcomas tend to be more solid with less infiltration than right heart sarcomas and tend to metastasize later in the course of disease.[133] Left-sided sarcomas are most often located in the LA and tend to grow into the wall. Diminution of blood flow quickly results in life-threatening heart failure. Neoadjuvant chemotherapy can rarely be used because of this presentation. Most left atrial sarcomas are initially clinically diagnosed as myxomas, have a positive resection margin, rapidly recur, and require repeat resection.

Primary malignant cardiac tumors arise sporadically, showing no inherited linkage. Although they may span the entire age spectrum, they usually occur in adults more than 40 years of age. The patients usually present with symptoms of congestive heart failure, pleuritic chest pain, malaise, anorexia, and weight loss.[124,134] The most common symptom has been dyspnea (**Table 6.3**).[135] Some develop refractory arrhythmias, syncope, pericardial effusion, and tamponade.[135] The chest radiograph may be abnormal and even show a mass lesion, but the definite diagnosis usually is made with cardiac echocardiography.[134,136] Right atrial lesions are more frequently malignant (usually angiosarcoma) than

TABLE 6.3
Symptoms of primary malignant cardiac tumors

Symptom	Number	Percentage
Dyspnea	13/21	61.9
Chest pain	6/21	28
Congestive heart failure	6/21	28
Palpitations	5/321	24
Fever	3/21	14
Myalgia	2/21	10

Data from Murphy MC, Sweeney MS, Putnam JB Jr, et al. Surgical treatment of cardiac tumors: a 25-year experience. Ann Thorac Surg 1990;49:612–8.

left-sided lesions (usually myxoma but, when malignant, often malignant fibrous histiocytoma [MFH]). If malignancy is suspected, chest CT or MRI may suggest histology and provide detailed anatomy and help in staging and assessing resectability. The current status of PET scans in evaluating these patients remains controversial. The authors perform cardiac catheterization on all patients older than 40 years of age presenting with intracardiac masses and on all patients with large right atrial masses. Malignancy may be suggested and coronary involvement suspected by tumor blush. This tumor blush is not pathognomonic because the authors have seen a large feeding vessel and tumor blush in a histologically confirmed myxoma.

Unfortunately, primary cardiac malignancy may grow to a large size before detection and involve portions of the heart not amenable to resection. Some of these patients have been considered for transplantation and are discussed later. Otherwise, palliative medical therapy can be attempted with radiation therapy, although success in both symptom relief and longevity has been somewhat limited. Whether the tumor is primary or secondary, the decision to resect is based on tumor size and location and an absence of metastatic spread seen on complete evaluation. Unfortunately, most primary cardiac malignancies that have been referred to the authors' center were considered to be benign initially and were resected incompletely at presentation. If malignancy is suspected or confirmed, and if the lesion appears anatomically resectable and there is no metastatic disease, then resection should be considered. Complete resection will depend on the location of the tumor, the extent of involvement of the myocardium and/or fibrous skeleton of the heart, and histology. If complete resection is possible, surgery provides better palliation and potentially can double survival.[137] After resection, the authors recommend adjuvant chemotherapy and believe that this can improve survival.[125,137] Even with resection and subsequent chemotherapy, survival remains severely limited for primary malignant cardiac tumors (median survival <2 years, 5-year survival 21%) as illustrated in a Mayo Clinic series of 19 patients, including 8 leiomyosarcomas, 6 angiosarcomas, 3 malignant fibrohistiosarcomas, and 2 rhabdomyosarcomas (see Fig. 6.8).

Angiosarcoma

Angiosarcomas are 2 to 3 times more common in men than in women and have a predilection for the right side of the heart. Eighty percent arise in the right atrium.[135,138,139] These tumors tend to be bulky and aggressively invade adjacent structures, including the great veins, tricuspid valve, right ventricular free wall, interventricular septum, and right coronary artery.[138] Obstruction and right-sided heart failure are not uncommon. Pathologic examination of resected specimens demonstrates anastomosing vascular channels lined with typical anaplastic epithelial cells. Unfortunately, most of these tumors have spread by the time of presentation, usually to the lung, liver, and brain.[135] Without resection, 90% of the patients are dead within 9 to 12 months of diagnosis despite radiation or chemotherapy.[7,135] The authors have seen carefully selected patients without evidence of spread on metastatic evaluation who have undergone complete surgical resection with subsequent chemotherapy. In addition to surgical resection of the right atrium, right coronary bypass and even tricuspid valve repair or replacement may be undertaken. The authors have had no hospital mortality in this small group, and most patients die from metastasis rather than recurrence at the local site.[140]

Malignant Fibrous Histiocytoma

MFH is the most common soft tissue sarcoma in adults. Its occurrence as a cardiac primary malignancy has been relatively recently accepted as a specific entity. It is characterized histologically by a mixture of spindle cells in a storiform pattern, polygonal cells resembling histiocytes, and malignant giant cells. The cell of origin is the fibroblast or histioblast.[136,141] It usually occurs in the LA and often mimics myxoma. In fact, every left atrial MFH referred to the authors' institution has been previously incompletely resected when thought to represent a myxoma. The tendency to metastasize early is not as prominent as with angiosarcoma. Several reports document rapid symptomatic recurrence after incomplete resection despite chemotherapy. These patients often die of local cardiac disease before the development of metastases. The authors believe that if complete resection can be obtained (particularly if the malignant nature is recognized and complete resection can be done at the original operation) and adequate chemotherapy can be provided, survival may be improved in this otherwise dismal disease.

Rhabdomyosarcoma

Rhabdomyosarcomas do not evolve from rhabdomyomas and occur equally in the sexes. The tumors are multicentric in 60% of patients and arise from either ventricle. These tumors frequently invade cardiac valves or interfere with valve function because of their intracavitary bulk. Microscopically, tumor cells demonstrate pleomorphic nuclei and spidery, wispy, streaming eosinophilic cytoplasm, usually in a musclelike pattern.

The tumors are aggressive and may invade pericardium. Surgical excision of small tumors may be rational, but local and distant metastases and poor response to radiation or chemotherapy limit survival to less than 12 months in most of these patients.[105,124,125,137,142]

Other Sarcomas and Mesenchymal-Origin Tumors

McAllister and Fenoglio[2] found that malignant mesotheliomas arising from the heart or pericardium and not from the surrounding pleura were the third most common malignant cardiac tumors and that fibrosarcomas were the fourth most common malignant cardiac tumors. However, in the 2 decades since their work, clinicians have rarely encountered these tumors. This apparent decrease in incidence may be related to changes in histologic criteria for classifying primary malignant neoplasms since their study (Table 6.4).[5,120,125,135–137,142,143]

The histology of these tumors can be ambiguous and difficult. These neoplasms can resemble other sarcomas, and some might be deemed fibrous histiocytomas today. The behavior of these tumors is more important, and as with other cardiac sarcomas, resection of small tumors in the absence of known metastasis perhaps is justified, but data are scarce.[7,135,137,142] That being said, it is important to rule out more diffuse thoracic involvement with mesothelioma before considering resection of an isolated cardiac or pericardial mesothelioma. A PET scan may be considered, and any suspicious pleural thickening or effusion should be evaluated carefully both radiographically and histologically.

TABLE 6.4
Primary malignant cardiac neoplasms in adults

Tumor	Number	Percentage
Angiosarcoma	39	33
Rhabdomyosarcoma	24	21
Mesothelioma	19	16
Fibrosarcoma	13	11
Lymphoma	7	6
Osteosarcoma	5	4
Thymoma	4	3
Neurogenic sarcoma	3	2
Leiomyosarcoma	1	<1
Liposarcoma	1	<1
Synovial sarcoma	1	<1
Total	117	100

Data from McAllister HA Jr, Fenoglio JJ Jr. Tumors of the cardiovascular system. In: Atlas of tumor pathology. Washington, DC: Armed Forces Institute of Pathology; 1978.

Myosarcoma, liposarcoma, osteosarcoma, chondromyxosarcoma, plasmacytoma, and carcinosarcoma arising from the heart all have been reported,[143–146] but by the time diagnosis is made, only palliative therapy usually can be offered, and surgery is indicated only occasionally. Regardless of therapy, it is unusual for patients with these diagnoses to survive more than a year.

Right-Sided Cardiac Sarcomas

The prognosis without surgery for right heart sarcoma is dismal, and surgical resection is the only treatment modality shown to increase survival. Complete surgical resection is complicated by both the bulky infiltrative nature of right heart sarcoma and the high incidence of metastatic disease at presentation. The authors' current approach to right heart sarcomas has been to begin with neoadjuvant chemotherapy once a definitive tissue diagnosis of sarcoma is made using a right heart catheterization biopsy. Occasionally, a diagnosis of lymphoma or other tumor is made. Multidisciplinary treatment planning based on the *correct* diagnosis is imperative. After 4 to 6 rounds of chemotherapy (with repeat imaging every other cycle to assess for tumor response), the patient is evaluated for surgical resection. This treatment regimen aims to improve on the current microscopic complete resection rate of 33%. The initial diagnostic test for right heart sarcomas is transthoracic echocardiography, which rarely misses these usually large tumors. Unlike large left atrial masses that are usually benign myxomas, most large right atrial masses are typically malignant. Most right heart sarcomas referred to the authors' specialty center have yet to undergo attempted resection, unlike left-sided heart tumors, which are typically resected under the presumption they are benign myomas. The primary reason for local failure of a right heart sarcoma is incomplete resection, typically because of surgical hesitancy to achieve complete resection because of involvement of the right coronary artery.

Most right heart sarcomas are angiosarcomas.[2] These tumors may occur in the right atrium or the right ventricle but far more commonly arise from the right atrium. They replace the right atrial wall and frequently grow into the cardiac chamber and into adjacent tissues. Right heart tumors tend to be infiltrative and form microscopic "fingers" of tumor extending beyond the margins of gross disease. Diffuse pericardial involvement, right ventricular involvement, or encasement of great vessels or veins often precludes surgical resection. The tricuspid valve, right coronary artery, and up to about 30% of the right ventricular muscle mass may be resected and replaced or reconstructed with reasonable risk to achieve a complete resection. Thus, all patients are evaluated preoperatively with coronary arteriography. In patients treated without surgical resection, the survival is approximately 10% at 12 months.[147] A microscopically negative surgical resection margin has been shown to extend survival[137] and remains standard therapy. Although some patients having a radical resection still locally recur, the leading cause of death is distant metastatic disease. Complete resection followed by adjuvant chemotherapy has been shown to extend survival.[137,147]

Patients with even limited metastatic disease that did not respond well to chemotherapy or who developed new metastatic disease while on treatment are not considered candidates for surgery. Patients with widely metastatic disease are not considered candidates unless palliative surgery because of severe symptoms. Every patient should be referred to oncology for potential continuation of chemotherapy after recovery from surgery.

Based on the anatomic extent of tumor and the needed margins for resection, venous cannulation for cardiopulmonary bypass must be carefully planned and individualized to each patient. Directly cannulating the high SVC for upper body drainage and cannulating directly into the IVC at the diaphragm usually allows adequate exposure for complete inferior resection, but occasionally femoral cannulation aids in exposing the more caudal structures of the right heart. Aortic cannulation is standard, because it is distant from the tumor. The right atrium can be completely resected and replaced with bovine pericardium. If the resection involves the SVC or IVC, a vascular stapler can be used to staple lengthwise, creating a tube from bovine pericardium to re-create the vein segment. One particular area of danger is at the right atrial junction with the root of the aorta, as overzealous resection in this area will result in damage to the fibrous skeleton of the heart, which is characteristically difficult to repair. Incomplete resection leaving gross disease rapidly leads to regrowth of the tumor and should be avoided if at all possible. When right coronary artery involvement is suspected, mobilization of the right internal mammary artery is performed at the beginning of the operation. The right ventricular wall can be simply partially replaced with bovine pericardium or incorporated into a prosthetic tricuspid valve used for valve replacement.

Left-Sided Cardiac Sarcomas

Surgical resection is the most effective therapeutic option for patients with malignant left-sided cardiac tumors. Delay can result in death from obstruction to flow within the heart or embolization, which may occur in as many as 8% of patients awaiting operation. The clinical presentation of patients with primary left heart sarcoma depends on the anatomic location and extent of the tumor and is not influenced by histology. Most primary left heart sarcomas are reported to occur in the LA, a concept supported by the authors' experience; 22/24 (92%) occurred in the LA and 2/24 (8%) occurred in the LV. Most left atrial masses seen by cardiac surgeons are mistaken to be benign myxomas. Every left atrial sarcoma patient referred to the authors' center previously underwent resection for a presumed myxoma that was later found to be a cardiac sarcoma. Each of these cases had rapid reappearance of the left atrial tumor at the site of resection likely representing regrowth of persistent incompletely resected sarcoma. Intracavitary left ventricular tumors are very uncommon and are rarely mistaken for a simple cardiac myxoma. Heart failure caused by obstruction of intracardiac blood flow is the most common and concerning presenting symptom. Heart block from local invasion, arrhythmia, pericardial effusion, distal embolus, fever, weight loss, and malaise are also seen. The mean age of presentation is reported to be 40 years of age.[136] Transthoracic echocardiography is the most common initial diagnostic test. TEE is specifically recommended for in all left-sided cardiac tumors because of increased resolution of left-sided structures. Cardiac MRI and PET/CT scans are also obtained in patients known or suspected to have sarcoma.

Once diagnosed, patients with primary cardiac sarcoma have an often dismal prognosis. When medically treated, the survival at 12 months is less than 10%.[147] Most reports in the literature are either autopsy series or individual case reports or small case series. Operative mortality usually exceeds 20%, and the mean survival is typically around 12 months.[148–150] Many published series focus on primary cardiac sarcoma in general without regard to anatomic location. The Mayo Clinic reported 34 patients over 32 years with a median survival of 12 months.[151] A combined series from the Texas Heart Institute and the MD Anderson Cancer Center reported an actuarial survival of 14% at 2 years in 21 patients over a 26-year period.[144] The authors have previously reported a combined multimodality approach and found a median survival of 23.5 months in 27 patients over 16 years with survival of 80.9% at 1 year and 61.9% at 2 years.[134] Subsequent analyses show histologic type does not influence survival or treatment approach.[152] The major determinant of clinical presentation and surgical approach is anatomic location. Currently, these tumors are grouped based on location, such as PA sarcomas, right heart sarcomas, or left heart sarcomas.[153,154]

The high rate of local recurrence and secondary resections reported in the literature[155] indicate the LA and ventricle present unique anatomic exposure challenges. Complete resection and reconstruction are complicated because of the left heart proximity to vital structures. Often, a surgeon's inability to adequately visualize vital structures and reconstruct leads to an inadequate resection with rapid regrowth of tumor. Typically, left atrial tumors are approached through the interatrial groove. The interatrial groove is often an adequate approach for benign tumors, but is limited for malignant tumors that are often larger and require a more generous margin of resection. The authors have considered complete cardiectomy and orthotopic cardiac transplantation for complete removal of these tumors. Although feasible, this approach requires the availability of a donor and postoperative immunosuppression, both of which present potential problems in patients with cancer. In addition, series using orthotopic cardiac transplantation for this purpose have only shown a median survival of 12 months.[156] Left ventricular tumors can be approached through the aortic valve, the mitral valve, or a ventriculotomy. A transaortic valve approach works nicely for benign tumors[67] but is inadequate for malignant tumors because of their size and the amount of resection needed. A ventriculotomy through normal ventricular muscle is possible, but not ideal. The authors' group adopted the approach of cardiac explantation, ex vivo tumor resection, cardiac reconstruction, and reimplantation of the heart (cardiac autotransplantation), which permits a radical tumor resection and accurate reconstruction.

Cardiac autotransplantation

The technique of cardiac autotransplantation was introduced for cardiac tumors by Cooley and colleagues[114] in 1985 to deal with a large left atrial pheochromocytoma. Although this case was not successful, it introduced the senior author (M.J.R.) to the technique and its potential use for cardiac tumors. The authors' group did the first successful cardiac autotransplant for cardiac sarcoma in 1998,[141] also reporting this for left atrial sarcoma and left ventricular sarcoma.[157] Working closely with the MD Anderson Cancer Center, the Methodist Hospital has now performed more than 35 cardiac autotransplants, with 26 of these for primary cardiac sarcoma.[158]

Cardiac autotransplantation has several fundamental differences from standard orthotopic heart transplantation.[159] In orthotopic heart transplantation, unless a domino procedure is being done, the explanted heart is not to be used and any damage to its structures is inconsequential. To see an autotransplant (including replacement of the mitral valve), please refer to Video 1. Therefore, the cardiectomy can be performed leaving a wide margin of remaining tissue to use in tailoring the heart to be implanted without regard to cutting critical structures such as the CS. Similarly, the donor heart can usually be harvested with extra tissue at its margins to be used to help tailor the implantation, unlike traditional orthotopic heart transplant surgery. The heart must be excised in cardiac autotransplantation in a manner that does not damage any structures that cannot be repaired, cannot be replaced, or are vital to cardiac function. In addition, if the heart is simply excised and reimplanted, loss of workable tissue makes reimplantation more challenging than orthotopic heart transplantation. Cannulation techniques must take into consideration planned explantation. The aorta can be cannulated distally in the transverse arch. Venous cannulation must be directly into the SVC and IVC just below the right atrial junction. This cannulation technique requires greater exposure and mobilization of the

SVC and IVC. After commencing CPB, further mobilization of the SVC and IVC is performed until each is completely free and surrounded with umbilical tapes on a tourniquet. Wide mobilization of the interatrial groove and circumferential mobilization of the ascending aorta and PA follow cannulation. This surgical dissection facilitates both accurate excision of the heart and reimplantation. The ascending aorta is cross-clamped and antegrade cold blood potassium cardioplegia is given (10 cc/kg) to achieve cardiac arrest. The LA is opened at the beginning of cardioplegia, and a sump drain placed to decompress the heart. After cardioplegia and cardiac quiescence, the LA is opened to confirm pathology and appropriateness of autotransplantation. The SVC first divided beyond the right atrial junction. SVC division is followed by IVC division, which should be transected near the right atrial and SVC junction. For each transection, it is important to note the rim of tissue being left behind retracts substantially toward the venous cannulae and an extraordinarily wide rim must be left or reimplantation at the IVC can be exceedingly difficult. The ascending aorta is divided about 1 cm distal to the sinotubular junction, and the PA is divided just proximal to its bifurcation. The LA transection is then completed, dividing the atrium just anterior to the pulmonary veins and on the left side equal distant between the pulmonary veins and the mitral valve and left atrial appendage. Complete left atrial division then allows for removal of the heart, which is placed into a basin of ice slush. The posterior LA is then inspected, and any tumor is widely excised. Bovine pericardium is used for reconstruction, and the pulmonary veins may be individually reimplanted into new orifices cut in the bovine pericardium or left as a cuff, if pathology permits. The anterior LA can be entirely removed, including the mitral valve, leaving only a mitral annulus.

Bovine pericardial reconstruction starts by cutting a hole to match the mitral annulus opening. Mitral valve replacement using pledgeted 2-0 Ticron sutures begins with pledgets placed on the left ventricular side of the annulus, passing through the annulus, through the bovine pericardium, and then through the prosthetic mitral valve. When the sutures are tied, the neo atrial wall is sealed to the valve and annulus. The anterior and posterior bovine pericardium can then be tailored by cutting darts and sewing them together before reanastomosis. Reimplantation is similar to standard cardiac transplantation, beginning with the LA anastomosis. The right atrium is then attached to the IVC, and the right atrium is attached to the SVC. If either of these anastomoses appear to be under excess tension, an interposition graft of Gore-Tex (WL Gore, Flagstaff, Arizona) (expanded polytetrafluoroethylene, ePTFE), Dacron, or crafted pericardial tube graft can be used to bridge the defect successfully. The PA and aorta are reanastomosed in a standard fashion using Prolene suture; warm-blood potassium cardioplegia is given antegrade, and the aortic cross-clamp is removed. The procedure for left ventricular tumors is similar and occasionally requires mitral valve excision or partial excision of the interventricular septum. The interventricular septum can be reconstructed with bovine pericardium, and valve replacement is typically done with a tissue valve. Although these patients are young, a tissue valve is often chosen to avoid anticoagulation. Issues with structural valve deterioration are of less concern because survival is counted now in years rather than decades.

Because of poor survival, lesions requiring a pneumonectomy in addition to cardiac autotransplant should be considered a contraindication to surgery. The need for pneumonectomy can usually be determined preoperatively with cardiac MRI to evaluate restriction of blood flow through the pulmonary veins.

Lymphomas

Lymphomas may arise from the heart, although this is rare.[160] Most of these tumors respond to radiation and chemotherapy, and surgical resection is rarely indicated.[140] Even when complete resection is not possible, incomplete resection has been performed to relieve acute obstructive systems and, when followed with radiation and chemotherapy, has allowed for extended survival in selected patients.

Pulmonary Artery Sarcomas

Most PA sarcomas are classified as pleomorphic or angiosarcoma. The most frequent presenting symptom is shortness of breath and peripheral edema from concomitant right-sided heart failure.[161] The diagnostic modalities of choice for both the initial evaluation and monitoring for recurrence after resection for PA sarcomas are chest CT or MRI.

PA sarcomas are very rare tumors that are often confused with acute or chronic pulmonary embolus. This confusion has led to both delay in diagnosis and many being treated with a tumor thromboendarterectomy approach rather than radical resection. These tumors usually are discovered after they have grown to considerable size. PA sarcoma can present with cough, dyspnea, hemoptysis, and chest pain that may mimic pulmonary embolus (PE). Constitutional symptoms often include fever, anemia, and weight loss, which are more consistent with malignancy than PE, and these mass lesions will not decrease in size with anticoagulation. These tumors tend to arise from the dorsal surface of the main PA just beyond the pulmonary valve.[162] They form from multipotential mesenchymal cells from the muscle remnant of the bulbus cordis[163] in the intimal and subintimal surfaces.[152] The tumor then tends to grow distally along the artery, rarely penetrating the actual wall of the artery but rather distending it. This characteristic is important to note when planning surgical resection. Distal extension can go to the lung parenchyma itself as emboli, infarction, or metastasis.[164] Although survival difference based on cell histology is found in limited cases, that has not been the authors' experience in cardiac sarcoma in general.[161] Surgical resection remains the primary method of treatment in patients with PA sarcoma and the only method shown to increase survival. A staging system has been developed to further classify these patients and determine who should be offered surgical therapy (Table 6.5).

Resection often requires replacement of a portion of the pulmonary root and branch PAs using a pulmonary homograft with or without artificial graft. Pneumonectomy may be required to resect the tumor completely. Because exposure of the right main PA may require division of the aorta and possibly the SVC, one may plan surgical cannulation for cardiopulmonary bypass by using dual venous cannulation with direct SVC cannulation and normal IVC cannulation via the right atrium. Arterial cannulation via the ascending aorta is routine. Both SVC and IVC are isolated with tourniquets to control blood flow into the right heart. Cardiopulmonary arrest is achieved with cold potassium blood cardioplegia. Fortunately, these tumors rarely penetrate the PA wall, allowing reasonable mobilization. The main PA has always been involved in the authors' experience, and the pulmonary valve is involved 30% of the time.[161] The main PAs can be resected out to their first branch points on each side from a median approach. In cases where one PA is relatively free and the other is involved deep into the lung, a pneumonectomy may be required. In this case, the pulmonary veins and main bronchus are dissected and divided before CPB is instituted to avoid bleeding while heparinized. The branch PAs and main PA are mobilized; CPB is instituted, and the involved main PA is divided. In such cases, the involved lung with little blood flow once resected may result in improved hemodynamics, especially after removal of tumor obstructing the contralateral PA. Once each PA has been divided, or in the case of pneumonectomy the lung and main PA are removed, the main PA trunk can be assessed for pulmonary valve involvement. If the pulmonary valve is involved, the entire PA trunk must be removed and replaced by a pulmonary allograft. Removal of the entire PA trunk and replacement by an allograft is similar to mobilization and replacement techniques for a Ross procedure.[164] If the resection of the right and/or left main PA is limited, then the allograft branches may be adequate to span the defect. When tumor extension is too distal for this, a Gore-Tex graft can be used to interpose between the distal right PA resection point to distal left PA resection point and then implantation of the pulmonary allograft into the side of the ePTFE graft is performed. Despite the extensive nature of the resection, separation from CPB has not been difficult. The surgery relieves the patient of severe PA obstruction that is present preoperatively.

TABLE 6.5
Staging system for primary pulmonary artery sarcomas

Stage I	Tumor limited to the main PA
Stage II	Tumor involving one lung plus a main PA
Stage III	Bilateral lung involvement
Stage IV	Extrathoracic spread

The authors have successfully resected PA sarcomas in 10 patients, 3 of whom required concomitant pneumonectomy. There were no in-hospital or 30-day deaths, and all patients were discharged home. The longest survivor currently has lived more than 100 months and has no known disease. In most cases, adjuvant chemotherapy is used, even in the face of clear surgical margins. Radical PA resection is safe and appears to prolong survival compared with minimal or palliative resection. Resection in conjunction with chemotherapy also appears to prolong survival. Currently, recommendations to record such rare tumors in a national registry may allow better analysis of long-term outcomes.

Heart Transplantation

Malignant primary cardiac tumors may grow to a large size before detection. In addition, extensive myocardial involvement or location affecting the fibrous trigone of the heart may make complete resection impossible. Because complete resection yields better results than incomplete resection, orthotopic cardiac transplantation has been considered as a treatment option. Reports of transplantation for several cardiac tumors, including sarcoma,[164–167] pheochromocytoma,[160] lymphoma,[161] fibroma,[121] and myxoma, have appeared. However, the long-term results are uncertain because some patients die from recurrent metastatic disease despite transplantation.[160,161,163] As of 2000, 28 patients had been reported involving orthotopic transplantation for primary cardiac tumors, and of these, 21 had malignant tumors.[163] The mean survival for patients with primary cardiac malignancy was 12 months. Although technically feasible in some cases, orthotopic transplantation is hindered by a scarcity of donor organs and coupled with an extensive recipient list of patients without cancer. In addition, the large size of the tumor when diagnosed often necessitates rapid intervention for progressive congestive heart failure. Finally, the effect of immunosuppression on any remaining malignancy is unknown. In most cases, orthotopic transplantation is reserved for unresectable benign tumors, such as cardiac fibroma.

SECONDARY METASTATIC TUMORS

Approximately 10% of metastatic tumors eventually reach the heart or pericardium, and almost every type of malignant tumor has been known to do so.[2] Secondary neoplasms are 20 to 40 times more common than primary neoplasms.[4,164] Up to 50% of patients with leukemia develop cardiac lesions. Other cancers that commonly involve the heart include breast cancer, lung cancer, lymphoma, melanoma, and various sarcomas.[2,165,166] Metastases involving the pericardium, epicardium, myocardium, and endocardium roughly follow that order of frequency[2] as well (Table 6.6).

TABLE 6.6
Metastatic cardiac disease

Tumor	Total (No.)	Cardiac (%)	Pericardial (%)
Leukemia	420	53.9	22.4
Melanoma	59	34.0	23.7
Lung cancer	402	10.2	15.7
Sarcoma	207	9.2	9.2
Breast cancer	289	8.3	11.8
Esophageal cancer	65	7.7	7.7
Ovarian cancer	115	5.7	7.0
Kidney cancer	95	5.3	0.0
Gastric cancer	3.8	3.6	3.2
Prostate cancer	186	2.7	1.0
Colon cancer	214	0.9	2.8
Lymphoma	75	—	14.6

Data from Perry MC. Cardiac metastasis. In: Kapoor AS, editor. Cancer and the heart. New York: Springer-Verlag Publishers; 1986.

The most common means of spread, particularly for melanoma, sarcoma, and bronchogenic carcinoma, is hematogenous and ultimately via coronary arteries. In addition, metastasis can reach the heart through lymphatic channels; through direct extension from adjacent lung, breast, esophageal, and thymic tumors; and from the subdiaphragmatic vena cava. The pericardium is involved most often by direct extension of thoracic cancer; the heart is the target of hematologous and/or retrograde lymphatic metastasis.[5] Cardiac metastases rarely are solitary and nearly always produce multiple microscopic nests and discrete nodules of tumor cells.[2] Cardiac metastases produce clinical symptoms in only about 10% of afflicted patients.[167,168] The most common symptom is pericardial effusion or cardiac tamponade. Occasionally, patients develop refractory arrhythmias or congestive heart failure. Chest radiographs and electrocardiograms tend to show nonspecific changes, but echocardiography is particularly useful for diagnosis of pericardial effusion, irregular pericardial thickening, or intracavity masses interfering with blood flow.

Surgical therapy is limited to relief of recurrent pericardial effusions or, occasionally, cardiac tamponade. In most instances, these patients have widespread disease with limited life expectancies. Surgical therapy is directed at providing symptomatic palliation with minimal patient discomfort and hospital stay. Drainage of pericardial effusion is most readily accomplished via subxiphoid pericardiotomy, which can be accomplished under local anesthesia if necessary with reliable relief of symptoms, a recurrence rate of about 3%, and little mortality.[166] Alternatively, a large pericardial window in the left pleural space can be created using thoracoscopy, but the authors recommend this only under unusual circumstances.[169] Thoracoscopy can be accomplished with minimal patient discomfort but does require general anesthesia with single-lung ventilation and may be poorly tolerated by patients with hemodynamic deterioration secondary to large effusions.

The mainstay of treatment of metastatic disease is systemic chemotherapy, for example, for renal cell carcinoma and malignant melanoma (Fig. 6.9). Similarly, systemic chemotherapy is the treatment modality of choice for leukemia

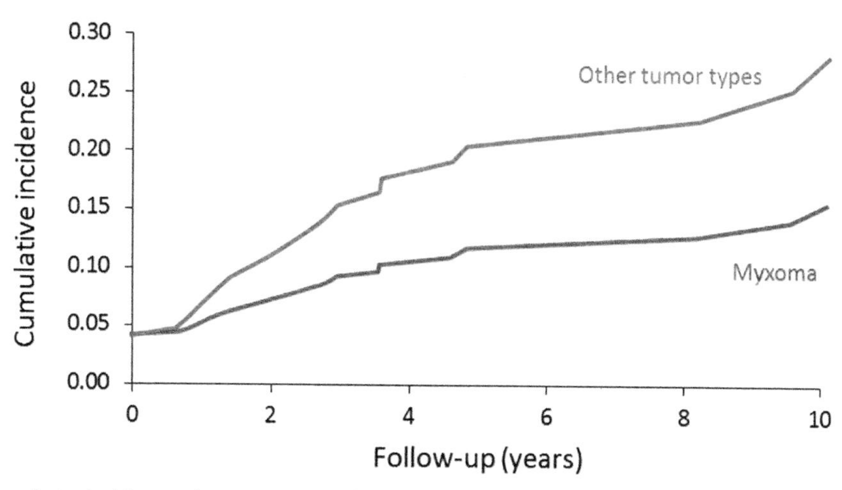

Fig. 6.9 Cumulative incidence of recurrence (number included in the analysis = 288). (*From* Elbardissi AW, Dearani JA, Daly RC, et al. Survival after resection of primary cardiac tumors: a 48-year experience. Circulation 2008;118(Suppl 14):S14; with permission.)

and lymphoma involving the heart, even with curative intent (Figs. 6.10 and 6.11). These hematological lesions are amendable to catheter-based biopsies, which may prove challenging for highly vascularized tumors (Fig. 6.12).

RIGHT ATRIAL EXTENSION OF SUBDIAPHRAGMATIC TUMORS

Abdominal and pelvic tumors on occasion may grow in a cephalad direction via the IVC to reach the right atrium. Subdiaphragmatic tumors are frequently renal carcinomas, although hepatic, adrenal, and uterine tumors occasionally have exhibited this behavior. Up to 10% of renal cell carcinomas invade the IVC, and nearly 40% of these reach the right atrium.[170] Radiation and chemotherapy are not effective in relieving the obstruction of blood flow. If the kidney can be fully removed, as well as the tail of the tumor thrombus, survival can approach 75% at 5 years.[81,171]

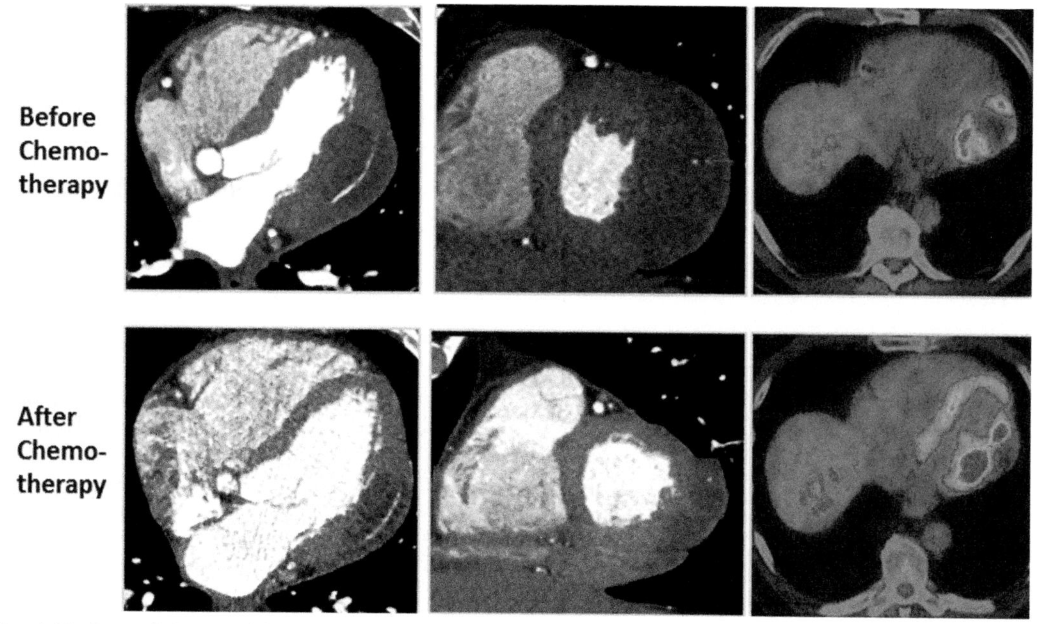

Fig. 6.10 Case of 55-year-old man with malignant melanoma metastatic to the left ventricular lateral wall, embedding the left circumflex artery (*arrow*). Treatment with pembrolizumab proved successful in accomplishing considerable size reduction. (*Courtesy of* Joerg Herrmann, Mayo Clinic, Rochester, MN.)

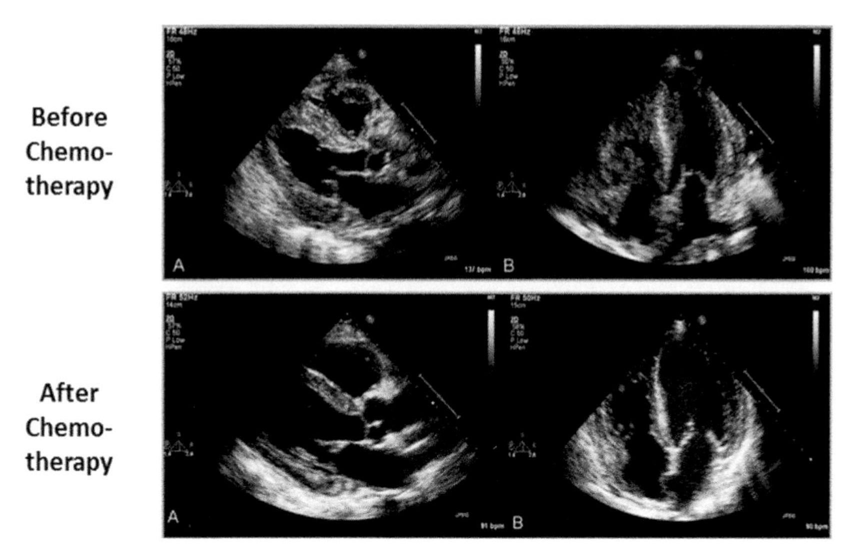

Fig. 6.11 Example of diffuse left ventricular involvement in the setting of cardiac lymphoma with a remarkable response to systemic chemotherapy. (*From* Gaspar A, Salomé N, Nabais S, et al. Echocardiographic assessment of a cardiac lymphoma: beyond two-dimensional imaging. Eur J Echocardiogr 2009;10(8):976; with permission.)

Renal cell tumors with atrial extension typically are resected with abdominal dissection to ensure resectability of the renal tumor. Initially, the authors performed a concomitant median sternotomy and often used cardiopulmonary bypass with hypothermic circulatory arrest when treating these patients. However, they changed the approach and now work closely with liver transplant surgeons who have extensive experience in the area of the retrohepatic vena cava. The authors found that they can expose the vena cava up to the right atrium through an abdominal incision. With ligation of the arterial inflow, the tumor tail often shrinks below the diaphragm, and in almost all circumstances, this can be removed without the use of cardiopulmonary bypass. Occasionally, venovenous bypass as used in hepatic transplantation is necessary to occlude inflow through the IVC, but this is unusual. If the tumor is too complex for this maneuver, then a median sternotomy is performed, and cardiopulmonary bypass with hypothermic circulatory arrest can be used to remove the tumor from the cardiac chambers down into the IVC. Perfusion can be restarted, followed by removal of the rest of the tumor. Although it leads to adequate exposure, significant problems with coagulopathy are often apparent after cardiopulmonary bypass and profound hypothermia.

A 5-year survival rate of 75% has been achieved following nephrectomy with resection of right atrial tumor extension.[171,172] Other subdiaphragmatic tumors with atrial extension that have been resected successfully include hepatic and adrenal carcinoma, as well gynecologic tumors.[108,173–176]

MOLECULAR- AND BIOLOGIC-BASED DIAGNOSIS AND THERAPY FOR CARDIAC TUMORS

This is an exciting time for investigators involved in the search for novel therapies for tumors such

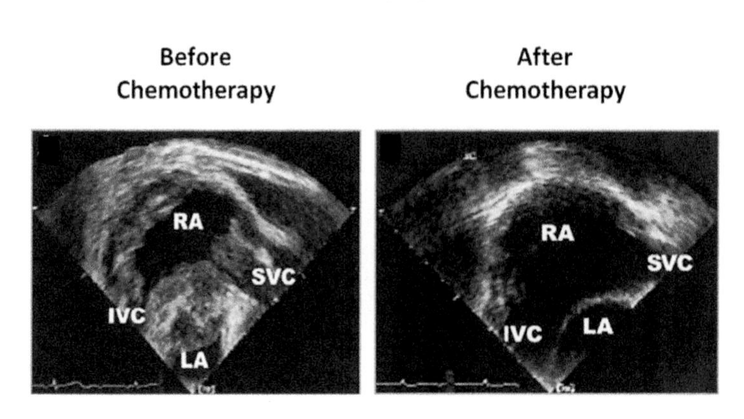

Fig. 6.12 Biatrial masses, confirmed to be cardiac lymphoma, with response to systemic chemotherapy. (*From* Kang SM, Rim SJ, Chang HJ, et al. Primary cardiac lymphoma diagnosed by transvenous biopsy under transesophageal echocardiographic guidance and treated with systemic chemotherapy. Echocardiography 2003;20(1):101–3; with permission.)

as many of those discussed in this chapter. A "new biology" is being developed in laboratories around the world working in these areas, and this is supplanted by the knowledge that is being obtained from the concerted Human Genome Project and the subsequent development of proteomics.[133] It is incumbent on the thoracic surgeon involved in the care of patients with cardiac tumors to have some degree of familiarity with the terms and promise of these advances because significant additional improvement in survival of many of these patients is unlikely to result from further advances in surgical technique.

Interestingly, many sarcomas demonstrate reproducible translocations that allow for the production of novel chimeric genes that may code for a variety of fusion proteins. Many of these proteins have been found to engender cellular phenotypic malignant changes, resistance to apoptosis, and unfettered growth.[170] Although not associated with cardiac involvement, the fusion proteins EWS-FL11 and EWS-ERG are noted in Ewing sarcoma. When full-length antisense oligonucleotide constructs are used to target the mRNA of these proteins, protein expression is downregulated, and an 8-fold increase in apoptosis sensitivity is noted.[177] These fusion proteins have been noted in some forms of rhabdomyosarcoma, and the most common is PAX3-FKHR. This oncoprotein combines components of 2 strong transcriptional activators and may increase the production of the downstream antiapoptotic protein BCL-XL. Antisense oligonucleotides directed at this oncoprotein mRNA have led to apoptosis in rhabdomyosarcoma cells.[178,179] A similar translocation and fusion protein has been noted in fibrosarcoma. This translocation [t(12;15)(p13q25)] brings together genes from chromosomes 12 and 15, which combines a transcription factor with a tyrosine kinase receptor. The resulting fusion protein is a tyrosine kinase that has oncogenic potential.[180] Reproducible translocations and fusion proteins with downstream effectors of malignant behavior have not been described for angiosarcoma, but they are actively being sought.[176] Antisense treatment has been maligned in the past owing to problems with both delivery and stability of therapeutic constructs. However, sophisticated biochemical alteration of these molecules has improved stability, and 2 recent solid tumor trials using antisense therapy for salvage have demonstrated positive results.[181] Additional methods of delivering antisense to tumor cells, including viral vector delivery, have been developed. Finally, in addition to antisense methods, small molecule inhibition of many of these fusion proteins should be possible.

Angiosarcoma is an obvious target for therapies based on antiangiogenesis. The weak antiangiogenic properties of interferon-α are presumed to be the mechanism that accounts for responses to this agent in this tumor.[182] Multiple new antiangiogenic agents are being evaluated currently in phase I and II trials, and several noncardiac angiosarcoma patients have been treated at the authors' institution on this basis. They have noted several to develop stabilized disease, but no definitive data are yet published. Certainly, the use of these agents in these vascular-origin tumors is theoretically attractive.

Viral vector–mediated gene therapy has been evaluated for various sarcomas in the preclinical setting. Several potential targets exist for these sorts of therapies. Although *p53* is not commonly mutated or absent, *mdm-2* is often overexpressed in many sarcomas, including angiosarcoma. This gene is a known oncogene that is able to directly induce cellular transformation. Importantly, when overexpressed, it binds to and inhibits *p53* activity, even though expression of *p53* may appear normal. Overexpression of *mdm-2* also has been associated with vascular endothelial growth factor (VEGF) overproduction and angiogenesis.[182] Preclinical studies of adenoviral *vector p53* transduction of sarcoma in severe combined immunodeficiency mice have demonstrated growth delay, tumor regression, and decreases in VEGF expression.[183] Many other targets for this approach, including inhibition of NF-κB expression using an adenoviral-dominant negative Iκ-βα construct and prodrug-mediated gene therapy using a doxorubicin prodrug and adenoviral transfer of a metabolizing enzyme in sarcoma cells, have been shown to be effective.[173] Unfortunately, the application of viral-mediated gene therapy paradigms to this tumor suffers the same problems of targeting, transgene expression durability, and immune response that are problematic for the field in general.

In regard to molecular diagnosis, there are no reproducible familial patterns for development of most malignant tumors. However, familial cardiac myxoma, rhabdomyoma, and fibroma may exhibit reproducible genetic abnormalities that lend themselves to the development of genetic testing to identify individuals at risk. Familial myxoma syndrome, or Carney complex, has been associated with mutations in the 17q24 gene *PRKAR1a* that codes for the R1 *a* regulatory subunit of cyclic adenosine monophosphate–dependent protein kinase A.[183] Although not widely available, genetic diagnosis of this syndrome is now technically achievable.[184] Reproducible mutations in the *TSC-1* and *TSC-2* genes in patients with tuberous sclerosis and cardiac rhabdomyoma, as well as mutations in the *PTC* gene of patients with the Gorlin syndrome and cardiac fibroma, have been noted.[185–188] It is hoped that in the near future we will be able to predict who is at particular risk for these and other cardiac tumors. Predicting who is at particular risk could allow for more intense surveillance, earlier detection, and a higher rate of surgical or multimodality cure for these patients.

IMPORTANT POINTS

- Complete excision and radical resection are recommended to prevent local recurrence of cardiac tumors.
- All benign cardiac tumors are potentially curable with current surgical techniques.
- Multimodality therapy and multidisciplinary planning should be incorporated into the care of cardiac tumor patients.
- Cardiac sarcomas are best classified by anatomic location rather than histologic subtype, and the former dictates their presentation, treatment, and prognosis.
- Right heart sarcomas tend to be more bulky and infiltrative, metastasize earlier, and are usually amenable to neoadjuvant chemotherapy.
- Left heart sarcomas tend to be more solid, less infiltrative, and metastasize later.
- PA sarcomas usually present with obstruction and right heart failure and tend to grow distally within the confinement of the PA.
- Cardiac tumors located in the anterior left atrial wall may require autotransplantation for complete excision of the tumor, reconstruction, and reimplantation.
- Cardiac autotransplant and concomitant pneumonectomy carry an unacceptable 50% mortality.
- Systemic chemotherapy is the treatment modality of choice for metastatic cardiac lesions and cardiac leukemia/lymphoma.

SUPPLEMENTARY DATA

Supplementary data related to this article can be found online at http://dx.doi.org/10.1016/j.chtm.2016.07.005.

REFERENCES

1. Smith C. Tumors of the heart. Arch Pathol Lab Med 1986;110:371.
2. McAllister HA, Fenoglio JJ Jr. Tumors of the cardiovascular system, in Atlas of tumor pathology, Series 2. Washington, DC: Armed Forces Institute of Pathology; 1978.
3. Straus R, Merliss R. Primary tumors of the heart. Arch Pathol 1945;39:74.
4. Reynen K. Cardiac myxomas. N Engl J Med 1995; 333:1610.
5. Wold LE, Lie JT. Cardiac myxomas: a clinicopathologic profile. Am J Pathol 1980;101:219.
6. Silverman NA. Primary cardiac tumors. Ann Surg 1980;91:127.
7. Waller R, Grider L, Rohr T, et al. Intracardiac thrombi: frequency, location, etiology and, complications: a morphologic review, part I. Clin Cardiol 1995;18:477.
8. Gertner E, Leatherman J. Intracardiac mural thrombus mimicking atrial myxoma in the antiphospholipid syndrome. J Rheumatol 1992;19:1293.
9. Balasundaram S, Halees SA, Duran C. Mesothelioma of the atrioventricular node: first successful follow-up after excision. Eur Heart J 1992; 13:718.
10. Ali SZ, Susin M, Kahn E, et al. Intracardiac teratoma in a child simulating an atrioventricular nodal tumor. Pediatr Pathol 1994;14:913.
11. Carney JA. Differences between nonfamilial and familial cardiac myxoma. Am J Surg Pathol 1985; 64:53.
12. Gelder HM, O'Brian DJ, Styles ED, et al. Familial cardiac myxoma. Ann Thorac Surg 1992;53:419.
13. McCarthy PM, Schaff HV, Winkler HZ, et al. Deoxyribonucleic acid ploidy pattern of cardiac myxomas. J Thorac Cardiovasc Surg 1989;98:1083.
14. Kuroda H, Nitta K, Ashida Y, et al. Right atrial myxoma originating from the tricuspid valve. J Thorac Cardiovasc Surg 1995;109:1249.
15. McAllister HA. Primary tumors of the heart and pericardium. Pathol Annu 1979;14:325.
16. Jones DR, Hill RC, Abbott AE Jr, et al. Unusual location of an atrial myxoma complicated by a secundum atrial septal defect. Ann Thorac Surg 1993;55:1252.
17. Bortolotti U, Faggian G, Mazzucco A, et al. Right atrial myxoma originating from the inferior vena cava. Ann Thorac Surg 1990;49:1000.
18. King YL, Dickens P, Chan ACL. Tumors of the heart. Arch Pathol Lab Med 1993;117:1027.
19. St. John Sutton MG, Mercier LA, Guiliana ER, et al. Atrial myxomas: a review of clinical experience in 40 patients. Mayo Clin Proc 1980;55:371.
20. Burke AP, Virmani R. Cardiac myxoma: a clinicopathologic study. Am J Clin Pathol 1993; 100:671.
21. Peters MN, Hall RJ, Cooley DA, et al. The clinical syndrome of atrial myxoma. JAMA 1974; 230:695.

22. Carney JA, Hruska LS, Beauchamp GD, et al. Dominant inheritance of the complex of myxomas, spotty pigmentation, and endocrine overactivity. Mayo Clin Proc 1986;61:165.
23. Imperio J, Summels D, Krasnow N, et al. The distribution patterns of biatrial myxoma. Ann Thorac Surg 1980;29:469.
24. Kuroki S, Naitoh K, Katoh O, et al. Increased interleukin-6 activity in cardiac myxoma with mediastinal lymphadenopathy. Intern Med 1992; 31:1207.
25. Reddy DJ, Rao TS, Venkaiah KR, et al. Congenital myxoma of the heart. Indian J Pediatr 1956; 23:210.
26. Prichard RW. Tumors of the heart: review of the subject and report of one hundred and fifty cases. Arch Pathol 1951;51:98.
27. Merkow LP, Kooros MA, Macgovern G, et al. Ultrastructure of a cardiac myxoma. Arch Pathol 1969; 88:390.
28. Lie JT. The identity and histogenesis of cardiac myxomas: a controversy put to rest. Arch Pathol Lab Med 1989;113:724.
29. Ferrans VJ, Roberts WC. Structural features of cardiac myxomas: histology, histochemistry, and electron microscopy. Hum Pathol 1973;4:111.
30. Krikler DM, Rode J, Davies MJ, et al. Atrial myxoma: a tumor in search of its origins. Br Heart J 1992;67:89.
31. Glasser SP, Bedynek JL, Hall RJ, et al. Left atrial myxoma: report of a case including hemodynamic, surgical, and histologic characteristics. Am J Med 1971;50:113.
32. Saji T, Yanagawa E, Matsuura H, et al. Increased serum interleukin-6 in cardiac myxoma. Am Heart J 1991;122:579.
33. Senguin JR, Beigbeder JY, Hvass U, et al. Interleukin-6 production by cardiac myxoma may explain constitutional symptoms. J Thorac Cardiovasc Surg 1992;103:599.
34. Buchanan RC, Cairns JA, Krag G, et al. Left atrial myxoma mimicking vasculitis: echocardiographic diagnosis. Can Med Assoc J 1979;120:1540.
35. Currey HLF, Matthew JA, Robinson J. Right atrial myxoma mimicking a rheumatic disorder. Br Med J 1967;1:547.
36. Byrd WE, Matthew OP, Hunt RE. Left atrial myxoma presenting as a systemic vasculitis. Arthritis Rheum 1980;23:240.
37. Hattler BG, Fuchs JCA, Coson R, et al. Atrial myxomas: an evaluation of clinical and laboratory manifestations. Ann Thorac Surg 1970;10:65.
38. Bulkley BH, Hutchins GM. Atrial myxomas: a fifty-year review. Am Heart J 1979;97:639.
39. Panidas IP, Kotler MN, Mintz GS, et al. Clinical and echocardiographic features of right atrial masses. Am Heart J 1984;107:745.
40. Meller J, Teichholz LE, Pichard AD, et al. Left ventricular myxoma: echocardiographic diagnosis and review of the literature. Am J Med 1977;63:81.
41. Desousa AL, Muller J, Campbell RL, et al. Atrial myxoma: a review of the neurological complications, metastases, and recurrences. J Neurol Neurosurg Psychiatr 1978;41:1119.
42. Suzuki T, Nagai R, Yamazaki T, et al. Rapid growth of intracranial aneurysms secondary to cardiac myxoma. Neurology 1994;44:570.
43. Chen HJ, Liou CW, Chen L. Metastatic atrial myxoma presenting as intracranial aneurysm with hemorrhage: case report. Surg Neurol 1993;40:61.
44. Browne WT, Wijdicks EF, Parisi JE, et al. Fulminant brain necrosis from atrial myxoma showers. Stroke 1993;24:1090.
45. Lewis JM. Multiple retinal occlusions from a left atrial myxoma. Am J Ophthalmol 1994;117:674.
46. Eriksen UH, Baandrup U, Jensen BS. Total disruptions of left atrial myxoma causing cerebral attack and a saddle embolus in the iliac bifurcation. Int J Cardiol 1992;35:127.
47. Carter AB, Lowe K, Hill I. Cardiac myxomata and aortic saddle embolism. Br Heart J 1960;22:502.
48. Hashimoto H, Tikahashi H, Fukiward Y, et al. Acute myocardial infarction due to coronary embolization from left atrial myxoma. Jpn Circ J 1993;57:1016.
49. Rajpal RS, Leibsohn JA, Leikweg WG, et al. Infected left atrial myxoma with bacteremia simulating infective endocarditis. Arch Intern Med 1979;139:1176.
50. Whitman MS, Rovito MA, Klions D, et al. Infected atrial myxoma: case report and review. Clin Infect Dis 1994;18:657.
51. Martinez-Lopez JI. Sounds of the heart in diastole. Am J Cardiol 1974;34:594.
52. Harvey WP. Clinical aspects of heart tumors. Am J Cardiol 1968;21:328.
53. Case records of the Massachusetts General Hospital, weekly clinicopathological exercises: case 14-1978. N Engl J Med 1978;298:834.
54. Mundinger A, Gruber HP, Dinkel E, et al. Imaging cardiac mass lesions. Radiol Med 1992;10:135.
55. Ensberding R, Erbel DR, Kaspar W, et al. Diagnosis of heart tumors by transesophageal echocardiography. Eur Heart J 1993;14:1223.
56. Samdarshi TE, Mahan EF 3rd, Nanda NC, et al. Transesophageal echocardiographic diagnosis of multicentric left ventricular myxomas mimicking a left atrial tumor. J Thorac Cardiovasc Surg 1992; 103:471.
57. Bleiweis MS, Georgiou D, Brungage BH. Detection of intracardiac masses by ultrafast computed tomography. Am J Card Imaging 1994;8:63.
58. Symbas PN, Hatcher CR Jr, Gravanis MB. Myxoma of the heart: clinical and experimental observations. Ann Surg 1976;183:470.

59. McCarthy PM, Piehler JM, Schaff HV, et al. The significance of multiple, recurrent, and "complex" cardiac myxoma. J Thorac Cardiovasc Surg 1986; 91:389.
60. Dato GMA, Benedictus M, Dato AA, et al. Long-term follow-up of cardiac myxomas (7–31 years). J Cardiovasc Surg 1993;34:141.
61. Bertolotti U, Mazzucco A, Valfre C, et al. Right ventricular myxoma: review of the literature and report of two patients. Ann Thorac Surg 1983;33:277.
62. Attum AA, Johnson GS, Masri Z, et al. Malignant clinical behavior of cardiac myxomas and "myxoid imitators." Ann Thorac Surg 1987;44:217.
63. Ravikumar E, Pawar N, Gnanamuthu R, et al. Minimal access approach for surgical management of cardiac tumors. Ann Thorac Surg 2000;70:1077.
64. Ko PJ, Chang CH, Lin PJ, et al. Video-assisted minimal access in excision of left atrial myxoma. Ann Thorac Surg 1998;66:1301.
65. Gulbins H, Reichenspurner H, Wintersperger BJ. Minimally invasive extirpation of a left-ventricular myxoma. Thorac Cardiovasc Surg 1999;47:129.
66. Espada R, Talwalker NG, Wilcox G, et al. Visualization of ventricular fibroelastoma with a video-assisted thoracoscope. Ann Thorac Surg 1997;63:221.
67. Walkes JC, Bavare C, Blackmon S, et al. Transaortic resection of an apical left ventricular fibroelastoma facilitated by a thoracoscope. J Thorac Cardiovasc Surg 2007;134(3):793–4.
68. Greco E, Mestres CA, Cartañá R, et al. Video-assisted cardioscopy for removal of primary left ventricular myxoma. Eur J Cardiothorac Surg 1999;16:667.
69. Reyes CV, Jablokow VR. Lipomatous hypertrophy of the atrial septum: a report of 38 cases and review of the literature. Am J Clin Pathol 1979;72:785.
70. McAllister HA. Primary tumors and cysts of the heart and pericardium. In: Harvey WP, editor. Current problems in cardiology. Chicago: Year Book Medical; 1979. p. 76–9.
71. Reece IJ, Cooley DA, Frazier OH, et al. Cardiac tumors: clinical spectrum and prognosis of lesions other than classic benign myxoma in 20 patients. J Thorac Cardiovasc Surg 1984;88:439.
72. Markel ML, Armstrong WF, Waller BF, et al. Left atrial myxoma with multicentric recurrence and evidence of metastases. Am Heart J 1986;111:409.
73. Castells E, Ferran KV, Toledo MCO, et al. Cardiac myxomas: surgical treatment, long-term results and recurrence. J Cardiovasc Surg 1993;34:49.
74. Seidman JD, Berman JJ, Hitchcock CL, et al. DNA analysis of cardiac myxomas: flow cytometry and image analysis. Hum Pathol 1991;22:494.
75. Attum AA, Ogden LL, Lansing AM. Atrial myxoma: benign and malignant. J Ky Med Assoc 1984;82:319.
76. Seo S, Warner TFCS, Colyer RA, et al. Metastasizing atrial myxoma. Am J Surg Pathol 1980;4:391.
77. Hirsch BE, Sehkar L, Kamerer DB. Metastatic atrial myxoma to the temporal bone: case report. Am J Otol 1991;12:207.
78. Kotani K, Matsuzawa Y, Funahashi T, et al. Left atrial myxoma metastasizing to the aorta, with intraluminal growth causing renovascular hypertension. Cardiology 1991;78:72.
79. Diflo T, Cantelmo NL, Haudenschild DD, et al. Atrial myxoma with remote metastasis: case report and review of the literature. Surgery 1992;111:352.
80. Hannah H, Eisemann G, Hiszvzynskyj R, et al. Invasive atrial myxoma: documentation of malignant potential of cardiac myxomas. Am Heart J 1982; 104:881.
81. Rankin LI, Desousa AL. Metastatic atrial myxoma presenting as intracranial mass. Chest 1978;74:451.
82. Burton C, Johnston J. Multiple cerebral aneurysm and cardiac myxoma. N Engl J Med 1970;282:35.
83. Harjola PR, Ala-Kulju K, Ketonen P. Epicardial lipoma. Scand J Thorac Cardiovasc Surg 1985; 19:181.
84. Arciniegas E, Hakimi M, Farooki ZQ, et al. Primary cardiac tumors in children. J Thorac Cardiovasc Surg 1980;79:582.
85. Isner J, Swan CS II, Mikus JP, et al. Lipomatous hypertrophy of the interatrial septum: in vivo diagnosis. Circulation 1982;66:470.
86. Simons M, Cabin HS, Jaffe CC. Lipomatous hypertrophy of the atrial septum: diagnosis by combined echocardiography and computerized tomography. Am J Cardiol 1984;54:465.
87. Basu S, Folliguet T, Anselmo M, et al. Lipomatous hypertrophy of the interatrial septum. Cardiovasc Surg 1994;2:229.
88. Zeebregts CJAM, Hensens AG, Timmermans J, et al. Lipomatous hypertrophy of the interatrial septum: indication for surgery? Eur J Cardiothorac Surg 1997;11:785.
89. Vander Salm TJ. Unusual primary tumors of the heart. Semin Thorac Cardiovasc Surg 2000;2:89.
90. Edwards FH, Hale D, Cohen A, et al. Primary cardiac valve tumors. Ann Thorac Surg 1991;52:1127.
91. Grandmougin D, Fayad G, Moukassa D, et al. Cardiac valve papillary fibroelastomas: clinical, histological and immunohistochemical studies and a physiopathogenic hypothesis. J Heart Valve Dis 2000;9:832.
92. Israel DH, Sherman W, Ambrose JA, et al. Dynamic coronary ostial occlusion due to papillary fibroelastoma leading to myocardial ischemia and infarction. Am J Cardiol 1991;67:104.
93. Grote J, Mugge A, Schfers HJ. Multiplane transesophageal echocardiography detection of a papillary fibroelastoma of the aortic valve causing myocardial infarction. Eur Heart J 1995; 16:426.

94. Gallas MT, Reardon MJ, Reardon PR, et al. Papillary fibroelastoma: a right atrial presentation. Tex Heart Inst J 1993;20:293.
95. Grinda JM, Couetil JP, Chauvaud S, et al. Cardiac valve papillary fibroelastoma: surgical excision for revealed or potential embolization. J Thorac Cardiovasc Surg 1999;117:106.
96. Shing M, Rubenson DS. Embolic stroke and cardiac papillary fibroelastoma. Clin Cardiol 2001; 24:346.
97. Mazzucco A, Bortolotti U, Thiene G, et al. Left ventricular papillary fibroelastoma with coronary embolization. Eur J Cardiothorac Surg 1989;3:471.
98. Topol EJ, Biern RO, Reitz BA. Cardiac papillary fibroelastoma and stroke: echocardiographic diagnosis and guide to excision. Am J Med 1986;80:129.
99. Mann J, Parker DJ. Papillary fibroelastoma of the mitral valve: a rare cause of transient neurologic deficits. Br Heart J 1994;71:6.
100. Ragni T, Grande AM, Cappuccio G, et al. Embolizing fibroelastoma of the aortic valve. Cardiovasc Surg 1994;2:639.
101. Nicks R. Hamartoma of the right ventricle. J Thorac Cardiovasc Surg 1967;47:762.
102. Bass JL, Breningstall GN, Swaiman DF. Echocardiographic incidence of cardiac rhabdomyoma in tuberous sclerosis. Am J Cardiol 1985;55:1379.
103. Fenoglio JJ, McAllister HA, Ferrans VJ. Cardiac rhabdomyoma: a clinicopathologic and electron microscopic study. Am J Cardiol 1976;38:241.
104. Garson A, Smith RT, Moak JP, et al. Incessant ventricular tachycardia in infants: myocardial hamartomas and surgical cure. J Am Coll Cardiol 1987;10:619.
105. Burke AP, Rosado-de-Christenson M, Templeton PA, et al. Cardiac fibroma: clinicopathologic correlates and surgical treatment. J Thorac Cardiovasc Surg 1994;108:862.
106. Yamaguchi M, Hosokawa Y, Ohashi H, et al. Cardiac fibroma: long-term fate after excision. J Thorac Cardiovasc Surg 1992;103:140.
107. Jamieson SA, Gaudiani VA, Reitz BA, et al. Operative treatment of an unresectable tumor on the left ventricle. J Thorac Cardiovasc Surg 1981;81:797.
108. Weinberg BA, Conces DJ Jr, Waller BF. Cardiac manifestation of noncardiac tumors: I. Direct effects. Clin Cardiol 1989;12:289.
109. Valente M, Cocco P, Thiene G, et al. Cardiac fibroma and heart transplantation. J Thorac Cardiovasc Surg 1993;106:1208.
110. Nishida K, Kaijima G, Nagayama T. Mesothelioma of the atrioventricular node. Br Heart J 1985;53:468.
111. Jebara VA, Uva MS, Farge A, et al. Cardiac pheochromocytomas. Ann Thorac Surg 1991;53:356.
112. Orringer MB, Sisson JC, Glazer G, et al. Surgical treatment of cardiac pheochromocytomas. J Thorac Cardiovasc Surg 1985;89:753.
113. Weir I, Mills P, Lewis T. A case of left atrial hemangioma: echocardiographic, surgical, and morphologic features. Br Heart J 1987;58:665.
114. Cooley DA, Reardon MJ, Frazier OH, et al. Human cardiac explantation and autotransplantation: application in a patient with a large cardiac pheochromocytoma. J Tex Heart Inst 1985;2:171.
115. Mirza M. Angina-like pain and normal coronary arteries: uncovering cardiac syndromes that mimic CAD. Postgrad Med 2005;117:41.
116. Pac-Ferrer J, Uribe-Etxebarria N, Rumbero JC, et al. Mediastinal paraganglioma irrigated by coronary vessels in a patient with an atypical chest pain. Eur J Cardiothorac Surg 2003;24:662.
117. Turley AJ, Hunter S, Stewart MJ. A cardiac paraganglioma presenting with atypical chest pain. Eur J Cardiothorac Surg 2005;28:352.
118. Can KM, Pontefract D, Andrews R, et al. Paraganglioma of the left atrium. J Thorac Cardiovasc Surg 2001;122:1032.
119. Ramlawi B, David EA, Kim MP, et al. Contemporary surgical management of cardiac paragangliomas. Ann Thorac Surg 2012;93(6):1972–6.
120. Bizard C, Latremouille C, Jebara VA, et al. Cardiac hemangiomas. Ann Thorac Surg 1993;56:390.
121. Grenadier E, Margulis T, Plauth WH, et al. Huge cavernous hemangioma of the heart: a completely evaluated case report and review of the literature. Am Heart J 1989;117:479.
122. Soberman MS, Plauth WH, Winn KJ, et al. Hemangioma of the right ventricle causing outflow tract obstruction. J Thorac Cardiovasc Surg 1988;96:307.
123. Palmer TC, Tresch DD, Bonchek LI. Spontaneous resolution of a large cavernous hemangioma of the heart. Am J Cardiol 1986;58:184.
124. Thomas CR, Johnson GW, Stoddard MF, et al. Primary malignant cardiac tumors: update 1992. Med Pediatr Oncol 1992;20:519.
125. Poole GV, Meredith JW, Breyer RH, et al. Surgical implications in malignant cardiac disease. Ann Thorac Surg 1983;36:484.
126. Castleman B, Iverson L, Menendez VP. Localized mediastinal lymph node hyperplasia resembling thymoma. Cancer 1956;9:822.
127. Keller AR, Hochholzer L, Castleman B. Hyaline-vascular and plasma-cell types of giant lymph node hyperplasia of the mediastinum and other locations. Cancer 1972;29:670–83.
128. Malaisrie SC, Loebe M, Walkes JC, et al. Coronary pseudoaneurysm: an unreported complication of Castleman's disease. Ann Thorac Surg 2006;82(1): 318–20.
129. Ko SF, Wan WL, Ng SH, et al. Imaging features of atypical thoracic Castleman's disease. Clin Imaging 2004;28:280.
130. Samuels LE. Castleman's disease: surgical implications. Surg Rounds 1997;20:449.

131. Murphy MC, Sweeney MS, Putnam JB Jr, et al. Surgical treatment of cardiac tumors: a 25-year experience. Ann Thorac Surg 1990;49:612.
132. Bakaeen F, Jaroszewski DE, Rice DC, et al. Outcomes after surgical resection of cardiac sarcoma in the multimodality treatment era. J Cardiovasc Surg 2009;137:1454–60.
133. Caccavale RJ, Newman J, Sisler GE, et al. Pericardial disease. In: Kaiser LR, Daniel TM, editors. Thorascopic surgery. Boston: Brown; 1993. p. 177.
134. Blackmon SH, Patel A, Reardon MJ. Management of primary cardiac sarcomas. Expert Rev Cardiovasc Ther 2008;6(9):1217–22.
135. Bear PA, Moodie DS. Malignant primary cardiac tumors: the Cleveland Clinic experience, 1956–1986. Chest 1987;92:860.
136. Burke AP, Cowan D, Virmani R. Primary sarcomas of the heart. Cancer 1922;69:387.
137. Putnam JB, Sweeney MS, Colon R, et al. Primary cardiac sarcomas. Ann Thorac Surg 1991;51:906.
138. Rettmar K, Stierle U, Shiekhzadeh A, et al. Primary angiosarcoma of the heart: report of a case and review of the literature. Jpn Heart J 1993;34:667.
139. Hermann MA, Shankerman RA, Edwards WD, et al. Primary cardiac angiosarcoma: a clinicopathologic study of six cases. J Thorac Cardiovasc Surg 1992; 102:655.
140. Wiske PS, Gillam LD, Blyden G, et al. Intracardiac tumor regression documented by two-dimensional echocardiography. Am J Cardiol 1986;58:186.
141. Reardon MJ, DeFelice CA, Sheinbaum R, et al. Cardiac autotransplant for surgical treatment of a malignant neoplasm. Ann Thorac Surg 1999;67: 1793.
142. Miralles A, Bracamonte MD, Soncul H, et al. Cardiac tumors: clinical experience and surgical results in 74 patients. Ann Thorac Surg 1991; 52:886.
143. Winer HE, Kronzon I, Fox A, et al. Primary chondromyxosarcoma: clinical and echocardiographic manifestations: a case report. J Thorac Cardiovasc Surg 1977;74:567.
144. Torsveit JF, Bennett WA, Hinchcliffe WA, et al. Primary plasmacytoma of the atrium: report of a case with successful surgical management. J Thorac Cardiovasc Surg 1977;74:563.
145. Nzayinambabo K, Noel H, Brobet C. Primary cardiac liposarcoma simulating a left atrial myxoma. J Thorac Cardiovasc Surg 1985;40:402.
146. Burke AP, Virmani R. Osteosarcomas of the heart. Am J Surg Pathol 1991;15:289.
147. Neragi-Miandoab S, Kim J, Vlahakes GJ. Malignant tumours of the heart: a review of tumour type, diagnosis and therapy. Clin Oncol (R Coll Radiol) 2007;19:748–56.
148. Centofani P, Di Rosa E, Deorsola L, et al. Primary cardiac tumors: early and late results of surgical treatment in 91 patients. Ann Thorac Surg 1999; 68:1236–41.
149. Zhang PJ, Brooks JS, Goldblum JR, et al. Primary cardiac sarcomas: a clinicopathologic analysis of a series with follow-up information in 17 patients and emphasis on long-term survival. Hum Pathol 2008;39:1385–95.
150. Bossert Torsten B, Gummert JF, Battellini, et al. Surgical experience with 77 primary cardiac tumors. Interact Cardiovasc Torac Surg 2005;4:311–5.
151. Simpson L, Kumar SK, Okuno SH, et al. Malignant primary cardiac tumors: review of a single institution experience. Cancer 2008;112(11): 2440–6.
152. Kim CH, Dancer JY, Coffey D, et al. Clinicopathologic study of 24 patients with primary cardiac sarcomas: a 10-year single institution experience. Hum Pathol 2008;39:933–8.
153. Blackmon SH, Patel AR, Bruckner BA, et al. Cardiac autotransplantation for malignant or complex primary left heart tumors. Tex Heart Inst J 2008; 35(3):296–300.
154. Ramlawi B, Leja MJ, Abu Saleh WK, et al. Surgical treatment of primary cardiac sarcomas: review of a single-institution experience. Ann Thorac Surg 2016 Feb;101(2):698–702.
155. Gabelman C, Al-Sadir J, Lamberti J, et al. Surgical treatment of recurrent primary malignant tumor of the left atrium. J Thorac Cardiovasc Surg 1979; 77(6):914–21.
156. Gowdamarajan A, Michler RE. Therapy for primary cardiac tumors: is there a role for heart transplantation? Curr Opin Cardiol 2000;15:121.
157. Reardon MJ, Walkes JC, DeFelice CA, et al. Cardiac auto-transplant for surgical resection of a primary malignant left ventricular tumor. Tex Heart Inst J 2006;33(4):495–7.
158. Ramlawi B, Al-Jabbari O, Blau LN, et al. Autotransplantation for the resection of complex left heart tumors. Ann Thorac Surg 2014;98:863–8.
159. Conklin LD, Reardon MJ. Autotransplantation of the heart for primary cardiac malignancy: development and surgical technique. Tex Heart Inst J 2002;29(2):105–8.
160. Takagi M, Kugimiya T, Fuii T, et al. Extensive surgery for primary malignant lymphoma of the heart. J Cardiovasc Surg 1992;33:570.
161. Blackmon SH, Rice DR, Correa AM, et al. Management of primary main pulmonary artery sarcomas. Ann Thorac Surg 2009;87(3):977–84.
162. Baker PB, Goodwin RA. Pulmonary artery sarcomas: a review and report of a case. Arch Pathol Lab Med 1985;109:35–9.
163. Schmookler BM, Marsh HB, Roberts WC. Primary sarcoma of the pulmonary trunk and/or right or left main pulmonary artery: a rare cause of obstruction to right ventricular outflow: report on two

patients and analysis of 35 previously described patients. Am J Med 1977;63:263–72.
164. Conklin LD, Reardon MJ. The technical aspects of the Ross procedure. Tex Heart Inst J 2001;28(3):186–9.
165. Golstein DJ, Oz MC, Rose EA, et al. Experience with heart transplantation for cardiac tumors. J Heart Lung Transplant 1995;14:382.
166. Baay P, Karwande SV, Kushner JP, et al. Successful treatment of a cardiac angiosarcoma with combined modality therapy. J Heart Lung Transplant 1994;13:923.
167. Crespo MG, Pulpon LA, Pradas G, et al. Heart transplantation for cardiac angiosarcoma: should its indication be questioned? J Heart Lung Transplant 1993;12:527.
168. Jeevanandam V, Oz MC, Shapiro B, et al. Surgical management of cardiac pheochromocytoma: resection versus transplantation. Ann Surg 1995; 221:415.
169. Yuh DD, Kubo SH, Francis GS, et al. Primary cardiac lymphoma treated with orthotopic heart transplantation: a case report. J Heart Lung Transplant 1994;13:538.
170. Prager RL, Dean R, Turner B. Surgical approach to intracardial renal cell carcinoma. Ann Thorac Surg 1982;33:74.
171. Aburto J, Bruckner BA, Blackmon SH, et al. Renal cell carcinoma, metastatic to the left ventricle. Tex Heart Inst J 2009;36(1):48–9.
172. Pillai R, Blauth C, Peckham M, et al. Intracardiac metastasis from malignant teratoma of the testis. J Thorac Cardiovasc Surg 1986;92:118.
173. Hallahan ED, Vogelzang NJ, Borow KM, et al. Cardiac metastasis from soft-tissue sarcomas. J Clin Oncol 1986;4:1662.
174. Press OW, Livingston R. Management of malignant pericardial effusion and tamponade. JAMA 1987;257:1008.
175. Hanfling SM. Metastatic cancer to the heart: review of the literature and report of 127 cases. Circulation 1960;2:474.
176. Cooper MM, Guillem J, Dalton J, et al. Recurrent intravenous leiomyomatosis with cardiac extension. Ann Thorac Surg 1992;53:139.
177. Goldstein DJ, Oz MC, Michler RE. Radical excisional therapy and total cardiac transplantation for recurrent atrial myxoma. Ann Thorac Surg 1995;60:1105.
178. Vaislic CD, Puel P, Grondin P, et al. Cancer of the kidney invading the vena cava and heart: results after 11 years of treatment. J Thorac Cardiovasc Surg 1986;91:604.
179. Shahian DM, Libertino JA, Sinman LN, et al. Resection of cavoatrial renal cell carcinoma employing total circulatory arrest. Arch Surg 1990;125:727.
180. Theman TE. Resection of atriocaval adrenal carcinoma (letter). Ann Thorac Surg 1990;49:170.
181. Phillips MR, Bower TC, Orszulak TA, et al. Intracardiac extension of an intracaval sarcoma of endometrial origin. Ann Thorac Surg 1995;59:742.
182. Tomescu O, Barr F. Chromosomal translocations in sarcomas: prospects for therapy. Trends Mol Med 2001;7:554.
183. Graadt van Roggen JF, Bovee JVMG, Morreau J, et al. Diagnostic and prognostic implications of the unfolding molecular biology of bone and soft tissue tumors. J Clin Pathol 1999;52:481.
184. Waters JS, Webb A, Cunningham D, et al. Phase I clinical and pharmacokinetic study of BCL-2 antisense oligonucleotide therapy in patients with non-Hodgkin's lymphoma. J Clin Oncol 2000;18: 1812.
185. Casey M, Vaughan CJ, He J, et al. Mutations in the protein kinase R1α regulatory subunit cause familial cardiac myxomas and Carney complex. J Clin Invest 2000;106:R31.
186. Goldstein MM, Casey M, Carney JA, et al. Molecular genetic diagnosis of the familial myxoma syndrome (Carney complex). Am J Med Genet 1999; 86:62.
187. Van Siegenhorst M, de Hoogt R, Hermans C, et al. Identification of the tuberous sclerosis gene TSC1 on chromosome 9q34. Science 1997;277:805.
188. The European Chromosome 16 Tuberous Sclerosis Consortium. Identification and characterization of the tuberous sclerosis gene on chromosome 16. Cell 1993;75:1305.

CHAPTER 7

Subtypes of Cancer Involving the Heart

Richard M. Steingart, MD*, Carol Chen, MD, Jennifer Liu, MD

CARCINOID

Introduction

Carcinoid tumors are rare, slow-growing malignancies originating from neuroendocrine cells usually within the gastrointestinal tract.[1] Surgical resection of localized tumors is considered curative, and hepatic cytoreduction via surgery or embolization for metastatic disease improves survival and quality of life over medical therapy.[2,3] Carcinoid syndrome (CS) due to the release of vasoactive hormones, predominantly serotonin, by tumor cells is characterized by episodes of flushing, hypertension, hypotension, diarrhea, and bronchospasm. CS occurs in 50% of patients with carcinoid tumors. Medical treatment is mainly limited to the use of a somatostatin analogue, such as depot octreotide, which binds to somatostatin receptors on tumor cells, slowing growth and decreasing hormone release. Circulating vasoactive hormones cause fibrosis of the valvular apparatus, which defines carcinoid heart disease (CHD). Severe tricuspid regurgitation from retracted tricuspid leaflets, pulmonic stenosis, and regurgitation is the most common valvular finding. These hormones are deactivated in the pulmonary bed, and thus, left-sided valvular dysfunction is seen in less than 10% of CHD. The presence of left-sided CHD suggests a patent foramen ovale (PFO) with right-to-left shunt or very high hormone levels.

Carcinoid Heart Disease

The diagnosis of CHD is important because its presence negatively impacts clinical outcome.[4–6] Patients who have significant CS symptoms suggesting high serum serotonin levels generally develop CHD within 1 to 2 years of the onset of CS. Fifty percent to 60% of patients with CS will develop CHD, and 20% may present with cardiac involvement at diagnosis.[7] Severe tricuspid regurgitation is a main predictor of an overall poor prognosis.[8] In one study, mean survival was decreased by 3 years in patients with CHD compared with those without.[4] Serotonin is thought to mediate CHD, and elevated levels of serum or urine 5-HIAA, its main metabolite, may indicate those who are at increased risk of progression or development of CHD. Several studies have shown that patients with increased levels of 5-HIAA (urine values >300 umol/24 hours or 50% increase over baseline serum value) and greater than 3 flushing episodes daily should be assessed for the development and progression of CHD.[9–11]

Clinical Findings

Clinical symptoms of worsening dyspnea, exercise tolerance, and peripheral edema despite good CS symptom control should increase suspicion for right heart compromise as a result of CHD. Significant tricuspid regurgitation may manifest as complaints of fullness in the neck and abdomen. On physical examination, a prominent V wave in jugular venous pulsation, holosystolic murmur at the right sternal border, and pulsatile hepatomegaly are consistent with severe tricuspid regurgitation. As the right ventricle dilates and fails, a right ventricular heave at the sternum and lower extremity edema occur.

Diagnostic Testing

A detailed transthoracic echocardiogram (TTE) is the gold standard for diagnosis and serial follow-up of CHD (Box 7.1). Several groups propose baseline echocardiography with a follow-up study if a new murmur or symptoms of right heart dysfunction are detected.[4,12] Some advocate for percutaneous closure of all PFO due to worsened prognosis of left-sided valve involvement.[12,13] Transesophageal echocardiography may be

Memorial Sloan Kettering Cancer Center, Weill Medical College of Cornell University, New York, NY, USA
* Corresponding author. 1275 York Avenue. New York, NY 10065
E-mail address: steingar@mskcc.org

BOX 7.1
Echocardiography findings of carcinoid heart disease

Tricuspid valve

Fixed, retracted thickening of leaflets, failure to coapt. Doppler signs of severe tricuspid regurgitation: early peaking, dagger-shaped profile

Pulmonic valve

Shortened and retracted leaflets. Stenosis: peak velocity >4 m/s. May be underestimated in the presence of low cardiac output and severe tricuspid regurgitation. Regurgitation: Short deceleration time

Right ventricle

Chamber enlargement and systolic dysfunction

PFO

Agitated venous saline injection with Valsalva maneuver. May become evident as right atrium enlarges

Left sided

Fibrosis and retraction of leaflets unusual, look for PFO

performed if TTE imaging is insufficient for diagnosis. Several echocardiographic and clinical scoring systems have been proposed to improve recognition of disease progression, decrease interobserver variability, and improve timing of referral for surgery; however, all seem equivalent in sensitivity and specificity.[8,14–16] Biomarkers, such as NT proBNP, chromogranin A, and 5-HIAA levels, are also being suggested as a more cost-efficient way to screen for CHD.[16] Cardiac MRI may be a useful adjunct imaging modality to more accurately assess and follow right heart size and function as well as assess for endocardial metastases, which may be resected during cardiac surgery.[17]

Treatment

Mild CHD symptoms can generally be treated with diuretics, salt restriction, and compression stockings. Decreasing tumor burden by hepatic resection appears to improve overall quality of life, slow progression of malignancy, and may possibly also decrease the risk of progression of CHD by reducing circulating hormones.[11,18] Treatment with octreotide has not been shown to slow or reverse CHD.[10,15] Worsening exercise capacity, progressive fatigue, and progressive decline in right ventricular function in the setting of controlled tumor burden are indications to consider valve surgery.[19] It is imperative to confirm control of patient's tumor burden and CS with the patient's oncologist before considering valve surgery. The mortality and morbidity of cardiac surgery for CHD are higher than general cardiac surgery, up to 20% in recent studies.[20,21] A Mayo Clinic study shows a decrease in morbidity from 25% in the 1980s to 8% in 2000, likely due to increased experience managing perioperative carcinoid crisis as well as improved patient selection.[6] This finding supports the overall shift to identify patients with early CHD to offer valvular surgery before development of severe right heart failure (HF), which increases surgical mortality.[21] A contemporary study of cardiac surgery in CHD showed that late deaths were due to metastatic carcinoid disease not HF, and patients experienced significant improvement in functional class.[21] Tricuspid valve replacement and not repair is recommended due to destruction of subvalvular apparatus and leaflets. Both tricuspid and pulmonic valves should be carefully assessed to plan the optimal surgery. In earlier times, mechanical prosthesis was recommended because of concern for bioprosthetic valve destruction by vasoactive peptides. The coagulopathy of hepatic disease and frequency of repeated hepatic surgery increase the risks associated with mechanical prostheses. With the use of octreotide, longevity of bioprostheses in this population has been deemed acceptable.[21] Valvular surgery for patients with right HF has allowed for safer hepatic resection because high right-sided pressures often preclude surgery because of increased bleeding risk in the hepatic bed.[22] As the right heart dilates, a PFO may allow for right-to-left shunting. If a PFO is present, this may also be closed during cardiac surgery to decrease shunting and left heart involvement.

Anesthesia for any surgery, but especially cardiac surgery, is complex for these patients because of risk of carcinoid crisis. Histamine-releasing neuromuscular relaxants, such as atracurium, mivacurium, succinylcholine; barbiturates, such as thiopental; opioids, such as morphine and meperidine; and vasopressors, such as epinephrine, norepinephrine, and dopamine, are known to precipitate carcinoid crisis with potentially fatal consequences, such as hypotension, flushing, tachycardia, arrhythmia, bronchoconstriction, and low cardiac output syndrome. Alternate anesthetic agents should be used. Usual anesthesia treatments for intraoperative hypotension may worsen patient status. A bolus of 50 to 100 μg octreotide before any anesthesia with a continuous infusion at 50 μg per hour for up to 48 or 72 hours is recommended. Any clinical signs of carcinoid crisis should be treated with additional boluses of octreotide. Octreotide may suppress insulin, and blood glucose levels should be followed in patients who have diabetes or obesity. Phenylephrine is the preferred vasopressor if necessary.[23–25] All of these precautions should also be used for patients undergoing tumor ablation or embolization as well.

CARDIAC AMYLOID

Cardiac amyloidosis refers to a condition characterized by extracellular amyloid deposition throughout the heart caused by different types of amyloid. The frequency and severity of cardiac involvement vary by amyloid fibril precursor. Cardiac involvement occurs invariably in familial or senile (ATTR) amyloidosis and in 50% of cases of light-chain (AL) amyloidosis.[26] This section is devoted exclusively to cardiac amyloid associated with light chain disease.

Extent and severity of cardiac involvement are often strong determinants of prognosis. Prompt recognition of the disease and initiation of therapy are critical for survival prognosis but often do not occur. Establishing the diagnosis of amyloidosis is frequently delayed due to the insidious development of multisystemic symptoms because patients often see multiple specialists before undergoing the tissue biopsy that leads to the diagnosis.

Diagnosis of Cardiac Amyloidosis

Endomyocardial biopsy is the gold standard for the diagnosis of cardiac amyloid, although not routinely performed as a first-line test. Cardiac involvement can be reasonably inferred in many cases based on clinical features and typical noninvasive test appearance of cardiac amyloidosis, provided that the histologic diagnosis has been made from another tissue.

Noninvasive evaluation

Electrocardiographic abnormalities occur frequently in patients with cardiac amyloid. Low-voltage and pseudo-infarct pattern, which represent myocardial replacement with electrically inactive amyloid fibrils, most commonly occur in 50% of cases of AL cardiac amyloidosis. Other abnormalities include 1° atrioventricular (AV) block, nonspecific intraventricular delay, and 2° or 3° AV block. In a large electrocardiographic series, atrial fibrillation was present in 20% and ventricular tachycardia in 5% of patients with AL amyloidosis and biopsy-proven cardiac involvement.[27]

Echocardiography is the diagnostic test of choice for cardiac amyloidosis and should be obtained as early as possible if amyloid is suspected. Classic echocardiographic findings, which include increased left ventricular (LV) wall thickness, normal or decreased LV cavity size, and dilated atria, are commonly present only in the later stages of cardiac amyloidosis (Fig. 7.1). However, these findings may also exist in hypertensive heart disease, hypertrophic cardiomyopathy, and other forms of infiltrative cardiac disease (glycogen storage disease, sarcoidosis, hemochromatosis). Low

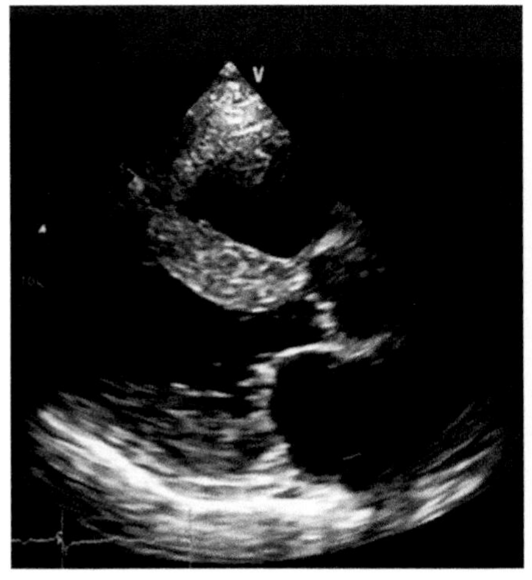

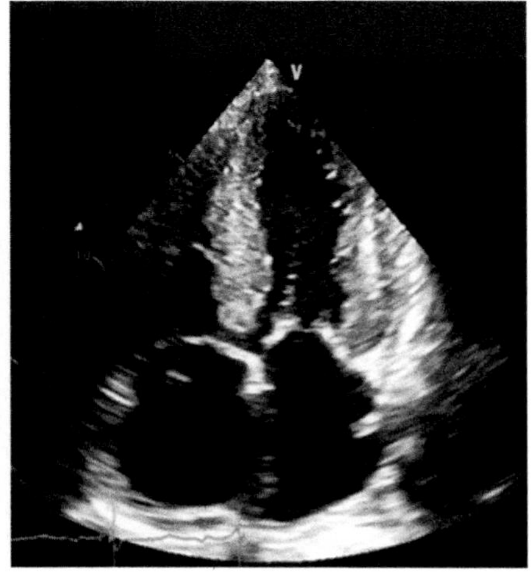

Fig. 7.1 Echocardiographic images from a patient with AL cardiac amyloid. (*left*) Parasternal long axis shows concentric LV thickening with echogenic-appearing myocardium and minimal pericardial effusion. (*right*) Apical 4-chamber view shows mildly reduced LV cavity size with biatrial enlargement.

voltage on the electrocardiogram coupled with LV hypertrophy by echocardiography or MRI is characteristic of cardiac amyloid involvement. Speckled or granular appearance of the myocardium is often associated with amyloid heart disease but is nonspecific and dependent on echocardiographic machine settings. Thus, it is not useful as a diagnostic feature for cardiac amyloid. Diastolic dysfunction is a hallmark of amyloid cardiomyopathy. Restrictive filling pattern (E/A ratio >2, deceleration time <140 ms, increased E/E′, and small A wave) is often associated with advance stages and portends a poor prognosis (Fig. 7.2).[28] Although systolic function assessed by standard measurements often appears normal (ejection fraction >50%), assessment of longitudinal function often reveals significant impairment as demonstrated by strain imaging. Moreover, global longitudinal strain based on 2-dimensional speckle tracking echocardiography has been shown to be a robust independent predictor of survival with incremental value over biomarkers and other clinical variables.[29] Strain imaging can also play a role in differentiating cardiac amyloid from other causes of cardiac hypertrophic syndrome. The amyloid heart has been characterized by reduced basal strain with regional variation of strain from base to apex creating a distinct appearance of the bull's-eye map (Fig. 7.3). This pattern of relative sparing of the apex has been shown to be an accurate method of differentiating amyloid from hypertrophic cardiomyopathy in a study involving a limited number of patients.[30] Thus, strain is a promising tool that provides diagnostic as well as prognostic value in the evaluation of patients with cardiac amyloid.

Other echocardiographic features of cardiac amyloid include thickened valves, thickened interatrial septum, and a small pericardial effusion. Atrial dysfunction is also very common due to infiltration with amyloid leading to blood stasis and thrombus formation, regardless of rhythm. Atrial thrombi have been seen in 30% of patients with cardiac amyloidosis, both at autopsy and during life, as noted on transesophageal echocardiography.[31]

Cardiac biomarkers

NT-proBNP and cardiac troponin are often elevated and are markers of poor prognosis in patients with AL amyloidosis.[32–34] A staging system was developed by the Mayo Clinic based on NT-BNP (cutoff value <332 ng/L; BNP <100 mg/L) and cardiac troponin (cTnT <0.035, cTnI <0.1 μg/L) to standardize staging and risk stratification of patients with AL amyloidosis. Patients are stratified into 3 groups: stage I (lowest risk), BNP and troponin both negative; stage II (intermediate risk), BNP or troponin positive; stage III (highest risk), BNP and troponin both positive (Fig. 7.4). This system has been widely adapted by the medical community and validated for overall survival in patients with AL amyloidosis.[35] More recently, the free light chain differential has been added to the prognostic model.[36]

Cardiac MRI

Cardiac MRI is often performed when cardiac amyloid is suspected because of its ability to provide tissue characterization and elucidate the cause of the apparent LV hypertrophy, particularly in differentiating amyloid cardiomyopathy from hypertensive heart disease. The appearance of global, subendocardial late gadolinium enhancement is highly suggestive of cardiac amyloid and correlates with prognosis.[37,38] This typical MRI finding however is generally seen only in advanced stages of the disease. The pattern of late gadolinium enhancement can be atypical and patchy, especially in early disease.

Nuclear imaging

Bone imaging agents, such as ^{99m}Technetium-3,3-diphosphono-1,2-propanodicarboxylic acid (^{99m}Tc-DPD) and ^{99m}Tc-pyrophosphate (^{99m}Tc-PYP), were introduced to diagnose cardiac ATTR

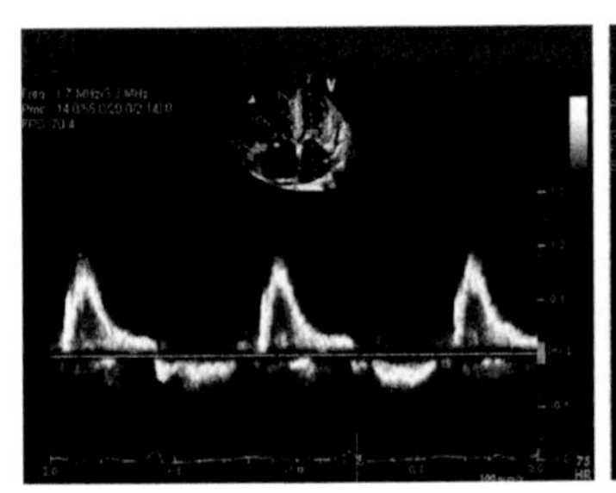
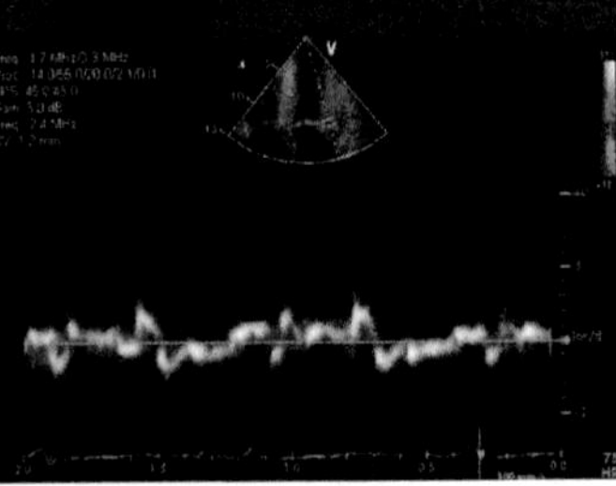
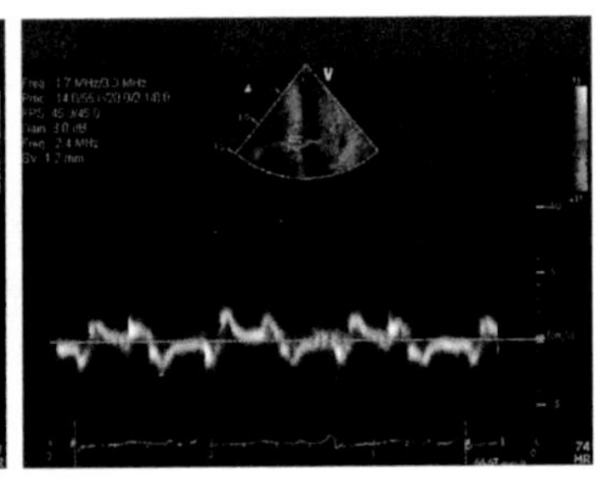

Fig. 7.2 (*left*) Left transmitral flow showing restrictive filling pattern with very low A-wave velocity. (*middle and right*) Tissue Doppler of the septal and lateral annuli reveals reduced myocardial velocity throughout systole and diastole.

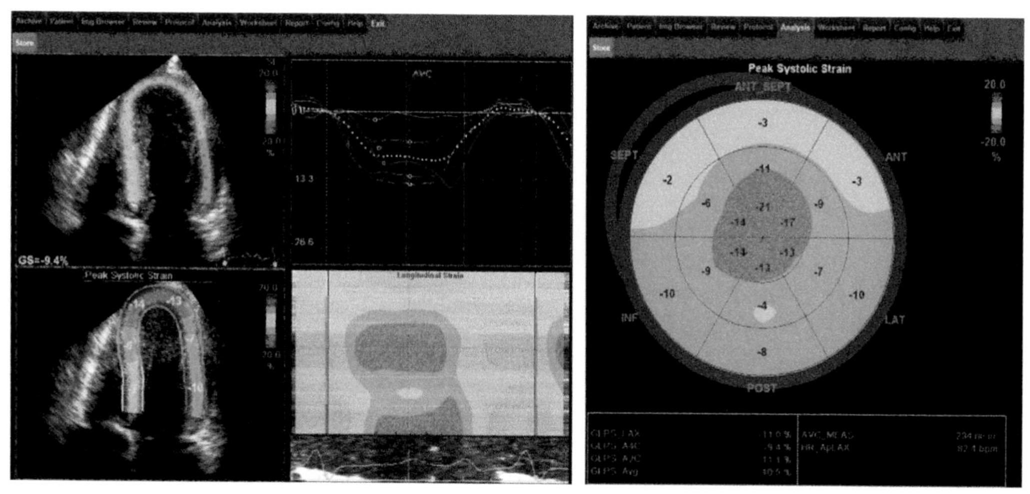

Fig. 7.3 Global longitudinal strain imaging in cardiac amyloidosis. Apical 4-chamber peak systolic strain (*left*) and the bull's-eye plot (*right*) showing classic strain pattern of relatively preserved apical strain with significantly reduced basal segments.

amyloidosis, leveraging on the high calcium levels in amyloid deposits. In the United States, ^{99m}Tc-pyrophosphate is more easily available, but both tracers yield similar results (near 100% sensitivity and specificity for ATTR). Compared with radionuclide imaging, MRI may underestimate the infiltration burden. Furthermore, there is suggestion that ^{99m}Tc-DPD and ^{99m}Tc-PYP may diagnose cardiac involvement before the appearance of characteristic abnormalities on echocardiography. However, although mild uptake can be seen in AL amyloidosis, these tracers are not for AL amyloidosis imaging. In this context, a new tracer, ^{18}F-florbetapir, might be useful, especially in combination with bone imaging agents (dual isotope imaging) to identify and type cardiac amyloid.[38]

In summary, diagnosis of cardiac amyloid remains difficult. The first step is to suspect the presence of amyloidosis based on the totality of the clinical presentation. Once amyloidosis is considered in the differential diagnosis, thinking about the possibility of cardiac involvement follows naturally. There are many noninvasive features common in amyloid, although no individual feature is highly specific for the diagnosis. Combining several noninvasive features with the clinical findings may facilitate differentiating cardiac amyloidosis from other diagnoses. A practical approach to the diagnosis of cardiac

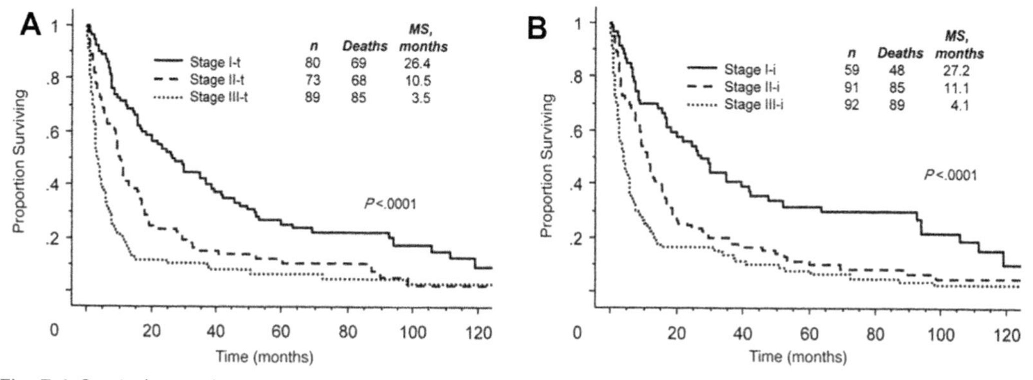

Fig. 7.4 Survival according to stage. Thresholds for cTnT, cTnI, and NT-proBNP are less than 0.035 μg/L, less than 0.1 μg/L, and less than 332 ng/L, respectively. (*A*) cTnT+NT-proBNP stage (stage I-t, both < threshold; stage II-t, either ≥ threshold; and stage III-t, both ≥ threshold). (*B*) cTnI+NT-proBNP stage (stage I-i, both < threshold; stage II-i, either ≥ threshold; and stage III-i, both ≥ threshold). cTnT, cardiac troponin T; cTnI, cardiac troponin I; NT-proBNP, N-terminal pro-brain natriuretic peptide; MS, median survival. (*From* Dispenzieri A, Gertz MA, Kyle RA, et al. Serum cardiac troponins and N-terminal pro-brain natriuretic peptide: a staging system for primary systemic amyloidosis. J Clin Oncol 2004;22(18):3755; with permission.)

amyloidosis is presented in Fig. 7.5. It is highly recommended that tissue be obtained to verify the diagnosis of amyloid. The origin of the amyloid (eg. AL vs TTYR) can be determined in some cases by immunohistology but amino acid sequencing or mass spectroscopy available at select centers are more reliable methods.

Management of Cardiac Amyloidosis

There are 2 aims in the management of cardiac amyloidosis: elimination of amyloid protein production and treatment of cardiac-related complications due to amyloid deposition. This section focuses on the supportive cardiac care for patients with cardiac amyloidosis.

Normalization of the precursor protein to amyloid has been shown to be an important predictor of survival in patients with AL amyloidosis.[39–41] In addition to preventing further accumulation of amyloid, it may also lead to reversal of organ dysfunction, possibly by promoting breakdown of amyloid in tissue.[42] Chemotherapy used to control light chains can often worsen HF due to fluid retention and hypertension associated with high-dose corticosteroids, and less commonly, due to the direct toxic effects of the chemotherapy. High-dose melphalan followed by autologous stem cell transplant is considered the first line of therapy for AL amyloid but is generally prescribed only to a select group of patients with adequate cardiac, renal, and pulmonary function. Patients with advanced cardiac involvement have often been excluded from stem cell transplant due to the high transplant-related mortality of 10% to 15%, although better outcomes have been reported with careful patient selection.[43–45] Cardiac issues and management during transplant are discussed in a later section. Less toxic regimens with immunomodulating agents, such as thalidomide and lenalidomide, have shown clear effects in patients with advanced AL amyloidosis without significant adverse cardiac effects.[46] Proteosome inhibitors, including bortezomib and carfilzomib, which are cornerstones for the management of multiple myeloma, are also established as targeted therapy for AL amyloidosis. Bortezomib, which has been used clinically for more than a decade, has not been shown to be particularly cardiotoxic. However, carfilzomib, which is a second-generation proteasome inhibitor approved for treatment of refractory multiple myeloma, is associated with significant cardiovascular side effects. These significant side effects include new onset or worsening of HF, pulmonary edema, decreased LV ejection fraction, restrictive cardiomyopathy, myocardial ischemia, and myocardial infarction. Cardiovascular events with carfilzomib were typically observed during the first 5 cycles, and furthermore, reports of sudden cardiac death within 24 hours of administration have led to US Food and Drug Administration warnings. The reported average incidences are

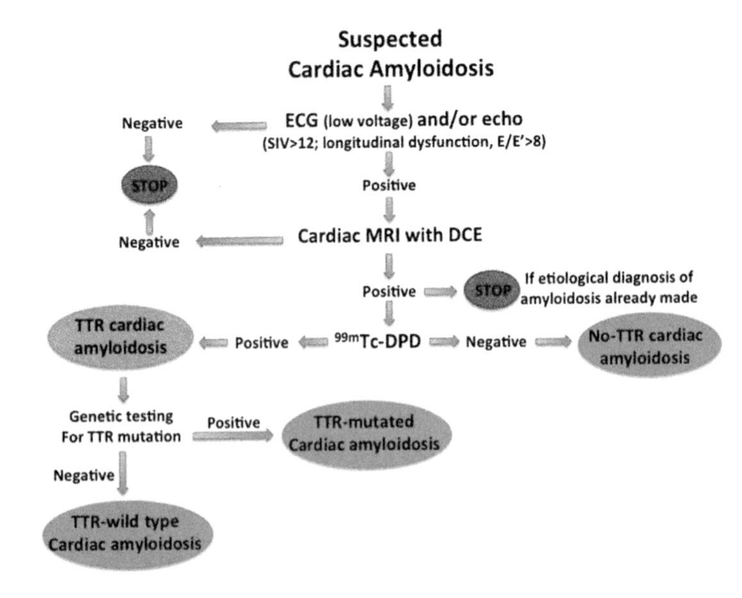

Fig. 7.5 Suggested work-flow diagram in the noninvasive diagnostic imaging workup of suspected cardiac amyloidosis. Note that non-TTR cardiac amyloidosis includes many diseases (multiple myeloma, non-Hodgkin lymphoma, Waldenstrom macroglobulinemia, monoclonal gammopathy of unknown significance, chronic arthritis, ankylosing spondylitis, Crohn disease, hereditary periodic fevers, acquired or inherited immunodeficiencies, chronic renal failure, and long-term history of hemodialysis). After finding evidence of cardiac amyloidosis using cardiac imaging, if there are no etiologic data, a large series of examinations are needed to confirm systemic amyloidosis and to diagnose the cause of cardiac amyloidosis. The mosaic of the cardiac amyloidosis diagnosis: role of imaging in subtypes and stages of the disease. DCE, delayed contrast enhancement; SIV=interventricular septal thickness >12 mm; ^{99m}Tc-DPD, ^{99m}Tc-3,3,-diphosphono-1,2-propano-dicarboxylic acid. (*From* Kang SM, Rim SJ, Chang HJ, et al. Primary cardiac lymphoma diagnosed by transvenous biopsy under transesophageal echocardiographic guidance and treated with systemic chemotherapy. Echocardiography 2003;20(1):101–3; with permission.)

7% for HF, 2% for pulmonary hypertension, and 35% for dyspnea (5% grade 3, <1% grade 4). Little is known regarding this cardiovascular toxicity profile when used in patients with cardiac amyloidosis, which may be more severe given the presence of baseline abnormal myocardial substrate.[47] Thus, a comprehensive cardiovascular evaluation before carfilzomib therapy is recommended, and the development of new dyspnea during therapy warrants immediate evaluation for cardiotoxicity. A phase I dose escalation trial of carfilzomib in patients with previously treated AL amyloidosis is currently in progress.

Signs and symptoms of HF are often the first clinical manifestation of cardiac amyloid. Treatment of HF due to cardiac amyloid differs from other forms of systolic and diastolic HF. The hemodynamic hallmark of cardiac amyloid is diastolic dysfunction with restrictive physiology causing high LV filling pressures and low stroke volume due to the stiff, noncompliant ventricle and reduced end-diastolic volume. The clinical and prognostic importance of the low stroke volume in cardiac amyloidosis cannot be overemphasized. That said, diuresis and salt restriction form the mainstay of therapy. Angiotensin-converting enzyme inhibitors have been prescribed in an attempt to limit cardiac fibrosis in the presence of myocardial amyloid, but often are not tolerated because they may induce severe hypotension, particularly when there is accompanying amyloid-related autonomic neuropathy. Calcium channel blockers can bind to the amyloid fibrils, which may have significant negative ionotropic and bradycardic effects leading to HF and hemodynamic instability. Their use should be avoided if at all possible. Digoxin can also bind to the amyloid fibrils and should be avoided due to increased risk of digoxin toxicity.[48] β-Blocker therapy has not been shown to be beneficial but may be considered in patients with atrial fibrillation for heart rate control. Amiodarone has been used safely for management of atrial fibrillation without significant adverse effects. Although not uncommonly used for control of ventricular arrhythmias, the impact of amiodarone on survival is not established. In the authors' experience, it seems to be helpful for symptomatic control of ventricular arrhythmias.

Patients will often develop hypotension, often accompanied by orthostasis, as a result of their low cardiac output, autonomic dysfunction, or altered vascular tone. Treatment with midodrine or mineralocorticoids can lead to modest improvement. Fluid boluses and salt supplementation may be useful in select patients. Support stockings and leg exercises are prescribed but not often helpful.

Patients with cardiac amyloid are at high risk for thromboembolic events. Atrial fibrillation in patients with cardiac amyloidosis is a strong indication for anticoagulation regardless of the CHADS2 score risk for stroke.[49] Anticoagulation is also indicated when thrombus has been demonstrated in the heart and can be carefully considered when there is sinus rhythm with evidence of atrial dysfunction on echocardiography.[50,51] However, it is also important to be aware of the increased bleeding risk when anticoagulating patients with extensive systemic amyloid due to widespread vascular fragility as well as possible gastrointestinal involvement and Factor X deficiency.[52]

Rhythm abnormalities including bradycardia with AV block are frequent in cardiac amyloid. Tachyarrhythmias, atrial and ventricular, are also seen. In the absence of evidence specific for cardiac amyloidosis, indications for permanent pacemaker placement are extrapolated from the general clinical guidelines on the subject. That is, there are no specific guidelines for device use in the presence of cardiac amyloidosis. Biventricular pacing is preferred to avoid further impairment of stroke volume due to dyssynchrony from right ventricular pacing. In a small series of patients undergoing stem cell transplant, nonsustained ventricular arrhythmia was commonly seen and inversely associated with stroke volume.[53] Syncope and sudden death are common in patients with advanced cardiac involvement, but prophylactic automatic implantable cardioverter-defibrillator (AICD) placement has not been shown to prolong survival.[54] Some studies have indicated that the terminal event in patients with advanced cardiac amyloid is typically electromechanical dissociation in some cases preceded by complete AV block. Whether bradycardia and tachyarrhythmias represent a preterminal event due to end-stage disease of the amyloid infiltrated heart versus a potentially salvageable event by intervention remains unclear. The authors advocate cardiac rhythm device therapy when it is likely to improve symptoms in cardiac amyloidosis (eg, symptomatic bradycardia). Whether device therapy including pacemakers and AICDs will prolong survival in cardiac amyloidosis is a highly controversial clinical conundrum.[55]

Cardiac transplantation in cardiac amyloid has been disappointing with a 5-year survival of only 20% to 30%, which is only marginally improved if followed by chemotherapy. However, a retrospective study showed that cardiac transplant can lead to a significantly improved survival when followed by high-dose chemotherapy and stem cell transplant in carefully selected patients.[56] The decision to perform cardiac transplant should incorporate the need for high-dose chemotherapy and autologous stem cell transplant after cardiac transplant and be limited to relatively young patients with isolated cardiac involvement who will likely be eligible for stem cell transplant after cardiac transplant.

PHEOCHROMOCYTOMA

Pheochromocytoma is a rare tumor with an incidence of about 2 to 8 per million people. The tumor may arise from the adrenal medulla (≈ 90%) or from the sympathetic ganglia along the sympathetic chain, overwhelmingly but not exclusively in the abdomen and can be associated with epinephrine, norepinephrine, or dopamine excess.[57] Pheochromocytomas usually arise spontaneously, but may be part of 1 of 4 known autosomal-dominant genetic syndromes: MEN2, VHL, neurofibromatosis type 1, and familial paraganglioma.[58]

DIAGNOSIS

Pheochromocytoma is an exceedingly rare cause for hypertension. The classic clinical triad of tachycardia, sweating, and headaches occurs only in a minority of patients. The clinical presentation is markedly heterogenous, often subtle. Presenting signs and symptoms include orthostatic hypotension and "spells" of anxiety, tachycardia, hypertension or hypotension, and/or diaphoresis precipitated by medical procedures, foods, drugs, or abdominal manipulation. Because of the nonspecific nature of the presentation, it is estimated that the diagnosis is confirmed in at most 1 in 300 patients evaluated for the condition.[57]

That said, biochemical evaluation for the possibility of pheochromocytoma is encouraged for patients with hypertension resistant to multiple drugs, for patients with paroxysmal anxiety, palpitations, and/or diaphoresis, for patients with an incidentally discovered adrenal tumor, and for patients with a family history for the disease or a predisposing genetic syndrome. Confirmation of the presence of pheochromocytoma is achieved through urine and/or blood testing, with confirmatory imaging for diagnosis and localization. Genetic testing should be considered.[58] The conditions needed for appropriate diagnostic testing and for the proper interpretation of results are sufficiently complex that the authors recommend that an experienced endocrinologist coordinate the evaluation.[59,60]

Treatment

Surgery is the treatment of choice for patients with pheochromocytoma.[57,61] The cardiologist's role is to assess the patient's suitability and to help prepare the patient for surgery. A careful history is of course required, with particular attention to the family history that could suggest a genetic syndrome. As with all preoperative evaluations, preserved exercise tolerance and freedom from uncontrolled HF, acute coronary syndromes, and uncontrolled arrhythmias should be assured.[62–65] Were the history and physical examination to suggest instability in these domains, further diagnostic testing is indicated as appropriate to develop a preoperative plan to stabilize the patient's condition. Routine 12-lead resting electrocardiography is reasonably indicated in all patients. There should be a low threshold for resting echocardiography if the presentation suggests LV dysfunction, sometimes related to catecholamine excess. Such LV dysfunction not uncommonly improves upon removal of the tumor.[63]

To prevent a catecholamine crisis in the perioperative period, α-adrenergic blockage is the established treatment of choice, usually with phenoxybenzamine started as an outpatient some 2 weeks before surgery and gradually uptitrated. Heart rate and blood pressure, including orthostatic blood pressures, should be monitored at home, the goal being controllable orthostatic hypotension. Once it is assured that the patient is adequately α blocked, a nonselective β-blocker, such as propranolol, can be given to blunt any α-blocker–related tachycardia and to further control the blood pressure. This addition of the β-blocker to the α-blocker will ensure that β-blockade does not precipitate a hypertensive crisis caused by unopposed α-adrenergic receptor stimulation. β-Blockers should be used cautiously if there is suspicion for a catecholamine-related cardiomyopathy with systolic LV dysfunction because they can precipitate flash pulmonary edema under these circumstances.[57] Concern about LV systolic dysfunction is another reason for performing a baseline echocardiogram. The patient should be encouraged to hydrate adequately during the perioperative period to minimize the consequences of orthostatic hypotension and the profound hypotension that can occur intraoperatively once the tumor is removed under anesthesia with residual α-blocker on board. As a further caution against perioperative hypotension, intravenous salt and water infusions are recommended on hospital admission before the operation.[66] Some advocate calcium channel blockers as an alternative to α- blockade preoperatively, but there is greater experience with favorable results with α-blockade.

Hypoglycemia is a concerning complication in the postoperative period, related to depletion of glycogen stores and hyperinsulinemia. The signs and symptoms of hypoglycemia can be masked by anesthesia and β-blockade. Careful glucose monitoring is indicated postoperatively, for at least 24 hours, although later hypoglycemia has been reported.[57]

Hypertension may persist in as many as 50% of patients postoperatively. Tumor recurrences have been reported in 17% of patients in one series with half the patients showing malignant disease. Recurrences were seen more often in extra-adrenal disease and in those with genetic tumors.[67]

About 10% of pheochromocytomas are malignant. Paragangliomas in patients with SDHB mutations (familial paraganglioma) have a particularly high rate of malignant disease. Histologically, benign and malignant tumors are indistinguishable; only the presence of metastases of chromaffin tissue at sites where no chromaffin tissue should be expected establishes a diagnosis of malignancy. Common metastatic sites are the bones, lungs, liver, and lymph nodes.[68,69] The clinical course of malignant pheochromocytoma is highly variable, making interpretation of the response of the limited number of patients difficult. Chemotherapy or MIBG (metaiodobenzylguanidine) radiotherapy has been used in patients who show signs of more than very slow progression. Tumor responses to therapy are highly variable, and positive responses can be associated with less of a need for antihypertensive medications.[70]

REFERENCES

1. Modlin IM, Sandor A. An analysis of 8305 cases of carcinoid tumors. Cancer 1997;79(4):813–29.
2. Sarmiento JM, Que FG. Hepatic surgery for metastases from neuroendocrine tumors. Surg Oncol Clin N Am 2003;12(1):231–42.
3. McEntee GP, Nagorney DM, Kvols LK, et al. Cytoreductive hepatic surgery for neuroendocrine tumors. Surgery 1990;108(6):1091–6.
4. Pellikka PA, Tajik AJ, Khandheria BK, et al. Carcinoid heart disease. Clinical and echocardiographic spectrum in 74 patients. Circulation 1993;87(4):1188–96.
5. Fox DJ, Khattar RS. Carcinoid heart disease: presentation, diagnosis, and management. Heart 2004;90(10):1224–8.
6. Moller JE, Pellikka PA, Bernheim AM, et al. Prognosis of carcinoid heart disease: analysis of 200 cases over two decades. Circulation 2005;112(21):3320–7.
7. Anderson AS, Krauss D, Lang R. Cardiovascular complications of malignant carcinoid disease. Am Heart J 1997;134(4):693–702.
8. Westberg G, Wängberg B, Ahlman H, et al. Prediction of prognosis by echocardiography in patients with midgut carcinoid syndrome. Br J Surg 2001;88(6):865–72.
9. Bhattacharyya S, Toumpanakis C, Chilkunda D, et al. Risk factors for the development and progression of carcinoid heart disease. Am J Cardiol 2011;107(8):1221–6.
10. Moller JE, Connolly HM, Rubin J, et al. Factors associated with progression of carcinoid heart disease. N Engl J Med 2003;348(11):1005–15.
11. Dobson R, Burgess MI, Valle JW, et al. Serial surveillance of carcinoid heart disease: factors associated with echocardiographic progression and mortality. Br J Cancer 2014;111(9):1703–9.
12. Mansencal N, Mitry E, Forissier JF, et al. Assessment of patent foramen ovale in carcinoid heart disease. Am Heart J 2006;151(5):1129.e1-6.
13. Mansencal N, Mitry E, Pillière R, et al. Prevalence of patent foramen ovale and usefulness of percutaneous closure device in carcinoid heart disease. Am J Cardiol 2008;101(7):1035–8.
14. Dobson R, Cuthbertson DJ, Jones J, et al. Determination of the optimal echocardiographic scoring system to quantify carcinoid heart disease. Neuroendocrinology 2014;99(2):85–93.
15. Denney WD, Kemp WE Jr, Anthony LB, et al. Echocardiographic and biochemical evaluation of the development and progression of carcinoid heart disease. J Am Coll Cardiol 1998;32(4):1017–22.
16. Bhattacharyya S, Toumpanakis C, Caplin ME, et al. Usefulness of N-terminal pro-brain natriuretic peptide as a biomarker of the presence of carcinoid heart disease. Am J Cardiol 2008;102(7):938–42.
17. Sandmann H, Pakkal M, Steeds R. Cardiovascular magnetic resonance imaging in the assessment of carcinoid heart disease. Clin Radiol 2009;64(8):761–6.
18. Bernheim AM, Connolly HM, Rubin J, et al. Role of hepatic resection for patients with carcinoid heart disease. Mayo Clin Proc 2008;83(2):143–50.
19. Raja SG, Bhattacharyya S, Davar J, et al. Surgery for carcinoid heart disease: current outcomes, concerns and controversies. Future Cardiol 2010;6(5):647–55.
20. Castillo JG, Filsoufi F, Rahmanian PB, et al. Early and late results of valvular surgery for carcinoid heart disease. J Am Coll Cardiol 2008;51(15):1507–9.
21. Bhattacharyya S, Raja SG, Toumpanakis C, et al. Outcomes, risks and complications of cardiac surgery for carcinoid heart disease. Eur J Cardiothorac Surg 2011;40(1):168–72.
22. Lillegard JB, Fisher JE, Mckenzie TJ, et al. Hepatic resection for the carcinoid syndrome in patients with severe carcinoid heart disease: does valve replacement permit safe hepatic resection? J Am Coll Surg 2011;213(1):130–6 [discussion: 136–8].

23. Mancuso K, Kaye AD, Boudreaux JP, et al. Carcinoid syndrome and perioperative anesthetic considerations. J Clin Anesth 2011;23(4):329–41.
24. Castillo JG, Milla F, Adams DH. Surgical management of carcinoid heart valve disease. Semin Thorac Cardiovasc Surg 2012;24(4):254–60.
25. Castillo JG, Silvay G, Solis J. Current concepts in diagnosis and perioperative management of carcinoid heart disease. Semin Cardiothorac Vasc Anesth 2013;17(3):212–23.
26. Falk RH. Diagnosis and management of the cardiac amyloidoses. Circulation 2005;112(13):2047–60.
27. Murtagh B, Hammill SC, Gertz MA, et al. Electrocardiographic findings in primary systemic amyloidosis and biopsy-proven cardiac involvement. Am J Cardiol 2005;95(4):535–7.
28. Klein AL, Hatle LK, Burstow DJ, et al. Doppler characterization of left ventricular diastolic function in cardiac amyloidosis. J Am Coll Cardiol 1989;13(5):1017–26.
29. Buss SJ, Emami M, Mereles D, et al. Longitudinal left ventricular function for prediction of survival in systemic light-chain amyloidosis: incremental value compared with clinical and biochemical markers. J Am Coll Cardiol 2012;60(12):1067–76.
30. Phelan D, Collier P, Thavendiranathan P, et al. Relative apical sparing of longitudinal strain using two-dimensional speckle-tracking echocardiography is both sensitive and specific for the diagnosis of cardiac amyloidosis. Heart 2012;98(19):1442–8.
31. Feng D, Edwards WD, Oh JK, et al. Intracardiac thrombosis and embolism in patients with cardiac amyloidosis. Circulation 2007;116(21):2420–6.
32. Apridonidze T, Steingart RM, Comenzo RL, et al. Clinical and echocardiographic correlates of elevated troponin in amyloid light-chain cardiac amyloidosis. Am J Cardiol 2012;110(8):1180–4.
33. Capone R, Amsterdam EA, Mason DT, et al. Systemic amyloidosis, functional coronary insufficiency, and autonomic impairment. Ann Intern Med 1972; 76(4):599–603.
34. Takemura G, Takatsu Y, Doyama K, et al. Expression of atrial and brain natriuretic peptides and their genes in hearts of patients with cardiac amyloidosis. J Am Coll Cardiol 1998;31(4):754–65.
35. Dispenzieri A, Gertz MA, Kyle RA, et al. Serum cardiac troponins and N-terminal pro-brain natriuretic peptide: a staging system for primary systemic amyloidosis. J Clin Oncol 2004;22(18):3751–7.
36. Kumar S, Dispenzieri A, Lacy MQ, et al. Revised prognostic staging system for light chain amyloidosis incorporating cardiac biomarkers and serum free light chain measurements. J Clin Oncol 2012; 30(9):989–95.
37. Syed IS, Glockner JF, Feng D, et al. Role of cardiac magnetic resonance imaging in the detection of cardiac amyloidosis. JACC Cardiovasc Imaging 2010;3(2):155–64.
38. Di Bella G, Pizzino F, Minutoli F, et al. The mosaic of the cardiac amyloidosis diagnosis: role of imaging in subtypes and stages of the disease. Eur Heart J Cardiovasc Imaging 2014; 15(12):1307–15.
39. Lachmann HJ, Goodman HJ, Gilbertson JA, et al. Natural history and outcome in systemic AA amyloidosis. N Engl J Med 2007;356(23):2361–71.
40. Gertz MA, Lacy MQ, Dispenzieri A, et al. Effect of hematologic response on outcome of patients undergoing transplantation for primary amyloidosis: importance of achieving a complete response. Haematologica 2007;92(10):1415–8.
41. Wilczek HE, Larsson M, Ericzon BG, et al. Long-term data from the Familial Amyloidotic Polyneuropathy World Transplant Registry (FAPWTR). Amyloid 2011;18(Suppl 1):193–5.
42. Palladini G, Barassi A, Klersy C, et al. The combination of high-sensitivity cardiac troponin T (hs-cTnT) at presentation and changes in N-terminal natriuretic peptide type B (NT-proBNP) after chemotherapy best predicts survival in AL amyloidosis. Blood 2010;116(18):3426–30.
43. Gertz MA, Lacy MQ, Dispenzieri A, et al. Refinement in patient selection to reduce treatment-related mortality from autologous stem cell transplantation in amyloidosis. Bone Marrow Transplant 2013;48(4): 557–61.
44. Saba N, Sutton D, Ross H, et al. High treatment-related mortality in cardiac amyloid patients undergoing autologous stem cell transplant. Bone Marrow Transplant 1999;24(8):853–5.
45. Seldin DC, Andrea N, Berenbaum I, et al. High-dose melphalan and autologous stem cell transplantation for AL amyloidosis: recent trends in treatment-related mortality and 1-year survival at a single institution. Amyloid 2011;18(Suppl 1):127–9.
46. Gatt ME, Palladini G. Light chain amyloidosis 2012: a new era. Br J Haematol 2013;160(5):582–98.
47. Siegel D, Martin T, Nooka A, et al. Integrated safety profile of single-agent carfilzomib: experience from 526 patients enrolled in 4 phase II clinical studies. Haematologica 2013;98(11):1753–61.
48. Rubinow A, Skinner M, Cohen AS. Digoxin sensitivity in amyloid cardiomyopathy. Circulation 1981; 63(6):1285–8.
49. Feng D, Syed IS, Martinez M, et al. Intracardiac thrombosis and anticoagulation therapy in cardiac amyloidosis. Circulation 2009;119(18):2490–7.
50. Dubrey S, Pollak A, Skinner M, et al. Atrial thrombi occurring during sinus rhythm in cardiac amyloidosis: evidence for atrial electromechanical dissociation. Br Heart J 1995;74(5):541–4.
51. Modesto KM, Dispenzieri A, Cauduro SA, et al. Left atrial myopathy in cardiac amyloidosis: implications of novel echocardiographic techniques. Eur Heart J 2005;26(2):173–9.

52. Choufani EB, Sanchorawala V, Ernst T, et al. Acquired factor X deficiency in patients with amyloid light-chain amyloidosis: incidence, bleeding manifestations, and response to high-dose chemotherapy. Blood 2001;97(6):1885–7.
53. Goldsmith YB, Liu J, Chou J, et al. Frequencies and types of arrhythmias in patients with systemic light-chain amyloidosis with cardiac involvement undergoing stem cell transplantation on telemetry monitoring. Am J Cardiol 2009;104(7):990–4.
54. Kristen AV, Dengler TJ, Hegenbart U, et al. Prophylactic implantation of cardioverter-defibrillator in patients with severe cardiac amyloidosis and high risk for sudden cardiac death. Heart Rhythm 2008; 5(2):235–40.
55. Lin G, Dispenziere A, Kyle R, et al. Implantable cardioverter defibrillators in patients with cardiac amyloidosis. J Cardiovasc Electrophysiol 2013;24: 793–8.
56. Maurer MS, Raina A, Hesdorffer C, et al. Cardiac transplantation using extended-donor criteria organs for systemic amyloidosis complicated by heart failure. Transplantation 2007;83(5):539–45.
57. Hodin R, Lubitz C, Phitayakorn R, et al. Diagnosis and management of pheochromocytoma. Curr Probl Surg 2014;51(4):151–87.
58. Lenders JWM, Eisenhofer E, Mannelli M, et al. Phaeochromocytoma. Lancet 2005;366:665–75.
59. Neary NM, King KS, Pacak K. Drugs and pheochromocytoma–don't be fooled by every elevated metanephrine. N Engl J Med 2011;364(23):2268–70.
60. Jun JH, Ahn HJ, Lee SM, et al. Is preoperative biochemical testing for pheochromocytoma necessary for all adrenal incidentalomas? Medicine (Baltimore) 2015;94(45):e1948.
61. Shen WT, Grogan R, Vriens M, et al. One hundred two patients with pheochromocytoma treated at a single institution since the introduction of laparoscopic adrenalectomy. Arch Surg 2010;145(9):893–7.
62. Jones G, Evans PH, Vaidya B. Phaeochromocytoma. BMJ 2012;344:e1042.
63. Agarwal G, Sadacharan D, Kapoor A, et al. Cardiovascular dysfunction and catecholamine cardiomyopathy in pheochromocytoma patients and their reversal following surgical cure: results of a prospective case-control study. Surgery 2011;150(6): 1202–11.
64. Shah NH, Ruan DT. Pheochromocytoma: a devious opponent in a game of hide-and-seek. Circulation 2014;130(15):1295–8.
65. Pacak K. Preoperative management of the pheochromocytoma patient. J Clin Endocrinol Metab 2007;92:4069–79.
66. Namekawa T, Utsumi T, Kawamura K, et al. Clinical predictors of prolonged postresection hypotension after laparoscopic adrenalectomy for pheochromocytoma. Surgery 2016;159(3):763–70.
67. Press D, Akyuz M, Dural C, et al. Predictors of recurrence in pheochromocytoma. Surgery 2014;156(6): 1523–7.
68. Ghayee HK. Strategic chemotherapy for pheochromocytoma? Endocrinology 2015;156(11):3880–1.
69. Scholz T, Eisenhofer G, Pacak K, et al. Clinical review: current treatment of malignant pheochromocytoma. J Clin Endocrinol Metab 2007;92(4): 1217–25.
70. Ayala-Ramirez M, Feng L, Habra MA. Clinical benefits of systemic chemotherapy for patients with metastatic pheochromocytomas or extra-adrenal paragangliomas. Cancer 2012;118:2804–12.

CHAPTER 8

Chemotherapy-Induced Cardiomyopathy

Rohit Moudgil, MD, PhD[a,*], Edward T.H. Yeh, MD[b]

INTRODUCTION

Over the last few decades, collective efforts of the basic science research, anticancer drug development, clinical trial, and patient care have culminated in improved mortality and morbidity outcomes. Recent statistics released by the American Cancer Society (http://www.cancer.org/research/cancerfactsstatistics/cancerfactsfigures2015/) highlighted that the 5-year relative survival rate for all cancers diagnosed in 2004 to 2010 was 68%, up from 49% in 1975 to 1977. By extrapolation, roughly more than a million new patients will be joining an already existing 14.5 million cancer survivors. These numbers reflect a commendable success of anticancer therapies; however, cardiotoxicity related to these therapies has become a feared and recognizable consequence. Although the traditional therapies have shown cardiovascular consequence, the newly targeted therapies are also joining the ranks of eliciting cardiotoxicity. Therefore, it is important to learn and hone the skills to treat cancer survivors who are presenting with a premature cardiovascular disease.

Much of the initial studies looking at the incidence and the prevalence of cardiovascular disease in cancer survivorship were derived from patients treated with the anthracyclines. Von Hoff and colleagues[1] did a retrospective analysis of more than 4000 patients treated with doxorubicin (DOX) and found that 2.2% of the patients developed clinical signs and symptoms of heart failure (HF). Because the study was based on clinical diagnosis, incorporation of subclinical left ventricular (LV) dysfunction would have resulted in higher incidence of the cardiovascular disease in DOX patients, as acknowledged by the investigators themselves.[1] Although initial upsurge in the interest of cardiotoxicity mediated by the anticancer drugs has been due to an increased incidence of cardiomyopathy and consequent HF in oncologic patients,[2] newer antioncologic agents have sparked concerns into a new array of cardiovascular dysfunction. This effort has culminated in the inception of a new field in cardiology: onco-cardiology, or cardio-oncology. Although many other cardiovascular effects have been identified as a side-effect profile of the anticancer medications such as myocardial infarction, hypertension, arrhythmias, and thromboembolic events, cardiomyopathy still remains the most prevalent and the most studied entity in onco-cardiology (Fig. 8.1).

This review focuses its efforts on cardiomyopathy as it pertains to chemotherapy treatment. The clinical and the molecular mechanisms behind the 2 subtypes of the cardiomyopathies and their potential therapies are identified. The chapter concludes with a look into the interaction between these 2 subtypes and how this interplay can lead to a greater risk and incidence of developing HF.

CARDIOMYOPATHIES

Since the word "cardiomyopathy" was coined by Brigden over half a century ago,[3] it has been scrutinized for decades. A simple Google search defines it as "a chronic disease of the heart muscle," whereas the free medical dictionary states "cardiomyopathy is a chronic disease of the heart muscle (myocardium), in which the muscle is abnormally enlarged, thickened, and/or stiffened." The World Health Organization defines cardiomyopathy as "a disease of the myocardium with associated cardiac dysfunction" with the incorporation of a classification scheme.[4] Finally, in 2006, the American Heart Association (AHA) defined cardiomyopathy as "a heterogeneous group of diseases of the myocardium associated

[a] Department of Cardiology, The University of Texas MD Anderson Cancer Center, Unit 1451, 1515 Holcombe Boulevard, Houston, TX, USA; [b] Department of Internal Medicine, University of Missouri, School of Medicine, One Hospital Drive, MA412, Columbia, MO 65212, USA
* Corresponding author.
E-mail address: RMoudgil@mdanderson.org

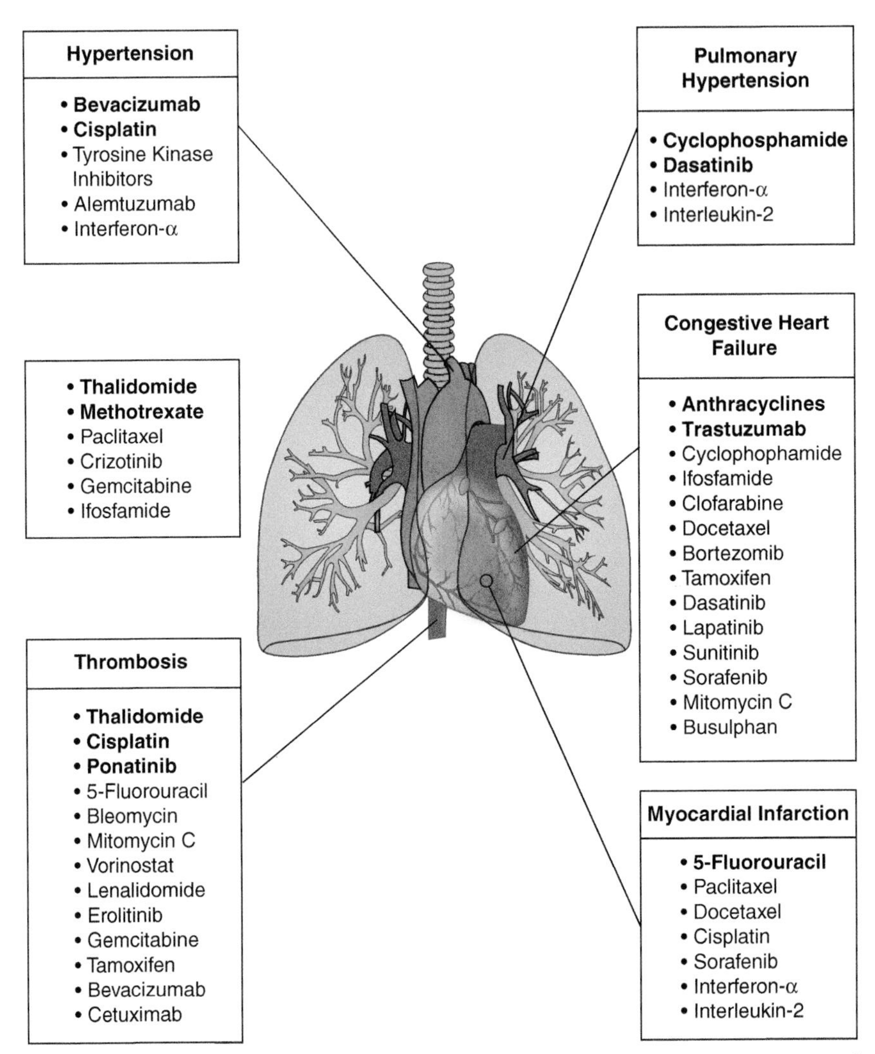

Fig. 8.1 Cardiotoxic effects of various currently known chemotherapeutic agents on various aspects of physiologic heart function.

with mechanical and/or electrical dysfunction, which usually (but not invariably) exhibit inappropriate ventricular hypertrophy or dilatation, due to a variety of etiologies that frequently are genetic. Cardiomyopathies are either confined to the heart or are part of generalized systemic disorders, and often lead to cardiovascular death or progressive heart failure–related disability."[5]

In onco-cardiology, or cardio-oncology, the first "consensus" clinical description of cardiomyopathy was formulated by the cardiac review and evaluation committee supervising trastuzumab clinical trials, who defined drug-associated cardiotoxicity as one or more of the following: (1) cardiomyopathy characterized by a decrease in left ventricular ejection fraction (LVEF) globally or because of regional changes in interventricular septum contraction; (2) symptoms associated with congestive heart failure (CHF); (3) signs associated with HF, such as S3 gallop, tachycardia, or both; (4) decline in initial LVEF of at least 5% to less than 55% with signs and symptoms of HF or asymptomatic decrease in LVEF of at least 10% to less than 55%.[6] This definition has a limited scope, because it does not include subclinical cardiovascular damage that may occur early in response to some of the chemotherapeutic agents. Other cardiovascular factors such as coronary artery disease, rhythm disturbances, and pulmonary hypertension are also not considered. Thus, this definition does not encompass the broader scope of unwanted cardiovascular effects of the anticancer drugs, that is, "cardiotoxicity"; however, it is suitable for describing cardiomyopathy.

Chemotherapy-related cardiomyopathy is conceptually divided into 2 subtypes (Fig. 8.2, Table 8.1). Anthracyclines are the prototype for

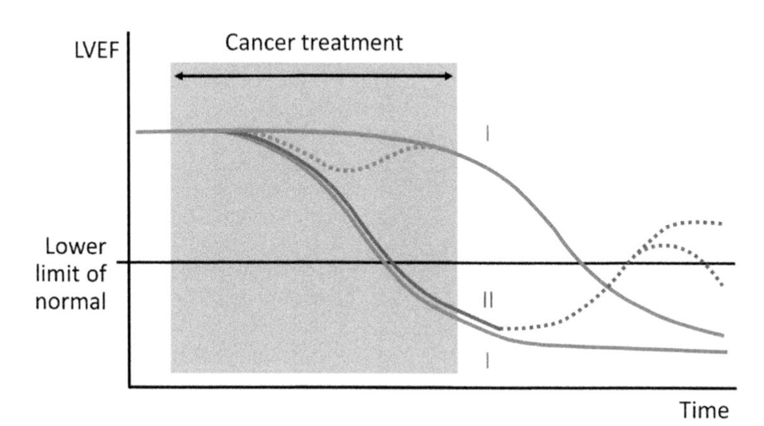

Fig. 8.2 LVEF dynamics for type I and type II chemotherapy-induced cardiotoxicity. (*Modified from* Altena R, Perik PJ, van Veldhuisen DJ, et al. Cardiovascular toxicity caused by cancer treatment: strategies for early detection. Lancet Oncol 2009;10:391.)

type I chemotherapy–related cardiac dysfunction, characterized by irreversible, dose-dependent myocardial injury.[7] Under the microscope, myofibrillar disarray, necrosis, and vacuoles formation can be seen before any biological or phenotypic manifestations (Fig. 8.3).[8] Oxidative stress via free radical formation and double-stranded breaks via topoisomerase IIβ are the mechanisms involved in myocardial injury resulting in a decrease in ejection fraction with global hypokinesis.[9] In contrast, type II chemotherapy–related cardiac dysfunction has been primarily seen with targeted therapies such as those directed against the human epidermal growth factor receptor-2 (HER2), for example, trastuzumab (see Table 8.1; Table 8.2).[8] Unlike type I cardiac dysfunction, type II cardiac dysfunction shows no dose-dependent response,

TABLE 8.1
Subtypes of chemotherapy-induced cardiotoxicity

	Type I (Damage)	Type II (Dysfunction)
Prototype	DOX	Trastuzumab
Ultrastructure	Vacuoles, necrosis Microfibrillar disarray	No abnormalities
Mechanism	Topoisomerase II Beta	ErbB2 signaling inhibition
Clinical course	Likely irreversible	Likely reversible
Rechallenge	Likely progressive	Likely safe
Late sequential stress	Likely not tolerated	Likely tolerated

Data from Ewer MS, Lippman SM. Type II chemotherapy-related cardiac dysfunction: time to recognize a new entity. J Clin Oncol 2005;23:2900–2.

results in no ultrastructural changes, and poses a favorable prognosis owing to its reversibility (see Fig. 8.2, Table 8.1).

Although there is overlap, there are also notable differences in the risk factors between these 2 subtypes. A recent meta-analysis of 18 studies with more than 22,815 patients confirmed cumulative anthracycline dose as the strongest risk factor for cardiotoxicity. In agreement, in a predictive scoring algorithm for cardiotoxicity risk of patients with breast cancer undergoing anthracycline therapy, more than half of the points are allocated to cumulative anthracycline dose.[10] The clinical outcomes are in agreement with the subcellular findings of worsening myocardial tissue injury as a function of cumulative anthracycline dose with a certain threshold phenomenon (see Fig. 8.4). Of further note, although myocardial damage is proportional to the degree of cytotoxic insult (dose), noninvasive and invasive studies of cardiac function are not over the current dose spectrum, but there are noticeable interindividual differences.

Chest radiation therapy, young (<5 years) or old (>60–70 years) age, high or low body weight, African American ethnicity, and comorbidities, including diabetes and hypertension, are among other significant risk factors.[11,12] With respect to pediatric population, their are some similarities and differences in risk factor profile. Higher cumulative anthracycline dose is still the predominant risk factor, and chest radiation and African American ethnicity are other common risk factors. However, younger age at diagnosis,[13,14] female sex,[15] and trisomy 21[15] are unique to the pediatric population.

On the other hand, risk factors for type II chemotherapy–related cardiac dysfunction are much more patient-specific. For instance, the incidence of trastuzumab-related cardiotoxicity is more common in elderly population by 30% (mean age in the seventh decade).[16–18] Traditional risk factors for cardiomyopathy, such as hypertension and coronary artery disease, also weigh in, as

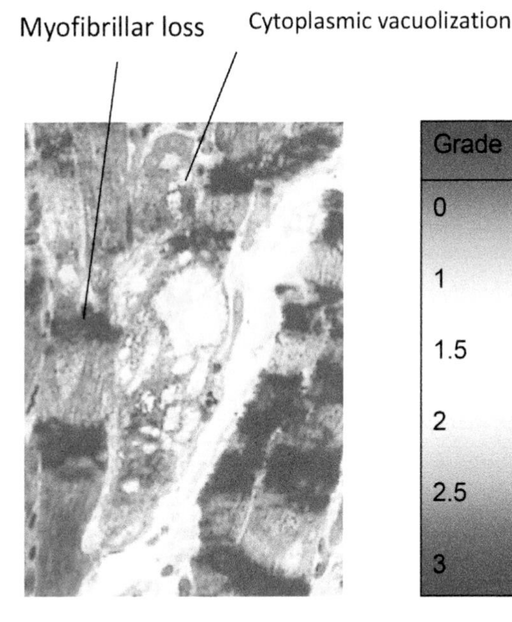

Grade	% myocytes
0	none
1	<5
1.5	5–15
2	16–25
2.5	26–35
3	>35

Fig. 8.3 Example of the histology of anthracycline cardiotoxicity and its grading by the percentage of myocytes involved with evidence of myofibrillar loss and cystoplasmic vacuolization due to swelling of the sacroplasmatic reticulum and the mitochondria. Disruption of these organelles leads to cardiomyocyte loss. The section is 0.5 μm thick and embedded in Epon resin (toluidine blue stain, ×40) (*From* Singal PK, Iliskovic N. Doxorubicin-induced cardiomyopathy. N Engl J Med 1998;339:900–5; with permission. Copyright © 1998, Massachusetts Medical Society.)

do shorter intervals between trastuzumab administrations.[17] In a risk prediction model for trastuzumab-related cardiomyopathy, a higher risk of cardiotoxicity was observed in patients with older age, adjuvant chemotherapy, coronary artery disease, atrial fibrillation or flutter, diabetes, hypertension, and renal failure (Fig. 8.5). However, caution is advised because the prediction model was derived from the Surveillance Epidemiology and End Result database, and the dataset lacks the accurate assessment of cardiac function, such as ejection fraction. Nevertheless, it provides a glimpse of risk factors to be vigilant about when assessing patients for trastuzumab therapy and associated risks of cardiotoxicity.[19]

ANTHRACYCLINES

Clinical Perspective

Acute morbidity is defined by events occurring during or shortly after the drug infusion. Most commonly, these include arrhythmias (supraventricular tachycardia, ventricular ectopy), and in some cases, HF and/or pericarditis-myocarditis syndrome (Fig. 8.6).[20,21] The subacute cardiac toxicity occurs within few weeks. This event clinically resembles myocarditis with edema and thickening of the LV walls and is associated with diastolic dysfunction and increased mortality (Fig. 8.7).[22] In contrast to the late anthracycline-mediated cardiotoxicity, improvement in LV function has been noted to occur in these subacute patients (see Fig. 8.7).[21,23,24] Furthermore, the mechanism responsible for the acute toxicity may involve an inflammatory response, which differs from the generally accepted cause of the chronic anthracycline cardiotoxicity (see Fig. 8.6). Clinically, the most significant effect of anthracyclines is late cardiac damage leading to LV dysfunction and CHF (Fig. 8.8).[24,25] This late anthracycline-mediated cardiac dysfunction has been correlated with diffuse replacement fibrosis and hypertrophy of the remaining cardiomyocytes (Fig. 8.9). The dogma of anthracycline-mediated cardiotoxicity has been that each temporal event has its own mechanism; therefore, they differ in outcomes.[20]

TABLE 8.2
Drugs associated with type I and type II chemotherapy-induced cardiotoxicity

	Type I (Damage)	Type II (Dysfunction)
Prototype	DOX	Trastuzumab
Other drugs	Epirubicin Idarubicin Mitoxantone	Pertuzumab Bevacizumab Lapatinib Sorafenib Sunitinib

Initial studies on chemotherapy-related cardiomyopathy focused on DOX, and the question remained if related compounds could have similar oncologic efficacy at lower cardiovascular toxicity. Over the past 5 decades, more than 2000 anthracycline derivatives have been synthesized and tested; several were evaluated in clinical trials,[26] but only epirubicin[27] and idarubicin[28] received approval for clinical use. Unfortunately, clinical

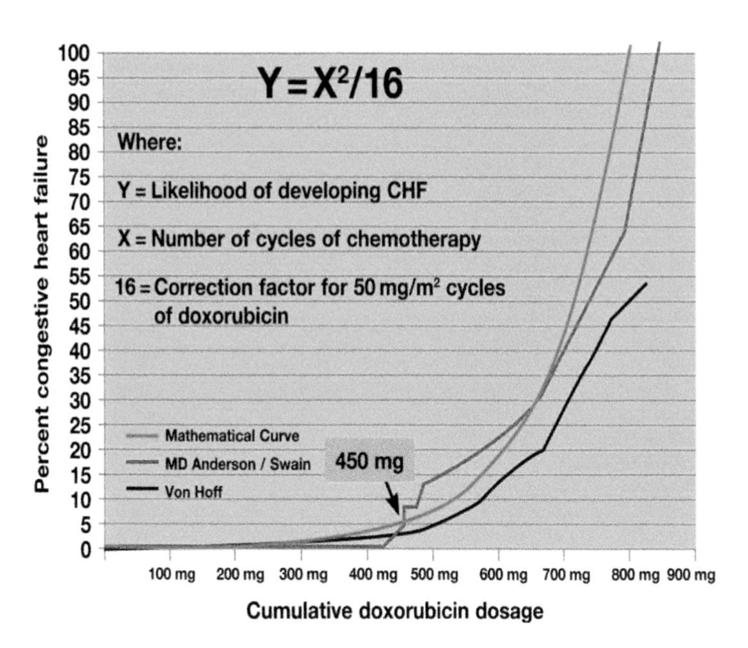

Fig. 8.4 Mathematical model predicting the likelihood of DOX-induced HF according to dose accumulation: cardiotoxicity is a quadratic function of DOX dose ($Y = X^2/16$). X is the number of cycles of chemotherapy undergone by patients, with a correction factor of 16 applied with the assumption of a DOX dose of 50 mg/m^2 per cycle of chemotherapy. Historically, a cumulative dose of 450 mg/m^2 was considered a fair compromise of benefit in terms of anticancer therapy at a risk of HF of 5%. (*Reproduced from* Ewer MS, Yeh ETH. Cancer and the Heart. 2nd Edition. People's Medical Publishing House - USA, Ltd., 2013.)

trials have not confirmed a lower cardiotoxicity risk with epirubicin or idarubicin.[28]

Epidoxorubicin, or in short, epirubicin, is an analogue of DOX, which was initially regarded as equally effective and less cardiotoxic on a milligram-to-milligram comparison.[29–31] In a prospective randomized trial in patients with breast cancer, epirubicin was associated with a longer median duration of response than DOX (11.9 months vs 7.1 months).[32] The cumulative dose at which CHF occurred was 1134 mg/m^2 with epirubicin and 492 mg/m^2 with DOX.[32] This dose was further confirmed in a meta-analysis of 13 studies comparing DOX with epirubicin. The trials were done predominantly in women with advanced or metastatic breast cancer. In these cohorts, epirubicin was associated with a significant decrease in the risk of clinical and subclinical cardiotoxicity, and any other cardiac event when compared with DOX.[33] Epirubicin-induced cardiotoxicity is also dose dependent, and therefore, the US Food and Drug Administration recommends a maximum cumulative dose of 900 mg/m^2.[34] However, in an analysis of 1097 patients, the safe maximum cumulative dosage was found to be lower when risk factors, such as age, radiation, and underlying cardiac risk factors, were taken into account.[35] In addition, a

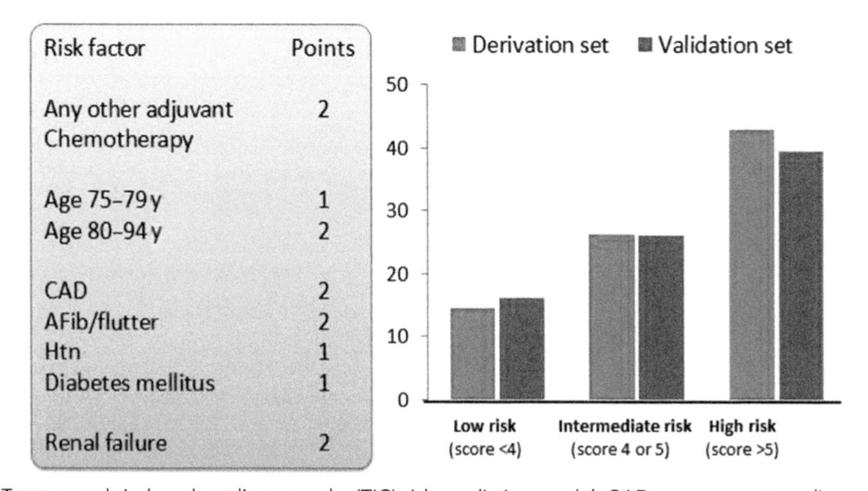

Fig. 8.5 Trastuzumab induced cardiomyopathy (TIC) risk prediction model. CAD, coronary artery disease; Htn, hypertension. (*From* Ezaz G, Long JB, Gross CP, et al. Risk prediction model for heart failure and cardiomyopathy after adjuvant trastuzumab therapy for breast cancer. J Am Heart Assoc 2014;3:e000472; with permission.)

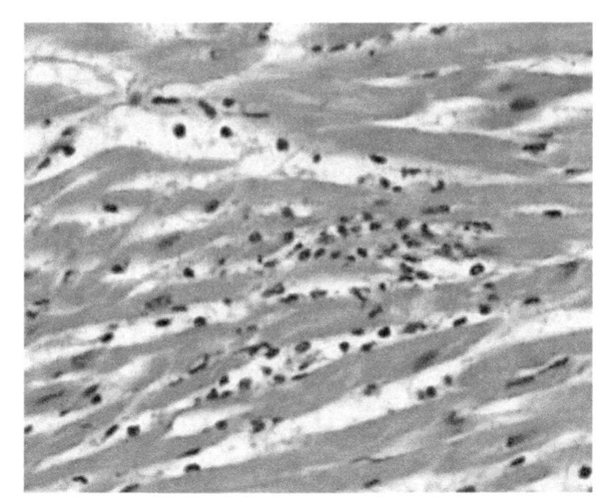

Fig. 8.6 Acute anthracycline-induced cardiotoxicity resembling acute toxic myocarditis with cardiomyocyte damage (pyknotic debris) and inflammatory infiltrate (H&E stain). (*From* Berry GJ, Jorden M. Pathology of radiation and anthracycline cardiotoxicity. Pediatr Blood Cancer 2005:44:630–7; with permission.)

Cochrane database analysis did not identify any difference in cardiotoxicity risk between epirubicin and DOX at equipotent doses.[36] In essence, for equipotent therapeutic efficacy, epirubicin has a similar profile of cardiotoxicity as DOX. Numerous other trials have reached similar conclusions, and DOX fared even better than its familial counterpart.[36,37] Thus, the severity of anthracycline-related cardiomyopathy remains similar within its group.

Pathophysiologic Mechanisms

Anthracycline-mediated cardiomyopathy has been studied extensively. The leading view historically has been that of production of reactive oxygen species (ROS)[38,39] and formation of iron complexes resulting in intracellular damage.[40–42] However, the authors identified a direct target of DOX that provides a unifying mechanism encompassing most of the implicated pathways (Fig. 8.10).[9]

It has been well studied that one of the cancer-toxic mechanisms of DOX is mediated by topoisomerase IIαinhibition.[43] Toposiomerase IIα is an enzyme that regulates the overwinding or underwinding of DNA during its reparative process. These twisting processes also play an important role in regulating cellular processes, such as replication, transcription, and chromosomal segregation by altering DNA topology.[44] On the other hand, topoisomerase II beta (Top II B) serves the same function in quiescent cells. Because they share catalytic mechanisms and have a high degree of amino acid similarity (~70% identity at

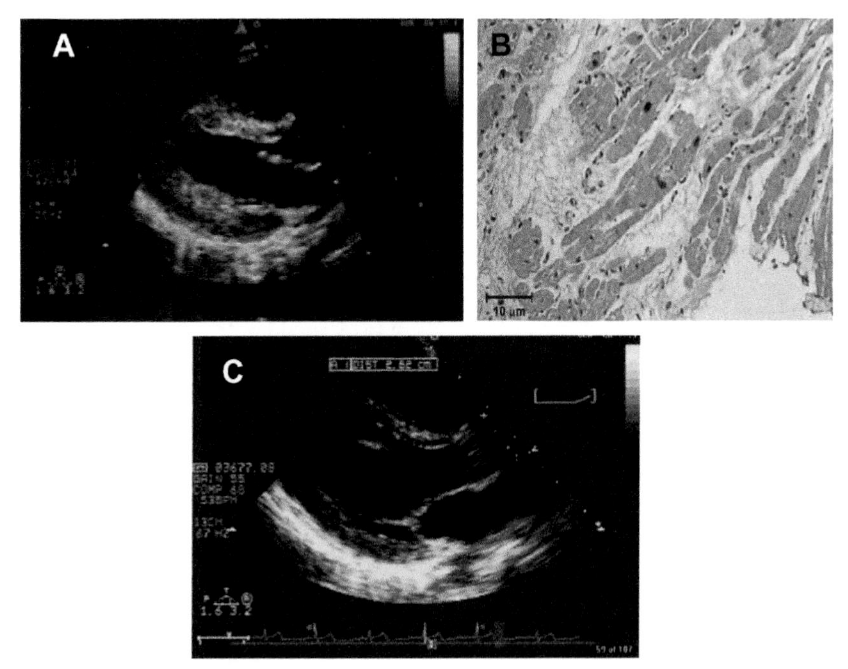

Fig. 8.7 Subacute anthracycline-induced cardiotoxicity of a 25-year-old man with acute myeloid leukemia, presenting with a myopericarditis syndrome 17 days after consolidation chemotherapy with high-dose cytarabine and idarubicin. TTE showed marked transient increased LV wall thickness associated with normal systolic contraction but diastolic dysfunction (*A*). Endomyocardial biopsy showed severe interstitial myocardial edema but no cellular infiltrate or myofiber damage (*B*; hematoxylin and eosin). Follow-up echocardiogram at 1 month shows resolution of abnormalities (*C*). (*From* Hengel CL, Russell PA, Gould PA, et al. Subacute anthracycline cardiotoxicity. Heart Lung Circ 2006;15:59–61; with permission.)

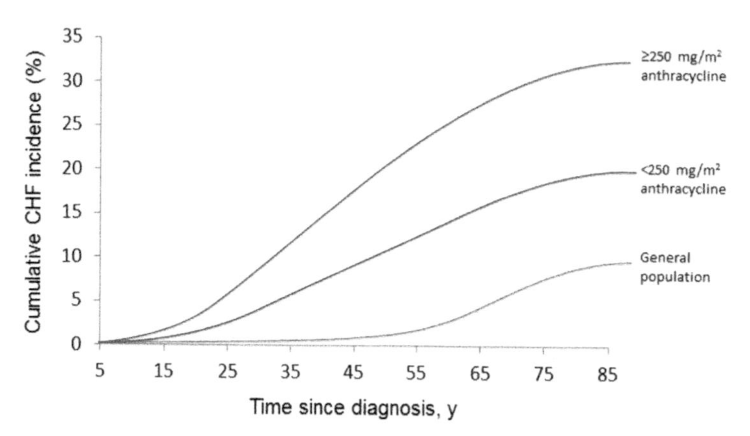

Fig. 8.8 Cumulative incidence of HF in pediatric cancer survivors stratified by cumulative anthracycline dose. (*Data from* Yeh JM, Nohria A, Diller L. Routine echocardiography screening for asymptomatic left ventricular dysfunction in childhood cancer survivors: a model-based estimation of the clinical and economic effects. Ann Intern Med 2014;160:661–71.)

the amino acid level),[45] the authors embarked on a project to study the role of Top II B in murine cardiac cells treated with DOX. They successfully demonstrated that[9]: (1) in rats, the molecular phenotype of acute and chronic DOX cardiomyopathy is characterized by the formation of a ternary DNA–Top II B–DOX cleavage complex, which triggers double-strand breaks in the DNA; (2) the acute stage is characterized by the upregulation of the apoptotic pathway signaling, specifically *Apaf-1*, *Bax*, *Mdm-2*, and *Fas*. Under chronic condition, (3) the genes implicated in the mitochondrial dysfunction and oxidative phosphorylation were activated by downregulation of peroxisome proliferator activated receptor γ, coactivator 1 α(*Ppargc-1a*), and β(*Ppargc-1b*).[9] This downregulation resulted in (4) decrease in the key components of the electron transport chain such as *Ndufa3*, *Sdha*, and *Atp5a1*, thus culminating into (5) ultrastructural mitochondrial damage with vacuolization.[9] There was also (6) mitochondrial dysfunction as measured by oxygen consumption and changes in the mitochondrial membrane potential. The end result was (7) an increase in end-systolic and end-diastolic volumes and a decrease in ejection fraction.[9] The formation of the ternary complex is also responsible for the production of most of the DOX-induced ROS (70%). Therefore, oxidative stress is preferentially the result of DOX-induced DNA damage and its consequences on the transcriptome rather than of the redox-cycling of DOX. Transgenic mice with cardiomyocyte-specific deletion of Top II B were indeed protected from the acute and progressive or chronic DOX-induced HF and did not exhibit the severe cardiomyopathic phenotype seen in wild-type mice. Therefore, Top II B is required to initiate the entire phenotypic cascade of DOX-induced cardiomyopathy.[9] Other studies also identified the activation of the p53 pathway to DNA damage and the consequent apoptosis and mitochondrial dysfunction in cultured cardiomyocytes treated with DOX.[46,47]

Support for the theory of Top II B as the leading mechanism is provided by the use of dexrazoxane (DEX). In vivo, DEX has shown significant cardioprotection against DOX in various preclinical models, such as mouse, rat, hamster, rabbit, and dog.[48–51] In addition, the

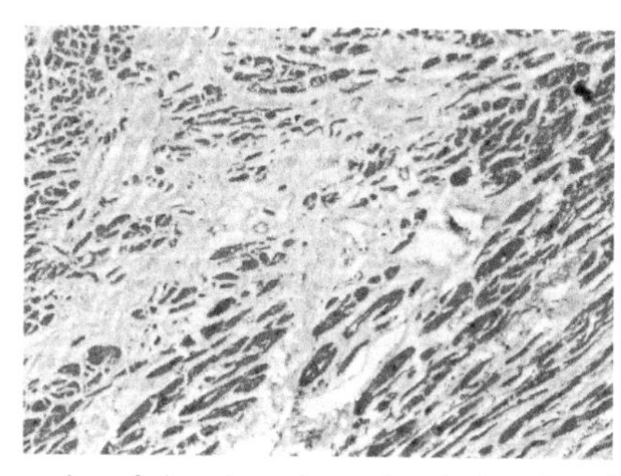
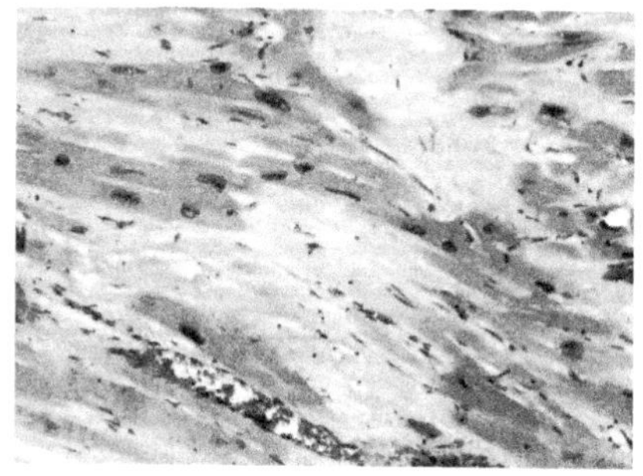

Fig. 8.9 Examples of chronic anthracycline-induced cardiotoxicity showing myocyte loss with replacement fibrosis (*left*) and hypertrophy of the remaining myocytes (*right*). (*From* Steinherz LJ, Steinherz PG, Tan C. Cardiac failure and dysrhythmias 6-19 years after anthracycline therapy: a series of 15 patients. Med Pediatr Oncol 1995;24:352–61; with permission.)

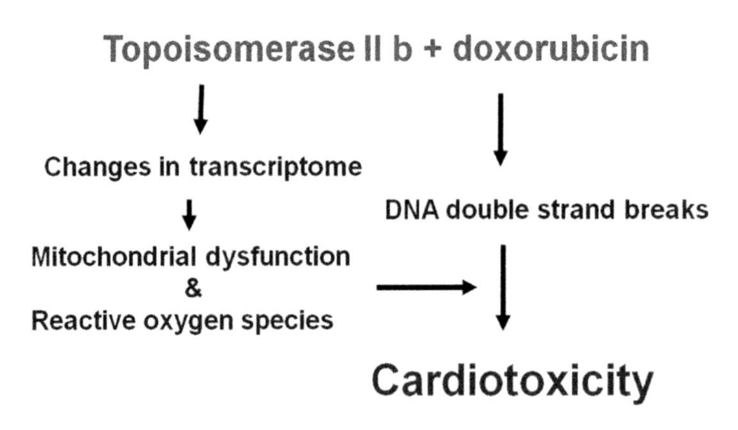

Fig. 8.10 Interaction of DOX with topoisomerase II b resulting in changes in the transcriptome, DNA damage, mitochondrial dysfunction, and ROS production culminating into cardiotoxicity.

cardioprotective effects were evident in both acute and chronic models of DOX-induced cardiomyopathy.[52,53] These findings were extended to human subjects in various clinical trials also.[54–57] It appears that DEX can block ATP hydrolysis and inhibit the reopening of the ATPase domain, thereby trapping the topoisomerase complex on DNA and blocking enzyme turnover,[58] which may be its predominant mechanism. Therefore, DEX inhibits DOX's activity on TOP II B catalytic site, thereby providing cardioprotection. In essence, DOX/DNA/Top II B ternary complex may be the prime mediator of anthracycline-mediated cardiomyopathy.

Current Therapies

Continuous infusion

Replacing bolus administration with slow infusions does not significantly affect anthracycline area under the curve but diminishes anthracycline maximum serum concentration (C_{max}) and anthracycline accumulation in the heart.[59] A *Cochrane Review*[60] identified 7 randomized controlled trials (RCTs) and showed a significantly lower rate of clinical HF with an infusion duration of 6 hours or longer as compared with a shorter infusion duration (relative risk = 0.27; 95% confidence interval [CI] 0.09–0.81; 5 studies; 557 patients). As far as the peak dose is concerned, neither less than 60 mg/m^2 DOX versus 60 mg/m^2 or more (2 RCTs), liposomal DOX at 25 mg/m^2 versus 50 mg/m^2 (1 RCT), and epirubicin peak dose of 83 mg/m^2 versus 110 mg/m^2 (1 RCT) showed promise for a lower incidence of clinical HF.[60] Thus, only prolongation of the anthracycline infusion to 6 hours or longer reduces the risk of clinical HF and subclinical cardiac damage to some extent.[60] It is important to consider that the review was only performed in adult population inflicted by solid tumors.

In pediatric populations, the results of infusion of anthracycline have been disappointing. A randomized trial in children with high-risk acute lymphoblastic leukemia (ALL) found that continuous infusion offered no additional cardiac protection over bolus administration in a median follow-up of 8 years after diagnosis.[61] A follow-up at 10 years also revealed no incremental therapeutic efficacy for infusion.[62] This finding is further supported by other studies, which also looked at cardiovascular outcomes in patients 5 to 7 years after treatment.[63,64] However, despite a lack of evidence for cardioprotection, anthracycline administration by continuous infusion is still incorporated into pediatric treatment protocols for cardioprotection.[62]

PEGylated liposomal doxorubicin

PEGylated liposomal DOX comprises an aqueous core of DOX hydrochloride encapsulated in liposomes with a protective hydrophilic outer coating of surface-bound methoxypolyethylene glycol.[65,66] Delivery of DOX in a PEGylated liposomal form decreases the circulating concentrations of free DOX and results in selective uptake of the agent in tumor cells.

In preclinical studies, PEGylated liposomal DOX demonstrated antitumor activity in several animal models of colon, breast, ovarian, lung, and other types of cancer, markedly inhibiting tumor growth rates and improving survival rates.[67] Furthermore, in a mouse mammary carcinoma (MC2) model, PEGylated liposomal DOX displayed efficacy against both high- and low-growth fraction tumor variants.[68] In 3 randomized,[69–71] open-label, multicenter trials, monotherapy conducted with PEGylated liposomal DOX showed that it is as effective as DOX or capecitabine in the first-line treatment of metastatic breast cancer, and as effective as vinorelbine or a combination mitomycin plus vinblastine in taxane-refractory metastatic breast cancer. PEGylated liposomal DOX alone was also as effective as topotecan or gemcitabine alone in patients with progressive ovarian cancer–resistant or refractory to platinum- or paclitaxel-based therapy.[72–74]

Although an effective antitumor activity has led to the development and sustainability of PEGylated liposomal DOX, this appears reinforced by the lower risk of symptomatic cardiotoxicity. In several studies, there was no evidence of symptomatic cardiotoxicity when PEGylated liposomal DOX was administered as a monotherapy or as part of combination therapy, irrespective of patients' prior exposure to anthracyclines, including high cumulative doses.[71,75,76] In the pivotal trial in patients with metastatic breast cancer, PEGylated liposomal DOX 50 mg/m^2 every 4 weeks was associated with a significantly (P<.001) lower risk of LVEF-defined cardiotoxicity than DOX 60 mg/m^2 every 3 weeks (hazard ratio [HR] 3.16; 95% CI 1.58, 6.31); this effect was observed irrespective of cardiovascular risk factors, including advanced age (65 years or older) and prior anthracycline exposure.[71] Ten of 254 recipients of PEGylated liposomal DOX (median cumulative anthracycline dose 293 mg/m^2) developed LVEF-defined cardiotoxicity compared with 48 of 255 recipients of conventional DOX (median cumulative anthracycline dose 361 mg/m^2). Of the patients who experienced cardiotoxicity, none in the PEGylated liposomal DOX group and 10 in the DOX group developed signs or symptoms of CHF.[71] Furthermore, high cumulative doses of PEGylated liposomal DOX were associated with a low risk of clinically significant cardiac dysfunction in patients with malignancies.[75,76] In a pooled analysis of patients with solid tumors (n = 418), the incidence of clinically significant cardiac dysfunction was low in PEGylated liposomal DOX 50 mg/m^2 recipients (lifetime cumulative anthracycline doses up to 1532 mg/m^2).[77] Thirteen (15%) of 88 patients who received cumulative anthracycline doses of greater than 400 mg/m^2 had at least one clinically significant change in LVEF; however, only one patient discontinued treatment because of clinical symptoms of HF. In a subset of 8 patients who received cumulative anthracycline doses of 509 to 1680 mg/m^2, endomyocardial biopsies demonstrated mild or no cardiotoxicity (Billingham cardiotoxicity scores of grades 0–1.5).[77]

PEGylated liposomal DOX exhibited a favorable cardiac safety profile compared with conventional DOX and other available chemotherapy agents. The most common treatment-related adverse events included myelosuppression, palmar-plantar erythrodysesthesia, and stomatitis, although these are manageable with appropriate supportive measures.[77] Thus, PEGylated liposomal DOX is a useful option in the treatment of various malignancies, including metastatic breast cancer, ovarian cancer, multiple myeloma, and AIDS-related Kaposi sarcoma.[78] However, the cost associated with administering the drug has prevented its widespread adoption as conventional anthracycline therapy.[79]

Dexrazoxane

DEX (ICRF-187, ADR-529) and the corresponding racemic mixture, razoxane (ICRF-159, ADR-159), belong to the bisdioxopiperazine agents originally developed by Creighton and Birnie[80] as potential anticancer agents. The investigators aimed to find cell-permeable EDTA prodrugs that may target biometals of vital importance within the cancer cells.[80] However, anticancer effects of DEX and razoxane have been later attributed to Top II inhibition.[81,82] Razoxane has passed through extensive preclinical development as an anticancer drug. DEX and other bisdioxopiperazines (ICRF-159, ICRF-193, and IRCF-194) have shown cytotoxicity in leukemic cells and cause DNA damage and apoptosis in various hematologic cell lines at clinically achievable (4–5 μM) concentrations.[48,80] DEX has some clinical anticancer activity as a single agent. Work reviewed by Kovacevic and colleagues[83] has shown that DEX can induce DNA double-stranded breaks as measured by the formation of the phosphorylated forms of the histone H2AX (termed serine 139 phosphorylated histone H2A [c-H2AX]) in cancer cells. Although it was being developed as anticancer agent, using H9c2 myoblasts and fibroblasts from TOP II B knockout (KO) mice, Lyu and colleagues[84] have suggested that the parent compound DEX may be protective through inhibition of anthracycline-induced and TOP II B-mediated DNA damage, thus opening a window of DEX as a protective agent for anthracycline-induced cardiotoxicity.

More evidence of support emerged when DEX was shown to be cardioprotective in DOX-treated populations. The salient effects of DEX against anthracycline-induced cardiotoxicity have been unanimously demonstrated in numerous clinical trials and in both adults and children.[56,57,85,86] Importantly, significant cardioprotection has been achieved in various chemotherapy regimens, using different DEX-to-anthracycline ratios and different subtypes of anthracyclines in clinical use. Cardioprotective potential of DEX has been evaluated by clinical examination (incidence of cardiac events and symptoms of CHF), using cardiac function examinations (echocardiography or radionuclide ventriculography), by analysis of biochemical markers (eg, plasma concentrations of cardiac troponins), and/or endomyocardial biopsy. Today, DEX has passed all stages of preclinical and clinical research and has been finally approved in Europe and the United States for cardioprotection in patients treated with anthracyclines (Cardioxane and Zinecard) with several generic preparations recently available (Procard and Cardynax). More recently, DEX has been also approved for treatment of accidental extravasation of anthracyclines (Savene). Thus, DEX's role as protective agent against anthracycline-induced cardiotoxicity has been firmly established.

Significant, although not well evidenced, suspicion on potential interference of DEX with anticancer effects of anthracycline has arisen from one of the phase III trials.[57] In this trial (n = 293), a significant difference in objective response has been reported (47% vs 61%, respectively, $P = .019$). Although high response in the placebo group was quite unusual; no other endpoints (including survival or time to progression) were affected in either of these studies. DEX nevertheless, became scrutinized for potentially negative effects on tumor response.[57,87] Careful meta-analyses of all available RCT data have, however, found no evidence for this hypothesis.[88,89] Still, the American Society of Clinical Oncology, Chemotherapy, and Radiotherapy Expert Panel remained cautious and recommended using DEX only in very limited conditions (eg, patients who have already received more than 300 mg/m^2 for metastatic breast cancer and who may benefit from continued DOX treatment).[90] The time has come to revisit this cautionary note.

Another controversial issue about DEX pertains to an increased risk of second malignancies; this was observed in survivors of Hodgkin lymphoma who had received DOX in combination with etoposide. As DOX, etoposide, and DEX inhibited topoisomerase IIα, albeit by different mechanisms and with different efficacies, it was postulated that combining the 3 drugs could exceed a threshold above which topoisomerase inhibitors may cause genetic instability in normal tissues.[91] This report led the European Medicine Agency to conclude that DEX should not be used in children due to increased risk of second malignancies. Two studies of survivors of childhood ALL reached opposite conclusions and did not detect an increased risk of second malignancies from DEX.[92,93] Thus, risk:benefit analyses support a wider clinical usage of DEX with the possible exception of conditions in which patients received etoposide or etoposide-anthracycline combinations. In essence, a cautionary note should be limited to the studied population only. Despite these isolated studies, DEX is a bona fide cardioprotective agent against anthracycline-induced cardiotoxicity, and as such, should be used as a part of anthracycline-based chemotherapy regimen (Table 8.3).

Preventive strategies. Close monitoring is required for patients with cancer who are undergoing treatment with cardiotoxic chemotherapy or have pre-existing cardiac disease, and the collaborative work between cardiologists and oncologists is particularly important in these patients. Of note, only 31% of patients receiving chemotherapy with an asymptomatic decrease in LVEF receive an angiotensin-converting enzyme (ACE) inhibitor or angiotensin receptor blocker (ARB); 35% receive a β-blocker, and 42% are referred for cardiology consultation (Table 8.4).[94] These cardiovascular medications have been shown to yield benefits in patients with cancer as well.

β-Blocker. β-Blockers are an integral element in the treatment of various cardiovascular diseases. Therefore, it is not surprising that initial investigations were done to demonstrate the beneficial effects of β-blockers for anthracycline cardiotoxicity, although they are limited. In a small, randomized, placebo-controlled study, patients treated with carvedilol at anthracycline initiation had preserved systolic and diastolic function

TABLE 8.3
Cost comparison of efforts of prevention of (acute) anthracycline cardiotoxicity

	US$
Enalapril 20 mg PO/d × 6 mo	90 (20)[a]
Carvedilol 12.5 mg PO BID × 6 mo	300 (20)[a]
Nebivolol 5 mg PO/d × 6 mo	420[a]
Atorvastatin 40 mg PO/d × 6 mo	600[a]
Continuous DOX infusion (48–72 h), 60 mg/m^2, max 500 mg	670[b]
DEX 10:1 dose ratio to DOX (ie, 5000 mg for 500 mg)	3,620[b]
Liposomal DOX, 500 mg	28,510[b]

Abbreviations: BID, twice a day; PO, orally.
[a] Based on Consumer Reports Health (US $10 3-month plan).
[b] Vejpongsa P, Yeh ET. Prevention of anthracycline-induced cardiotoxicity: challenges and opportunities. J Am Coll Cardiol 2014;64:938.

TABLE 8.4
Summary recommendations for the prevention of (acute) anthracycline cardiotoxicity

Clinical Setting	Primary Prevention	Level of Evidence	Class of Recommendation
High-risk profile from genetic testing	DEX Liposomal DOX Continuous infusion	C	IIb
Breast cancer (metastatic >300 mg/m^2)	DEX	A	I
Sarcoma	DEX Continuous infusion	A	IIa
High-risk pediatric ALL	DEX	A	IIa
All patients receiving anthracyclines	β-Blockers, ACE-I, ARB	C	IIb
Clinical Setting	**Secondary Prevention**	**Level of Evidence**	**Class of Recommendation**
Abnormal strain/LV function ± ↑ cardiac biomarkers	β-Blockers, ACE-I, ARB	B	IIa

Data from Vejpongsa P, Yeh ET. Prevention of anthracycline-induced cardiotoxicity: challenges and opportunities. J Am Coll Cardiol 2014;64:938–45.

at 6 months.[95] Similarly, patients with breast cancer who were randomized to nebivolol versus placebo (to be initiated 7 days before anthracycline-based chemotherapy and continued for 6 months) had preservation of LVEF at 6 months.[96] Recent data from the OVERCOME (preventiOn of left Ventricular dysfunction with Enalapril and caRvediolol in patients submitted to intensive ChemOtherapy for the treatment of Malignant hEmopathies) trial have also shown that β-blocker therapy, in combination with ACE inhibitor therapy, may be beneficial in preventing anthracycline-induced cardiotoxicity, evident in less significant changes in LVEF and a lower incidence of death or HF compared with placebo.[97] Similarly, a randomized controlled trial in 50 children diagnosed with ALL, assigned to receive the anthracycline DOX with or without carvedilol pretreatment, showed a significant increase in LV fractional shortening and global peak-systolic strain after the last dose compared with values before treatment in the pretreated group, whereas the DOX-only group had significant decreases in both parameters.[98] Furthermore, in the pretreated group, a significant decrease in plasma cardiac troponin I and lactic dehydrogenase was seen after the last dose, compared with values before treatment, whereas the DOX-only group saw significant increases in these same parameters.[98]

The PRADA (PRevention of cArdiac Dysfunction during Adjuvant breast cancer therapy) trial was designed as the largest clinical trial thus far to look at the chemotherapy-mediated cardiotoxicity. It was a randomized, placebo-controlled, 2 × 2 factorial, double-blind trial to assess whether LV dysfunction and injury are preventable, completely or partly, by the concomitant administration of the ARB, candesartan, and the β-blocker, metoprolol, during postoperative chemotherapy and radiotherapy.[99] The important finding in PRADA was that unlike the ARB candesartan, metoprolol, a β blocker, did not prevent the early drop in LVEF commonly seen in patients with breast cancer treated with anthracyclines and trastuzumab, even though both classes of heart medications are at the hub of treating ischemic and hypertensive cardiomyopathy.[100] This finding may be due to some of the study limitations. A foremost concern was the small number of participants in the study, even though it is the largest clinical trial in chemotherapy-mediated cardiotoxicity. Another limitation is that this was an extremely low-cardiovascular-risk patient cohort: the baseline prevalence of diabetes was less than 4% per group, and fewer than 7% of patients had hypertension. Therefore, the incidence of moderate and severe HF was extremely low and thereby hard to extrapolate to the authors' symptomatic population. Furthermore, the incidence of cardiomyopathy following breast cancer therapy is known to increase over time; the short duration of follow-up in the study was also concerning from β-blocker perspective.[96]

Cumulatively, preservation or limited decrease of LVEF has been seen in studies of carvedilol (α1- and β1–2-adrenoceptor blocker)[95] and nebivolol (β1-blocker with nitric oxide [NO]-potentiating effects).[96] Conversely, less or no protection has been seen with metoprolol (β1-blocker).[101] The rationale for using carvedilol or nebivolol can possibly been attributed to their additional cardioprotective roles. In addition to blocking adrenergic receptors, carvedilol diminishes ROS formation in isolated cardiomyocytes exposed to DOX.[102] Nebivolol induces endothelial NO synthase expression, thereby favoring NO-mediated vasodilation[103]; nebivolol also prevents NO synthase uncoupling, inappropriate generation of peroxynitrite, and nitroxidative stress.[104] It has also been hypothesized that certain β-blockers (carvedilol, nebivolol, alprenolol) inhibit β-adrenergic receptor–mediated G protein–coupled receptor signaling while preserving β-adrenergic receptor recruitment of β-arrestin and transactivation of ErbB1 (or epidermal growth factor receptor).[105,106] β-Arrestin is cardioprotective under long-term catecholamine stimulation, and activation of prosurvival signaling via the ErbB receptor pathway, and related downstream mediators have been associated with an attenuation of anthracycline-induced cardiotoxicity.[107] The available evidence nonetheless suggests that beneficial effects from one β-blocker or another eventually depends on its affinity and selectivity for β1 receptors [Ki(β2)/Ki(β1)] and on the consequent effects such as reductions in rate-pressure products and its subsequent role in myocardial remodeling.[108]

Angiotensin converting enzyme inhibitors and angiotensin receptor (type 1) inhibitor. The role of enalapril was studied in 114 patients with a normal baseline LVEF but an elevated troponin I level within 72 hours after high-dose anthracycline administration. These patients were then randomized to enalapril or placebo after completion of chemotherapy and followed for 12 months.[109] Roughly half of the control cohort (43%) and none of the ACE inhibitor–treated patients met the primary end point (decrease in LVEF of >10%). In addition, there were 30 cardiac events in the control patients and only 1 cardiac event in ACE inhibitor–treated patients.[109] Thus, early administration of enalapril proved to be cardioprotective.[5] In another observational study, patients with an LVEF ≤45% attributed to anthracycline cardiotoxicity were treated with enalapril with the addition of carvedilol as tolerated.[110] Interestingly, they observed that there seems to be a correlation with the institution of enalapril. Patients who received enalapril showed normalization of LVEF in 42% of patients, whereas no response was observed in patients in whom therapy was initiated greater than 6 months after completion of chemotherapy.[110] These findings suggest that the prompt administration of angiotensin-converting enzyme inhibitors (ACEI) was important in the LVEF recovery.[110] However, these patients were not randomized; therefore, the enalapril effect could be also due to pre-existing cardiac condition. A prospective study examined the effects of ACE inhibitors in patients with breast cancer treated with epirubicin. Patients receiving ACEI inhibitors had an increase in their LVEF, suggesting that ACEI should be part of the treatment of LV dysfunction in patients with cancer.[111] These studies paved the way for the OVERCOME trial, which showed beneficial effects with ACEI.

Conversely, in younger populations, such as DOX-treated long-term childhood cancer survivors, improvement in LV function with enalapril treatment was lost 10 years after treatment, suggesting that the effects of ACEI are transient.[112] In 2004, Silber and colleagues[113] reported the results of a randomized, double-blind, controlled clinical trial comparing enalapril with placebo in 135 long-term survivors of pediatric cancer who had at least 1 cardiac abnormality identified at any time after anthracycline exposure. There was no difference in the rate of change in maximal cardiac index per year between enalapril and placebo groups (0.30 L/min/m^2 vs 0.18 L/min/m^2; $P = .55$). However, the rate of change in LV end-systolic wall stress was greater in the enalapril group than in the placebo group (−8.59 g/cm^2 vs 1.85 g/cm^2; $P = .033$), and this difference was maintained over the study period, resulting in a 9% reduction in estimated LV end-systolic wall stress by the enalapril group.[113] However, this study only observed patients for 5 years.[112]

One possible explanation is that ACE inhibitors do not provide long-term protection in children because of the restrictive nature of anthracycline-induced cardiomyopathy.[114] In addition to the lack of evidence of a long-term benefit in children, compliance may be an issue with this cohort. In pediatric cancer populations who are undergoing chemotherapy, adverse effects of ACEI therapy are well known, including hypotension, dizziness, fatigue, and chronic neurohormonal suppression.[115] Thus, ACEI's effects may be limited in pediatric cancer population over the long term.

From a molecular biology standpoint, multiple animal studies have shown a beneficial effect of ACE inhibitor therapy on anthracycline-induced cardiotoxicity.[116–118] Possible key mechanisms supporting the benefit of ACE inhibition in chemotherapy-induced cardiotoxicity include a reduction in interstitial fibrosis,[119] attenuation of oxidative stress,[116,120] improved intracellular calcium handling,[121] and alterations in gene expression that affect cardiomyocyte metabolism and mitochondrial function.[122]

ARBs have also been studied as cardioprotective agents in patients receiving anthracycline therapy. Valsartan was found to have a protective effect against acute cardiotoxicity in a small study of patients who received DOX for Hodgkin lymphoma.[123] In a randomized control trial, patients who received telmisartan with epirubicin also showed preserved systolic function by LVEF and strain rate.[124] Overall, ARBs seem to have the same efficacy of cardioprotection as ACEIs.

Spironolactone. The cardioprotective role of spironolactone was identified in one study.[125] Female patients with breast cancer were randomized to either 25 mg/d spironolactone (n = 43, mean age 50 ± 11 years) or placebo (n = 40, mean age 51 ± 10 years). LVEF decreased from 67.0 ± 6.1% to 65.7 ± 7.4% (P = .094) in the spironolactone group, and from 67.7 ± 6.3% to 53.6 ± 6.8% in the control group (P<.001).[125] The intergroup LVEF decrease was significantly lower in the spironolactone group than in the control group (P<.001), and the diastolic function grade remained preserved in the spironolactone group (P = .096), whereas it deteriorated in the control group (P<.001).[125] A future clinical trial, NCT01708798, is being conducted where the potential ability of the aldosterone antagonist, eplerenone, to prevent DOX-induced cardiotoxicity, will be explored in a randomized controlled trial in the patients with breast cancer.

Statins. Clinical data regarding statin therapy for anthracycline-induced cardiotoxicity in humans have emerged. In a retrospective observational study of 201 patients with breast cancer treated with anthracyclines, concomitant statin use for other indications was associated with a reduced risk of HF hospitalization compared with propensity-matched controls (HR 0.3, 95% CI 0.1–0.9, P<.03).[126] In a small trial, 40 patients receiving anthracycline-containing chemotherapy regimens were randomized to receive atorvastatin or no intervention. The control but not the atorvastatin group showed statistically significant worsening of LVEF and change in LV dimensions, and the incidence of an LVEF less than 50% was lower (although not statistically significant) in patients on atorvastatin as compared with those in the control group (5% vs 25%, P<.18).[127]

Initial work in animal studies showed promising results for the use of statins in anthracycline-mediated cardiotoxicity. It was found that lovastatin reduced DOX-induced cardiomyocyte cell death[128] and reduced Top II B-mediated DNA damage via Rac1 signaling.[129] Activation of Rac1 signaling attenuated troponin I elevation and cardiac fibrosis after exposure to DOX.[129] In addition, lovastatin may potentiate the antitumor effects of DOX in vitro and in vivo in human fibrosarcoma cells.[129] Similarly, mice treated with fluvastatin had an attenuation of LV dysfunction after DOX exposure.[130] Therefore, statins should be considered in patients with cardiac toxicity secondary to chemotherapy, although it requires more evidence to be adopted as a part of conventional therapy.

HUMAN EPIDERMAL GROWTH FACTOR RECEPTOR-2/EPIDERMAL GROWTH FACTOR RECEPTOR-2 TARGETED THERAPIES

Clinical Perspective

Trastuzumab is a monoclonal antibody against the HER2-ErbB2, which is a member of a receptor tyrosine kinase family that regulates cell growth and intracellular repair.[131] Overexpression of HER2 is seen in approximately 25% of breast cancers and confers increased proliferative and metastatic potential. Trastuzumab has been used in HER2$^+$ breast cancers with significant reductions in recurrence rates and overall mortality. In agreement, a pivotal study in the metastatic setting demonstrated a 33% reduction in mortality at 1 year and an increase in median survival of 5 months.[132]

The cardiac side effect of trastuzumab was first noticed following the trials, leading to its approval by the US Food and Drug Administration in 1998.[6] In these trials, trastuzumab was administered on top of standard therapy, which consisted of either paclitaxel or DOX and cyclophosphamide. Post-hoc analyses revealed an incidence of "cardiotoxicity" of up to 11% in patients receiving trastuzumab on top of paclitaxel compared with only 1% to 4% in those who received paclitaxel alone.[132] There was an even greater incidence of cardiotoxicity in patients receiving the combination of trastuzumab and anthracyclines. Anthracyclines, such as DOX,[133] are themselves cardiotoxic, but the addition of trastuzumab leads to a synergistic increase in the incidence of cardiotoxicity from 13% to 27%. Moreover, severe HF (New York Heart Association [NYHA] class III and IV) occurred in 16% of patients treated with this combination.[6] Subsequently, several large clinical trials confirmed the importance of trastuzumab in increasing disease-free survival from cancer, but also established traztuzumab's association with HF.[134,135] The incidence of cardiomyopathy dropped to 13% when anthracyclines were not administered concurrently with trastuzumab, although these patients were previously treated with anthracycline. In the adjuvant trials, 1.7% to 4.1% of trastuzumab-treated patients developed CHF[134] when anthracycline was not part of the therapeutic regimen. Thus, trastuzumab carries a black box warning for cardiotoxicity.

Trastuzumab-related cardiac damage includes various degrees of LV systolic dysfunction, occasionally leading to CHF. Electrocardiographic changes are not seen.[136] Symptoms are usually mild or moderate and improve following medical management and termination of drug administration.[137,138] The improvement is usually seen in about 6 weeks after trastuzumab withdrawal but can be noted even earlier.[139] After symptomatic improvement, the reinstitution of trastuzumab treatment is usually possible.[137–139] The reversibility of trastuzumab-induced cardiac toxicity may be explained by the fact that this compound does not cause cell death but only temporary dysfunction by inducing changes in the structure of contractile proteins.[140] In further agreement, the risk of cardiotoxicity is confined to the time of administration, as illustrated in randomized controlled trials (Fig. 8.11). Because of these structural changes, trastuzumab belongs to the subgroup of type II chemotherapy-mediated cardiac dysfunction characteristics of type II chemotherapy-related cardiac damage.[8]

Pathophysiologic Mechanisms

Early studies indicated that the murine Erb-B2 Receptor Tyrosine Kinase 2 (ERBB2), and its activating ligand, neuregulin-1 (NRG-1), play an integral role in the cardiac development. Germline deletion of ERBB2[141] or NRG-1[142] resulted in midgestational lethality owing to dysmorphic ventricular development. The mid-gestational lethality suggests that ERBB2 signaling is required for cardiomyocyte proliferation and cardiac development. After cardiac development, mice with the cardiac-specific deletion of ERBB2 were viable, but developed dilated cardiomyopathy as they aged and had decreased survival when subjected to pressure overload induced by aortic banding.[143–145] Cardiomyocytes from these mice also exhibited enhanced sensitivity to the anthracyclines, thus alluding to a synergistic mechanism between anthracyclines and trastuzumab.

ERBB2 activation activates the ERK and PI3K/Akt pathways promoting cardiomyocyte survival.[146] Expression of the antiapoptotic protein Bcl-XL in the hearts of mice with cardiospecific ERBB2 deletion partially prevented the heart chamber dilation and the impaired contractility seen in the adulthood and suggests that ERBB2 signaling is important for normal cardiomyocyte function per se.[143] Unlike trastuzumab, however, lapatinib, a small molecule tyrosine kinase inhibitor of ERBB2 and EGFR, causes limited depression of cardiac function.[147,148] The same is true for pertuzumab, which inhibits ligand-mediated heterodimer formation.[149] Whether this mechanism of action yields cardioprotective effects, similar to what has been discussed for the activation of adenosine monophosphate-activated protein kinase with lapatinib, is unknown.[150,151] Regardless, these observations have questioned the mechanisms involved in trastuzumab-mediated cardiotoxicity.

Another school of thought exists regarding the actions of targeted Her-2 inhibitors on different

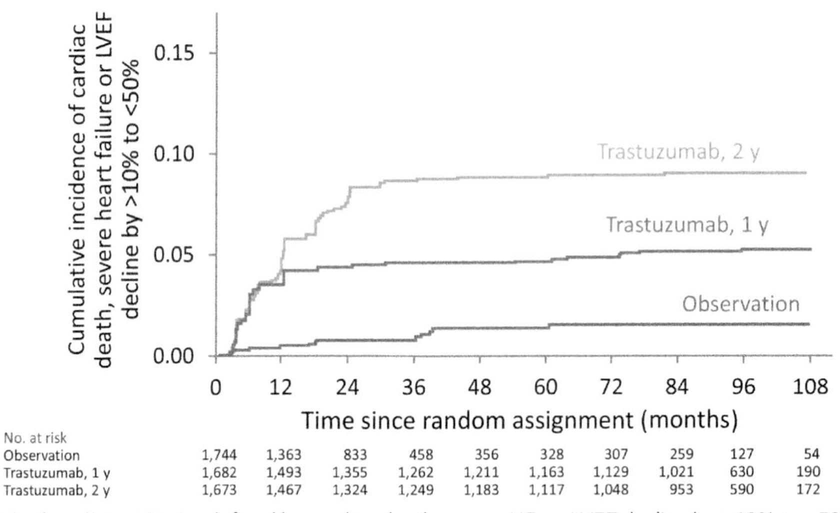

Fig. 8.11 Risk of cardiotoxicity (as defined by cardiac death, severe HF, or LVEF decline by >10% to <50%) over the course of trastuzumab therapy in the HERA trial. Note the confinement of risk to the duration of therapy. (*Data from* de Azambuja E, Procter MJ, Veldhuisen DJ. Trastuzumab-associated cardiac events at 8 years of median follow-up in the Herceptin Adjuvant trial (BIG 1-01). J Clin Oncol 2014;32(20):2159–65.)

aspects of Erb2 signal transduction possibly conferring a differential response. Trastuzumab is a humanized monoclonal antibody to the subdomain IV of ErbB2.[152] The antibody leads to disruption of ErbB2- ErbB3 complexes, which are preferentially formed when ErbB2 is overexpressed in the absence of ligand binding to ErbB3.[152] The exact mechanisms of this disruption are still unclear. Disruption of these complexes inhibits PI3K signaling and Akt activation and explains the antiproliferative effects of trastuzumab in ErbB2-amplified tumor cells. Hence, trastuzumab inhibits only ligand-independent signaling.[153] On the other hand, pertuzumab is a humanized monoclonal antibody to subdomain II, the dimerization arm of ErbB2.[154] Pertuzumab leads to inhibition of ligand-induced ErbB2 signaling, not of ligand-independent ErbB2 signaling, thus inhibiting the signal transduction mechanism only in the presence of a ligand.[153] Alternatively, lapatinib is a small molecule tyrosine kinase inhibitor of ErbB1 and ErbB2.[155] Lapatinib blocks tyrosine kinase activity, independently of whether this activity has been triggered by a ligand or not, thus inhibiting both ligand-dependent and -independent mechanisms.[153,156,157] With this assertion then, lapatinib should cause a similar, if not greater, incidence of cardiomyopathy, which is not the case clinically. Thus, precise mechanisms are not clearly delineated yet.

Current Therapies

In a Cardiac Review and Evaluation Committee analysis of 82 women with trastuzumab-induced cardiomyopathy,[8] 79% responded to conventional therapy, including ACEIs, diuretics, cardiac glycosides, and other inotropic agents. There was a significant difference in the recovery potential between patients with and without additional anthracycline therapy and those with and without cardiac troponin elevation, which was noted at baseline or during the first 2 cycles of trastuzumab, suggestive of an interactive phenomenon, as further outlined in later discussion.[8,28] Withdrawal of trastuzumab resulted in complete recovery in ejection fraction in 84% of the patients within a mean time of 1.5 months. More than 75% of patients in this cohort were reintroduced to traztuzumab, and 88% of these showed no further change in cardiac parameters.[8]

In 2009, the United Kingdom National Cancer Research Institute released recommendations for management of cardiac health in trastuzumab-treated patients with breast cancer. The readers are referred to this clinical resource for an effective management of trastuzumab-induced cardiomyopathy.[158]

Preventative strategies

Cardiovascular comorbidities certainly bode adverse outcomes in patients who are subjected to cardiotoxic chemotherapies. The disease and treatment burden has been shown to contribute to both weight gain[159] and a decrease in physical activity,[160,161] thus potentially raising cardiovascular disease risk. In 5721 asymptomatic women who underwent baseline evaluation in the St. James Women Take Heart Project, exercise tolerance measured by metabolic equivalents on treadmill testing predicted a 17% increase in Framingham Risk Score–adjusted mortality with each unit decline in metabolic equivalent of task (MET) level.[162] The decline in MET can be attenuated by exercise training in women because it improves cardiovascular function, especially in patients with breast cancer.[163,164] Furthermore, a *Cochrane Review* in 2012 showed benefit of a regular exercise program on quality of life in patients with cancer.[165] Taken together, these reports underscore the importance of cardiovascular fitness. Therefore, prevention and treatment should be centered around these adverse risk factors.

Before starting a chemotherapeutic regimen, it is important to be aware of patient comorbidities, such as hypertension or coronary artery disease, to precisely design therapeutic strategy specific for the patients. During cancer treatment, close cardiovascular monitoring should be applied for the early detection of cardiac toxicity, evaluation of the initial therapeutic plan, and treatment of cardiac dysfunction. Toxic agents such as alcohol consumption, drug abuse, and cigarette smoking should be avoided. Patients should follow a healthy lifestyle with a diet low in saturated fat and with restriction of salt intake, maintaining their body mass index near ideal range. Physical exercise, such as swimming or running, with different intensities (high, moderate, or low), should be performed before, during, or after chemotherapy to increase cardiovascular reserve.[166] Unfortunately, no clinical trials have been performed to prove its potential role to prevent chemotherapy-induced cardiac toxicity. An ongoing trial is testing the efficacy of acute exercise 24 hours before every chemotherapy treatment (NCT02006979).

It is recommended that all patients undergo baseline screening transthoracic echocardiography (TTE) before initiation of chemotherapy with agents known to cause cancer therapeutics–related cardiac dysfunction (grade IA from European Society for Medical Oncology [ESMO] guidelines).[167] This recommendation identifies patients with pre-existing compromised cardiac function so that their treatment regimen may be modified. Other methodologies, such as biomarkers and risk prediction models, can be used to risk stratify the patients. However, use of biomarkers and risk prediction model has not been integrated in the standard of practice. ESMO guidelines recommend assessment of cardiac function at baseline and at 3, 6, and 9 months during treatment as well as at 12 and 18 months after initiation of treatment (grade IA).[167] Thereafter, recommended monitoring with TTE is annual or biannual depending on the clinical indication.[167] A TTE should include assessment of LVEF, wall motion, diastolic dysfunction, and strain. American Society of Echocardiography and European Association of Echocardiography both recommend calculating LVEF using the modified biplane Simpson's technique in combination with the wall motion score index.[6,168,169] Although these recommendations are largely based on studies stemming from anthracycline treatments, the data on trastuzumab are sparse.

The Canadian Trastuzumab Working Group recommends that LVEF should be assessed using echocardiography or multigated acquisition scan at least every 3 months until trastuzumab therapy is completed, with annual follow-ups only for patients with cardiac symptoms or LVEF decline.[170] Long-term monitoring guidelines from the Children's Oncology Group can be considered for survivors of pediatric malignancies.[171,172] It is also unclear whether certain HF therapies are more suitable for specific cancer populations. Drug choice is usually based on clinical presentation and standard HF guidelines. Although there are some discrepancies regarding their effectiveness, these drugs have been recommended for use in at-risk patients undergoing systemic treatment, and these patients should be treated as per HF guidelines.[173] At present, studies are ongoing to evaluate cardioprotective agents in larger prospective randomized controlled trials. NCT01009918, the largest randomized controlled trial to date, is currently being conducted and will involve 468 patients undergoing trastuzumab chemotherapy to study the cardioprotective effects of lisinopril. Therefore, the recommendations for the traztuzumab group are different than the anthracycline counterpart, and it has been long awaited for some of the ongoing trials to dictate the therapeutic strategies.

In addition, prophylactic treatment in patients with high-dose chemotherapy may be a prudent therapeutic strategy in anthracycline-treated patients; however, the same concept cannot be extended to traztusumab-treated patients. Primary prevention is defined by early surveillance of at-risk patients using either biomarkers, imaging, or a combination of both. Because many of the patients who develop trastuzumab-induced cardiotoxicity have a chance to recover spontaneously, patients treated with trastuzumab will not be served well if they are started on cardioprotective agents prophylactically as a general rule. If patients have risk factors for type II cardiomyopathy (which includes hypertension, pre-existing coronary artery disease, and so forth; as noted above), then they should be on proper cardioprotective medications even before the cancer treatment, A more objective evidence-based data will be available after the trial NCT01009918 is published.

For secondary prevention in women with early breast cancer, treatment with a cardiotoxic agent should be discontinued and noncardiotoxic therapy substituted whenever possible. For women with metastatic HER-2-amplified breast cancer, temporarily discontinuing HER-2-targeted agents, treatment with blockers and ACEIs, and then cautious reintroduction of the HER-2-targeted agent is often successful with continued indefinite use of the β-blocker and ACE inhibitor.[174] Furthermore, for the general population experience, it is clear that individuals with an asymptomatic ejection fraction less than 50% have a ~3.5-fold increase in all-cause mortality over the ensuing 9 to 10 years.[175] Therefore, as per ESMO guidelines, use of ACEI should be considered in asymptomatic woman with LVEF of less than 50%. Furthermore, a combination of ACEI and β-blockers is recommended for both symptomatic and asymptomatic patients with LVEF less than 40%.[167] In addition, algorithms have also been proposed by the ESMO Clinical Practice Guideline for when to hold or discontinue treatment with trastuzumab based on serial LVEF measures.[167] Therefore, decisions to modify or stop cancer therapy should be made by the treating team comprising cardiologist, oncologist, other health care participants, and the patient.

ANTHRACYCLINES AND HUMAN EPIDERMAL GROWTH FACTOR RECEPTOR-2/EPIDERMAL GROWTH FACTOR RECEPTOR-2 TARGETED THERAPIES

Clinical Perspective

Since its introduction, trastuzumab has improved the clinical course of HER2-positive breast cancer in the metastatic, adjuvant, and neoadjuvant settings. The joint analysis of the National Surgical Adjuvant Breast and Bowel (NSABP) B-31 and North Central Cancer Treatment Group (NCCTG) N9831 trials demonstrated that the sequential addition of a year of trastuzumab therapy to the standard anthracycline-taxane regimen reduces the risk of recurrence by approximately half (HR, 0.48) and the risk of death by one-third (HR, 0.67).[176] These mortality and morbidity gains are substantial, but they are at the expense of developing cardiomyopathies.

In the anthracycline-trastuzumab arm in HER2-positive metastatic breast cancer trial, traztuzumab was given concurrently with 6 cycles of anthracycline (cumulative anthracycline dose 360 mg/m^2) with further cycles administered at investigator discretion. The resultant incidence of cardiac dysfunction and NYHA classes III–IV cardiotoxicity (ie, symptomatic CHF) was 27% and 16%, respectively,[6,132,137] as previously mentioned. Cardiotoxicity rates were lower in subsequent trials conducted in patients with metastatic breast cancer after the risk of cardiotoxicity was recognized, and concurrent administration with anthracyclines was avoided (Fig. 8.12). In an analysis of pooled data from 6 metastatic breast cancer trials, 11.6% of patients treated with trastuzumab after prior anthracyclines experienced a decrease in LVEF of 15 points or greater to a level less than 50%.[177]

Russell and colleagues[178] retrospectively reviewed patients with CHF in the NSABPB-31 and NCCTGN9831 studies. This analysis was a joint initiative of oncologists and cardiologists and was carried out in a blinded fashion. CHF was defined by symptoms, physical signs, and objective findings and included an LVEF decrease of 10% or a decrease to an absolute LVEF of less than 50% by locally obtained multigated radionuclide angiography or echocardiogram. The study showed that the addition of trastuzumab to anthracycline-based chemotherapy increased the incidence of CHF nearly 4-fold, from 0.45% to 2.0%, at a median follow-up of 1.9 and 2.0 years, respectively.[178] Among those assigned to trastuzumab, 133 (7.4%) patients with possible cardiac events were reviewed, yielding 36 that were deemed to have definitely suffered a cardiac event.[178] Most importantly, roughly 86% of these patients had some degree of recovery in function with more than two-thirds showing complete regain of baseline cardiac function.[178]

Procter and colleagues[179] report a similar analysis from the Herceptin Adjuvant (HERA) study. As expected, the most common cardiac event noted was a "significant" LVEF decrease, defined as an absolute decline of at least 10 percentage points from baseline to less than 50%. The LVEF decrease occurred in 164 (9.8%) trastuzumab-treated patients compared with 49 (2.9%) controls.[179] However, these changes in LVEF rarely translated into symptomatic CHF, which occurred in 32 (1.9%) trastuzumab-treated patients versus 2 (0.1%) controls.[179]

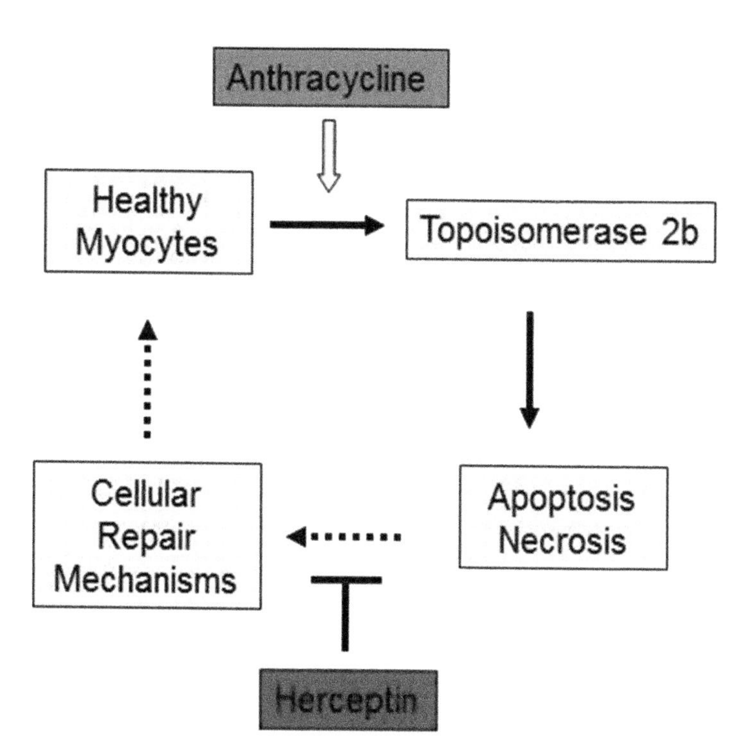

Fig. 8.12 Incidence of HF with trastuzumab as a function of time from anthracycline therapy. (*Data from* Ewer MS, Ewer SM. Cardiotoxicity of anticancer treatments: what the cardiologist needs to know. Nat Rev Cardiol 2010;7(10):564.)

Pathophysiologic Mechanisms

The precise mechanism(s) responsible for the toxic synergistic interaction(s) of trastuzumab with anthracyclines has not been fully elucidated yet. Earlier studies speculated that the interference(s) of trastuzumab with cardiac tissue repair mechanisms mediated by HER2 during DOX toxicity, primarily in the form of a HER2:HER4 heterodimer might be the cause of synergism.[132,138,177] The idea of HER2 being cardioprotective was largely inferred when gene-targeting studies in mice show that HER2 is essential for cardiac development.[143] Moreover, conditional deletion of HER2 leads to a dilated cardiomyopathy.[143] Thus, earlier observation indicates that the HER2 receptor and associated intracellular signaling are important determinants of normal cardiac structure and function. The link between the physiologic function of HER2 in the heart and the enhancement of DOX-induced cardiotoxicity was elucidated in KO mice for NRG-1, a well-defined ligand for the HER2:HER4 heterodimer.[180] These studies showed that under normal conditions the wild-type and KO mice exhibited comparable total levels of HER2 in the left ventricle; however, DOX administration caused much more HER2 phosphorylation in wild-type mice as compared with KO mice, consistent with the hypothesis that NRG-1 modulation of HER2 activation represents an important adaptive response to the stress induced by anthracyclines.[180]

Subsequent studies indicated that sequential stress might provide a plausible explanation of traztuzumab-enhanced anthracycline cardiomyopathy. Studies done by Pentassuglia and colleagues[181] showed that PKI166, which is a specific inhibitor of Erb1-Erb2 heterodimer, resulted in myofibrillar structural damage that was additive to that induced by DOX at clinically relevant doses. These changes were associated with an inhibition of the excitation-contraction coupling mediated via mitogen-activated protein–kinase signaling pathway.[181] In addition, the cross-talk between anthracycline and HER2 receptors was also identified at the miRNA level. Horie and colleagues[182] showed that DOX treatment resulted in overexpression of miR-146a, which in turn inhibited ErbB4 expression, thereby inducing cell death in cardiomyocytes. Re-expression of ErbB4 in miR-146a–overexpressing cardiomyocytes ameliorated DOX-induced cell death as did the use of "decoy" genes with tandem complementary sequences for miR-146a.[182] The concept of anthracycline and traztuzumab interaction was also confirmed in human-induced pluripotent stem cell–derived cardiomyocytes (hiPSC-CMs).[183] Activation of ErbB signaling with NRG, or inhibition with trastuzumab in hiPSC-CMs, alleviated or aggravated DOX-induced cardiomyocyte damage, respectively, as assessed by a real-time cellular impedance analysis and ATP measurement.[183] Thus, it is plausible that inhibition of reparative pathways by trastuzumab may exacerbate the damage instilled by DOX in keeping with the concept of a synergistic sequential stress response (see Fig. 8.12).

Current Therapies

The main crux of minimizing trastuzumab-enhanced anthracycline cardiotoxicity lies in the sequential administration of these chemotherapies. The metastatic breast cancer trial showed that concurrent treatment of trastuzumab and anthracycline had detrimental cardiac outcomes.[6,132] However, as the time duration was increased between the anthracycline and trastuzumab administration, the incidence of CHF drastically reduced (Fig. 8.13). In the N9831 trial, the incidence of NYHA class III/IV CHF or cardiac

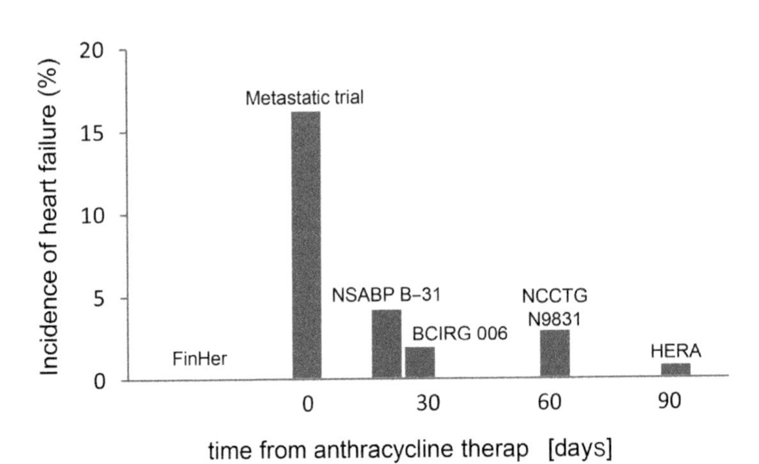

Fig. 8.13 The sequential stress. The interaction of anthracycline and topoisomerase 2b results in apoptosis and necrosis. Under ideal conditions, some of the reparative process is done by HER2 signaling. When herceptin inhibits this reparative process, the population of healthy cardiomyocytes decrease, leading to an exaggerated cardiotoxic response.

TABLE 8.5
Guideline recommendations for cardiac monitoring

Guideline	Year	Recommendation	Level of Evidence
Cardiology			
American College of Cardiology/AHA Management of Heart Failure[37]	2013	The incidence and reversibility of chemotherapy-related cardiotoxicity are not well documented, and meaningful interventions to prevent injury have not yet been elucidated	Not stated
European Society of Cardiology[38]	2012	Preevaluation and postevaluation of EF is essential in patients receiving cardiotoxic chemotherapy Patients developing LVSD should not receive further chemotherapy and should receive standard treatment for HFrEF	Not stated
American Society of Echocardiography[40]	2003	Baseline and re-evaluation examinations in patients receiving cardiotoxic chemotherapeutic agents	Class 1
Oncology			
Canadian Trastuzumab Working Group[31]	2008	Cardiac imaging (Echo or MUGA) at baseline and 3-mo intervals until completion of therapy at minimum with more frequent/stringent monitoring for higher risk patients	Not stated
American Society of Clinical Oncology: Cardiac and Pulmonary Late Effects[10]	2007	The optimal duration, frequency, and method of cardiac monitoring during trastuzumab and anthracycline treatment remains unknown	Not stated
Position statements			
American Society of Echocardiography/European Association of Cardiovascular Imaging: Multimodality Imaging Evaluation[24]	2014	Treatment with anthracycline → baseline LVEF assessment with 3D or 2D Echo, GLS, and troponin I measurement. If abnormal, cardiology consultation. Follow-up at completion of therapy and 6 mo later for doses <240 mg/m^2 Treatment with trastuzumab → baseline LVEF assessment with 3D or 2D Echo, GLS, and TROPONIN I measurement. If abnormal, cardiology consultation. Follow-up every 3 and 6 mo.	Not stated
ESMO Clinical Practice Guidelines[25]	2012	In patients receiving anthracyclines ± trastuzumab → serial monitoring of cardiac function at baseline, 3, 6, and 9 mo during treatment, 12 and 18 mo after start of treatment	Level 1, grade A
		In patients with metastatic diseases → monitor EF at baseline and infrequently in absence of symptoms	Level II, grade A
		Measurement of troponin, BNP at baseline, and periodically during therapy	Level III, grade B
		Cardiac function assessment 4–10 y after anthracycline in patients treated at <15 y of age or >15 y with cumulative dose DOX >240 mg/m^2	Level II, grade B
		LVEF drop <50% during anthracycline-containing → reassess in 3 wk. If confirmed, hold chemotherapy and consider therapy for LVSD	Level II, grade B
		LVEF drop <50% during trastuzumab therapy → reassess in 3 wk. If confirmed, continue trastuzumab and consider therapy for LVSD	Level II, grade B

(continued on next page)

Table 8.5
(*continued*)

Guideline	Year	Recommendation	Level of Evidence
Heart Failure Association of the European Society of Cardiology: Cardiovascular Side Effects of Cancer Therapies[36]	2011	Regular cardiovascular evaluation should be part of routine care in patients receiving treatment regimens known to be associated with cardiotoxicity Follow-up beyond completion of therapy should be considered, particularly in those receiving high doses of anthracyclines. Use of troponin and BNP should be strongly considered	Not stated

Abbreviations: EF, ejection traction; GLS, global longitudinal strain; HFrEF, heart failure reduced ejection fraction; LVSD, left ventricular systolic dysfunction; MUSA, multigated acquisition scan.

Data from Hamo CE, Bloom MW, Cardinale D, et al. Cancer therapy–related cardiac dysfunction and heart failure: part 2: prevention, treatment, guidelines, and future directions. Circ Heart Fail 2016;9:e002843.

deaths was 0% in the control arm, and 3.3% in the concurrent trastuzumab arm (1 cardiac death).[16] In the B-31 study, these toxic effects occurred in 0.8% of the control group (1 cardiac death) and 4.1% of the trastuzumab arm (no cardiac deaths).[184] The results of both studies were in marked distinction from the 27% incidence rate of CHF in the original metastatic trials. Better results were seen in the FinHer trial.[185] A subset of 232 patients with HER2 amplification was randomized to receive chemotherapy (either docetaxel or vinorelbine) followed by fluorouracil, epirubicin, and cyclophosphamide (FEC) in all groups and a further randomization to 9 weeks trastuzumab or docetaxel or vinorelbine in those with HER2 amplification.[185] Thus, 58 patients were randomized to docetaxel followed by FEC, 54 to docetaxel and trastuzumab followed by FEC, 58 to vinorelbine followed by FEC without trastuzumab, and finally, 62 to vinorelbine and trastuzumab followed by FEC. A significant improvement in disease-free survival and a borderline-significant overall survival advantage were seen even with only 9 weeks of trastuzumab therapy, but contrary to previous studies, there were no CHF cases with trastuzumab, and a negligible LVEF effect. Caution, however, is to be exercised given the small number of participants in this trial. Overall, nevertheless, one may conclude that nonconcurrent administration of traztuzumab and anthracycline yields oncologic benefits with lower on-treatment cardiotoxicity risk.

Other Chemotherapeutics with Cardiotoxicity Potential

Although this chapter exclusively dealt with anthracycline and trastuzumab-associated cardiomyopathies, there are numerous chemotherapeutic agents that have reported cardiotoxicity. The reader is referred to Fig. 8.1 for some of the known cardiotoxic effects of various chemotherapy agents. Furthermore, in-depth clinical readings are also available elsewhere.[167,186,187]

APPROACH TO HEART FAILURE IN THE PATIENTS WITH CANCER

Tremendous strides have been made in last few decades on the management of cancer, which has culminated into improved mortality and morbidity outcomes. However, this has come at the cost of various cardiovascular toxicities such as HF. A comprehensive approach to HF has thus become an essential aspect of oncology practice. The current approach is divided into 4 distinct pathways.

Primordial prevention is defined by prophylactic therapy given before or during adjuvant therapy to prevent anticipated injury.[188] Recent small trials involving β-blockers,[95,101] ACEI,[101] ARBs,[123,189] and statins[127] have shown the preemptive strike with medications in high cardiovascular risk population may be beneficial in attenuating the LV dysfunction and/or remodeling of the heart. Although these were small studies, the results are anticipated from some of the big trials (such as NCT01724450 and NCT00236806), which may identify at-risk populations in which this strategy can be deployed. With the exception of the statin trial,[127] most of the above-mentioned trials either had no change in cardiac functional parameters or changes were noticed only in analysis where the anthracycline dose used was at a relevant level as per ESMO guidelines.[95]

Primary prevention is a therapeutic modality whereby patients at risk of developing toxicity are closely monitored and/or therapy is administered at the onset of signs of injury. For the purposes of this chapter, the main objective is to identify the patients with cancer who are at risk for cardiotoxicity. Therefore, evaluation of patients for known risk factors (as noted above), or presence of pre-existing cardiac disease, is essential in formulating the treatment and follow-up plan. Furthermore, use of biomarkers and cardiac imaging modalities can be used for monitoring purposes. Numerous risk scores[19,190,191] have been designed to stratify cardiac patients; however, rigorous evaluation is needed before these risk assessment scores are integrated in the normal clinical practices. Nevertheless, these risk scores do identify some of the biomarkers, pre-existing conditions, and/or chemotherapeutic plan that may pose added risk of developing cardiotoxicity.

Secondary prevention encompasses deployment of therapeutic strategies once the impairment is noted. As noted above, numerous clinical trials outline the use of β-blockers,[95,97] ACEI,[109,111] ARBs,[123,124] statins,[126,127] and some evidence with respect to aldosterone receptor antagonists in patients with cancer[125] with cardiotoxicities. Although the time of initiation or guidelines as to when combination therapy (such as β-blocker and ACEI vs b-b locker + ACEI + angiotensin receptor antagonist +) should be used is lacking, the ideal management strategy used is similar to treating the HF population. In the MD Anderson Cancer Center, they have developed their own clinical practice guide based on experiences, which is available in video and paper-book format for free to the interested parties. These practice guidelines are developed based on the authors' experiences of treating patients with cancer afflicted with cardiac disease since 2000. In addition, numerous guidelines and position statements have been published and are outlined in Table 8.5.

Patients with symptomatic and/or overt HF should be treated as per AHA HF guideline.[192] This guideline includes managing patients with medications, cardiac devices, and inotropes. Patients with end-stage HF should be evaluated and appropriately treated with mechanical circulatory support and/or heart transplant.

SUMMARY

Anthracyclines are heralded as old drugs with unwavering beneficial effects. Their application has been widespread and forms an integral part of cancer therapy regimens. However, the widespread use has been hampered by its cardiomyopathic effect. Understanding and delineating the mechanisms is the first step in ameliorating the side effects of anthracyclines, and therefore, we should be vigorous in our pursuit. A similar approach should also be exercised with newer chemotherapies such as trastuzumab, which also causes cardiomyopathy but with significant differences with regards to molecular pathways and prognosis. Thus, we cannot paint all the cardiomyopathies/cardiotoxicity with the same brush, and there is a need still to advance our knowledge in this area to identify, understand, and thereby attenuate if not ameliorate chemotherapy-induced cardiomyopathy.

REFERENCES

1. Von Hoff DD, Layard MW, Basa P, et al. Risk factors for doxorubicin-induced congestive heart failure. Ann Intern Med 1979;91:710–7.
2. Yeh ET, Bickford CL. Cardiovascular complications of cancer therapy: incidence, pathogenesis, diagnosis, and management. J Am Coll Cardiol 2009; 53:2231–47.
3. Brigden W. Uncommon myocardial diseases: the non-coronary cardiomyopathies. Lancet 1957; 273:1243–9.
4. Richardson P, McKenna W, Bristow M, et al. Report of the 1995 World Health Organization/International Society and Federation of Cardiology Task Force on the Definition and Classification of cardiomyopathies. Circulation 1996;93: 841–2.
5. Maron BJ, Towbin JA, Thiene G, et al. Contemporary definitions and classification of the cardiomyopathies: an American Heart Association Scientific Statement from the Council on Clinical Cardiology, Heart Failure and Transplantation Committee; Quality of Care and Outcomes Research and Functional Genomics and Translational Biology Interdisciplinary Working Groups; and Council on Epidemiology and Prevention. Circulation 2006; 113:1807–16.
6. Seidman A, Hudis C, Pierri MK, et al. Cardiac dysfunction in the trastuzumab clinical trials experience. J Clin Oncol 2002;20:1215–21.
7. Theodoulou M, Seidman AD. Cardiac effects of adjuvant therapy for early breast cancer. Semin Oncol 2003;30:730–9.
8. Ewer MS, Lippman SM. Type II chemotherapy-related cardiac dysfunction: time to recognize a new entity. J Clin Oncol 2005;23:2900–2.
9. Zhang S, Liu X, Bawa-Khalfe T, et al. Identification of the molecular basis of doxorubicin-induced cardiotoxicity. Nat Med 2012;18:1639–42.
10. Balducci L, Extermann M. Cancer and aging. An evolving panorama. Hematol Oncol Clin North Am 2000;14:1–16.
11. Lotrionte M, Biondi-Zoccai G, Abbate A, et al. Review and meta-analysis of incidence and clinical predictors of anthracycline cardiotoxicity. Am J Cardiol 2013;112:1980–4.

12. Tashakkor AY, Moghaddamjou A, Chen L, et al. Predicting the risk of cardiovascular comorbidities in adult cancer survivors. Curr Oncol 2013;20: e360–70.
13. Lipshultz SE, Lipsitz SR, Sallan SE, et al. Chronic progressive cardiac dysfunction years after doxorubicin therapy for childhood acute lymphoblastic leukemia. J Clin Oncol 2005;23:2629–36.
14. Swain SM, Whaley FS, Ewer MS. Congestive heart failure in patients treated with doxorubicin: a retrospective analysis of three trials. Cancer 2003; 97:2869–79.
15. Krischer JP, Epstein S, Cuthbertson DD, et al. Clinical cardiotoxicity following anthracycline treatment for childhood cancer: the Pediatric Oncology Group experience. J Clin Oncol 1997; 15:1544–52.
16. Romond EH, Jeong JH, Rastogi P, et al. Seven-year follow-up assessment of cardiac function in NSABP B-31, a randomized trial comparing doxorubicin and cyclophosphamide followed by paclitaxel (ACP) with ACP plus trastuzumab as adjuvant therapy for patients with node-positive, human epidermal growth factor receptor 2-positive breast cancer. J Clin Oncol 2012;30:3792–9.
17. Chavez-MacGregor M, Zhang N, Buchholz TA, et al. Trastuzumab-related cardiotoxicity among older patients with breast cancer. J Clin Oncol 2013;31:4222–8.
18. Chen J, Long JB, Hurria A, et al. Incidence of heart failure or cardiomyopathy after adjuvant trastuzumab therapy for breast cancer. J Am Coll Cardiol 2012;60:2504–12.
19. Ezaz G, Long JB, Gross CP, et al. Risk prediction model for heart failure and cardiomyopathy after adjuvant trastuzumab therapy for breast cancer. J Am Heart Assoc 2014;3:e000472.
20. Bristow MR, Mason JW, Billingham ME, et al. Doxorubicin cardiomyopathy: evaluation by phonocardiography, endomyocardial biopsy, and cardiac catheterization. Ann Intern Med 1978;88: 168–75.
21. Hayek ER, Speakman E, Rehmus E. Acute doxorubicin cardiotoxicity. N Engl J Med 2005;352: 2456–7.
22. Lenihan DJ. Progression of heart failure from AHA/ ACC stage A to stage B or even C: can we all agree we should try to prevent this from happening? J Am Coll Cardiol 2012;60:2513–4.
23. Bristow MR, Thompson PD, Martin RP, et al. Early anthracycline cardiotoxicity. Am J Med 1978;65: 823–32.
24. Dazzi H, Kaufmann K, Follath F. Anthracycline-induced acute cardiotoxicity in adults treated for leukaemia. Analysis of the clinico-pathological aspects of documented acute anthracycline-induced cardiotoxicity in patients treated for acute leukaemia at the University Hospital of Zurich, Switzerland, between 1990 and 1996. Ann Oncol 2001;12:963–6.
25. Slordal L, Spigset O. Heart failure induced by non-cardiac drugs. Drug Saf 2006;29:567–86.
26. Sterba M, Popelova O, Vavrova A, et al. Oxidative stress, redox signaling, and metal chelation in anthracycline cardiotoxicity and pharmacological cardioprotection. Antioxid Redox Signal 2013;18: 899–929.
27. Poole CJ, Earl HM, Hiller L, et al. Epirubicin and cyclophosphamide, methotrexate, and fluorouracil as adjuvant therapy for early breast cancer. N Engl J Med 2006;355:1851–62.
28. Li X, Xu S, Tan Y, et al. The effects of idarubicin versus other anthracyclines for induction therapy of patients with newly diagnosed leukaemia. Cochrane Database Syst Rev 2015;(6):CD010432.
29. Brambilla C, Rossi A, Bonfante V, et al. Phase II study of doxorubicin versus epirubicin in advanced breast cancer. Cancer Treat Rep 1986;70:261–6.
30. Jain KK, Casper ES, Geller NL, et al. A prospective randomized comparison of epirubicin and doxorubicin in patients with advanced breast cancer. J Clin Oncol 1985;3:818–26.
31. Kaklamani VG, Gradishar WJ. Epirubicin versus doxorubicin: which is the anthracycline of choice for the treatment of breast cancer? Clin Breast Cancer 2003;4(Suppl 1):S26–33.
32. Blanco JG, Sun CL, Landier W, et al. Anthracycline-related cardiomyopathy after childhood cancer: role of polymorphisms in carbonyl reductase genes–a report from the Children's Oncology Group. J Clin Oncol 2012;30:1415–21.
33. Smith LA, Cornelius VR, Plummer CJ, et al. Cardiotoxicity of anthracycline agents for the treatment of cancer: systematic review and meta-analysis of randomised controlled trials. BMC Cancer 2010; 10:337.
34. Ryberg M, Nielsen D, Skovsgaard T, et al. Epirubicin cardiotoxicity: an analysis of 469 patients with metastatic breast cancer. J Clin Oncol 1998;16: 3502–8.
35. Ryberg M, Nielsen D, Cortese G, et al. New insight into epirubicin cardiac toxicity: competing risks analysis of 1097 breast cancer patients. J Natl Cancer Inst 2008;100:1058–67.
36. van Dalen EC, Michiels EM, Caron HN, et al. Different anthracycline derivates for reducing cardiotoxicity in cancer patients. Cochrane Database Syst Rev 2010:CD005006.
37. Hohloch K, Zwick C, Ziepert M, et al. Significant dose Escalation of Idarubicin in the treatment of aggressive Non- Hodgkin Lymphoma leads to increased hematotoxicity without improvement in efficacy in comparison to standard CHOEP-14: 9-year follow

up results of the CIVEP trial of the DSHNHL. Springerplus 2014;3:5.
38. Davies KJ, Doroshow JH, Hochstein P. Mitochondrial NADH dehydrogenase-catalyzed oxygen radical production by adriamycin, and the relative inactivity of 5-iminodaunorubicin. FEBS Lett 1983; 153:227–30.
39. Doroshow JH, Davies KJ. Comparative cardiac oxygen radical metabolism by anthracycline antibiotics, mitoxantrone, bisantrene, 4′-(9-acridinylamino)-methanesulfon-m-anisidide, and neocarzinostatin. Biochem Pharmacol 1983;32:2935–9.
40. Hershko C, Link G, Tzahor M, et al. Anthracycline toxicity is potentiated by iron and inhibited by deferoxamine: studies in rat heart cells in culture. J Lab Clin Med 1993;122:245–51.
41. Link G, Tirosh R, Pinson A, et al. Role of iron in the potentiation of anthracycline cardiotoxicity: identification of heart cell mitochondria as a major site of iron-anthracycline interaction. J Lab Clin Med 1996;127:272–8.
42. Myers CE, Gianni L, Simone CB, et al. Oxidative destruction of erythrocyte ghost membranes catalyzed by the doxorubicin-iron complex. Biochemistry 1982;21:1707–12.
43. Bodley A, Liu LF, Israel M, et al. DNA topoisomerase II-mediated interaction of doxorubicin and daunorubicin congeners with DNA. Cancer Res 1989;49:5969–78.
44. Schoeffler AJ, Berger JM. DNA topoisomerases: harnessing and constraining energy to govern chromosome topology. Q Rev Biophys 2008;41: 41–101.
45. Corbett KD, Berger JM. Structure of the topoisomerase VI-B subunit: implications for type II topoisomerase mechanism and evolution. EMBO J 2003;22:151–63.
46. L'Ecuyer T, Sanjeev S, Thomas R, et al. DNA damage is an early event in doxorubicin-induced cardiac myocyte death. Am J Physiol Heart Circ Physiol 2006;291:H1273–80.
47. Liu J, Mao W, Ding B, et al. ERKs/p53 signal transduction pathway is involved in doxorubicin-induced apoptosis in H9c2 cells and cardiomyocytes. Am J Physiol Heart Circ Physiol 2008;295: H1956–65.
48. Hasinoff BB, Hellmann K, Herman EH, et al. Chemical, biological and clinical aspects of dexrazoxane and other bisdioxopiperazines. Curr Med Chem 1998;5:1–28.
49. Herman EH, el-Hage A, Ferrans VJ. Protective effect of ICRF-187 on doxorubicin-induced cardiac and renal toxicity in spontaneously hypertensive (SHR) and normotensive (WKY) rats. Toxicol Appl Pharmacol 1988;92:42–53.
50. Herman EH, Ferrans VJ, Myers CE, et al. Comparison of the effectiveness of (+/-)-1,2-bis(3,5-dioxopiperazinyl-1-yl)propane (ICRF-187) and N-acetylcysteine in preventing chronic doxorubicin cardiotoxicity in beagles. Cancer Res 1985;45:276–81.
51. Herman EH, Zhang J, Chadwick DP, et al. Comparison of the protective effects of amifostine and dexrazoxane against the toxicity of doxorubicin in spontaneously hypertensive rats. Cancer Chemother Pharmacol 2000;45:329–34.
52. Herman EH, Ferrans VJ. Timing of treatment with ICRF-187 and its effect on chronic doxorubicin cardiotoxicity. Cancer Chemother Pharmacol 1993; 32:445–9.
53. Rao VA, Zhang J, Klein SR, et al. The iron chelator Dp44mT inhibits the proliferation of cancer cells but fails to protect from doxorubicin-induced cardiotoxicity in spontaneously hypertensive rats. Cancer Chemother Pharmacol 2011;68:1125–34.
54. Imondi AR. Preclinical models of cardiac protection and testing for effects of dexrazoxane on doxorubicin antitumor effects. Semin Oncol 1998; 25:22–30.
55. Lipshultz SE, Colan SD, Gelber RD, et al. Late cardiac effects of doxorubicin therapy for acute lymphoblastic leukemia in childhood. N Engl J Med 1991;324:808–15.
56. Marty M, Espie M, Llombart A, et al. Multicenter randomized phase III study of the cardioprotective effect of dexrazoxane (Cardioxane) in advanced/metastatic breast cancer patients treated with anthracycline-based chemotherapy. Ann Oncol 2006;17:614–22.
57. Swain SM, Whaley FS, Gerber MC, et al. Cardioprotection with dexrazoxane for doxorubicin-containing therapy in advanced breast cancer. J Clin Oncol 1997;15:1318–32.
58. Nitiss JL. Targeting DNA topoisomerase II in cancer chemotherapy. Nat Rev Cancer 2009;9:338–50.
59. Minotti G, Menna P, Salvatorelli E, et al. Anthracyclines: molecular advances and pharmacologic developments in antitumor activity and cardiotoxicity. Pharmacol Rev 2004;56:185–229.
60. van Dalen EC, van der Pal HJ, Caron HN, et al. Different dosage schedules for reducing cardiotoxicity in cancer patients receiving anthracycline chemotherapy. Cochrane Database Syst Rev 2009:CD005008.
61. Lipshultz SE, Miller TL, Lipsitz SR, et al. Continuous Versus Bolus Infusion of Doxorubicin in Children With ALL: Long-term Cardiac Outcomes. Pediatrics 2012;130:1003–11.
62. Lipshultz SE, Cochran TR, Franco VI, et al. Treatment-related cardiotoxicity in survivors of childhood cancer. Nat Rev Clin Oncol 2013;10: 697–710.
63. Gupta M, Steinherz PG, Cheung NK, et al. Late cardiotoxicity after bolus versus infusion

anthracycline therapy for childhood cancers. Med Pediatr Oncol 2003;40:343–7.
64. Levitt GA, Dorup I, Sorensen K, et al. Does anthracycline administration by infusion in children affect late cardiotoxicity? Br J Haematol 2004;124:463–8.
65. Pignata S, Scambia G, Ferrandina G, et al. Carboplatin plus paclitaxel versus carboplatin plus pegylated liposomal doxorubicin as first-line treatment for patients with ovarian cancer: the MITO-2 randomized phase III trial. J Clin Oncol 2011;29: 3628–35.
66. Sharpe M, Easthope SE, Keating GM, et al. Polyethylene glycol-liposomal doxorubicin: a review of its use in the management of solid and haematological malignancies and AIDS-related Kaposi's sarcoma. Drugs 2002;62:2089–126.
67. Vail DM, Amantea MA, Colbern GT, et al. Pegylated liposomal doxorubicin: proof of principle using preclinical animal models and pharmacokinetic studies. Semin Oncol 2004;31:16–35.
68. Vaage J, Donovan D, Mayhew E, et al. Therapy of mouse mammary carcinomas with vincristine and doxorubicin encapsulated in sterically stabilized liposomes. Int J Cancer 1993;54:959–64.
69. Al-Batran SE, Guntner M, Pauligk C, et al. Anthracycline rechallenge using pegylated liposomal doxorubicin in patients with metastatic breast cancer: a pooled analysis using individual data from four prospective trials. Br J Cancer 2010;103: 1518–23.
70. Keller AM, Mennel RG, Georgoulias VA, et al. Randomized phase III trial of pegylated liposomal doxorubicin versus vinorelbine or mitomycin C plus vinblastine in women with taxane-refractory advanced breast cancer. J Clin Oncol 2004;22: 3893–901.
71. O'Brien ME, Wigler N, Inbar M, et al. Reduced cardiotoxicity and comparable efficacy in a phase III trial of pegylated liposomal doxorubicin HCl (CAELYX/Doxil) versus conventional doxorubicin for first-line treatment of metastatic breast cancer. Ann Oncol 2004;15:440–9.
72. Gordon AN, Fleagle JT, Guthrie D, et al. Recurrent epithelial ovarian carcinoma: a randomized phase III study of pegylated liposomal doxorubicin versus topotecan. J Clin Oncol 2001;19:3312–22.
73. Mutch DG, Orlando M, Goss T, et al. Randomized phase III trial of gemcitabine compared with pegylated liposomal doxorubicin in patients with platinum-resistant ovarian cancer. J Clin Oncol 2007; 25:2811–8.
74. Pujade-Lauraine E, Wagner U, Aavall-Lundqvist E, et al. Pegylated liposomal Doxorubicin and Carboplatin compared with Paclitaxel and Carboplatin for patients with platinum-sensitive ovarian cancer in late relapse. J Clin Oncol 2010;28: 3323–9.
75. Kesterson JP, Odunsi K, Lele S. High cumulative doses of pegylated liposomal doxorubicin are not associated with cardiac toxicity in patients with gynecologic malignancies. Chemotherapy 2010;56:108–11.
76. Yildirim Y, Gultekin E, Avci ME, et al. Cardiac safety profile of pegylated liposomal doxorubicin reaching or exceeding lifetime cumulative doses of 550 mg/m2 in patients with recurrent ovarian and peritoneal cancer. Int J Gynecol Cancer 2008;18:223–7.
77. Agency C. Caelyx (Doxorubicin hydrochloride in a pegylated liposomal doxorubicin formulation). Available at: http://www.ema.europa.eu/docs/en_GB/document_library/EPAR_product_information/human/000089/WU500020180.pdf Accessed April 2, 2015.
78. Duggan ST, Keating GM. Pegylated liposomal doxorubicin: a review of its use in metastatic breast cancer, ovarian cancer, multiple myeloma and AIDS-related Kaposi's sarcoma. Drugs 2011; 71:2531–58.
79. Smith DH, Adams JR, Johnston SR, et al. A comparative economic analysis of pegylated liposomal doxorubicin versus topotecan in ovarian cancer in the USA and the UK. Ann Oncol 2002; 13:1590–7.
80. Creighton AM, Birnie GD. The effect of bisdioxopiperazines on the synthesis of deoxyribonucleic acid, ribonucleic acid and protein in growing mouse-embryo fibroblasts. Biochem J 1969;114:58P.
81. Classen S, Olland S, Berger JM. Structure of the topoisomerase II ATPase region and its mechanism of inhibition by the chemotherapeutic agent ICRF-187. Proc Natl Acad Sci U S A 2003;100: 10629–34.
82. Tanabe K, Ikegami Y, Ishida R, et al. Inhibition of topoisomerase II by antitumor agents bis(2,6-dioxopiperazine) derivatives. Cancer Res 1991;51: 4903–8.
83. Kovacevic Z, Kalinowski DS, Lovejoy DB, et al. Iron Chelators: Development of Novel Compounds with High and Selective Anti-Tumour Activity. Curr Drug Deliv 2010;7:194–207.
84. Lyu YL, Kerrigan JE, Lin CP, et al. Topoisomerase IIbeta mediated DNA double-strand breaks: implications in doxorubicin cardiotoxicity and prevention by dexrazoxane. Cancer Res 2007;67: 8839–46.
85. Lipshultz SE, Rifai N, Dalton VM, et al. The effect of dexrazoxane on myocardial injury in doxorubicin-treated children with acute lymphoblastic leukemia. N Engl J Med 2004;351:145–53.
86. Lipshultz SE, Scully RE, Lipsitz SR, et al. Assessment of dexrazoxane as a cardioprotectant in doxorubicin-treated children with high-risk acute lymphoblastic leukaemia: long-term follow-up of

a prospective, randomised, multicentre trial. Lancet Oncol 2010;11:950–61.
87. Swain SM, Vici P. The current and future role of dexrazoxane as a cardioprotectant in anthracycline treatment: expert panel review. J Cancer Res Clin Oncol 2004;130:1–7.
88. Seymour L, Bramwell V, Moran LA. Use of dexrazoxane as a cardioprotectant in patients receiving doxorubicin or epirubicin chemotherapy for the treatment of cancer. The Provincial Systemic Treatment Disease Site Group. Cancer Prev Control 1999;3:145–59.
89. van Dalen EC, Caron HN, Dickinson HO, Kremer LC. Cardioprotective interventions for cancer patients receiving anthracyclines. Cochrane Database Syst Rev 2008:CD003917.
90. Schuchter LM, Hensley ML, Meropol NJ, et al, American Society of Clinical Oncology Chemotherapy and Radiotherapy Expert Panel. 2002 update of recommendations for the use of chemotherapy and radiotherapy protectants: clinical practice guidelines of the American Society of Clinical Oncology. J Clin Oncol 2002;20:2895–903.
91. Tebbi CK, London WB, Friedman D, et al. Dexrazoxane-associated risk for acute myeloid leukemia/myelodysplastic syndrome and other secondary malignancies in pediatric Hodgkin's disease. J Clin Oncol 2007;25:493–500.
92. Salzer WL, Devidas M, Carroll WL, et al. Long-term results of the pediatric oncology group studies for childhood acute lymphoblastic leukemia 1984-2001: a report from the children's oncology group. Leukemia 2010;24:355–70.
93. Vrooman LM, Neuberg DS, Stevenson KE, et al. The low incidence of secondary acute myelogenous leukaemia in children and adolescents treated with dexrazoxane for acute lymphoblastic leukaemia: a report from the Dana-Farber Cancer Institute ALL Consortium. Eur J Cancer 2011;47: 1373–9.
94. Yoon GJ, Telli ML, Kao DP, et al. Left ventricular dysfunction in patients receiving cardiotoxic cancer therapies are clinicians responding optimally? J Am Coll Cardiol 2010;56:1644–50.
95. Kalay N, Basar E, Ozdogru I, et al. Protective effects of carvedilol against anthracycline-induced cardiomyopathy. J Am Coll Cardiol 2006;48: 2258–62.
96. Kaya MG, Ozkan M, Gunebakmaz O, et al. Protective effects of nebivolol against anthracycline-induced cardiomyopathy: a randomized control study. Int J Cardiol 2013;167:2306–10.
97. Bosch X, Rovira M, Sitges M, et al. Enalapril and carvedilol for preventing chemotherapy-induced left ventricular systolic dysfunction in patients with malignant hemopathies: the OVERCOME trial (preventiOn of left Ventricular dysfunction with Enalapril and caRvedilol in patients submitted to intensive ChemOtherapy for the treatment of Malignant hEmopathies). J Am Coll Cardiol 2013;61: 2355–62.
98. El-Shitany NA, Tolba OA, El-Shanshory MR, et al. Protective effect of carvedilol on adriamycin-induced left ventricular dysfunction in children with acute lymphoblastic leukemia. J Card Fail 2012;18:607–13.
99. Heck SL, Gulati G, Ree AH, et al. Rationale and design of the prevention of cardiac dysfunction during an Adjuvant Breast Cancer Therapy (PRADA) Trial. Cardiology 2012;123:240–7.
100. Gulati G, Heck SL, Ree AH, et al. Prevention of cardiac dysfunction during adjuvant breast cancer therapy (PRADA): a 2 x 2 factorial, randomized, placebo-controlled, double-blind clinical trial of candesartan and metoprolol. Eur Heart J 2016; 37:1671–80.
101. Georgakopoulos P, Roussou P, Matsakas E, et al. Cardioprotective effect of metoprolol and enalapril in doxorubicin-treated lymphoma patients: a prospective, parallel-group, randomized, controlled study with 36-month follow-up. Am J Hematol 2010;85:894–6.
102. Spallarossa P, Garibaldi S, Altieri P, et al. Carvedilol prevents doxorubicin-induced free radical release and apoptosis in cardiomyocytes in vitro. J Mol Cell Cardiol 2004;37:837–46.
103. Moen MD, Wagstaff AJ. Nebivolol: a review of its use in the management of hypertension and chronic heart failure. Drugs 2006;66:1389–409 [discussion: 1410].
104. Mason RP, Kalinowski L, Jacob RF, et al. Nebivolol reduces nitroxidative stress and restores nitric oxide bioavailability in endothelium of black Americans. Circulation 2005;112:3795–801.
105. Erickson CE, Gul R, Blessing CP, et al. The beta-blocker Nebivolol Is a GRK/beta-arrestin biased agonist. PLoS One 2013;8:e71980.
106. Kim IM, Tilley DG, Chen J, et al. Beta-blockers alprenolol and carvedilol stimulate beta-arrestin-mediated EGFR transactivation. Proc Natl Acad Sci U S A 2008;105:14555–60.
107. Tilley DG, Kim IM, Patel PA, et al. beta-Arrestin mediates beta1-adrenergic receptor-epidermal growth factor receptor interaction and downstream signaling. J Biol Chem 2009;284:20375–86.
108. Salvatorelli E, Menna P, Cantalupo E, et al. The concomitant management of cancer therapy and cardiac therapy. Biochim Biophys Acta 2015;1848: 2727–37.
109. Cardinale D, Colombo A, Sandri MT, et al. Prevention of high-dose chemotherapy-induced cardiotoxicity in high-risk patients by angiotensin-converting enzyme inhibition. Circulation 2006;114:2474–81.

110. Cardinale D, Colombo A, Lamantia G, et al. Anthracycline-induced cardiomyopathy: clinical relevance and response to pharmacologic therapy. J Am Coll Cardiol 2010;55:213–20.
111. Jensen BV, Skovsgaard T, Nielsen SL. Functional monitoring of anthracycline cardiotoxicity: a prospective, blinded, long-term observational study of outcome in 120 patients. Ann Oncol 2002;13: 699–709.
112. Lipshultz SE, Lipsitz SR, Sallan SE, et al. Long-term enalapril therapy for left ventricular dysfunction in doxorubicin-treated survivors of childhood cancer. J Clin Oncol 2002;20:4517–22.
113. Silber JH, Cnaan A, Clark BJ, et al. Enalapril to prevent cardiac function decline in long-term survivors of pediatric cancer exposed to anthracyclines. J Clin Oncol 2004;22:820–8.
114. Barry E, Alvarez JA, Scully RE, et al. Anthracycline-induced cardiotoxicity: course, pathophysiology, prevention and management. Expert Opin Pharmacother 2007;8:1039–58.
115. Sieswerda E, van Dalen EC, Postma A, et al. Medical interventions for treating anthracycline-induced symptomatic and asymptomatic cardiotoxicity during and after treatment for childhood cancer. Cochrane Database Syst Rev 2011;(9):CD008011.
116. Abd El-Aziz MA, Othman AI, Amer M, et al. Potential protective role of angiotensin-converting enzyme inhibitors captopril and enalapril against adriamycin-induced acute cardiac and hepatic toxicity in rats. J Appl Toxicol 2001;21:469–73.
117. Vaynblat M, Shah HR, Bhaskaran D, et al. Simultaneous angiotensin converting enzyme inhibition moderates ventricular dysfunction caused by doxorubicin. Eur J Heart Fail 2002;4:583–6.
118. Boucek RJ Jr, Steele A, Miracle A, et al. Effects of angiotensin-converting enzyme inhibitor on delayed-onset doxorubicin-induced cardiotoxicity. Cardiovasc Toxicol 2003;3:319–29.
119. Tokudome T, Mizushige K, Noma T, et al. Prevention of doxorubicin (adriamycin)-induced cardiomyopathy by simultaneous administration of angiotensin-converting enzyme inhibitor assessed by acoustic densitometry. J Cardiovasc Pharmacol 2000;36:361–8.
120. Okumura K, Jin D, Takai S, et al. Beneficial effects of angiotensin-converting enzyme inhibition in adriamycin-induced cardiomyopathy in hamsters. Jpn J Pharmacol 2002;88:183–8.
121. Maeda A, Honda M, Kuramochi T, et al. An angiotensin-converting enzyme inhibitor protects against doxorubicin-induced impairment of calcium handling in neonatal rat cardiac myocytes. Clin Exp Pharmacol Physiol 1997;24:720–6.
122. Cernecka H, Ochodnicka-Mackovicova K, Kucerova D, et al. Enalaprilat increases PPARbeta/delta expression, without influence on PPARalpha and PPARgamma, and modulate cardiac function in sub-acute model of daunorubicin-induced cardiomyopathy. Eur J Pharmacol 2013;714:472–7.
123. Nakamae H, Tsumura K, Terada Y, et al. Notable effects of angiotensin II receptor blocker, valsartan, on acute cardiotoxic changes after standard chemotherapy with cyclophosphamide, doxorubicin, vincristine, and prednisolone. Cancer 2005; 104:2492–8.
124. Dessi M, Madeddu C, Piras A, et al. Long-term, up to 18 months, protective effects of the angiotensin II receptor blocker telmisartan on Epirubin-induced inflammation and oxidative stress assessed by serial strain rate. Springerplus 2013; 2:198.
125. Akpek M, Ozdogru I, Sahin O, et al. Protective effects of spironolactone against anthracycline-induced cardiomyopathy. Eur J Heart Fail 2015;17:81–9.
126. Seicean S, Seicean A, Plana JC, et al. Effect of statin therapy on the risk for incident heart failure in patients with breast cancer receiving anthracycline chemotherapy: an observational clinical cohort study. J Am Coll Cardiol 2012;60:2384–90.
127. Acar Z, Kale A, Turgut M, et al. Efficiency of atorvastatin in the protection of anthracycline-induced cardiomyopathy. J Am Coll Cardiol 2011;58:988–9.
128. Damrot J, Nubel T, Epe B, et al. Lovastatin protects human endothelial cells from the genotoxic and cytotoxic effects of the anticancer drugs doxorubicin and etoposide. Br J Pharmacol 2006;149: 988–97.
129. Huelsenbeck J, Henninger C, Schad A, et al. Inhibition of Rac1 signaling by lovastatin protects against anthracycline-induced cardiac toxicity. Cell Death Dis 2011;2:e190.
130. Riad A, Bien S, Westermann D, et al. Pretreatment with statin attenuates the cardiotoxicity of Doxorubicin in mice. Cancer Res 2009;69:695–9.
131. Yarden Y. The EGFR family and its ligands in human cancer. Signalling mechanisms and therapeutic opportunities. Eur J Cancer 2001; 37(Suppl 4):S3–8.
132. Slamon DJ, Leyland-Jones B, Shak S, et al. Use of chemotherapy plus a monoclonal antibody against HER2 for metastatic breast cancer that overexpresses HER2. N Engl J Med 2001;344:783–92.
133. Chen B, Peng X, Pentassuglia L, et al. Molecular and cellular mechanisms of anthracycline cardiotoxicity. Cardiovasc Toxicol 2007;7:114–21.
134. Bird BR, Swain SM. Cardiac toxicity in breast cancer survivors: review of potential cardiac problems. Clin Cancer Res 2008;14:14–24.
135. Hudis CA. Trastuzumab–mechanism of action and use in clinical practice. N Engl J Med 2007;357:39–51.

136. Yavas O, Yazici M, Eren O, et al. The acute effect of trastuzumab infusion on ECG parameters in metastatic breast cancer patients. Swiss Med Wkly 2007;137:556–8.
137. Keefe DL. Trastuzumab-associated cardiotoxicity. Cancer 2002;95:1592–600.
138. Perez EA, Rodeheffer R. Clinical cardiac tolerability of trastuzumab. J Clin Oncol 2004;22:322–9.
139. Ewer MS, Vooletich MT, Durand JB, et al. Reversibility of trastuzumab-related cardiotoxicity: new insights based on clinical course and response to medical treatment. J Clin Oncol 2005;23:7820–6.
140. de Azambuja E, Bedard PL, Suter T, et al. Cardiac toxicity with anti-HER-2 therapies: what have we learned so far? Target Oncol 2009;4:77–88.
141. Lee KF, Simon H, Chen H, et al. Requirement for neuregulin receptor erbB2 in neural and cardiac development. Nature 1995;378:394–8.
142. Meyer D, Birchmeier C. Multiple essential functions of neuregulin in development. Nature 1995; 378:386–90.
143. Crone SA, Zhao YY, Fan L, et al. ErbB2 is essential in the prevention of dilated cardiomyopathy. Nat Med 2002;8:459–65.
144. Negro A, Brar BK, Lee KF. Essential roles of Her2/erbB2 in cardiac development and function. Recent Prog Horm Res 2004;59:1–12.
145. Ozcelik C, Erdmann B, Pilz B, et al. Conditional mutation of the ErbB2 (HER2) receptor in cardiomyocytes leads to dilated cardiomyopathy. Proc Natl Acad Sci U S A 2002;99:8880–5.
146. Zhao YY, Sawyer DR, Baliga RR, et al. Neuregulins promote survival and growth of cardiac myocytes. Persistence of ErbB2 and ErbB4 expression in neonatal and adult ventricular myocytes. J Biol Chem 1998;273:10261–9.
147. Bilancia D, Rosati G, Dinota A, et al. Lapatinib in breast cancer. Ann Oncol 2007;18(Suppl 6): vi26–30.
148. Geyer CE, Forster J, Lindquist D, et al. Lapatinib plus capecitabine for HER2-positive advanced breast cancer. N Engl J Med 2006;355:2733–43.
149. Lenihan D, Suter T, Brammer M, et al. Pooled analysis of cardiac safety in patients with cancer treated with pertuzumab. Ann Oncol 2012;23: 791–800.
150. Hervent AS, De Keulenaer GW. Molecular mechanisms of cardiotoxicity induced by ErbB receptor inhibitor cancer therapeutics. Int J Mol Sci 2012; 13:12268–86.
151. Spector NL, Yarden Y, Smith B, et al. Activation of AMP-activated protein kinase by human EGF receptor 2/EGF receptor tyrosine kinase inhibitor protects cardiac cells. Proc Natl Acad Sci U S A 2007;104:10607–12.
152. Junttila TT, Akita RW, Parsons K, et al. Ligand-independent HER2/HER3/PI3K complex is disrupted by trastuzumab and is effectively inhibited by the PI3K inhibitor GDC-0941. Cancer Cell 2009;15: 429–440.
153. De Keulenaer GW, Doggen K, Lemmens K. The vulnerability of the heart as a pluricellular paracrine organ: lessons from unexpected triggers of heart failure in targeted ErbB2 anticancer therapy. Circ Res 2010;106:35–46.
154. Badache A, Hynes NE. A new therapeutic antibody masks ErbB2 to its partners. Cancer Cell 2004;5: 299–301.
155. Cameron DA, Stein S. Drug Insight: intracellular inhibitors of HER2–clinical development of lapatinib in breast cancer. Nat Clin Pract Oncol 2008;5:512–20.
156. Rusnak DW, Lackey K, Affleck K, et al. The effects of the novel, reversible epidermal growth factor receptor/ErbB-2 tyrosine kinase inhibitor, GW2016, on the growth of human normal and tumor-derived cell lines in vitro and in vivo. Mol Cancer Ther 2001;1:85–94.
157. Xia W, Mullin RJ, Keith BR, et al. Anti-tumor activity of GW572016: a dual tyrosine kinase inhibitor blocks EGF activation of EGFR/erbB2 and downstream Erk1/2 and AKT pathways. Oncogene 2002;21:6255–63.
158. Jones AL, Barlow M, Barrett-Lee PJ, et al. Management of cardiac health in trastuzumab-treated patients with breast cancer: updated United Kingdom National Cancer Research Institute recommendations for monitoring. Br J Cancer 2009; 100:684–92.
159. Rock CL, Flatt SW, Newman V, et al. Factors associated with weight gain in women after diagnosis of breast cancer. Women's Healthy Eating and Living Study Group. J Am Diet Assoc 1999;99: 1212–21.
160. Koelwyn GJ, Khouri M, Mackey JR, et al. Running on empty: cardiovascular reserve capacity and late effects of therapy in cancer survivorship. J Clin Oncol 2012;30:4458–61.
161. Irwin ML, Crumley D, McTiernan A, et al. Physical activity levels before and after a diagnosis of breast carcinoma: the Health, Eating, Activity, and Lifestyle (HEAL) study. Cancer 2003;97: 1746–57.
162. Gulati M, Pandey DK, Arnsdorf MF, et al. Exercise capacity and the risk of death in women: the St James Women Take Heart Project. Circulation 2003;108:1554–9.
163. Giallauria F, Fattirolli F, Tramarin R, et al. Clinical characteristics and course of patients with diabetes entering cardiac rehabilitation. Diabetes Res Clin Pract 2015;107:267–72.
164. Giallauria F, Maresca L, Vitelli A, et al. Exercise training improves heart rate recovery in women with breast cancer. Springerplus 2015;4:388.

165. Mishra SI, Scherer RW, Snyder C, et al. Exercise interventions on health-related quality of life for people with cancer during active treatment. Cochrane Database Syst Rev 2012;(8):CD008465.
166. Scott JM, Khakoo A, Mackey JR, et al. Modulation of anthracycline-induced cardiotoxicity by aerobic exercise in breast cancer: current evidence and underlying mechanisms. Circulation 2011;124: 642–50.
167. Curigliano G, Cardinale D, Suter T, et al. Cardiovascular toxicity induced by chemotherapy, targeted agents and radiotherapy: ESMO Clinical Practice Guidelines. Ann Oncol 2012;23(Suppl 7): vii155–66.
168. Lang RM, Bierig M, Devereux RB, et al. Recommendations for chamber quantification: a report from the American Society of Echocardiography's Guidelines and Standards Committee and the Chamber Quantification Writing Group, developed in conjunction with the European Association of Echocardiography, a branch of the European Society of Cardiology. J Am Soc Echocardiogr 2005;18:1440–63.
169. Moja L, Tagliabue L, Balduzzi S, et al. Trastuzumab containing regimens for early breast cancer. Cochrane Database Syst Rev 2012;(4):CD006243.
170. Mackey JR, Clemons M, Cote MA, et al. Cardiac management during adjuvant trastuzumab therapy: recommendations of the Canadian Trastuzumab Working Group. Curr Oncol 2008;15:24–35.
171. Lipshultz SE, Adams MJ, Colan SD, et al. Long-term cardiovascular toxicity in children, adolescents, and young adults who receive cancer therapy: pathophysiology, course, monitoring, management, prevention, and research directions: a scientific statement from the American Heart Association. Circulation 2013;128:1927–95.
172. Landier W, Bhatia S, Eshelman DA, et al. Development of risk-based guidelines for pediatric cancer survivors: the Children's Oncology Group Long-Term Follow-Up Guidelines from the Children's Oncology Group Late Effects Committee and Nursing Discipline. J Clin Oncol 2004;22:4979–90.
173. Hunt SA, Abraham WT, Chin MH, et al. ACC/AHA 2005 Guideline Update for the Diagnosis and Management of Chronic Heart Failure in the Adult: a report of the American College of Cardiology/American Heart Association Task Force on Practice Guidelines (Writing Committee to Update the 2001 Guidelines for the Evaluation and Management of Heart Failure): developed in collaboration with the American College of Chest Physicians and the International Society for Heart and Lung Transplantation: endorsed by the Heart Rhythm Society. Circulation 2005;112:e154–235.
174. Vaz-Luis I, Keating NL, Lin NU, et al. Duration and toxicity of adjuvant trastuzumab in older patients with early-stage breast cancer: a population-based study. J Clin Oncol 2014;32:927–34.
175. Yeboah J, Rodriguez CJ, Stacey B, et al. Prognosis of individuals with asymptomatic left ventricular systolic dysfunction in the multi-ethnic study of atherosclerosis (MESA). Circulation 2012;126: 2713–9.
176. Morris PG, Hudis CA. Trastuzumab-related cardiotoxicity following anthracycline-based adjuvant chemotherapy: how worried should we be? J Clin Oncol 2010;28:3407–10.
177. Suter TM, Cook-Bruns N, Barton C. Cardiotoxicity associated with trastuzumab (Herceptin) therapy in the treatment of metastatic breast cancer. Breast 2004;13:173–83.
178. Russell SD, Blackwell KL, Lawrence J, et al. Independent adjudication of symptomatic heart failure with the use of doxorubicin and cyclophosphamide followed by trastuzumab adjuvant therapy: a combined review of cardiac data from the National Surgical Adjuvant breast and Bowel Project B-31 and the North Central Cancer Treatment Group N9831 clinical trials. J Clin Oncol 2010;28: 3416–21.
179. Procter M, Suter TM, de Azambuja E, et al. Longer-term assessment of trastuzumab-related cardiac adverse events in the Herceptin Adjuvant (HERA) trial. J Clin Oncol 2010;28:3422–8.
180. Liu FF, Stone JR, Schuldt AJ, et al. Heterozygous knockout of neuregulin-1 gene in mice exacerbates doxorubicin-induced heart failure. Am J Physiol Heart Circ Physiol 2005;289:H660–6.
181. Pentassuglia L, Graf M, Lane H, et al. Inhibition of ErbB2 by receptor tyrosine kinase inhibitors causes myofibrillar structural damage without cell death in adult rat cardiomyocytes. Exp Cell Res 2009; 315:1302–12.
182. Horie T, Ono K, Nishi H, et al. Acute doxorubicin cardiotoxicity is associated with miR-146a-induced inhibition of the neuregulin-ErbB pathway. Cardiovasc Res 2010;87:656–64.
183. Eldridge S, Guo L, Mussio J, et al. Examining the protective role of ErbB2 modulation in human-induced pluripotent stem cell-derived cardiomyocytes. Toxicol Sci 2014;141:547–59.
184. Tan-Chiu E, Yothers G, Romond E, et al. Assessment of cardiac dysfunction in a randomized trial comparing doxorubicin and cyclophosphamide followed by paclitaxel, with or without trastuzumab as adjuvant therapy in node-positive, human epidermal growth factor receptor 2-overexpressing breast cancer: NSABP B-31. J Clin Oncol 2005;23:7811–9.
185. Joensuu H, Kellokumpu-Lehtinen PL, Bono P, et al. Adjuvant docetaxel or vinorelbine with or without trastuzumab for breast cancer. N Engl J Med 2006;354:809–20.

186. Ewer MS, Ewer SM. Cardiotoxicity of anticancer treatments. Nat Rev Cardiol 2015;12:547–58.
187. Albini A, Pennesi G, Donatelli F, et al. Cardiotoxicity of anticancer drugs: the need for cardio-oncology and cardio-oncological prevention. J Natl Cancer Inst 2010;102:14–25.
188. Khouri MG, Douglas PS, Mackey JR, et al. Cancer therapy-induced cardiac toxicity in early breast cancer: addressing the unresolved issues. Circulation 2012;126:2749–63.
189. Cadeddu C, Piras A, Mantovani G, et al. Protective effects of the angiotensin II receptor blocker telmisartan on epirubicin-induced inflammation, oxidative stress, and early ventricular impairment. Am Heart J 2010;160:487.e481–7.
190. Dranitsaris G, Rayson D, Vincent M, et al. The development of a predictive model to estimate cardiotoxic risk for patients with metastatic breast cancer receiving anthracyclines. Breast Cancer Res Treat 2008;107:443–50.
191. Herrmann J, Lerman A, Sandhu NP, et al. Evaluation and management of patients with heart disease and cancer: cardio-oncology. Mayo Clin Proc 2014;89:1287–306.
192. Writing Committee Members, Yancy CW, Jessup M, et al. 2013 ACCF/AHA guideline for the management of heart failure: a report of the American College of Cardiology Foundation/American Heart Association Task Force on practice guidelines. Circulation 2013;128:e240–327.

CHAPTER 9

Vascular Toxicities of Cancer Therapies

Joerg Herrmann, MD*, Amir Lerman, MD

Although considerable attention has been directed toward cardiotoxicity, several other toxicities and complications can occur with cancer therapies and are important to know. Vascular toxicities are of particular significance for obvious reasons. In essence and as it will become apparent herein, there are three principle types of vascular toxicities that capture clinical attention: accelerated atherosclerosis, acute thrombosis, and acute vasospasm (Fig 9.1). The management strategies vary accordingly. It remains presently unresolved if screening and initiation of any preventive treatment is to be pursued to yield better clinical outcomes. Similar to the classification scheme for cardiac toxicities, one may distinguish between a sustained (type 1) and a transient (type 2) subtype (Fig. 9.2). Such classification scheme mainly serves an operational function, that is, to aid with the conceptual approach to any given patient knowing that a particular drug is associated with more permanent and progressive disease, even after discontinuation, versus reversibility of injury after its discontinuation (Table 9.1). The focus of this chapter is on ischemic heart disease, peripheral arterial disease (PAD), and cerebrovascular events. It also covers peripheral vasospasm and pulmonary hypertension but not systemic hypertension and thromboembolism as presented elsewhere. As a prerequisite, the main chemotherapeutics among those associated with vascular toxicity are reviewed first.

PART 1: CHEMOTHERAPEUTICS ASSOCIATED WITH VASCULAR TOXICITY

The classes of drugs with vascular toxicity potential as well as the spectrum of presentation are quite diverse (Fig. 9.3, Table 9.2). In keeping with a historical perspective, these drugs will be reviewed from the most traditional to the most recent.

5-Fluouracil and Capecitabine

5-Fluouracil (5-FU) was the first and still is the most notoriously known chemotherapeutic drug with a propensity for vascular side effects.[1] Related to differences in patient populations, treatment regimens, and outcome parameters, the incidence of ischemic heart disease events has been quite broad, ranging from 0.1% to 20%. The onset can be rather quickly, that is, within the first hours of infusion, likely due to evolving vasoconstriction.[2,3] The alteration in vascular reactivity does not appear to be the primary consequence of an alteration of endothelial function but rather of molecular signaling pathways that control vascular smooth muscle cell tone (Fig. 9.4).[1] In agreement with this theory, the propensity toward vasoconstriction can be prevented by direct vasodilators, such as nitroglycerin or calcium channel blockers. The presentation spectrum includes typical and atypical angina as well as acute coronary syndromes with and without arrhythmias and even sudden cardiac death.[4] Moreover, takotsubo cardiomyopathy (apical ballooning syndrome) can develop, possibly as a reflection of severe and diffuse vasoconstriction of the coronary microvasculature.[1,4–6] The documentation of profound coronary vasoconstriction in response to acetylcholine after infusion of 5-FU supports the "vasoreactivity theory" in general.[7]

Case scenarios of stable and acute angina similar to 5-FU but with an approximately 50% lower incidence have been observed with capecitabine, an oral pro-drug of 5-FU.[8,9] Intriguingly, thymidine phosphorylase, the enzyme that catalyzes the final metabolism step into the active compound, is expressed in atherosclerotic plaques.[10] For this reason, the assumption has been that patients with underlying coronary atherosclerosis are at an increased risk of cardiovascular toxicity with capecitabine as it has been

Department of Cardiovascular Diseases, Mayo Clinic, 200 First Street Southwest, Rochester, MN 55905, USA
* Corresponding author.
E-mail address: herrmann.joerg@mayo.edu

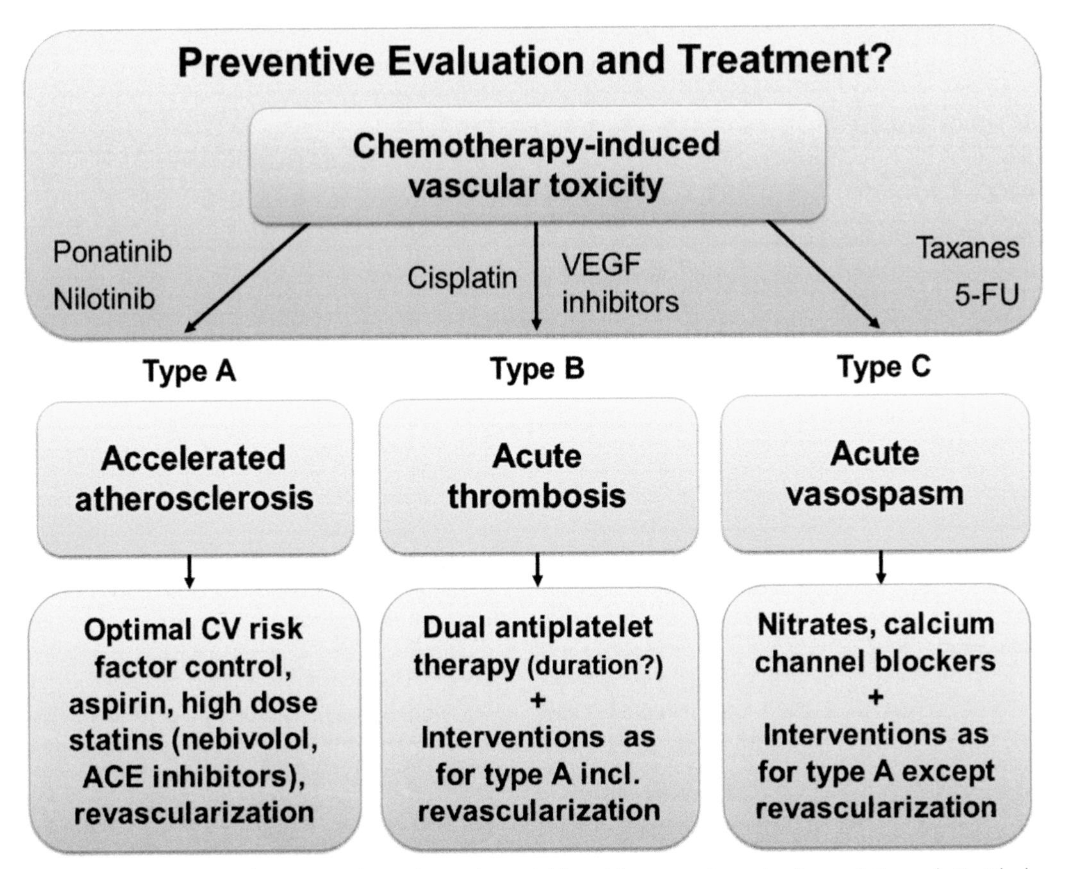

Fig. 9.1 The three principle presentations of vascular toxicities with cancer therapies (types A through C with drug examples) and recommendations for management. The value of preventive evaluation and treatment remains to be defined.

indicated for 5-FU. However, the benefit of screening for coronary artery disease (CAD) in these patients remain unknown. This being said, there seems to be merit in knowing about diseases characterized by abnormal vasoreactivity such as Raynaud disease and even CAD in preparing for potential aggravation and treatment of symptoms during treatment with 5-FU drugs.[11–13]

Taxanes (Paclitaxel and Docetaxel)

The administration of paclitaxel has been associated with stable and unstable presentations of myocardial ischemia at an incidence rate of 0.2% to 4%.[14–16] Similar to 5-FU and capecitabine, vasoconstriction (spasm) has been considered a key mechanism, and underlying, unrecognized CAD might be a predisposing factor. In

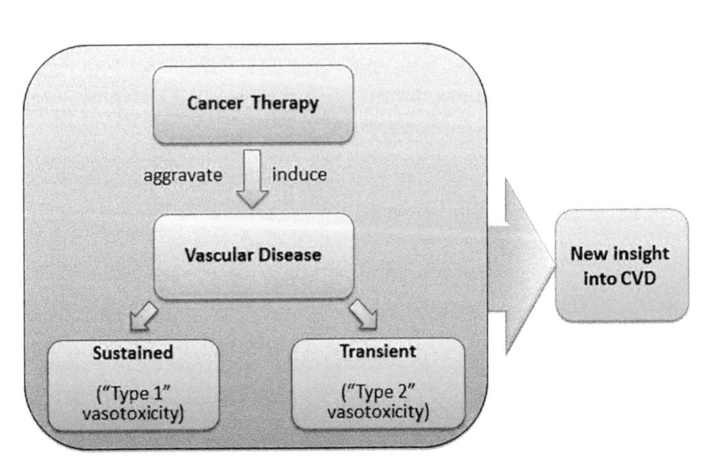

Fig. 9.2 Vascular toxicity concept within cardio-oncology.

distinction, cardiac rhythm disturbances are more common with taxanes.[14]

Cisplatin

Induction of acute single and even multivessel coronary thrombosis is a concern with cisplatin.[17–19] The underlying coronary vasculature appears benign and the appearance is that of erosion with subsequent thrombus development, which matches experimental data on the induction of endothelial damage and stimulation of thromboxane production, platelet activation, and platelet aggregation.[18,20–22] Furthermore unique, there is a 1.5 to 7 times increased risk of CAD and myocardial infarction (MI) long term in patients who received platinum-based chemotherapies, namely, testicular cancer survivors.[23–28] This sustained risk might relate to prolonged exposure, as circulating levels of cisplatin may remain detectable even more than 10 years after treatment, and/or additional injury to the endothelium and vasculature.[24] Consistent with the latter, the cardiovascular risk is higher in those who also underwent radiation therapy, and hyperlipidemia, hypertension, and vascular consequences of the metabolic syndrome are more commonly noted in these patients.[23,27–30] Whether any impairment in endothelial progenitor cells contributes to the ischemic risk and is unknown at this point, and the question remains if a particular emphasis on medications and cardiovascular risk factor control to improve endothelial and progenitor cell function should be given is unknown at this point.

Cyclophosphamide

Cyclophosphamide is another agent that exerts direct damage to the endothelium in a dose-dependent manner.[31] This toxicity followed by extravasation of blood is the mechanism of the most commonly known presentation of hemorrhagic perimyocarditis.[32,33] However, Raynaud, Prinzmetal angina, and even MI and stroke have been reported as well.[34,35] Considerations are similar to cisplatin.

Bleomycin, Vinca Alkaloids, and Gemcitabine

With the combination of bleomycin and vinca alkaloids with cisplatin or gemcitabine, the incidence of angina can be as high as 40%, and Raynaud can be seen in around 30% of patients.[34,36] Acute life-threatening events, including MI, can be encountered as well.[37–39] Intriguingly, the development of Raynaud may precede the occurrence of acute myocardial infarction (AMI). Mechanistically, bleomycin can cause endothelial dysfunction and activation, whereas vinblastine is capable of inducing endothelial apoptosis.[40] The incremental risk of gemcitabine is unknown. Only a few cases of AMI have been reported, and in fact, recent studies suggest that the risk of arterial thromboembolic events is lower with gemcitabine-based vascular endothelial growth factor (VEGF) inhibitor combination therapies.[41]

Vascular Endothelial Growth Factor Signaling Pathway Inhibitors

This heterogeneous group of drugs is composed of antibodies, such as bevacizumab, interfering with the interaction of VEGF with its receptor, and tyrosine kinase inhibitors (TKIs), such as sunitinib, sorafenib, and pozapanib, interfering with the activity of the catalytic domains of the VEGF receptor and the downstream signaling pathways. An almost universal response to these drugs is the induction or worsening of systemic hypertension. Chest pain episodes have been reported in 1% to 15% of patients, ranging from stable angina to ACS and even takotsubo/apical ballooning syndrome. The risk of acute thromboembolic events during treatment is in the order of 1.5 for bevacizumab and 2 to 3 for VEGF receptor TKIs overall.[41–45] The highest relative risks have been observed with sunitinib, pazopanib, and sorafenib (5.9, 4.6, and 2.3, respectively).[45]

Presumably central to these presentations is the role of VEGF for endothelial function and survival (Fig. 9.5).[46] Interference with VEGF receptor signaling impairs stimulation of endothelial nitric oxide (NO) synthase (eNOS) activity via the Akt/PKB pathway. In fact, eNOS uncoupling may occur with an increase in mitochondrial superoxide production, activation of the endothelin system, and increased endothelin-1 production as additional elements in the systemic vasoconstriction response.[47–50] Interference with Rho kinase activation in vascular smooth muscle cells in addition to the aforementioned effects on VEGF signaling on endothelial cell level might further contribute to potentially profound vasospasms, as reported especially for sorafenib (Fig. 9.6).[51–53] For bevacizumab and sunitinib, cases of takotsubo (apical ballooning syndrome) have been reported, and both of these drugs have been shown to impair microvascular function.[54,55] In fact, 70% of patients on sunitinib treatment have a reduced coronary flow reserve (on average 1.8 ± 0.4), especially with longer duration of therapy.[56] A reduction in coronary flow reserve has been recapitulated in experimental studies and related to a loss of pericytes in the microcirculation and interference with platelet-derived growth factor (PDGF) signaling pathways. As outlined in Fig. 9.7, endothelial cells produce PDGF

TABLE 9.1
Chemotherapeutics with a prominent vascular side effect profile

	HTN	Angina	AMI	Takotsubo	Raynauds	Stroke	PAD	Pulm HTN	DVT/PE
Antimetabolites									
5-Flourouracil		X	X	X	X				
Capecitabine		X	X	X	X				
Gemcitabine		X	X		X				
Anti-microtubule agents									
Paclitaxel	X	X	X						X
Alkylating agents									
Cisplatin	X	X	X		X	X	X		
Cyclophosphamide		X						X	
Antitumor antibiotics									
Bleomycin		X	X		X	X		X	
Vinca alkaloids									
Vincristine	X	X	X		X				
mTOR inhibitors									
Everolimus	X	X							X
Temsirolimus	X	X							X
Proteasome inhibitors									
Bortezomib			X			X		X	
Carfilzomib	X	X	X			X		X	X

Immunomodulatory imide Drugs									
Thalidomide								X	X
Lenalidomide	X	X	X			X		X	X
Vascular disrupting agents									
Combretastatin	X	X	X	X					
Monoclonal antibodies									
Bevacizumab	X	X	X	X		X			X
Ramucirumab	X	X	X			X			
Rituximab	X	X	X	X					
VEGF-receptor fusion molecules									
Aflibercept	X		X			X			X
Tyrosine kinase inhibitors									
Sorafenib	X	X	X			X			X
Sunitinib	X	X	X	X		X			X
Pazopanib	X	X	X			X			X
Axitinib	X	X	X			X			X
Regorafenib	X	X	X						
Cabozantinib	X		X			X			X
Vandetanib	X					X			
Lenvatinib	X		X			X			X
Nilotinib		X	X			X	X		X
Ponatinib	X	X	X			X	X		X
Dasatinib								X	
Miscellaneous									
Interferon-alpha	X	X	X		X	X	X	X	X
Thalidomide									X

Abbreviations: DVT, deep vein thrombosis; HTN, hypertension; PE, pulmonary embolism.

Modified from Herrmann J, Yang EH, Iliescu CA, et al. Vascular toxicities of cancer therapies: the old and the new-an evolving avenue. Circulation 2016;133(13):1272–89; with permission.

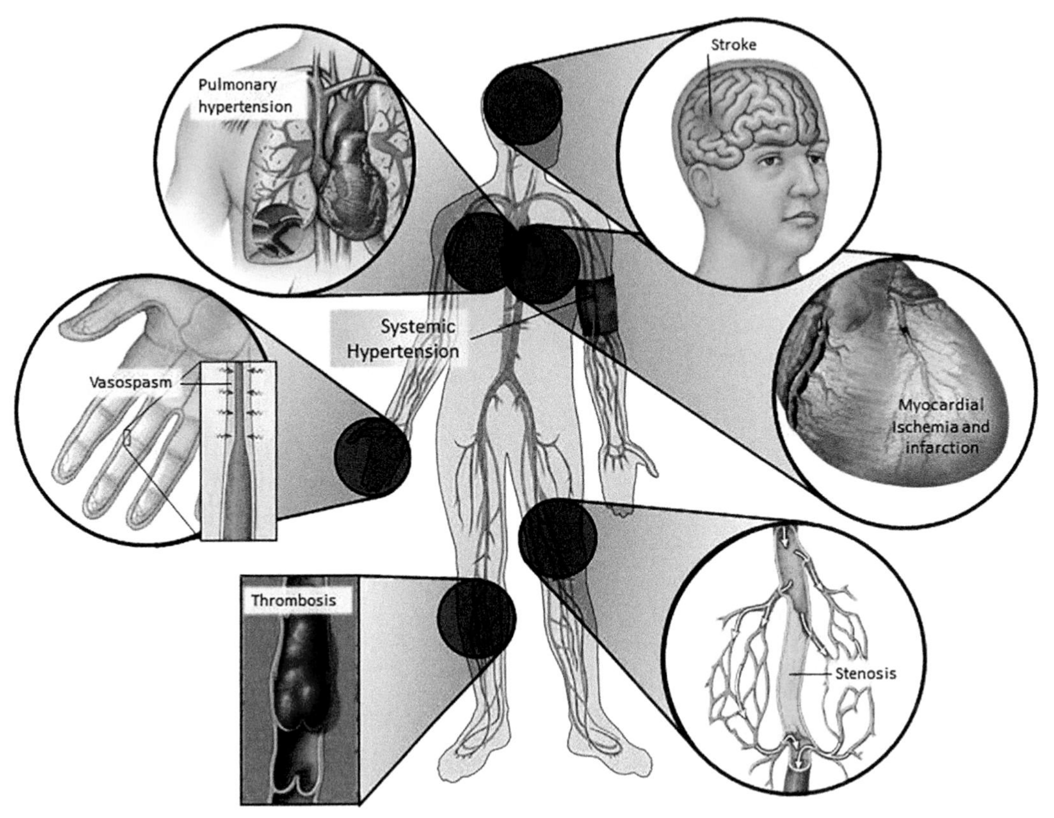

Fig. 9.3 Clinical spectrum of vascular toxicity. (*From* Herrmann J, Yang EH, Iliescu CA, et al. Vascular toxicities of cancer therapies: the old and the new—an evolving avenue. Circulation 2016;133(13):1272–89; with permission.)

to maintain the survival of pericytes, which produce VEGF and angiopoietin-1 to maintain the function of endothelial cells.[57–59] Sunitinib blocks both PDGF and VEGF signaling pathways and leads to "pericyte-endothelial cell uncoupling" (see Fig. 9.7). Of further note, coupling of endothelial cells extends to the cardiomyocytes and links microvascular integrity to myocardial function (Fig. 9.8). It is furthermore of relevance that drugs that inhibit VEGF signaling intracellularly (eg, sunitinib) exert a more potent effect on endothelial cell survival than drugs that inhibit VEGF signaling from the extracellular domain (eg, bevacizumab) (Fig. 9.9).

TABLE 9.2
Type 1 and type 2 vasotoxicity agents

Type 1 (Sustained Vasotoxicity Risk)	Type 2 (Transient Vasotoxicity Risk)
Ciplatin	5-Fluorouracil
Bleomycin	Capecitabine
Nilotinib	Taxanes
Ponatinib	
Interferon-α	

Progression of CAD and plaque rupture has been reported for sorafenib and sunitinib, respectively[60,61]; this is particularly interesting in view of the discussions on the role of adventitial and plaque neovascularization in atherosclerosis. Studies indicated that the early/initiation stage of atherosclerosis is angiogenesis-independent, contrary to the progression phase, and raised concerns of plaque neovessel destabilization with VEGF inhibition for the complication stage.[62–65] However, in an experimental model, chronic systemic VEGF inhibitor treatment increases atherosclerotic lesion formation but not plaque vulnerability.[48] When started after the development of atherosclerosis, bevacizumab did not increase plaque complication but rather reduced plaque neovascularization and growth similar to the initial studies with angiogenesis inhibitors.[66] Other mechanisms for acute vascular events therefore need to be considered, among them the impact of VEGF inhibitors on platelet function. Indeed, a mechanism similar to heparin-induced thrombocytopenia was

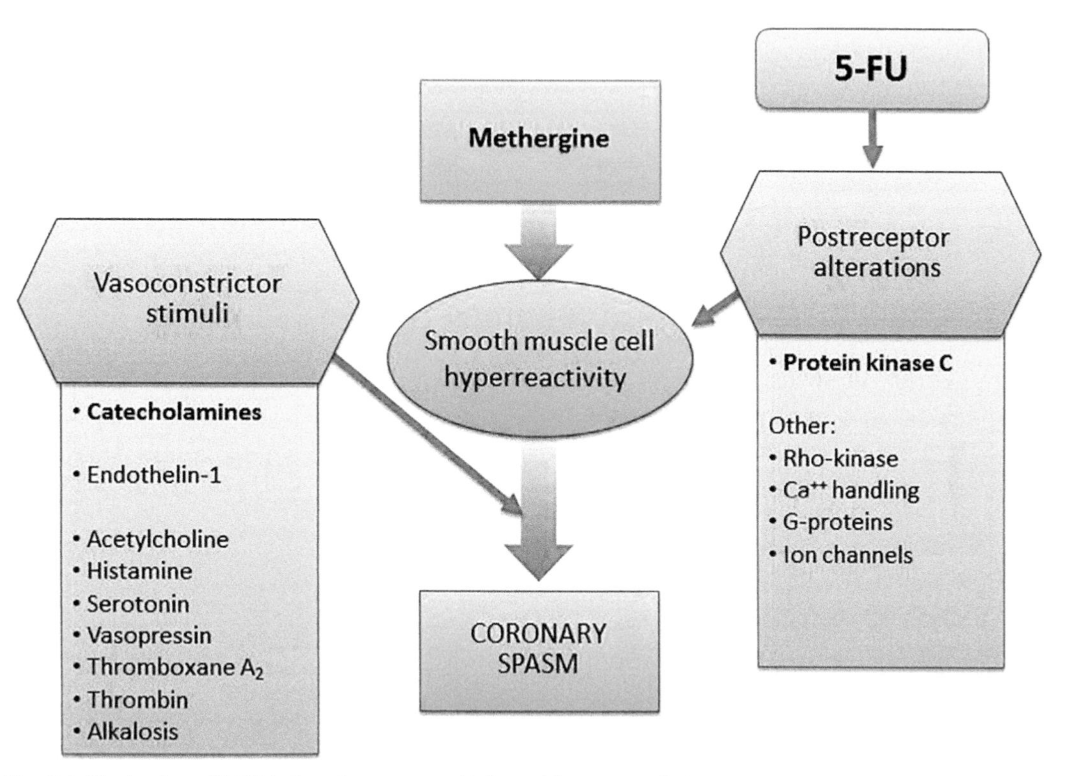

Fig. 9.4 Mechanism of 5-FU-induced vasospasm. (*Adapted from* Lanza G, Careri G, Crea F. Mechanisms of coronary artery spasm. Circulation 2011;124:1774–82.)

discovered. VEGF, like PF4, binds heparin, and in immune complexes with bevacizumab, can bind to FCyRIIa, inducing aggregation and procoagulant activity.[67]

Multitargeted Tyrosine Kinase Inhibitors

Recent reports on serious adverse cardiovascular events with TKIs designed to inhibit Bcr-Abl, the oncogenic tyrosine kinase fusion

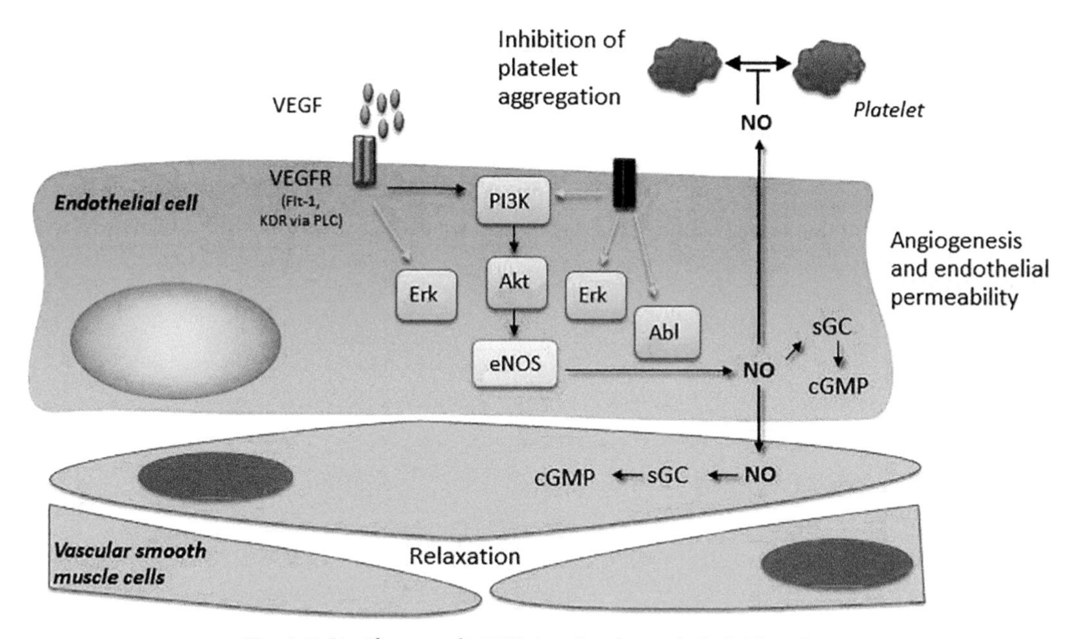

Fig. 9.5 Significance of VEGF signaling for endothelial function.

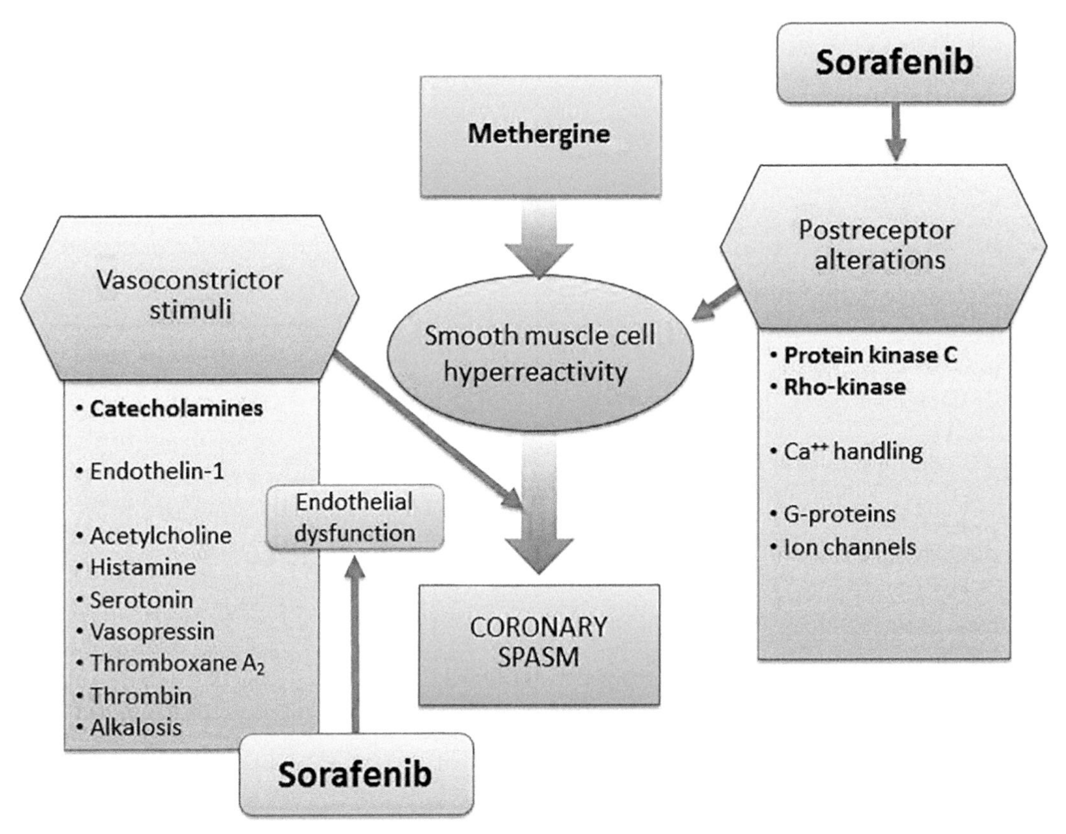

Fig. 9.6 Mechanism of sorafenib-induced vasospasm. (*Adapted from* Lanza G, Careri G, Crea F. Mechanisms of coronary artery spasm. Circulation 2011;124:1774–82.)

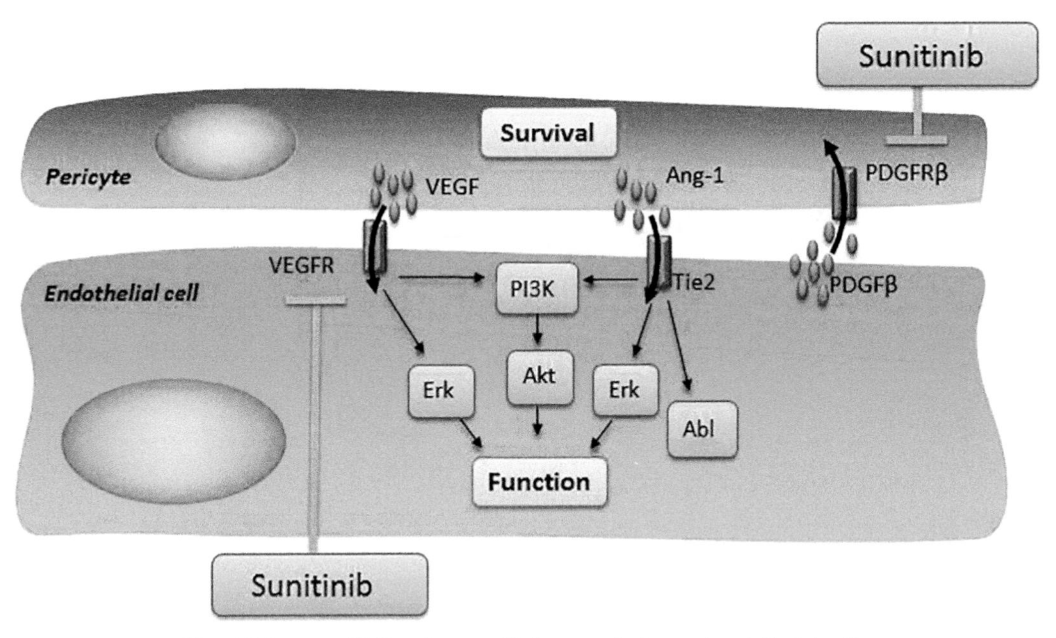

Fig. 9.7 Impact of TKI such as sunitinib on pericytes and endothelial cells.

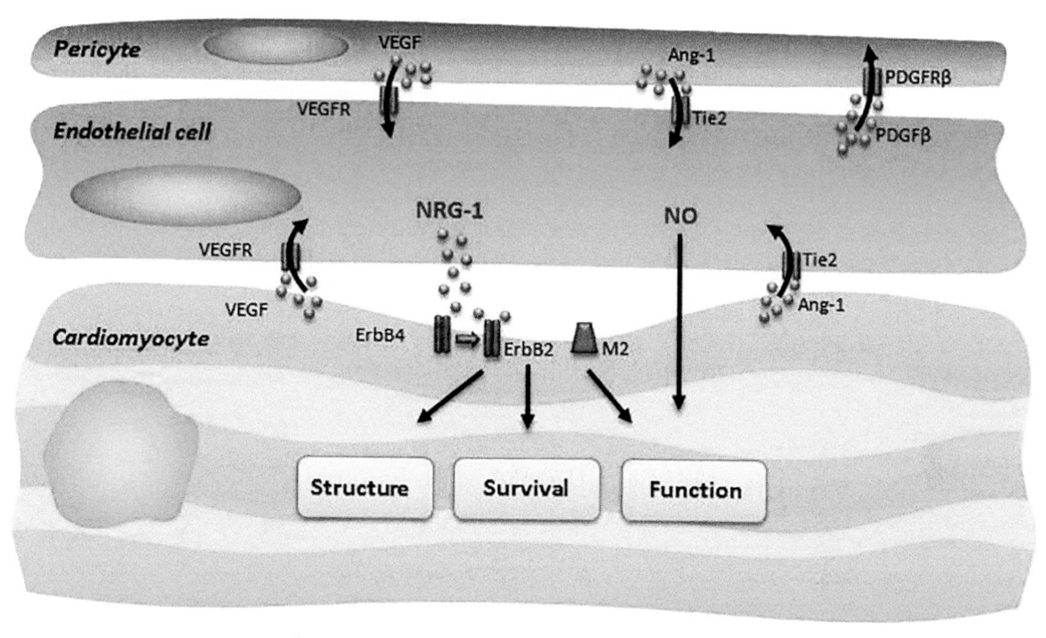

Fig. 9.8 Pericyte-endothelial-myocardial coupling.

product of a reciprocal gene translocation ("Philadelphia chromosome", Ph), especially nilotinib and ponatinib, have received greater attention. These cardiovascular events include rapidly progressive peripheral arterial occlusive disease (PAOD), acute ischemic events, and even sudden cardiac death with an overall incidence of 2% to 25% for nilotinib and 9% to 42% for ponatinib.[68–73] Importantly, multiple events in different vascular territories can evolve in the same patient, and these unfavorable dynamics can persist even when therapy is rapidly discontinued.[74–76] Although these events can occur in patients without any history of cardiovascular disease or risk factor exposure, some studies have suggested a higher risk of events in patients with a higher cardiovascular risk factor profile.[77] However, there is currently no understanding of the underlying mechanisms. Nilotinib can lead to hyperglycemia as a potentially contributing factor, whereas ponatinib causes hypertension. Dissecting the

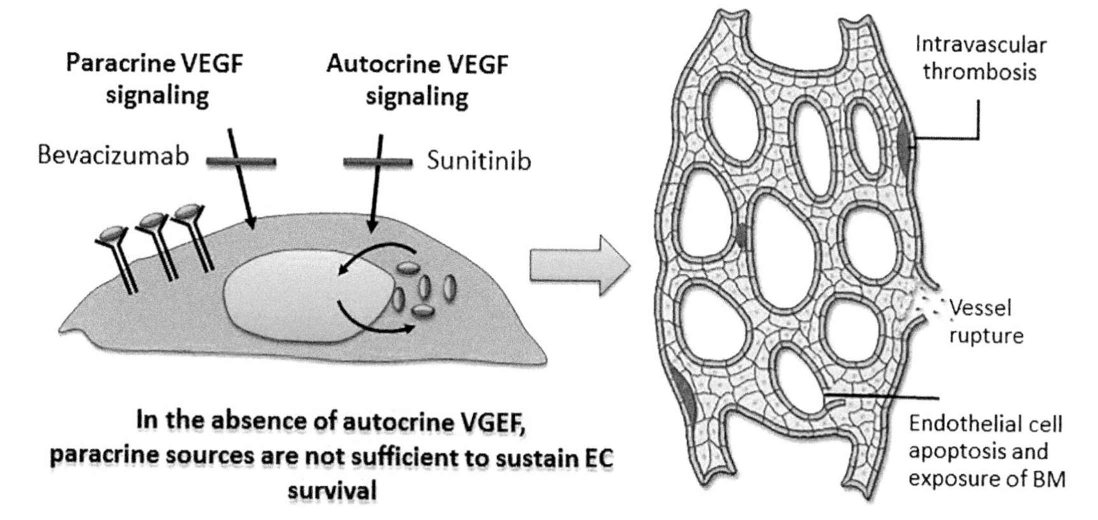

Fig. 9.9 Consequences of impairment of inhibition of VEGF signaling, which are notably worse with inhibition of VEGF signaling in endothelial cells.

differences between the different Bcr-Abl inhibitors is crucial, and the only commonality is inhibition of Abl, which is not explanatory but significant (Fig. 9.10). Loss of Abl activity impairs not only the formation of new vessels but also the function and stability of existing vessels as a result of endothelial cell damage. Indeed, endothelial Abl kinases are of crucial significance for Tie2 receptor signaling and angiopoietin-1–mediated endothelial cell survival and are themselves activated by this pathway in a positive feedback loop. VEGF stimulates Abl as well, and Abl seems to be involved in the prosurvival effects of VEGF on endothelial cells, especially under stress conditions such as serum starvation. Abl inhibition may therefore be even more so important under conditions that negatively impact endothelial function.[78]

Vascular-Disrupting Agents

These agents were developed to target and disrupt tumor vasculature and are classified into 2 main categories: flavonoids (eg, vadimezan [ASA404] and tubulin-binding molecules [similar but distinct from vinca alkaloids and taxanes]). These agents showed promise in preclinical studies but failed in clinical trials and have no role as single agents at present. Hypertension has been one of the most frequent observations (4%–40%), as has been myocardial ischemia; atypical chest pain occurred in as many as 16% of patients.[79] Non-ST-segment elevation and ST-segment elevations in MIs were reported in as many 4% of the patients in phase I trials.[79] Some of the events even occurred weeks after drug discontinuation.[80] An increase in circulating endothelial cell levels were noted in the hours after drug administration, indicating a toxic effect on endothelial cells in general and not just the tumor vasculature.[80] In addition to arterial thrombotic events, venous thromboembolic events also can occur, whereas bleeding events are rare.

Interferon-α

A black box warning was issued by the US Food and Drug Administration (FDA) in 2001 in view of various severe and potentially fatal side effects. For the cardiovascular system, the most notable were blood pressure derangements with hypertension and hypotension, arrhythmias (especially atrial fibrillation), cardiomyopathy (especially with longer-term use), and notably, ischemic events.[81,82] Chest pain has been noted in almost 30% related predominantly to vasospastic angina and/or microvascular angina.[81] Similarly, a vasospastic component has been related to digital ischemic events (Raynaud), which can reach severity grades of gangrene.[83,84] With regard to strokes, both hemorrhagic and ischemic events can occur. Furthermore, pulmonary vasculitis and hypertension can evolve.[84] Experimental studies suggest that type I interferons such as interferon-α contribute to endothelial dysfunction, vascular inflammation, platelet activation, and thrombosis.[85] Of note, some of these events can occur with a certain delay and not only during the active treatment phase and may not be reversible. It is therefore recommended that patients with any of the above conditions are to be very closely monitored even though events can occur even in those without a cardiovascular history or risk factors. In case of any signs or symptoms of vascular side effects, the need for interferon-α is to be re-evaluated, and it is definitively to be discontinued if any severe change is noted.

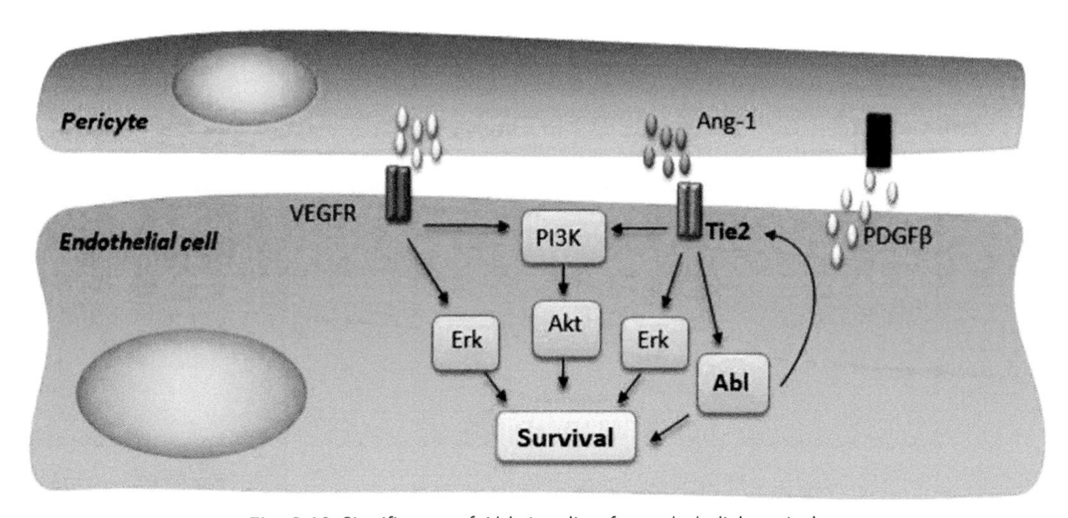

Fig. 9.10 Significance of Abl signaling for endothelial survival.

PART 2: CLINICAL PRESENTATIONS OF CHEMOTHERAPY-RELATED VASCULAR TOXICITIES

Typical and Atypical Chest Pain

Several different causes can account for chest pain in patients with cancer, including myocardial ischemia, which by itself can be due to various mechanisms. Abnormal (paradoxic) vasoconstriction and vasospasm can be provoked by chemotherapeutics, most notoriously 5-FU and its oral prodrug capecitabine.[13] Paclitaxel, docetaxel, and cisplatin, often in combination with bleomycin, as well as interferon-α are to be listed as well.[81,86–88] Effort angina and abnormal stress tests can be noted,[89] but not uncommonly symptoms can occur at rest, raising concerns for an acute coronary syndrome (ACS).

Another unique consideration in patients with cancer to account for chest pain episode is cardiac and primary noncardiac tumors, leading to coronary artery compression.[90] Location is an important aspect and external compression can be caused even by atrial tumors.[91] Mediastinal tumors such as lymphoma can lead to left main compromise.[92] On the other hand, involvement of the right ventricular grove by mediastinal diffuse large B-cell lymphoma and thymoma can lead to encasement but not necessarily compression of the right coronary artery, so-called "floating artery sign".[93] On the other hand, true invasion of coronary arteries should always raise concerns for angiosarcoma.

Management

The first step is to define the most likely cause of the chest pain episodes, for example, pulmonary embolism, pericarditis, and myocardial ischemia versus noncardiovascular pain, such as esophageal spasm. Myocardial ischemia can be stratified further into a functional/vasoreactive versus a structural/plaque or compression etiology. For chemotherapeutics, a distinction can be made between type I and type II vasotoxicity agents as outlined above, and management varies accordingly. Whereas it is more functionally directed for type II agents (eg, peripheral vasoreactivity testing), it is to include structural assessments for type I agents (eg, coronary angiography).

Administration of nitroglycerin and/or calcium channel blockers is the best initial diagnostic and therapeutic step for type II agents such as 5-FU (Box 9.1). Thereafter, one may decide on further testing for structural heart disease. A more comprehensive and definitive assessment is advised for patients at risk of developing progressive atherosclerosis, such as those on type I vasotoxicity agents, which are to be discontinued if concerns prevail. A complete cardiovascular risk and disease assessment is also recommended if continuation of treatment with the same or a similar drug is considered. The goal then would be to facilitate continuation of chemotherapy while managing and mitigating cardiovascular disease risk and side effects. Finally, comprehensive imaging should be pursued if there are any concerns of coronary artery compression.

BOX 9.1
Management of 5-fluorouracil/capecitabine cardiotoxicity

At the time of acute presentation
- Stop administration of the drug
- Use nitrates or calcium channel blockers (CCB)
- Cardiac monitoring, CCU for patients with cardiac biomarker elevation >2 times upper limit of normal for ≥72 hours

At the time of consideration of rechallenge
- 3-day course of nitrates or CCB, 24 hours before, during, and after rechallenge
- Continuous ECG monitoring on the day of drug administration
- Avoid use in patients with myocardial infarction as a prior complication of therapy

With regards to preventive efforts, it is recommended to reduce dosing in general and for 5-FU in particular to avoid continuous and high-dose infusions.[12,13] Pretreatment with nitrates and/or calcium channel blockers is an option when the risk of vasoconstriction is presumed to be high. No definite management recommendation can be given for those starting type I vasotoxicity agents, but dual antiplatelet therapy, statins, angiotensin-converting enzyme (ACE) inhibitor, and amlodipine may be considered.[94] Surveillance for patients with cancer while on and even after therapy of vasotoxic drugs is important, and one proposed algorithm is presented in Fig. 9.11.

Acute Coronary Syndrome

Patients with cancer can develop the full spectrum of ACS ranging from unstable angina to AMI and sudden cardiac death. One central mechanism is the aforementioned alteration in coronary vasoreactivity, which can lead to unstable angina, even MI (type II by the Universal Definition) and arrhythmic complications such as ventricular tachycardia and fibrillation. Such events have been

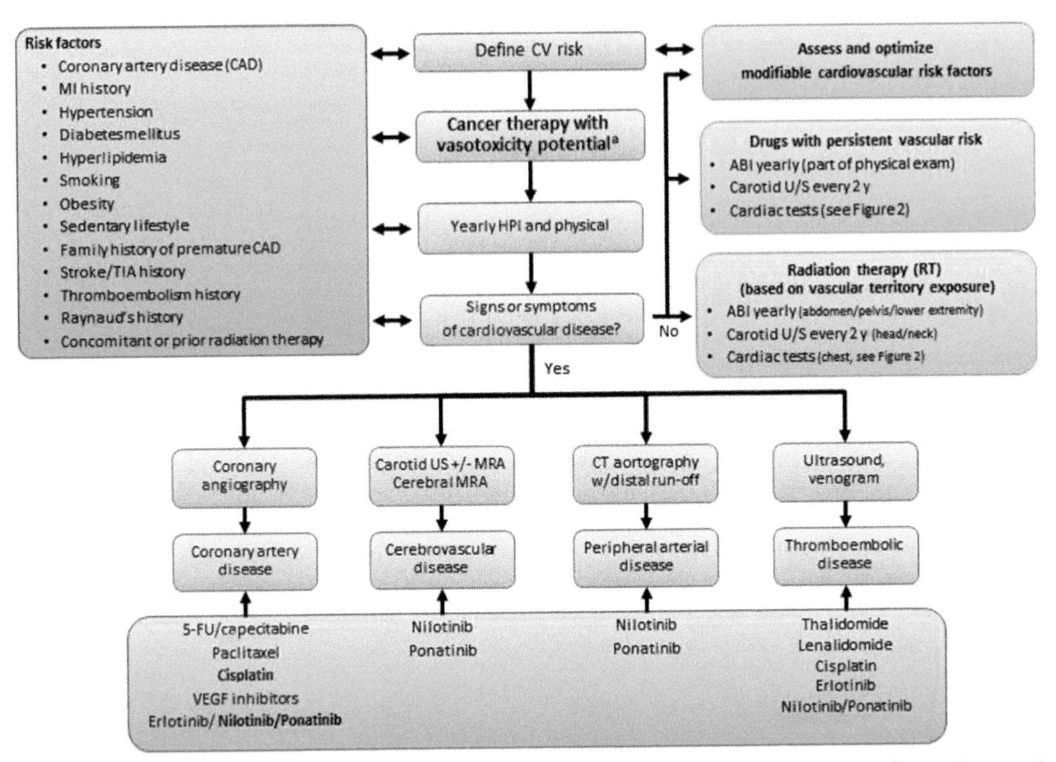

Fig. 9.11 Society for Cardiac Angiography and Interventions algorithm for vascular toxicity surveillance. [a] vasotaxic drugs by vascular territories (in bold: drug with peristent risk after therapy.)

reported for 5-FU and capecitabine, and the same seems to apply to paclitaxel, gemcitabine, rituximab, and sorafenib.[15,16,51,95–100] Tachycardia, hypotension, hypoxia, and anemia are additional contributing factors to ACS presentations in patients with cancer, especially with any additional predisposing reduction in myocardial reserve due to CAD or variants such as myocardial bridging.

In addition to the above, patients with cancer also develop type I ACS (MI) scenarios that need to be promptly recognized and acted upon. Given the toxic effect of chemotherapeutics on the endothelial cells, these patients might have a greater propensity toward erosion. This concept has been illustrated in patients receiving cisplatin, with and without bleomycin and/or vinca alkaloids, who developed single- and even multivessel coronary thrombosis without any evidence of underlying atherosclerosis.[17–22,37–39] Of further interest, cisplatin levels can remain detectable for years after therapy and so can the risk for chest pain episodes and acute ischemic events.[24] Plaque hemorrhage is another, at least theoretic, possibility in those patients receiving treatment with vascular disrupting agents given the fragility of the plaque neovessels.[101] Classical plaque rupture can also be encountered but might not be as frequent given the modulation of inflammation and immune response with cancer therapies. More common in patients with cancer than in the general population is a predisposition to thrombus formation. Thus, these patients might present more readily with ACS presentations in response to any of the outlined pathoanatomical scenarios. Moreover, thrombi forming elsewhere can lead to embolic coronary artery occlusion, for instance, paradoxic emboli via a patent foramen ovale, from the cardiac chambers and valves, and even tumor embolization or a combination thereof.[102,103] Another entity to consider in patients with cancer is spontaneous coronary artery dissection, which could be a reflection of the impact of cancer therapy on vascular remodeling.[104–106] Extrinsic compression by a tumor mass is usually a gradual phenomenon, but sudden growth could lead to unstable and acute presentations.

Management

The first step is to establish the diagnosis of ACS. Patients with signs and symptoms of myocardial ischemia should receive nitroglycerin to alleviate any possible coronary vasoconstriction. Cardiac catheterization is advisable (especially with any symptomatic, arrhythmic, or hemodynamic instability) to exclude any concomitant process that could account for an ACS presentation. Further management decisions are based on the angiographic results. If uncertainty remains with regards to vascular abnormality, further imaging with intravascular ultrasound and/or optical coherence tomography (OCT) can be used. PCI is to be pursued only if indicated. Aspirin may attenuate the ischemic event risk, at least with bevacizumab, and especially in those 65 years or older and with a prior history of an arterial thrombotic event (12.5% vs 22.9%), however, at a 1.3 times higher risk of grade 3 and 4 bleeding events.[107] In general, all patients should be treated with optimal guideline-directed therapy, unless there is a compelling prohibitive reason (Fig. 9.1).

Apical Ballooning Syndrome

Given the tremendous stress patients with cancer are exposed to, apical ballooning syndrome needs to be considered even more in these patients than in the general population.[6] Numerous chemotherapeutics can add to the risk, including 5-FU, capecitabine, cytarabine, axitinib, sunitinib, bevacizumab, rituximab, trastuzumab, and combretastatin.[54,55,108–115] Indeed, most of the events seem to occur in close temporal proximity to cancer surgery, stem cell transplantation, or chemotherapy, and mainly in women (76%), of advanced age (65.9 $\pm$ 9 years), and with advanced cancer.[116] The prognosis, however, does seem favorable, and two-thirds are seemingly able to resume chemotherapy (on cardioprotective agents) within 1 month of the event without the risk of (immediate) recurrence.

Although the exact pathophysiology is not known, induction of abnormal coronary vasoreactivity on the level of the coronary microcirculation generating the substrate for abnormal perfusion and contraction is one of the leading theories. This pathophysiology may apply to chemotherapies and/or the interaction with (stress) catecholamines.[1,4–7] Excitingly, the significant role of the pericyte for the coronary microcirculation, coronary flow reserve, and myocardial stress response was highlighted in experimental studies with sunitinb.[54,55] The evolving concept is that of pericyte-endothelial-myocardial coupling for microvascular and myocardial function with implications for apical ballooning syndrome. Importantly, a reduction in coronary flow reserve has been observed in patients on sunitinib.[56] Injury to the endothelium and the microvasculature also underlies the all-trans retinoic acid (ATRA) differentiation syndrome, and cardiac stunning has been reported in patients with acute promyelocytic leukemia who are developing this syndrome with retinoic acid treatment.[117]

Management

The first step is to follow published ACS guidelines. Patients with ST-segment elevation, hemodynamic instability, or persistent chest pain should undergo emergent catheterization. If these features are not present, but a high level of suspicion for apical ballooning syndrome exists, echocardiography and coronary computed tomography (CT) angiography may suffice for the diagnosis and to guide management in many cases, especially if there are additional factors favoring a noninvasive approach. Coronary angiography and left ventriculography, however, can be safely performed, even in patients with cancer with low platelet counts and higher bleeding risks via a radial or micropuncture femoral approach. If the findings are not typical for apical ballooning syndrome, plaque erosion or extreme vasoconstriction/vasospasm needs to be considered. Structural abnormalities, even of subtle extent such as erosions, can be revealed by adjunctive invasive techniques such as OCT. Functional abnormalities and predispositions can be recognized by vasoreactivity studies with acetylcholine (endothelial function), methergine (vascular smooth muscle cell function), and adenosine (microvascular function). Sometimes, the vasoactive agent needs to be combined with the cancer agent to reveal the vasofunctional abnormality.[7] Vasodilator therapy (and drugs with vasodilator properties such as carvedilol and ACE inhibitors) should be provided in the absence of a dynamic outflow tract obstruction. Otherwise, one should strive to optimize the volume status and administer β-blocker such as metoprolol. The best preventive strategy for recurrent apical ballooning syndrome has not been defined, but β-blocker, ACE inhibitors and aspirin have emerged as the "anecdotal standard of care."[118]

Claudication/Acute Limb Ischemia

The primary presentation of limb ischemia in patients with cancer has been Raynaud, which relates to digital vasospasm and can be of variable degree, even to the extent of gangrene. Depending on the circumstances, Raynaud can be noted in almost one-third of patients and may signal globally abnormal vasoreactivity and MI risk.[34,36] It should be thought of in the context of therapies with bleomycin, vinca alkaloids, cisplatin, carboplatin, gemcitabine, and interferon-α.[84,119–122] For some of these agents, for example, bleomycin, it can be noted as early as after the first dose, likely related to a direct effect on endothelial cells.[123]

For others, for example, interferon-α, it can be delayed and related to more complex mechanisms such as immune-mediated vasculitis.[124] Finally, it has to be kept in mind that Raynaud can occur as a paraneoplastic phenomenon, even before an initial or recurrent cancer diagnosis.[125]

With the emerging use of TKIs targeting the *Bcr-Abl* oncogenic fusion gene products, namely nilotinib and ponatinib, the new entity of chemotherapy-induced peripheral arterial occlusive disease (PAOD) was recognized.[126,127] This entity is characterized by rapidly progressive atherosclerosis to the point of total occlusion especially of the lower extremity circulation (see Fig. 9.4). The visceral and renal arteries can be involved as well, leading to a plethora of clinical presentations. The rate of acute ischemic events is as high as 2% to 25% for nilotinib and 9% to 48% for ponatinib.[68–73] Importantly, the risk may persist even after discontinuation of therapy and while on optimal medical therapy.[74–76,128] There is currently no proven concept of the underlying pathophysiology; acute thrombosis may not be the main mechanism.

Historically, thromboembolism is the most frequent mechanism of acute limb ischemia in patients with cancer and might be related to various causes.[129] For instance, acute arterial thrombosis is characteristic of acute promyelocytic leukemia.[130] Finally, aortic tumors such as intimal sarcoma are rare causes of limb ischemia.[131]

Management

The first step in the evaluation of patients with cancer with peripheral arterial changes is to confirm its nature such as vasoreactive, embolic/thrombotic, or progressively obstructive, related to chemotherapy or any other concomitant or pre-existing predisposition to functional or structural peripheral arterial disease with cancer therapy. A thorough clinical history is key as some studies have suggested higher event rates in patients with an unfavorable risk factor profile.[77] However, events can occur even in patients without any history of cardiovascular disease or risk factor exposure. The merit of assessing nontraditional risk factors and procoagulant states in these patients is unknown as is the role of provocative testing. One may argue for general surveillance with serial ankle-brachial indices and/or EndoPAT (see Fig. 9.11). General surveillance might be particularly worthwhile in the case of nilotinib and ponatinib as abnormalities of the peripheral vasculature preceded acute coronary and cerebrovascular events. Although events have occurred on antiplatelet and statin therapy, patients should still receive best practice vascular therapy, including (possibly dual) antiplatelet therapy (high dose), statins, ACE inhibitor, and amlodipine.[94]

Cerebrovascular Events

Transient ischemic attacks and stroke can occur in patients with cancer with patterns (ischemic, hemorrhagic) and risk factors (eg, atrial fibrillation) similar to patients without cancer. Although theoretically at higher risk, there have been essentially no hemorrhagic strokes reported in patients with cancer even with the use of vascular disrupting agents. Also, patients with cancer are seemingly not at higher risk of intracerebral hemorrhage when undergoing thrombolytic therapy for acute stroke.[132] On the contrary, patients with cancer are at higher risk of thromboembolic events of venous origin (paradoxic embolization) as well as arterial origin, for example, due to indwelling arterial catheters or atrial fibrillation.[133–136] Although there is insufficient evidence that hypercoagulability is a causal factor in general, it might be a contributing factor in some patients.[137] Likewise, not all but some chemotherapeutics have been associated with a risk of stroke.[138] These chemotherapeutics include 5-FU and especially platinum-based therapies in keeping with a general effect on the vasculature.[139–142] Endothelial cell death induced by cisplatin may generate not only local but also possibly even systemic vulnerability by the production of procoagulant microparticles,[143] possibly providing some explanation for cases of ischemic stroke for which no other cause could be identified.[144]

Concerns for stroke risk have been raised for VEGF signaling pathway inhibitors, particularly in view of the outlined side-effect profile of arterial thrombosis, bleeding, and hypertension.[145] In the initial phase I and II trials, the reported rate of ischemic stroke was 1.9% with bevacizumab and 0% with VEGF receptor TKIs and 1.9% and 3.8% for intracranial hemorrhage, respectively.[146] Ischemic strokes were seen with prolonged therapy (at a median time of 16.2 months), while intracranial hemorrhages were noted earlier (at a median time of 2.6 months), often in the setting of tumor progression, and with dismal survival prognosis. Based on an FDA MedWatch database review, cranial bleeds accounted for 12.9% of all bleeding events with bevacizumab (which were 6.8% of all adverse events) and were fatal in 50%.[147] Additional use of medications associated with bleeding and thrombocytopenia are the main risk factors, whereas central nervous system tumors and metastases do not seem to increase the risk.[148,149] With regards to arterial thromboembolic events, the combination of bevacizumab with 5-FU- or carboplatin-based therapies may more than double the risk, especially in patients 65 years of age or older or with a prior arterial thromboembolic event (15.7%).[107] Carotid atherosclerosis or dissections have rarely been reported as the underlying mechanisms of cerebrovascular events in these patients even though significant carotid artery disease has been seen in patients on sorafenib.[150–154]

Ischemic strokes have been reported with the use of nilotinib, even on optimal medial therapy and anticoagulation.[128] In some cases, no cause could be identified, whereas in others diffuse intracranial atherosclerosis and rapid progression of carotid artery disease (from 50%-60% to subtotal occlusion within 1 year) was noted with symptom development during episodes of hypotension.[75] Concerns for moyamoya disease and cerebral vasculitis were raised in a patient on ponatinib treatment. However, no pathologic substrate for this patient's cerebrovascular event was found on autopsy.[155] Similar mechanistic concerns have been raised for cerebrovascular events occurring with interferon-α therapy.[156]

In patients presenting with headache, confusion, visual symptoms, and seizures, especially in combination with high blood pressure, posterior reversible encephalopathy syndrome (PRES) needs to be considered as the cause of the neurologic presentation. Posterior cerebral white matter edema is the distinguishing pathognomonic feature on neuroimaging and reflects impaired autoregulation of the cerebral vasculature. PRES has been reported for several chemotherapy drugs, especially VEGF signaling pathway inhibitors and the proteasome inhibitor bortezomib.[157,158] Finally, any cerebrovascular event in a patient with cancer should raise concern for cerebral tumor development, namely cerebral metastases. Furthermore, opportunistic infections may account for some of these presentations as well.

Management

The first step with any signs or symptoms of stroke in a patient with cancer should be a emergent head CT scan to address the question of a hemorrhagic event or intracranial tumors (metastases).[159] If negative, and thus presumed ischemic, decisions on lytic therapy and endovascular approaches are to be made. Importantly, patients with cancer are not at a generally higher risk of intracerebral hemorrhage with thrombolytic therapy.[132] However, patients with cancer have not been rigorously studied in fibrinolysis trials. Noteworthy contraindications to lytic therapy for patients with cancer are platelet count less than 100,000 and plasma glucose less than 50 or greater than 400 mg/dL. Specific tests for thrombotic occlusion, critical stenosis, or dissections should be pursued as needed. A 12-lead electrocardiogram (ECG) should be obtained to assess for atrial flutter/fibrillation and an echocardiogram to assess for a patent foramen ovale, valve abnormalities, regional wall abnormalities, and aneurysms.[135] A Neurology consultation should always be obtained as soon as possible. Care decisions are to be made in the context of the patient's overall prognosis.

Pulmonary Hypertension

Dyspnea in patients with cancer encompasses a broad differential that includes cancer therapies. Dasatinib, a TKI of Bcr-Abl, used in patients with Philadelphia chromosome-positive (Ph+) leukemias, is the prime example. It can cause precapillary pulmonary hypertension (commonly moderate to severe degree, mean pulmonary artery 46 mm Hg, mean right ventricular systolic pressure 65) seemingly at any time during the active treatment.[160,161] The reported incidence is 1% to 12%,[160,161] but might be higher with routine screening. Importantly, the clinical course may not always be benign. As outlined in the original series, improvement in clinical, functional, and hemodynamic parameters was noted, but over the course of months after cessation of therapy and pulmonary pressures may never fully normalize. One-third of the patients required prolonged pulmonary hypertension-directed treatment, and 2 patients died. The first patient had persistent severe pulmonary hypertension, functional class III dyspnea, and right ventricular dilation. The second patient experienced functional improvement but sudden death.[160]

Intriguingly, the combination of a VEGF receptor 2 inhibitor with chronic hypoxia has been used as an experimental model of pulmonary hypertension.[162] Of further note, VEGF receptor 2 deficiency, even confined to endothelial cells, impairs vascularization and resolution of intrapulmonary artery thrombi, and combined with the right substrate, this has the propensity to contribute to chronic thromboembolic pulmonary hypertension.[163] Rho kinase–mediated vasoconstriction might play an additional role.[164] Not all TKIs (VEGF signaling pathway directed or not), however, have been associated with pulmonary hypertension. Moreover, the drug found to be most favorable in in vitro and in vivo studies for the treatment of pulmonary hypertension due to the concomitant inhibition of PDGF receptor and

Src kinases is the one found to cause most of the clinical events: dasatinib.[165] Oppositely, imatinib was found to be inferior in preclinical studies but efficacious in reducing pulmonary hypertension in clinical practices.[166] Thus, the mechanisms remain poorly understood. Potentially though, immune mechanisms are involved because dasatinib-induced pulmonary hypertension is often associated with exudative pleural effusions (and even pericardial effusion), and almost exclusively lymphocytic accumulations have been found on pleural and bronchoalveolar lavage and biopsies.[167]

Bleomycin is the chemotherapeutic historically associated with pulmonary hypertension. The overall risk is 10%, emerging gradually over the course of therapy and even years later.[168] A distinctive feature is the development of pulmonary fibrosis, which has been thought to be the consequence of the stimulation and transformation of fibroblasts into collagen-producing myofibroblasts by activated alveolar macrophages and epithelial cells in the context of a response to injury.[168] Inflammation, oxidative stress, and alternation in NO signaling play a role similar to atherosclerosis. Statin, Rho kinase inhibition, endothelin receptor antagonism, arginase inhibition, provision of inhaled or even dietary NO, and sildenafil have all been shown to ameliorate bleomycin-induced lung injury.[169–176]

Last but not least, interferon-α can induce pulmonary hypertension and pulmonary vasculitis, which has been related to immune mechanism even though the pathophysiology remains to be defined.[84] Pulmonary arterial pressures may also increase as the consequence of noninfectious pneumonitis with mammalian target of rapamycin (mTOR) inhibitors.[177]

Management

The first step is to define the nature of dyspnea in any given patient with cancer. The list of differential diagnoses is exceptionally broad and includes pulmonary and cardiac causes as well as anemia and deconditioning. It is extremely important to ask the patient to more specifically define the sensation of dyspnea. Additional signs and symptoms then direct the evaluation further. In general, it is recommended that all patients are evaluated for any cardiopulmonary disease before initiation and during treatment, especially with the drugs mentioned herein (Case Study, available on Expert Consult). Patients may become symptomatic at any time during and even years after their treatment, posing diagnostic challenges. Dyspnea, hypoxia, cough, chest pressure, reduced exercise tolerance, fatigue, and abdominal and lower extremity edema should prompt immediate re-evaluation. This re-evaluation should include an ECG, chest radiograph, and echocardiogram. Pulmonary function tests have their role in defining obstructive and restrictive lung disease and reductions in diffusion capacity. Potential disease processes such as pulmonary embolism and pneumonitis are well studied by contrast and high-resolution chest CT scans. Invasive right and left heart catheterization can be of further value, and treatment should be directed to the underlying cause and in keeping with published guidelines.[178]

REFERENCES

1. Polk A, et al. A systematic review of the pathophysiology of 5-fluorouracil-induced cardiotoxicity. BMC Pharmacol Toxicol 2014;15:47.
2. de Forni M, et al. Cardiotoxicity of continuous intravenous infusion of 5-fluorouracil: clinical study, prevention and physiopathology. Apropos of 13 cases. Bull Cancer 1990;77(5):429–38 [in French].
3. Sudhoff T, et al. 5-Fluorouracil induces arterial vasocontractions. Ann Oncol 2004;15(4):661–4.
4. Stewart T, Pavlakis N, Ward M. Cardiotoxicity with 5-fluorouracil and capecitabine: more than just vasospastic angina. Intern Med J 2010;40(4):303–7.
5. Grunwald MR, Howie L, Diaz LA Jr. Takotsubo cardiomyopathy and Fluorouracil: case report and review of the literature. J Clin Oncol 2012;30(2):e11–4.
6. Smith SA, Auseon AJ. Chemotherapy-induced takotsubo cardiomyopathy. Heart Fail Clin 2013;9(2):233–42, x.
7. Kobayashi N, et al. A case of Takotsubo cardiomyopathy during 5-fluorouracil treatment for rectal adenocarcinoma. J Nippon Med Sch 2009;76(1):27–33.
8. Cerny J, et al. Coronary vasospasm with myocardial stunning in a patient with colon cancer receiving adjuvant chemotherapy with FOLFOX regimen. Clin Colorectal Cancer 2009;8(1):55–8.
9. Ambrosy AP, et al. Capecitabine-induced chest pain relieved by diltiazem. Am J Cardiol 2012;110(11):1623–6.
10. Boyle JJ, et al. Expression of angiogenic factor thymidine phosphorylase and angiogenesis in human atherosclerosis. J Pathol 2000;192(2):234–42.
11. Coward J, Maisey N, Cunningham D. The effects of capecitabine in Raynaud's disease: a case report. Ann Oncol 2005;16(5):835–6.
12. Jensen SA, Sorensen JB. Risk factors and prevention of cardiotoxicity induced by 5-fluorouracil or capecitabine. Cancer Chemother Pharmacol 2006;58(4):487–93.

13. Polk A, et al. Cardiotoxicity in cancer patients treated with 5-fluorouracil or capecitabine: a systematic review of incidence, manifestations and predisposing factors. Cancer Treat Rev 2013; 39(8):974–84.
14. Rowinsky EK, et al. Cardiac disturbances during the administration of taxol. J Clin Oncol 1991; 9(9):1704–12.
15. Schrader C, et al. Symptoms and signs of an acute myocardial ischemia caused by chemotherapy with Paclitaxel (Taxol) in a patient with metastatic ovarian carcinoma. Eur J Med Res 2005;10(11): 498–501.
16. Shah K, et al. Acute non-ST elevation myocardial infarction following paclitaxel administration for ovarian carcinoma: a case report and review of literature. J Cancer Res Ther 2012;8(3):442–4.
17. Berliner S, et al. Acute coronary events following cisplatin-based chemotherapy. Cancer Invest 1990;8(6):583–6.
18. Jafri M, Protheroe A. Cisplatin-associated thrombosis. Anti Cancer Drugs 2008;19(9):927–9.
19. Karabay KO, Yildiz O, Aytekin V. Multiple coronary thrombi with cisplatin. J Invasive Cardiol 2014; 26(2):E18–20.
20. Togna GI, et al. Cisplatin triggers platelet activation. Thromb Res 2000;99(5):503–9.
21. Dieckmann KP, et al. Myocardial infarction and other major vascular events during chemotherapy for testicular cancer. Ann Oncol 2010; 21(8):1607–11.
22. Ito D, et al. Primary percutaneous coronary intervention and intravascular ultrasound imaging for coronary thrombosis after cisplatin-based chemotherapy. Heart Vessels 2012;27(6):634–8.
23. Meinardi MT, et al. Cardiovascular morbidity in long-term survivors of metastatic testicular cancer. J Clin Oncol 2000;18(8):1725–32.
24. Gietema JA, et al. Circulating plasma platinum more than 10 years after cisplatin treatment for testicular cancer. Lancet 2000;355(9209):1075–6.
25. Huddart RA, et al. Cardiovascular disease as a long-term complication of treatment for testicular cancer. J Clin Oncol 2003;21(8):1513–23.
26. van den Belt-Dusebout AW, et al. Long-term risk of cardiovascular disease in 5-year survivors of testicular cancer. J Clin Oncol 2006;24(3):467–75.
27. Haugnes HS, et al. Cardiovascular risk factors and morbidity in long-term survivors of testicular cancer: a 20-year follow-up study. J Clin Oncol 2010; 28(30):4649–57.
28. Feldman DR, Schaffer WL, Steingart RM. Late cardiovascular toxicity following chemotherapy for germ cell tumors. J Natl Compr Cancer Netw 2012;10(4):537–44.
29. Nuver J, et al. Microalbuminuria, decreased fibrinolysis, and inflammation as early signs of atherosclerosis in long-term survivors of disseminated testicular cancer. Eur J Cancer 2004;40(5): 701–6.
30. Oh JH, et al. Long-term complications of platinum-based chemotherapy in testicular cancer survivors. Med Oncol 2007;24(2):175–81.
31. Kachel DL, Martin WJ 2nd. Cyclophosphamide-induced lung toxicity: mechanism of endothelial cell injury. J Pharmacol Exp Ther 1994;268(1):42–6.
32. Gottdiener JS, et al. Cardiotoxicity associated with high-dose cyclophosphamide therapy. Arch Intern Med 1981;141(6):758–63.
33. Katayama M, et al. Fulminant fatal cardiotoxicity following cyclophosphamide therapy. J Cardiol 2009;54(2):330–4.
34. Stefenelli T, et al. Acute vascular toxicity after combination chemotherapy with cisplatin, vinblastine, and bleomycin for testicular cancer. Eur Heart J 1988;9(5):552–6.
35. Soultati A, et al. Endothelial vascular toxicity from chemotherapeutic agents: preclinical evidence and clinical implications. Cancer Treat Rev 2012; 38(5):473–83.
36. Schwarzer S, et al. Non-Q-wave myocardial infarction associated with bleomycin and etoposide chemotherapy. Eur Heart J 1991;12(6):748–50.
37. Doll DC, et al. Acute vascular ischemic events after cisplatin-based combination chemotherapy for germ-cell tumors of the testis. Ann Intern Med 1986;105(1):48–51.
38. Samuels BL, Vogelzang NJ, Kennedy BJ. Severe vascular toxicity associated with vinblastine, bleomycin, and cisplatin chemotherapy. Cancer Chemother Pharmacol 1987;19(3):253–6.
39. Panella M, et al. Cardiac sudden death as a result of acute coronary artery thrombosis during chemotherapy for testicular carcinoma. J Forensic Sci 2010;55(5):1384–8.
40. Gallagher H, et al. The effects of vinblastine on endothelial cells. Endothelium 2008;15(1):9–15.
41. Schutz FA, et al. Bevacizumab increases the risk of arterial ischemia: a large study in cancer patients with a focus on different subgroup outcomes. Ann Oncol 2011;22(6):1404–12.
42. Ranpura V, et al. Risk of cardiac ischemia and arterial thromboembolic events with the angiogenesis inhibitor bevacizumab in cancer patients: a meta-analysis of randomized controlled trials. Acta Oncol 2010;49(3):287–97.
43. Chen XL, et al. Angiogenesis inhibitor bevacizumab increases the risk of ischemic heart disease associated with chemotherapy: a meta-analysis. PLoS One 2013;8(6):e66721.
44. Choueiri TK, et al. Risk of arterial thromboembolic events with sunitinib and sorafenib: a systematic review and meta-analysis of clinical trials. J Clin Oncol 2010;28(13):2280–5.

45. Qi WX, et al. Risk of arterial thromboembolic events with vascular endothelial growth factor receptor tyrosine kinase inhibitors: An up-to-date meta-analysis. Crit Rev Oncol Hematol 2014.
46. Isenberg JS, et al. Regulation of nitric oxide signalling by thrombospondin 1: implications for antiangiogenic therapies. Nat Rev Cancer 2009;9(3): 182–94.
47. Kappers MH, et al. Hypertension induced by the tyrosine kinase inhibitor sunitinib is associated with increased circulating endothelin-1 levels. Hypertension 2010;56(4):675–81.
48. Winnik S, et al. Systemic VEGF inhibition accelerates experimental atherosclerosis and disrupts endothelial homeostasis–implications for cardiovascular safety. Int J Cardiol 2013;168(3): 2453–61.
49. Kappers MH, et al. The vascular endothelial growth factor receptor inhibitor sunitinib causes a preeclampsia-like syndrome with activation of the endothelin system. Hypertension 2011;58(2): 295–302.
50. Kappers MH, et al. Sunitinib-induced systemic vasoconstriction in swine is endothelin mediated and does not involve nitric oxide or oxidative stress. Hypertension 2012;59(1):151–7.
51. Arima Y, et al. Sorafenib-induced acute myocardial infarction due to coronary artery spasm. J Cardiol 2009;54(3):512–5.
52. Porto I, et al. A case of variant angina in a patient under chronic treatment with sorafenib. Nat Rev Clin Oncol 2010;7(8):476–80.
53. Naib T, Steingart RM, Chen CL. Sorafenib-associated multivessel coronary artery vasospasm. Herz 2011;36(4):348–51.
54. Franco TH, et al. Takotsubo cardiomyopathy in two men receiving bevacizumab for metastatic cancer. Ther Clin Risk Manag 2008;4(6):1367–70.
55. Numico G, et al. Takotsubo syndrome in a patient treated with sunitinib for renal cancer. J Clin Oncol 2012;30(24):e218–20.
56. Sen F, et al. Impaired coronary flow reserve in metastatic cancer patients treated with sunitinib. J BUON 2013;18(3):775–81.
57. Chintalgattu V, et al. Coronary microvascular pericytes are the cellular target of sunitinib malate-induced cardiotoxicity. Sci Transl Med 2013; 5(187):187ra69.
58. de Boer MP, et al. Sunitinib-induced reduction in skin microvascular density is a reversible phenomenon. Ann Oncol 2010;21(9):1923–4.
59. van der Veldt AA, et al. Reduction in skin microvascular density and changes in vessel morphology in patients treated with sunitinib. Anti Cancer Drugs 2010;21(4):439–46.
60. Pantaleo MA, et al. Development of coronary artery stenosis in a patient with metastatic renal cell carcinoma treated with sorafenib. BMC Cancer 2012;12:231.
61. Ropert S, et al. VEGF pathway inhibition by anticancer agent sunitinib and susceptibility to atherosclerosis plaque disruption. Invest New Drugs 2011;29(6):1497–9.
62. Moulton KS, et al. Angiogenesis inhibitors endostatin or TNP-470 reduce intimal neovascularization and plaque growth in apolipoprotein E-deficient mice. Circulation 1999;99(13):1726–32.
63. Moulton KS, et al. Inhibition of plaque neovascularization reduces macrophage accumulation and progression of advanced atherosclerosis. Proc Natl Acad Sci U S A 2003;100(8):4736–41.
64. Herrmann J, et al. Angiogenesis in atherogenesis. Arterioscler Thromb Vasc Biol 2006;26(9): 1948–57.
65. Holm PW, et al. Atherosclerotic plaque development and instability: a dual role for VEGF. Ann Med 2009;41(4):257–64.
66. Hu, S., et al. Bevacizumab for plaque stabilization: evaluation of its effect on vasa vasorum, lipid pool, and atheroma volume by multimodality imaging techniques in an atherosclerotic rabbit model. Circulation. 2012;126:A17934.
67. Meyer T, et al. Bevacizumab immune complexes activate platelets and induce thrombosis in FCGR2A transgenic mice. J Thromb Haemost 2009;7(1):171–81.
68. Aichberger KJ, et al. Progressive peripheral arterial occlusive disease and other vascular events during nilotinib therapy in CML. Am J Hematol 2011;86(7):533–9.
69. Quintas-Cardama A, Kantarjian H, Cortes J. Nilotinib-associated vascular events. Clin Lymphoma Myeloma Leuk 2012;12(5):337–40.
70. Levato L, et al. Progressive peripheral arterial occlusive disease and other vascular events during nilotinib therapy in chronic myeloid leukemia: a single institution study. Eur J Haematol 2013; 90(6):531–2.
71. Cortes JE, et al. A phase 2 trial of ponatinib in Philadelphia chromosome-positive leukemias. N Engl J Med 2013;369(19):1783–96.
72. Cortes JE, et al. Ponatinib in refractory Philadelphia chromosome-positive leukemias. N Engl J Med 2012;367(22):2075–88.
73. Nicolini FE, et al. Cardio-vascular events occurring on ponatinib in chronic phase chronic myeloid leukemia patients, preliminary analysis of a multicenter cohort. Blood 2013;122(21):4020.
74. Tefferi A. Nilotinib treatment-associated accelerated atherosclerosis: when is the risk justified? Leukemia 2013;27(9):1939–40.
75. Coon EA, et al. Nilotinib treatment-associated cerebrovascular disease and stroke. Am J Hematol 2013;88(6):534–5.

76. Tefferi A, Letendre L. Nilotinib treatment-associated peripheral artery disease and sudden death: yet another reason to stick to imatinib as front-line therapy for chronic myelogenous leukemia. Am J Hematol 2011;86(7):610–1.
77. Breccia M, et al. Cardiovascular risk assessments in chronic myeloid leukemia allow identification of patients at high risk of cardiovascular events during treatment with nilotinib. Am J Hematol 2015; 90(5):E100–1.
78. Chislock EM, Ring C, Pendergast AM. Abl kinases are required for vascular function, Tie2 expression, and angiopoietin-1-mediated survival. Proc Natl Acad Sci U S A 2013;110(30):12432–7.
79. Subbiah IM, Lenihan DJ, Tsimberidou AM. Cardiovascular toxicity profiles of vascular-disrupting agents. Oncologist 2011;16(8):1120–30.
80. Beerepoot LV, et al. Phase I clinical evaluation of weekly administration of the novel vascular-targeting agent, ZD6126, in patients with solid tumors. J Clin Oncol 2006;24(10):1491–8.
81. Teragawa H, et al. Adverse effects of interferon on the cardiovascular system in patients with chronic hepatitis C. Jpn Heart J 1996;37(6):905–15.
82. Senkus E, Jassem J. Cardiovascular effects of systemic cancer treatment. Cancer Treat Rev 2011; 37(4):300–11.
83. Kruit WH, Eggermont AM, Stoter G. Interferon-alpha induced Raynaud's syndrome. Ann Oncol 2000;11(11):1501–2.
84. Al-Zahrani H, et al. Vascular events associated with alpha interferon therapy. Leuk Lymphoma 2003; 44(3):471–5.
85. Thacker SG, et al. Type I interferons modulate vascular function, repair, thrombosis, and plaque progression in murine models of lupus and atherosclerosis. Arthritis Rheum 2012;64(9):2975–85.
86. Dixon A, et al. Angina pectoris and therapy with cisplatin, vincristine, and bleomycin. Ann Intern Med 1989;111(4):342–3.
87. Rodriguez J, et al. Angina pectoris following cisplatin, etoposide, and bleomycin in a patient with advanced testicular cancer. Ann Pharmacother 1995;29(2):138–9.
88. Fukuda M, et al. Vasospastic angina likely related to cisplatin-containing chemotherapy and thoracic irradiation for lung cancer. Intern Med 1999;38(5): 436–8.
89. Sestito A, et al. Coronary artery spasm induced by capecitabine. J Cardiovasc Med 2006;7(2): 136–8.
90. Weinberg BA, Conces DJ Jr, Waller BF. Cardiac manifestations of noncardiac tumors. Part I: direct effects. Clin Cardiol 1989;12(5):289–96.
91. Orban M, et al. Cardiac malignant tumor as a rare cause of acute myocardial infarction. Int J Cardiovasc Imaging 2004;20(1):47–51.
92. Zeymer U, Hirschmann WD, Neuhaus KL. Left main coronary stenosis by a mediastinal lymphoma. Clin Investig 1992;70(11):1024–6.
93. Juan YH, et al. Tumor encasement of the right coronary artery: role of anatomic and functional imaging in diagnosis and therapeutic management. Open Cardiovasc Med J 2014;8:110–2.
94. Herrmann J, et al. Complicated and advanced atherosclerosis in a young woman with Philadelphia chromosome-positive acute lymphoblastic leukemia: success and challenges of BCR/ABL1-targeted cancer therapy. Mayo Clin Proc 2015;90(8):1167–8.
95. Lu JI, et al. Acute coronary syndrome secondary to fluorouracil infusion. J Clin Oncol 2006;24(18): 2959–60.
96. Cardinale D, Colombo A, Colombo N. Acute coronary syndrome induced by oral capecitabine. Can J Cardiol 2006;22(3):251–3.
97. Frickhofen N, et al. Capecitabine can induce acute coronary syndrome similar to 5-fluorouracil. Ann Oncol 2002;13(5):797–801.
98. Gemici G, et al. Paclitaxel-induced ST-segment elevations. Clin Cardiol 2009;32(6):E94–6.
99. Ozturk B, et al. Gemcitabine-induced acute coronary syndrome: a case report. Med Princ Pract 2009;18(1):76–80.
100. Armitage JD, et al. Acute coronary syndromes complicating the first infusion of rituximab. Clin Lymphoma Myeloma 2008;8(4):253–5.
101. Michel JB, et al. Pathology of human plaque vulnerability: mechanisms and consequences of intraplaque haemorrhages. Atherosclerosis 2014; 234(2):311–9.
102. Kushiyama S, Ikura Y, Iwai Y. Acute myocardial infarction caused by coronary tumour embolism. Eur Heart J 2013;34(48):3690.
103. Diaz Castro O, Bueno H, Nebreda LA. Acute myocardial infarction caused by paradoxical tumorous embolism as a manifestation of hepatocarcinoma. Heart 2004;90(5):e29.
104. Mir MA, Patnaik MM, Herrmann J. Spontaneous coronary artery dissection during hematopoietic stem cell infusion. Blood 2013;122(19):3388–9.
105. Ghosh N, et al. An unusual case of chronic coronary artery dissection: did cisplatin play a role? Can J Cardiol 2008;24(10):795–7.
106. Abbott JD, et al. Spontaneous coronary artery dissection in a woman receiving 5-fluorouracil–a case report. Angiology 2003;54(6):721–4.
107. Scappaticci FA, et al. Arterial thromboembolic events in patients with metastatic carcinoma treated with chemotherapy and bevacizumab. J Natl Cancer Inst 2007;99(16):1232–9.
108. Dechant C, et al. Acute reversible heart failure caused by coronary vasoconstriction due to continuous 5-fluorouracil combination chemotherapy. Case Rep Oncol 2012;5(2):296–301.

109. Qasem A, et al. Capecitabine-induced takotsubo cardiomyopathy: a case report and literature review. Am J Ther 2014.
110. Gianni M, Dentali F, Lonn E. 5 Fluorouracil-induced apical ballooning syndrome: a case report. Blood Coagul Fibrinolysis 2009;20(4):306–8.
111. Baumann S, et al. Takotsubo cardiomyopathy after systemic consolidation therapy with high-dose intravenous cytarabine in a patient with acute myeloid leukemia. Oncol Res Treat 2014;37(9): 487–90.
112. Ovadia D, et al. Association between takotsubo cardiomyopathy and axitinib: case report and review of the literature. J Clin Oncol 2015;33(1):e1–3.
113. Ng KH, Dearden C, Gruber P. Rituximab-induced Takotsubo syndrome: more cardiotoxic than it appears? BMJ Case Rep 2015;2015. pii:bcr2014208203.
114. Khanji M, et al. Tako-Tsubo syndrome after trastuzumab—an unusual complication of chemotherapy for breast cancer. Clin Oncol 2013;25(5):329.
115. Bhakta S, et al. Myocardial stunning following combined modality combretastatin-based chemotherapy: two case reports and review of the literature. Clin Cardiol 2009;32(12):E80–4.
116. Vejpongsa P, et al. Takotsubo cardiomyopathy in cancer patients: triggers, recovery, and resumption of therapy. J Am Coll Cardiol 2015;65(10S):A927.
117. De Santis GC, et al. Cardiac stunning as a manifestation of ATRA differentiation syndrome in acute promyelocytic leukemia. Med Oncol 2012;29(1): 248–50.
118. Santoro F, et al. Lack of efficacy of drug therapy in preventing takotsubo cardiomyopathy recurrence: a meta-analysis. Clin Cardiol 2014;37(7):434–9.
119. Staff S, et al. Acute digital ischemia complicating gemcitabine and carboplatin combination chemotherapy for ovarian cancer. Acta Obstet Gynecol Scand 2011;90(11):1296–7.
120. Vogelzang NJ, et al. Raynaud's phenomenon: a common toxicity after combination chemotherapy for testicular cancer. Ann Intern Med 1981;95(3): 288–92.
121. Kuhar CG, Mesti T, Zakotnik B. Digital ischemic events related to gemcitabine: Report of two cases and a systematic review. Radiol Oncol 2010;44(4): 257–61.
122. Zeidman A, Dicker D, Mittelman M. Interferon-induced vasospasm in chronic myeloid leukaemia. Acta Haematol 1998;100(2):94–6.
123. McGrath SE, Webb A, Walker-Bone K. Bleomycin-induced Raynaud's phenomenon after single-dose exposure: risk factors and treatment with intravenous iloprost infusion. J Clin Oncol 2013;31(4):e51–2.
124. Raanani P, Ben-Bassat I. Immune-mediated complications during interferon therapy in hematological patients. Acta Haematol 2002;107(3):133–44.
125. Madabhavi I, et al. Paraneoplastic Raynaud's phenomenon manifesting before the diagnosis of lung cancer. BMJ Case Rep 2012;2012. pii:bcr0320125985.
126. Herrmann J, Lerman A. An update on cardio-oncology. Trends Cardiovasc Med 2014;24(7): 285–95.
127. Valent P, et al. Vascular safety issues in CML patients treated with BCR/ABL1 kinase inhibitors. Blood 2015;125(6):901–6.
128. Jager NG, et al. Cerebrovascular events during nilotinib treatment. Neth J Med 2014;72(2):113–4.
129. Tsang JS, et al. Acute limb ischemia in cancer patients: should we surgically intervene? Ann Vasc Surg 2011;25(7):954–60.
130. Kalk E, Goede A, Rose P. Acute arterial thrombosis in acute promyelocytic leukaemia. Clin Lab Haematol 2003;25(4):267–70.
131. Raj V, et al. An unusual cause of acute limb ischemia: aortic intimal sarcoma. Ann Thorac Surg 2011;91(3):e33–5.
132. Murthy SB, et al. Thrombolysis for acute ischemic stroke in patients with cancer: a population study. Stroke 2013;44(12):3573–6.
133. Ahn D, Brickner ME, Dowell J. Embolic stroke secondary to an indwelling catheter in a patient with a patent foramen ovale: a case report and review of the literature. Clin Adv Hematol Oncol 2012;10(5): 335–7.
134. Stefan O, et al. Stroke in cancer patients: a risk factor analysis. J Neurooncol 2009;94(2):221–6.
135. Farmakis D, Parissis J, Filippatos G. Insights into onco-cardiology: atrial fibrillation in cancer. J Am Coll Cardiol 2014;63(10):945–53.
136. Sanon S, Lenihan DJ, Mouhayar E. Peripheral arterial ischemic events in cancer patients. Vasc Med 2011;16(2):119–30.
137. Chaturvedi S, Ansell J, Recht L. Should cerebral ischemic events in cancer patients be considered a manifestation of hypercoagulability? Stroke 1994;25(6):1215–8.
138. Rogers LR. Cerebrovascular complications in patients with cancer. Semin Neurol 2010;30(3):311–9.
139. El Amrani M, et al. Brain infarction following 5-fluorouracil and cisplatin therapy. Neurology 1998; 51(3):899–901.
140. Serrano-Castro PJ, Guardado-Santervas P, Olivares-Romero J. Ischemic stroke following cisplatin and 5-fluorouracil therapy: a transcranial Doppler study. Eur Neurol 2000;44(1):63–4.
141. Meattini I, et al. Ischemic stroke during cisplatin-based chemotherapy for testicular germ cell tumor: case report and review of the literature. J Chemother 2010;22(2):134–6.
142. Kuan AS, et al. Risk of ischemic stroke in patients with ovarian cancer: a nationwide population-based study. BMC Med 2014;12:53.

143. Periard D, et al. Are circulating endothelial-derived and platelet-derived microparticles a pathogenic factor in the cisplatin-induced stroke? Stroke 2007;38(5):1636–8.
144. Martin GG, et al. Vertebral artery occlusion after chemotherapy. Stroke 2008;39(2):e38 [author reply: e39].
145. Seidel C, et al. A comprehensive analysis of vascular complications in 3,889 glioma patients from the German Glioma Network. J Neurol 2013;260(3):847–55.
146. Fraum TJ, et al. Ischemic stroke and intracranial hemorrhage in glioma patients on antiangiogenic therapy. J Neurooncol 2011;105(2):281–9.
147. Letarte N, Bressler LR, Villano JL. Bevacizumab and central nervous system (CNS) hemorrhage. Cancer Chemother Pharmacol 2013;71(6):1561–5.
148. Sandler A, et al. An evidence-based review of the incidence of CNS bleeding with anti-VEGF therapy in non-small cell lung cancer patients with brain metastases. Lung Cancer 2012;78(1):1–7.
149. Khasraw M, et al. Intracranial hemorrhage in patients with cancer treated with bevacizumab: the Memorial Sloan-Kettering experience. Ann Oncol 2012;23(2):458–63.
150. Mantia-Smaldone GM, et al. Vertebral artery dissection and cerebral infarction in a patient with recurrent ovarian cancer receiving bevacizumab. Gynecol Oncol Case Rep 2013;5:37–9.
151. Maraiki F, Aljubran A. Carotid and brachiocephalic arteries stenosis with long term use of sorafenib. Hematol Oncol Stem Cell Ther 2014;7(1):53–5.
152. Vandewynckel YP, et al. Cerebellar stroke in a low cardiovascular risk patient associated with sorafenib treatment for fibrolamellar hepatocellular carcinoma. Clin Case Rep 2014;2(1):4–6.
153. Lonergan MT, et al. Ischaemic stroke in a patient on sunitinib. BMJ Case Rep 2010;2010.
154. Saif MW, et al. Cerebrovascular accidents associated with sorafenib in hepatocellular carcinoma. Gastroenterol Res Pract 2011;2011:616080.
155. Mayer K, et al. Fatal progressive cerebral ischemia in CML under third-line treatment with ponatinib. Leukemia 2014;28(4):976–7.
156. Buchbinder D, et al. Moyamoya in a child treated with interferon for recurrent osteosarcoma. J Pediatr Hematol Oncol 2010;32(6):476–8.
157. Singer S, et al. Posterior reversible encephalopathy syndrome in patients with cancer. Oncologist 2015;20(7):806–11.
158. Foerster R, et al. Posterior reversible leukoencephalopathy syndrome associated with pazopanib. Case Rep Oncol 2013;6(1):204–8.
159. Seok JM, et al. Clinical presentation and ischemic zone on MRI in cancer patients with acute ischemic stroke. Eur Neurol 2012;68(6):368–76.
160. Montani D, et al. Pulmonary arterial hypertension in patients treated by dasatinib. Circulation 2012;125(17):2128–37.
161. Jeon Y-W, et al. Six-year follow-up of dasatinib-related pulmonary arterial hypertension (PAH) for chronic myeloid leukemia in single center. Blood 2013;122(21):4017.
162. Sakao S, Tatsumi K. The effects of antiangiogenic compound SU5416 in a rat model of pulmonary arterial hypertension. Respiration 2011;81(3):253–61.
163. Alias S, et al. Defective angiogenesis delays thrombus resolution: a potential pathogenetic mechanism underlying chronic thromboembolic pulmonary hypertension. Arterioscler Thromb Vasc Biol 2014;34(4):810–9.
164. Oka M, et al. Rho kinase-mediated vasoconstriction is important in severe occlusive pulmonary arterial hypertension in rats. Circ Res 2007;100(6):923–9.
165. Pullamsetti SS, et al. Role of Src tyrosine kinases in experimental pulmonary hypertension. Arterioscler Thromb Vasc Biol 2012;32(6):1354–65.
166. Hoeper MM, et al. Imatinib mesylate as add-on therapy for pulmonary arterial hypertension: results of the randomized IMPRES study. Circulation 2013;127(10):1128–38.
167. Bergeron A, et al. Lung abnormalities after dasatinib treatment for chronic myeloid leukemia: a case series. Am J Respir Crit Care Med 2007;176(8):814–8.
168. Reinert T, et al. Bleomycin-induced lung injury. J Cancer Res 2013;2013:9.
169. Lee AH, et al. Rho-kinase inhibitor prevents bleomycin-induced injury in neonatal rats independent of effects on lung inflammation. Am J Respir Cell Mol Biol 2014;50(1):61–73.
170. Bei Y, et al. Long-term treatment with fasudil improves bleomycin-induced pulmonary fibrosis and pulmonary hypertension via inhibition of Smad2/3 phosphorylation. Pulm Pharmacol Ther 2013;26(6):635–43.
171. Schroll S, et al. Effects of simvastatin on pulmonary fibrosis, pulmonary hypertension and exercise capacity in bleomycin-treated rats. Acta Physiol 2013;208(2):191–201.
172. Baliga RS, et al. Dietary nitrate ameliorates pulmonary hypertension: cytoprotective role for endothelial nitric oxide synthase and xanthine oxidoreductase. Circulation 2012;125(23):2922–32.
173. Van Rheen Z, et al. Lung extracellular superoxide dismutase overexpression lessens bleomycin-induced pulmonary hypertension and vascular remodeling. Am J Respir Cell Mol Biol 2011;44(4):500–8.
174. Schroll S, et al. Improvement of bleomycin-induced pulmonary hypertension and pulmonary fibrosis by

the endothelin receptor antagonist Bosentan. Respir Physiolo Neurobiol 2010;170(1):32–6.
175. Hemnes AR, Zaiman A, Champion HC. PDE5A inhibition attenuates bleomycin-induced pulmonary fibrosis and pulmonary hypertension through inhibition of ROS generation and RhoA/Rho kinase activation. Am J Physiol Lung Cell Mol Physiol 2008;294(1):L24–33.
176. Grasemann H, et al. Arginase inhibition prevents bleomycin-induced pulmonary hypertension, vascular remodeling, and collagen deposition in neonatal rat lungs. Am J Physiol Lung Cell Mol Physiol 2015;308(6):L503–10.
177. Atkinson BJ, et al. Mammalian target of rapamycin (mTOR) inhibitor-associated non-infectious pneumonitis in patients with renal cell cancer: predictors, management, and outcomes. BJU Int 2014; 113(3):376–82.
178. Galie N, et al. Guidelines for the diagnosis and treatment of pulmonary hypertension: the Task Force for the Diagnosis and Treatment of Pulmonary Hypertension of the European Society of Cardiology (ESC) and the European Respiratory Society (ERS), endorsed by the International Society of Heart and Lung Transplantation (ISHLT). Eur Heart J 2009;30(20):2493–537.

CHAPTER 10

Cardiovascular Complications from Cancer Therapy

Hypertension–Focus on Vascular Endothelial Growth Factor Inhibitors

Alan C. Cameron, BSc (Hons), MB ChB, MRCP*,
Ninian N. Lang, MB, ChB, PhD, MRCP, Rhian M. Touyz, MBBCh, PhD, FRCP, FRSE

INTRODUCTION

Developments in the treatment of cancer have improved the prognosis of patients with several malignancies, to the extent that cancer therapy is now often given with curative intent.[1,2] Angiogenesis, the process of new blood vessel formation, is essential for tumor growth and metastasis, and vascular endothelial growth factor (VEGF) is fundamental to this process.[3,4] Chemotherapy agents that inhibit the proangiogenic effects of VEGF signaling are therefore an ideal approach for reducing tumor growth and metastasis.[5] Indeed, VEGF inhibitors (VEGFI) have revolutionized therapy and substantially improved the prognosis for patients with several previously untreatable malignancies.[1]

Hypertension is a common complication that occurs in up to 80% of patients treated with VEGFI, and almost all patients have an absolute increase in blood pressure.[6–9] There is an acute, dose-dependent increase in blood pressure that occurs in the early period after starting VEGFI.[6,10–12] Patients are therefore at risk of acute hypertensive complications, such as transient ischemic attack or stroke, whereas those who survive their initial cancer diagnosis are at risk of developing hypertension-associated end-organ damage leading to ischemic heart disease, heart failure, renal failure, and stroke.[2,6] Indeed, with substantially increased cancer cure and survivorship, patients often survive long enough to allow cardiovascular morbidity to take precedent over their initial cancer diagnosis.[2]

As more potent VEGFIs are developed, as more patients with cancer are treated, and as the use of VEGFIs is extended to include older patients and those with pre-existing cardiovascular disease, the burden of hypertension as an acute and latent complication will increase.[6] The management of VEGFI-associated hypertension should aim to reduce cardiovascular morbidity and mortality while maintaining effective dosing of anti-angiogenic chemotherapy. This management requires a collaborative approach between oncologists and cardiovascular specialists to achieve a balance from both perspectives.[2,6,13]

This chapter provides a clinically relevant overview of VEGFI-induced hypertension. In particular, pathophysiologic mechanisms, strategies to predict those at greatest risk, and approaches to blood pressure monitoring and management are the focus. Future directions that aim to reduce the development of VEGFI-induced hypertension and novel therapeutic approaches are also discussed (Case Study, available on Expert Consult).

VASCULAR ENDOTHELIAL GROWTH FACTOR, VASCULAR ENDOTHELIAL GROWTH FACTOR RECEPTORS, AND SIGNALING

Vascular Endothelial Growth Factor

VEGF is a glycoprotein produced by many cell types, including endothelial cells, renal epithelial cells, podocytes, fibroblasts, macrophages, and various tumors.[3,4,6,14–16] It exerts potent

Institute of Cardiovascular and Medical Sciences, BHF Glasgow Cardiovascular Research Centre, University of Glasgow, 126 University Place, Glasgow G12 8TA, United Kindgom
* Corresponding author.
E-mail address: Alan.Cameron.2@glasgow.ac.uk

endothelial effects and plays a central role in the maintenance of vascular homeostasis and angiogenesis.[6,17]

VEGF gene expression is regulated by hypoxia-inducible factor 1α, reactive oxygen species (ROS), and inflammatory cytokines (tumor necrosis factor-α).[3,6,18,19] The VEGF gene undergoes alternative splicing to produce multiple isoforms of the protein that include VEGF-A, VEGF-B, VEGF-C, VEGF-D, and placental growth factors (PlGFs) 1 and 2.[3,6] However, VEGF-A is the most comprehensively characterized isoform and the most biologically active of the group.[6,20] This 45-kDa glycoprotein is usually referred to as VEGF.

Vascular Endothelial Growth Factor Receptors

VEGF interacts with 3 types of tyrosine kinase receptors, including VEGFR-1 (Flt-1), VEGFR-2 (Flk-1/KDR), and VEGFR-3 (Flt-4) (Fig. 10.1).[3,6,21] VEGFR-1 and VEGFR-2 are predominantly expressed on vascular endothelial cells, whereas VEGFR-3 is mainly expressed on lymphatic endothelial cells.[3,6] VEGFR-1 is also expressed in monocytes and macrophages.[22–25] These receptors consist of an extracellular region, a transmembrane, and a cytoplasmic tyrosine kinase domain with specific autophosphorylation tyrosine residues that act as docking and activation sites for proteins that include VEGFR-associated protein, Src, Sck, and phospholipase C (PLC).[3,6,26]

VEGF-A binds VEGFR-1 and VEGFR-2, whereas VEGF-B and PlGF bind only VEGFR-1.[22,27–29] VEGF-A exhibits a greater affinity for VEGFR-1 than VEGFR-2, although most of the biological effects of VEGF-A on endothelial cells are mediated by VEGFR-2. Indeed, VEGF-A and VEGFR-2 have been the primary focus in anticancer therapeutic targeting of the VEGF signaling pathway.[3,30]

Vascular Endothelial Growth Factor Receptor 1

Human VEGFR-1, also known as Fms-like tyrosine kinase-1 (Flt-1), has a high affinity for VEGF-A, being at least one order of magnitude higher than that of VEGFR-2.[29,31,32] The tyrosine kinase activity of VEGFR-1 is relatively weak, and it has been suggested to act as a negative regulator of VEGFR-2.[31]

Vascular Endothelial Growth Factor Receptor 2

VEGFR-2 has important functions in vascular endothelial cell survival and growth and regulation of angiogenesis. It is ubiquitously expressed in vascular endothelial progenitor cells during early embryogenesis before its expression declines during the later stages of vascular development. In pathologic angiogenesis, such as tumor growth and metastasis, expression is markedly increased.[22]

Binding of VEGF to VEGFR-2 stimulates tyrosine kinase–dependent phosphorylation signaling pathways that evoke vasodilatation and cell proliferation, survival, migration, and differentiation into mature blood vessels.[6,33] Activation of the phosphoinositide 3-kinase (PI3K)/Akt/protein kinase B–mammalian target of rapamycin (mTOR) pathways, as well as endothelial nitric oxide synthase (eNOS) and inducible NOS, results in downstream release of potent vasodilators, including nitric oxide (NO) and prostacyclin (PGI_2) (see Fig. 10.1; Fig. 10.2).[34,35] VEGFR-2 stimulation also leads to PLC-γ activation, which in turn stimulates protein kinase C (PKC), leading to inositol triphosphate generation and calcium mobilization.[22] These signaling changes are accompanied by activation of Raf-1, extracellular signal-regulated protein kinase (ERK1/2), focal adhesion kinase (FAK), and mitogen-activated protein kinase (MEK1/2) pathways, which

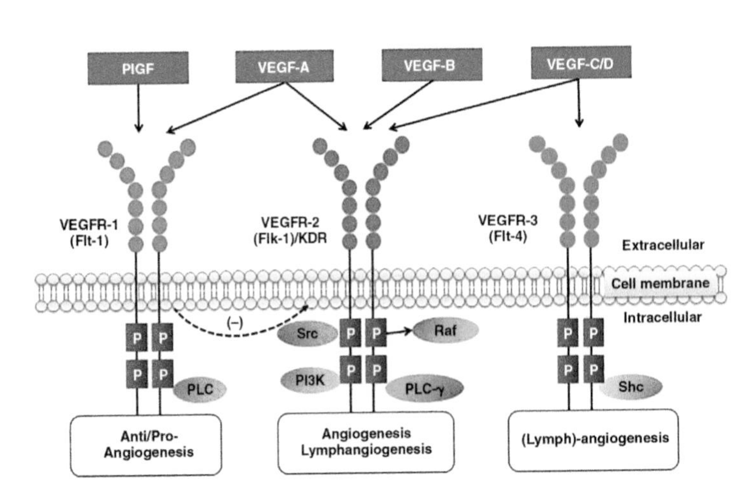

Fig. 10.1 Interacting VEGF ligands (VEGF-A/B/C) with VEGF receptors (VEGFR-1/2/3), resulting in angiogenesis and/or lymphangiogenesis. VEGFR1 may have both a positive and a negative regulatory role in angiogenesis depending on the biological conditions; it inhibits embryonic angiogenesis and stimulates pathologic angiogenesis. VEGFR1 may act as a negative regulator of VEGFR2, indicated by the (−) symbol. Flk-1, fetal liver kinase 1; Flt-1, Fms-like tyrosine kinase-1; KDR, kinase insert domain receptor.

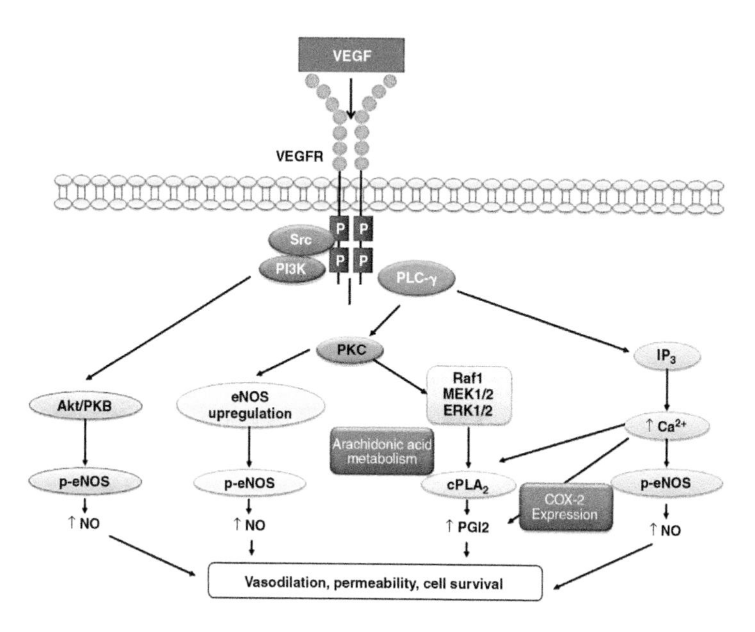

Fig. 10.2 VEGF/VEGFR signaling through tyrosine kinase-dependent phosphorylation pathways. Signaling pathways activated by ligand-binding to VEGFRs include PI3K/Akt/PKB, PLC-γ, and the Raf-1/MEK/ERK cascade, resulting in increased activation of eNOS and cyclo-oxygenase-2 (COX-2) activity with increased NO and PGI_2 production. These are important regulators of vascular tone and function. P, phosphorylation; p-eNOS, phosphorylated eNOS.

regulate endothelial cell survival, proliferation, migration, and permeability.[3,6] These pathways serve further to activate eNOS as well as stimulate PGI_2 release and consequent vasodilatation (see Figs. 10.1 and 10.2).[3]

Vascular Endothelial Growth Factor Receptor 3

VEGFR-3 is a specific receptor for the lymphatic growth factors VEGF-C and VEGF-D and regulates vascular and lymphatic endothelial cell function during embryogenesis.[22]

Although VEGFR-3 is involved in vascular development during early embryogenesis, its expression subsequently becomes relatively confined to lymphatic endothelial cells, monocytes, macrophages, and fenestrated capillaries and veins of endocrine organs.[22]

The VEGFR-3 signaling pathways remain relatively unexplored, although 5 tyrosine phosphorylation sites have been identified.[22,36] VEGF-C acts to promote the formation of VEGFR-2/VEGFR-3 heterodimers in primary endothelial cells, which may be involved in sprouting of lymphatic vessels.[22]

VASCULAR ENDOTHELIAL GROWTH FACTOR, VASCULAR FUNCTION, AND ANGIOGENESIS

Angiogenesis, the process of new blood vessel formation, is an essential physiologic process that is upregulated in tumor growth and metastasis.[3,4] VEGF is fundamental to this process (Fig. 10.3).

Acting via VEGFR-2, VEGF initiates tyrosine kinase–dependent phosphorylation pathways, including PLC-γ as well as the Raf-1/MEK/ERK cascade. These pathways are potent effectors of endothelial cell proliferation, migration, and differentiation into mature blood vessels.[3,6,33,37] These actions are central to pathologic angiogenesis that allows tumors to grow and spread without outstripping their own blood supply[38] and are therefore an obvious target for cancer chemotherapeutic agents.[6,39–41]

Vasomotion

The endothelium forms a single-cell layer that covers the luminal surface of all blood vessels under normal physiologic conditions and is intimately involved in the regulation of vasomotion and vascular smooth muscle cell function. Activation of VEGFR-2 on endothelial cells stimulates the release of NO via eNOS through calcium-dependent and calcium-independent mechanisms, including PI3K and Akt. NO plays a key role in the regulation of systemic blood vessel tone and blood pressure by stimulating the formation of cyclic guanosine 3′,5′-cyclic monophosphate (cGMP) through smooth muscle guanylyl cyclase, resulting in vascular smooth muscle cell relaxation and vasodilatation. The endothelium also releases PGI_2 in response to VEGF signaling, but it is not clear to what extent PGI_2 is relevant to human arterial vasorelaxation in vivo.

Endothelial VEGF-VEGFR-2 evokes vasodilatation via several tyrosine kinase-dependent phosphorylation pathways.[3,6] Activation of the PI3K/Akt/protein kinase B–mTOR pathway results in

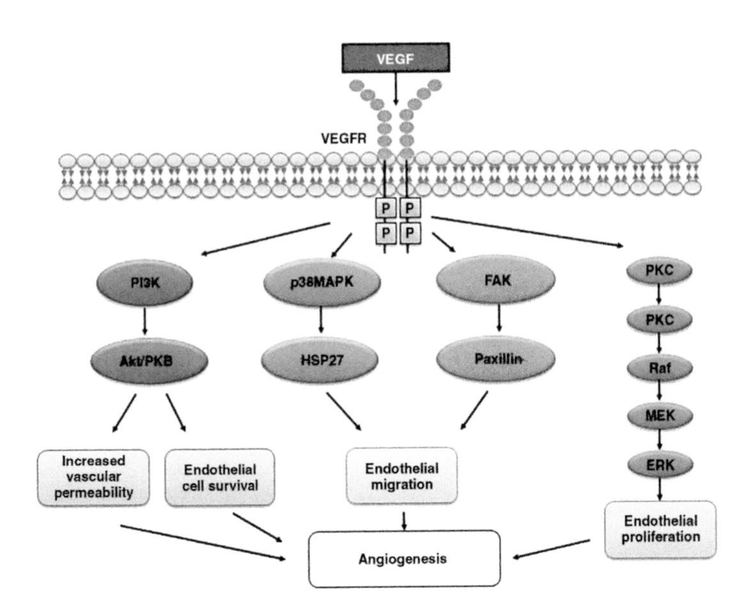

Fig. 10.3 Pathways through which VEGF signaling contributes to angiogenesis. VEGFR activation leads to stimulation of PI3K/Akt/PKB, p38MAP kinase (p38MAPK)/Heat shock protein 27 (HSP27), FAK/Paxillin, and Raf-1/MEK/ERK cascades, resulting in increased vascular permeability and endothelial cell survival, migration, and proliferation, processes important in angiogenesis.

NO release through eNOS activation. Other effects of VEGFR-2 stimulation include activation of PKC, PLC, ERK1/2, Raf-1, and FAK.[3,6] These pathways provide additional activation of eNOS and also stimulate PGI_2 release to cause vasodilatation.[3]

Following incubation of human umbilical vein endothelial cells with VEGF, NO production is increased both in the acute phase and also in the longer term.[3,42] Furthermore, VEGF causes relaxation of ex vivo human radial artery and internal mammary via NO and PGI_2. However, combined antagonism of NO and PGI_2 does not completely abolish the vasodilator effect of VEGF, and a contribution from endothelium-derived hyperpolarizing factor (EDHF) has been proposed.[43] The relative contributions of NO, PGI_2, and EDHF in VEGF-mediated vasodilatation may be variable between vascular bed and species. The Vascular Endothelial Growth Factor in Ischaemia for Vascular Angiogenesis trial assessed the potential for recombinant human VEGF as a treatment for patients with chronic angina.[44] When administered intracoronary and intravenously, recombinant human VEGF causes facial flushing and a dose-dependent reduction in blood pressure.[44,45]

Vascular Endothelial Growth Factor and Vascular Permeability

VEGF directly induces an acute and chronic increase in microvascular permeability 50,000 times greater than histamine.[21,38,46–50] These effects are mediated through opening of endothelial intracellular junctions and induction of fenestrae into the endothelia of venules and capillaries, which is, at least in part, NO dependent.[51] Increased vascular permeability allows plasma proteins to spill into the extravascular space, leading to the deposition of a fibrin-rich extracellular matrix with in-growth of fibroblasts and endothelial cells that transform the provisional matrix into a mature stroma. These changes occur in both physiologic and pathologic angiogenesis and are found throughout the circulatory tree, including in the renal vasculature.[46]

VASCULAR ENDOTHELIAL GROWTH FACTOR INHIBITORS AS ANTIANGIOGENIC THERAPY

Given the central role of angiogenesis in solid tumor growth and metastasis, interruption of the proangiogenic VEGF signaling pathway is an ideal target for reducing tumor growth and metastasis. This principle was first proposed by Folkman in 1971 and has become a major focus of antiangiogenic drug development.[5] Indeed, the use of VEGFI has revolutionized the treatment of a wide range of solid cancers as well as utility in the treatment of hematologic malignancy[3,6] and improved prognosis for various previously untreatable malignancies.[1] In addition to their use in cancer chemotherapeutics, VEGFIs are now also used in the treatment of age-related macular degeneration.

The VEGF signaling pathway can be interrupted at various levels by targeting VEGF itself,

VEGF tyrosine kinase receptors, or downstream signaling pathways,[6] and these constitute the main groups of VEGFIs (Table 10.1).[6,52]

Monoclonal Antibodies Against Circulating Vascular Endothelial Growth Factor

Bevacizumab is a recombinant humanized monoclonal antibody against VEGF[52] that selectively binds to VEGF and inhibits VEGF/VEGFR interaction.[6,8] Bevacizumab has traditionally been regarded as a "smart" or "clean" VEGFI because it acts only to target VEGF, which should minimize off-target effects. It was the first VEGFI to be approved by the US Food and Drug Administration for use in a solid tumor, including colon, renal, colorectal, and nonsquamous, non–small-cell lung cancers.

Small Molecule Tyrosine Kinase Inhibitors

Small molecule tyrosine kinase inhibitors cross the cell membrane and interact with the intracellular domain of receptors and signaling molecules, thus targeting intracellular VEGFR tyrosine kinase activity. Their actions are not specific to VEGFR-2, and they also block other targets involved in tumor angiogenesis, including platelet-derived growth factor (PDGF), c-Kit, and Flt-3.[52] Although this combined effect has broad antiangiogenic activity, it also increases the risk of cardiovascular side effects.[53–57]

TABLE 10.1
Summary of available vascular endothelial growth factor inhibitors, their antiangiogenic spectra, primary signaling targets, and cancers they have been used to treat

Antiangiogenic Spectrum	Drug Class	Agent	Principal Target(s)	Cancer Type(s)
Single target	Monoclonal antibody	Bevacizumab	VEGF-A	Colorectal cancer Nonsquamous non–small-cell lung cancer Glioblastoma Renal cell carcinoma
Multitargeted	Tyrosine kinase inhibitor	Axitinib	VEGFR-1/2/3 PDGFR c-Kit	Renal cell carcinoma
		Cediranib	VEGFR-1/2/3 PDGFR c-Kit	Colorectal cancer Recurrent glioblastoma Ovarian cancer Lung cancer
		Indetanib	VEGFR PDGFR	Non–small-cell lung cancer Ovarian cancer
		Pazopanib	VEGFR-1/2/3 PDGFR c-Kit	Renal cell carcinoma Soft tissue carcinoma
		Sorafenib	VEGFR-2/3 PDGFR Raf c-Kit FLT3	Hepatocellular carcinoma Renal cell carcinoma Melanoma
		Sunitinib	VEGFR-1/2/3 PDGFR c-Kit FLT3	Gastrointestinal stromal tumor Renal cell carcinoma Pancreatic neuroendocrine tumors
		Vandetanib	VEGFR-2 c-Kit	Non–small-cell lung cancer Medullary thyroid cancer
		Vatalanib	VEGFR-1/2/3 PDGFR c-Kit	Colorectal cancer
	VEGF-Trap	Aflibercept	VEGF-A/B PlGF	Colorectal cancer

Vascular Endothelial Growth Factor "Trap"

Aflibercept is the first soluble "VEGF-Trap," which is a VEGF ligand that displays a broader binding spectrum compared with bevacizumab and comprises the VEGF-binding regions of VEGFR-1 and VEGFR-2 fused to the Fc portion of human immunoglobulin G. This property allows aflibercept to function as a soluble "decoy" receptor and reduce binding of VEGF-A, VEGF-B, and PlGF to VEGF receptors.[52]

HYPERTENSION ASSOCIATED WITH ANTIANGIOGENIC THERAPY

Despite the rapid introduction, widespread and growing therapeutic use of VEGFIs, these agents are associated with several unwanted cardiovascular effects, including hypertension, thrombosis/thromboembolism, and left ventricular dysfunction. These effects appear primarily to be the result of an upset in the fine balance of VEGF-sensitive mechanisms. In addition to the direct effects of VEGF inhibition, off-target or bystander effects may be implicated in the development of toxicities and are discussed further later.

Hypertension is the most common cardiovascular complication associated with VEGFIs.[6] Almost all patients treated with these agents have an absolute increase in blood pressure with most clinical trials reporting increased blood pressure as an adverse effect (Fig. 10.4),[58] and up to 80% of patients developing hypertension. Furthermore, the resultant hypertension can be aggressive and difficult to treat.[2,6–9,59,60]

There is an acute, dose-dependent increase in blood pressure that occurs within hours to days of starting treatment with VEGFIs (Fig. 10.5).[6,10–12,53] This effect increases further if multiple antiangiogenic agents are used in combination.[6,61] The rapid increase in blood pressure in the early period of treatment increases the risk of acute complications, such as stroke and posterior reversible leukoencephalopathy in extreme cases, although this is rare and occurs in less than 1 in 100 patients treated with VEGFIs. However, this complication has been reported in patients receiving bevacizumab, sunitinib, vatalanib, and sorafenib.[6,62–64]

Patients who survive their initial cancer diagnosis after treatment with a VEGFI are at risk of developing chronic end-organ effects and complications associated with hypertension, including myocardial ischemia and infarction, heart failure, renal dysfunction, and stroke.[6]

The true prevalence of VEGFI-associated hypertension may be underestimated due to variation in definitions used in clinical trials with blood pressure thresholds often greater than those used in evidence-based guidelines.[2,6,65] Furthermore, patients with difficult-to-treat hypertension or a history of cardiovascular disease are usually excluded from clinical trials.[2,6] There have been efforts to improve consistency in the diagnosis and reporting of VEGFI-associated hypertension, with recent consensus statements recommending a threshold of 140/90 mm Hg on 2 to 3 occasions at least 1 week apart for most patients, and 130/80 mm Hg for patients with additional cardiovascular risk factors, such as diabetes mellitus or renal impairment.[6,13,66,67]

Risk factors for the development of VEGFI-associated hypertension include a history of previous hypertension, treatment with more than one VEGFI agent, age greater than 65 years, and possibly hypercholesterolemia.[6,68–72]

PATHOGENESIS OF HYPERTENSION INDUCED BY VASCULAR ENDOTHELIAL GROWTH FACTOR INHIBITION

The pathophysiologic mechanisms contributing to the development of VEGFI-associated

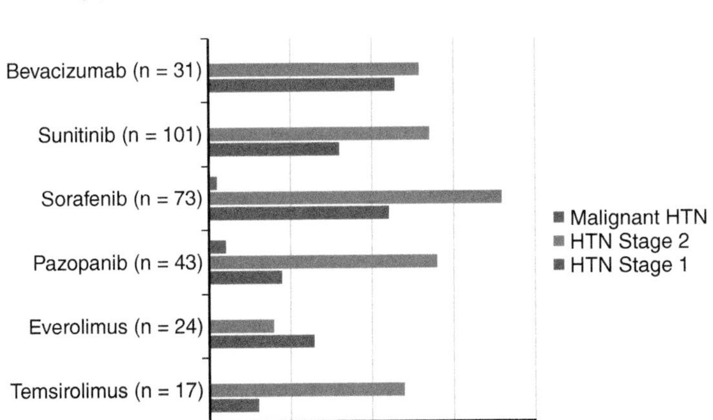

Fig. 10.4 The comparative incidence of hypertension observed with different antiangiogenic therapies in clinical practice. HTN, hypertension. (*Adapted from* Hall PS, Harshman LC, Srinivas S, et al. The frequency and severity of cardiovascular toxicity from targeted therapy in advanced renal cell carcinoma patients. JACC Heart Fail 2013; 1(1):72–8.)

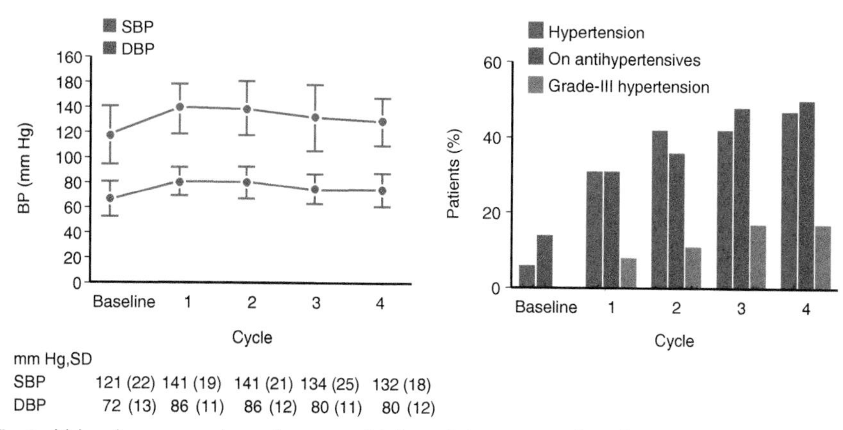

Fig. 10.5 Typical blood pressure dynamics on sunitinib and the extent of antihypertensive therapy escalation in a phase I/II trial of sunitinib in patients with imatinib-resistant, metastatic, gastrointestinal stromal tumors. DBP, diastolic blood pressure; SBP, systolic blood pressure. (*Adapted from* Chu TF, Rupnick MA, Kerkela R, et al. Cardiotoxicity associated with tyrosine kinase inhibitor sunitinib. Lancet 2007;70(9604):2011–9.)

hypertension include endothelial dysfunction, capillary rarefaction and vascular remodeling, and renal dysfunction with impaired sodium handling and increased salt sensitivity (Figs. 10.6 and 10.7).[6,68–70,72,73] There is a complex relationship between these pathophysiologic mechanisms, and the relative contribution of each mechanism may vary at different stages in the progression of acute hypertensive effects through to chronically elevated blood pressure.

Inhibition of Nitric Oxide Signaling

By impairing VEGF-mediated endothelial NO synthesis and release, it is clear that VEGFIs are well placed to have profound effects on endothelial vasomotor function. In combination with the promotion of vascular medial cell proliferation, this mechanism does appear to play an important role in the development of VEGFI-associated hypertension.[4,42,72–78] VEGFI-induced impairment of endothelial cell turnover and replacement may further contribute to altered vasorelaxation.

Experimental Evidence

The first direct experimental evidence to support a role for suppressed NO signaling in the development of VEGFI-associated hypertension came from Facemire and colleagues,[73] who demonstrated that blockade of VEGFR-2 in mice results in an acute increase in blood pressure that is prevented by administration of the eNOS inhibitor, L-N^{G}-Nitroarginine methyl ester.[73]

The small molecule tyrosine kinase inhibitor sunitinib reduces urinary excretion of NO metabolites in preclinical studies.[79] Robinson and colleagues[72] demonstrated a suppressed

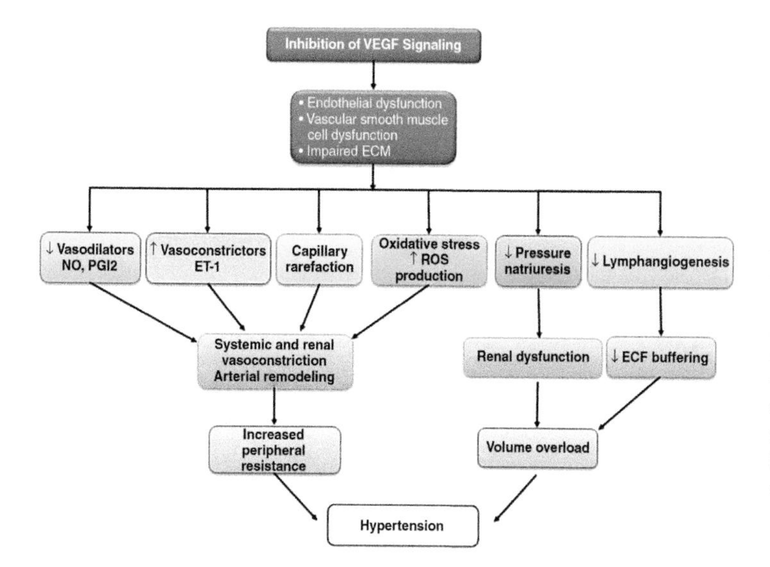

Fig. 10.6 Possible mechanisms through which VEGFIs contribute to the development of hypertension. These are primarily related to endothelial dysfunction and include reduced production of vasodilators (NO and PGI_2), increased production of vasoconstrictors (ET-1), oxidative stress, and capillary rarefaction, which lead to increased total peripheral resistance. Reduced pressure natriuresis and impaired lymphatic function contribute to volume overload, which could also promote blood pressure elevation. ECF, extracellular fluid; ECM, extracellular matrix.

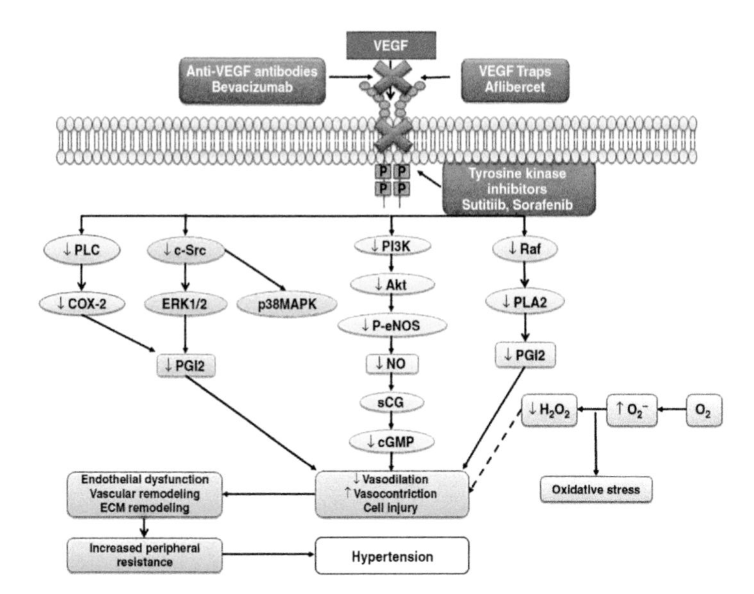

Fig. 10.7 The pathogenesis whereby inhibition of VEGF signaling leads to hypertension. Reduced production of vasodilators (NO and PGI_2) through disruption of the PI3K/Akt/PKB and Raf-1/MEK/ERK cascades and reduced eNOS and COX-2 activity, combined with increased oxidative stress, contribute to endothelial dysfunction, vascular remodeling, and hypertension.

cGMP/creatinine ratio and a trend toward suppressed nitrate/creatinine ratio in patients receiving VEGFIs for the treatment of metastatic renal cell cancer, consistent with reduced NO bioavailability. They did not however detect any significant changes in PGI_2 activity.

Thijs and colleagues[5] demonstrated that intra-arterial infusion of bevacizumab to healthy volunteers acutely and specifically reduces endothelium-dependent vasodilatation when assessed using forearm venous occlusion plethysmography. Importantly, endothelium-independent vasodilator responses were unaltered, refuting the potential for a nonspecific "toxic" effect of bevacizumab. The study also suggests that the hypertensive effects of bevacizumab occurs as a result of altered endothelial vasomotor pathways, in which NO signaling is central, rather than a structural arterial change, given that impaired vasodilator responses were noted within 15 minutes of the start of infusion. This correlates well with the rapid increase in blood pressure seen in patients receiving VEGFIs for the treatment of cancer.

Although these studies suggest a prominent effect of reduced NO bioavailability in the pathogenesis of VEGFI-induced hypertension, other studies have provided conflicting results. Patients receiving the small molecule tyrosine kinase inhibitor vandetanib displayed no alteration in brachial artery flow–mediated dilatation, a surrogate marker of NO vasomotor activity.[80] It should, however, be noted that the main regional vascular determinant of blood pressure lies in the resistance vasculature (which is better assessed using the forearm venous occlusion plethysmography technique) and not within conduit arteries (assessed using the brachial flow–mediated dilatation technique). Irrespective, these findings do throw some dubiety on the proposal that decreased NO bioavailability alone is enough to fully explain the hypertensive phenomenon associated with VEGF inhibition.

Reactive Oxygen Species and Oxidative Stress

Although oxidative stress itself induces the expression of VEGF in endothelial and vascular smooth muscle cells via hypoxia-inducible factor-1α, VEGF itself may further stimulate the production of ROS by activation of nicotinamide adenine dinucleotide phosphate (NADPH) oxidase (Fig. 10.8). Low, physiologic concentrations of ROS are required for physiologic angiogenesis, but excessive or pathophysiologic ROS production induces endothelial and stem cell senescence.[81,82]

Given the role that VEGF plays in the maintenance of ROS production, VEGFI agents may perturb this fine balance and shift the vascular milieu toward oxidative stress and a toxic environment.[82] Increased circulating ROS and oxidative stress may contribute further to hypertension by increasing the oxidation of NO to peroxynitrite with consequent reduction in NO bioavailability.[3,83]

However, animal models have failed to convincingly demonstrate evidence for increased ROS-mediated vasoconstriction with VEGFIs.[3,79,83,84] Kappers and colleagues[79,84] demonstrated that the administration of sunitinib to rats was associated with the development of hypertension. However, this was not associated with an increase in

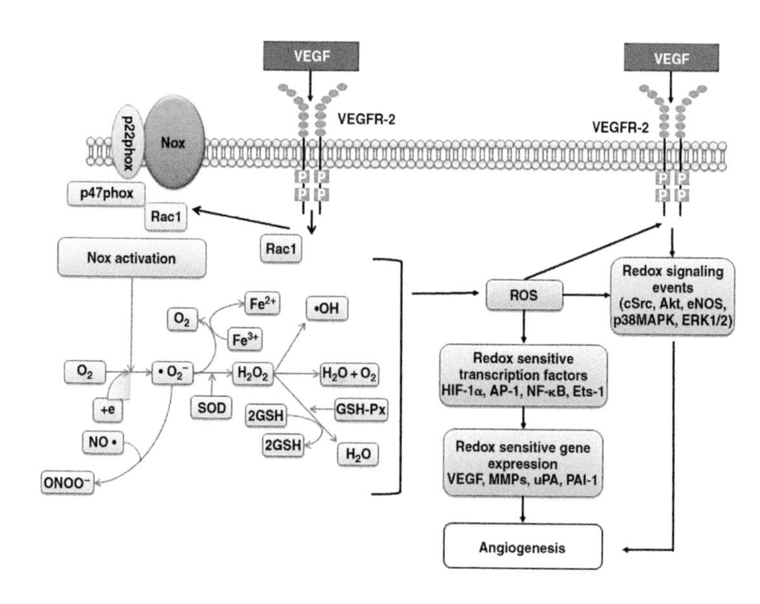

Fig. 10.8 VEGF signaling and generation of ROS via activation of NADPH oxidase (Nox). VEGFIs may perturb this fine balance of ROS production and shift the vascular milieu toward oxidative stress, leading to vascular dysfunction and molecular processes associated with angiogenesis.

biomarkers of oxidative stress. Furthermore, the antioxidant, superoxide dismutase mimetic 4-hydroxy-2,2,6,6-tetra-methylpiperidine-N-oxyl (tempol), produced only a marginal attenuation of the sunitinib-induced increase in blood pressure.[79,84] The overall contribution of oxidative stress to VEGFI-associated hypertension therefore remains unclear.

Activation of the Endothelin System

Endothelin-1 (ET-1) is the most potent endogenous vasoconstrictor and is strongly implicated in the pathogenesis of hypertension and endothelial dysfunction.[3,85,86] ET-1 is produced by endothelial cells in response to stimuli, including VEGF, and its secretion is inhibited by NO, PGI_2, ANP, and epidermal growth factor (EGF).[85,87,88] ET-1 mediates its effects through ET_AR and ET_BR, both of which are G-protein–coupled receptors. ET-1 generates ROS and contributes to oxidative stress through activation of the MAPK pathway and vascular NADPH oxidase.[87]

Activation of vascular smooth muscle ET_AR and ET_BR stimulates vasoconstriction and vascular remodeling.[86,88] ET_BR is also expressed on endothelial cells, where its activation mediates NO and PGI_2 secretion as well as prevents further endothelial cell activation.[3,86,88] ET_AR effects predominate with a net vasoconstrictor response to ET-1.

Given that VEGF increases ET-1 secretion, VEGFIs might be expected to downregulate the endothelin axis and be associated with relative vasorelaxation. However, inhibition of the VEGF signaling pathway is associated with increased levels of ET-1 in plasma and urine ET-1 that could contribute to the development of hypertension. Indeed, sunitinib treatment is associated with a 2-fold increase in the concentration of circulating ET-1 in humans, and, when administered to rats, causes similar increases in urinary and venous ET-1 concentrations.[3,4,79,89]

Administration of an experimental VEGF tyrosine kinase inhibitor to rats is associated with an increase in mean arterial pressure that can be prevented by the administration of a combined ET_AR/ET_BR antagonist.[3,90] In swine, sunitinib is associated with an increase in blood pressure that does not appear to be related to impaired NO bioavailability and is reversible with tezosentan, the combined ET_AR/ET_BR antagonist.[3,84]

The discrepancy between the physiologic, permissive effects of VEGF on ET-1 bioavailability and the increase in ET-1 seen in the presence of VEGFIs suggests that the ET-1 effects may be indirect. Indeed, elevated circulating ET-1 may be a reflection of VEGFI-induced endothelial dysfunction and loss of the negative feedback exerted by NO on ET-1 synthesis and release.[91–94] Furthermore, whether there is a temporal change in the relative roles of NO and ET-1 in the generation of hypertension associated with VEGFIs remains to be assessed.[84]

Activation of the Renin-Angiotensin-Aldosterone System

Activation of the renin-angiotensin-aldosterone system (RAAS) is arguably the key pathophysiologic mechanism in the development of essential hypertension. Indeed, agents that interrupt the

RAAS, such as angiotensin converting enzyme (ACE) inhibitors, angiotensin-II (AT-II) receptor antagonists, and mineralocorticoid receptor antagonists, are the cornerstone of treatment of essential hypertension.[95]

Given the central role of RAAS in essential hypertension, it is notable that clinical and preclinical studies suggest that RAAS activation is not fundamentally involved in the development of VEGFI-associated hypertension.[4] Clinical studies have examined the effects of sorafenib and sunitinib on blood pressure and correlation with circulating levels of plasma renin, aldosterone, and catecholamine. In patients with metastatic renal cell carcinoma or gastrointestinal stromal tumor, sunitinib is associated with an approximately 15-mm Hg increase in blood pressure and a loss of diurnal variation in blood pressure. In this group, Kappers and colleagues reported a 60% *decrease* in plasma renin concentrations, whereas plasma aldosterone levels remained unchanged. These findings have been taken to provide evidence that the renin-angiotensin system is not responsible for the blood pressure effect, but the investigators do accept that the findings do not exclude mineralocorticoid receptor activation, which remains a possible mechanism given the lack of effect of VEGFI on aldosterone.[89] In patients with metastatic solid tumors untreatable with standard therapy, sorafenib is associated with an approximately 20-mm Hg increase in blood pressure, and although a trend toward increased plasma renin has been observed in these patients, these changes did not reach statistical significance, nor was a change in aldosterone seen.[70] Furthermore, in this group, catecholamine levels *decreased* in correlation with increases in systolic blood pressure, suggesting that reductions in catecholamine levels may reflect a compensatory response to increased blood pressure.[70]

Animal models provide conflicting evidence for involvement of the RAAS in VEGFI-associated hypertension. The highly potent VEGF signaling pathway inhibitor, cediranib, induces marked increases in blood pressure of 35 to 50 mm Hg that are associated with a trend toward *decreased* plasma renin activity. Although the ACE inhibitor captopril was effective at reversing small increases (<10 mm Hg), it did not modulate more profound increases in blood pressure. This may be interpreted as RAAS downregulation as a compensatory mechanism in situations of increased blood pressure associated with VEGFIs.[96] Data from mice support this hypothesis because the administration of an anti-VEGFR-2 antibody induces acute and sustained increases in blood pressure that are associated with significant reductions in renin expression and urinary aldosterone excretion.[73]

Belcik and colleagues[97] demonstrated an approximately 10-mm Hg increase in blood pressure in mice treated with a monoclonal anti-VEGF antibody. Although this blood pressure effect was reversible with ACE inhibition, Lankhorst and colleagues[98] report that greater (approximately 30 mm Hg) increases in blood pressure induced by sunitinib in rats could not be prevented with an ACE inhibitor. It is conceivable that ACE inhibitors are effective in the prevention or reversal of small increases in blood pressure via their intrinsic antihypertensive effects but are unable to fully reverse larger increases that may stem from mechanisms unrelated to the RAAS axis.

On the whole, the available data do not provide convincing support to the hypothesis that upregulation of the RAAS is a key mechanism underpinning VEGFI-associated hypertension. Indeed, downregulation of the RAAS may occur as a compensatory mechanism in response to increases in blood pressure developing through alternative pathways, such as interference with NO signaling and upregulation of endothelin.

Vascular Rarefaction

Capillary rarefaction is characterized by a reduced density of microvascular networks (arterioles and capillaries) within a vascular bed and is a hallmark of essential hypertension.[92,99] Prolonged treatment with VEGFIs is associated with capillary rarefaction in preclinical models and in humans.[4,92,100–102]

Mice treated with a small molecule tyrosine kinase inhibitor against VEGF develop marked reductions in capillary density that rapidly regress after stopping therapy.[103] Furthermore, early features of capillary rarefaction can be identified within 24 hours of therapy with a VEGFI in mice, and more marked reductions are observed after 1 to 2 weeks.[8,104,105]

In patients treated for metastatic renal cell carcinoma, sunitinib induces an approximately 10-mm Hg increase in blood pressure that is associated with a significant reduction in capillary microdensity.[101] Interestingly, both blood pressure and capillary density recovered to baseline in some patients after stopping sunitinib.[101,102] Bevacizumab induces increases in blood pressure in patients with metastatic colorectal cancer that coincide with reductions in capillary density,[92] and this reduction in capillary density associated with bevacizumab has been demonstrated to be reversible following cessation of the drug.[106]

The pathophysiology of vascular rarefaction related to VEGFI is thought partially to reflect reduced endothelial cell survival. Furthermore, endothelial dysfunction associated with VEGFIs may precipitate thrombosis, evoking a further reduction in vascular perfusion, increased apoptosis, and obliteration of microvessels.[8,104] The consequences of these structural changes include increased vascular tone and afterload with impaired endothelium-dependent and endothelium-independent vasodilatation.

It remains unclear whether vascular rarefaction occurs as a cause or consequence of VEGFI-associated hypertension. Blood pressure changes occur acutely after starting VEGFIs, whereas microvascular changes are potentially reversible, suggesting that changes in the microvascular network occur as a consequence of VEGFI-induced hypertension.[4,5]

Renal Dysfunction and Salt Sensitivity

Renal dysfunction is frequently observed during the use of VEGFIs.[75] Proteinuria occurs as a dose-dependent side effect in up to 60% of patients treated with bevacizumab and, although most cases are not severe, grade 3 or 4 proteinuria occurs in up to 6%.[75,107] A meta-analysis of almost 2000 patients treated with bevacizumab demonstrated a 1.4- to 2.2-fold increased risk of proteinuria with low and high doses.[107] In a larger analysis of approximately 12,000 patients treated with bevacizumab, 13.3% developed proteinuria and 2.2% developed high-grade proteinuria.[108]

The small molecule tyrosine kinase inhibitors are associated with similarly high incidence of proteinuria. In a meta-analysis of almost 7000 patients, 18.7% developed proteinuria and 2.4% developed high-grade proteinuria.[109] The pathophysiologic changes include endotheliosis, mesangiolysis, endothelial swelling, red cell fragmentation, and thrombus.[110] The most common finding at renal biopsy is thrombotic microangiopathy,[87] although cryoglobulinemia, membranoproliferative and ischemic glomerulopathies, and interstitial nephritis have also been reported.[111]

The kidneys play a central role in physiologic responses to increased blood pressure through renal sodium excretion (the pressure-natriuresis relationship).[8] The kidneys regulate extracellular volume by increasing sodium excretion, thus mounting a compensatory response to increased blood pressure.[4] Indeed, impairments of renal sodium excretion and interruption of this response contribute to essential hypertension.[8]

VEGFIs are associated with a rightward shift of the renal pressure–natriuresis curve and impaired sodium excretion with consequent fluid retention and salt-dependent hypertension.[4,73,112,113] Gu and coworkers[112] demonstrated that VEGFIs cause salt-dependent hypertension in rats, whereas Facemire and colleagues[73] demonstrated that an anti-VEGFR-2 antibody causes a rightward shift of the renal pressure–natriuresis curve in mice. Endothelial dysfunction and reduced NO bioavailability may underpin these effects. Indeed, the hypertensive effect observed in these animals was accompanied by reduced renal expression of endothelial and neuronal NO synthases.[113] NO exerts direct effects on regulation of renal pressure natriuresis, which suggests that interruption of eNOS signaling by VEGFIs may contribute to sodium retention, increased extracellular fluid volume, and salt-dependent hypertension.[8,114]

BIOMARKERS TO PREDICT VASCULAR ENDOTHELIAL GROWTH FACTOR INHIBITION–ASSOCIATED HYPERTENSION

VEGFI-induced hypertension, like essential hypertension, is associated with significant morbidity and mortality.[115,116] *Prehypertension* reflects blood pressure measurements greater than normal but below diagnostic criteria for hypertension.[116–118] More than a third of such patients develop hypertension within 4 years,[119] and strategies for early intervention with pharmacologic therapy and/or lifestyle modifications have been proposed; this strategy can be extended to those with prehypertension who are under consideration for treatment with a VEGFI.[116,120,121]

Essential hypertension has a multifactorial pathogenesis that includes physiologic alterations, including endothelial dysfunction, neurohormonal and adrenergic overactivation, abnormalities of sodium handling, systemic inflammation, reduced endogenous fibrinolysis, and oxidative stress.[122] The early phases of these pathophysiologic changes can be evident via the assessment of a variety of biomarkers that may be important in the identification of patients at risk of hypertension. Plasma C-reactive protein (CRP), renin and aldosterone, and urinary microalbuminuria are all linked with the development of essential hypertension.[122] The relative contribution of individual biomarkers in isolation is difficult to accurately assess given that many co-correlate and individual biomarkers generally reflect a single biological pathway.[122] The use of a multiple biomarker model may therefore be more useful in predicting the development of essential hypertension.[116,122] There could be great utility for taking a similar approach to predict patients at greatest risk of developing VEGFI-associated hypertension to facilitate more intensive blood pressure monitoring and aggressive approaches to management.[8] However, the relative contributions of neurohormonal and proinflammatory biomarkers to the development of VEGFI-associated hypertension are less well defined than in essential hypertension.[8] Indeed, most descriptions of features predictive of VEGFI-induced hypertension have focused on conventional risk factors, such as age, body weight, gender, previous hypertension, smoking status, and hypercholesterolemia.[6,8,9,68–72,123]

Inflammatory Biomarkers

Hypertension is associated with systemic inflammation, which contributes to endothelial dysfunction, and elevated levels of CRP reflect this.[122,124,125] CRP also causes upregulation of the RAAS[122,125,126] and is therefore one of the principal biomarkers associated with the development of essential hypertension.[122] However, CRP is also often elevated as a result of malignancy,[127] and its utility to predict VEGFI-associated hypertension in patients with malignancy is consequently limited.

Urinary Biomarkers

Proteinuria, particularly albuminuria, predicts the development of essential hypertension to a greater extent than CRP.[122] Although the development of proteinuria in patients treated with VEGFIs is common[75] and often occurs in association with the development of hypertension,[128] there are relatively few data examining the effect of proteinuria before treatment with VEGFIs and the subsequent risk of hypertension. Clinical trials of VEGFIs have generally not screened for proteinuria at baseline[128–132] or have excluded patients with proteinuria.[133,134] Patients with a history of hypertension or renal dysfunction, who are more likely to have proteinuria, have also generally been excluded from clinical trials of VEGFIs.[6] This makes an assessment of the association between proteinuria before treatment with VEGFIs and the risk of developing hypertension challenging.

Renin-Angiotensin-Aldosterone System

Although activation of the RAAS is one of the key pathophysiologic mechanisms contributing to the development of essential hypertension,[135–137] there are relatively few data reporting associations between renin, Ang II, or aldosterone levels before treatment with VEGFIs and the risk of developing hypertension. However, in 2 relatively small clinical studies of sunitinib and Sorafenib, there was no correlation between levels of renin and aldosterone at baseline, or changes in renin and aldosterone levels during treatment, and risk of developing hypertension.[70,89] This observation may reflect the fact that upregulation of the RAAS does not appear to be a key mechanism underpinning VEGFI-associated hypertension.

Traditional Cardiovascular Risk Factors

Traditional cardiovascular risk factors that predispose to the development of VEGFI-associated hypertension include increasing age (older than 65 years), history of previous hypertension, smoking, and possibly hypercholesterolemia.[6,8,68–71] It is intriguing that elevated body mass index, reduced renal function, and family history of hypertension or cardiovascular disease were not predictive of hypertension in a study of the small molecule tyrosine kinase inhibitor cediranib in patients with recurrent epithelial ovarian cancer.[9] Furthermore, traditional cardiovascular risk factors, such as older age, gender, and increased weight, did not correlate with increases in blood pressure among patients treated with sorafenib.[8]

Clinical Implications

Although it is clear that there would be clinical value in the use of a stratified-risk prediction tool to identify patients at greatest risk of developing VEGFI-associated hypertension to facilitate more intensive blood pressure monitoring and early intervention, the use of biomarkers to identify such patients appears limited at present. Clarification of the associations between cardiovascular biomarkers and risk of developing VEGFI-associated hypertension is required. In the meantime, clinical focus should be on traditional cardiovascular risk factors that predispose to the development of VEGFI-associated hypertension and to those at greatest risk from the sequelae of both acute and chronic hypertensive effects.

MANAGEMENT AND THERAPY OF VASCULAR ENDOTHELIAL GROWTH FACTOR INHIBITOR–INDUCED HYPERTENSION

The main goal in the management of VEGFI-associated hypertension is to reduce morbidity and mortality because of conditions such as stroke, myocardial infarction, and heart failure, while minimizing the risk of end-organ damage and maintaining effective chemotherapy.[6,13,138,139] Effective blood pressure control can reduce attributable 10-year mortality by 9% with a number needed to treat of only 11 patients.[67,140] This approach remains relevant in both the acute "peritreatment" period when the hypertensive effect of VEGFIs can be severe and difficult to treat and the chronic phase following completion of cancer chemotherapy. Indeed, with substantially increased cancer cure and survivorship, cardiovascular morbidity now often takes precedent over the previous cancer diagnosis. The rationale for actively managing any increases in blood pressure before, during, and after therapy with VEGFIs is therefore clear. This requires a coordinated and collaborative approach between oncologists and cardiovascular specialists. There is an increasing recognition of this need for shared care of these complex patients who require thought and balance from both the oncologic and the cardiovascular perspectives.[2]

Maitland and colleagues[67] published a comprehensive commentary on the assessment, surveillance, and management of blood pressure in patients receiving VEGFIs in the *Journal of the National Cancer Institute* in 2010, and many of the recommendations within this subchapter are adapted from this commentary.

Screening Before Initiation of Vascular Endothelial Growth Factor Inhibitor Treatment

A formal assessment for pre-existing cardiovascular disease and cardiovascular risk factors should be performed before commencing a VEGFI. This assessment includes a detailed history, physical examination, and focused investigations to screen for risk factors and pre-existing end-organ damage.[2,6,67] It is important to identify any history of pre-existing hypertension or established cardiovascular disease, including ischemic heart disease, cerebrovascular disease, peripheral arterial disease, retinal disease, and heart failure. Additional cardiovascular risk factors including smoking history and family history of premature cardiovascular disease should also be identified. All patients should have blood taken for the measurement of serum cholesterol, triglycerides, and fasting plasma glucose, and an echocardiogram may also be indicated.[67]

The above assessment allows an evaluation of individual patients' risk of developing cardiovascular complications before treatment with a VEGFI. The rationale is not to exclude patients from treatment with a VEGFI but to provide a systematic means of identifying and addressing modifiable risk factors to reduce the likelihood of developing acute cardiovascular complications during treatment and long-term cardiovascular sequelae thereafter.[67]

Monitoring of Blood Pressure

Blood pressure should be measured before starting treatment with a VEGFI as well as at regular intervals during treatment. Measuring blood pressure at regular intervals is particularly relevant during the first cycle of chemotherapy when the risk of acute elevations in blood pressure is greatest. Blood pressure should be monitored weekly during the first cycle of chemotherapy and thereafter at least every 2 to 3 weeks.[6,13,67] Measurements should be made using an appropriately calibrated device with a correctly sized cuff and the patient sitting at rest for 5 minutes. A minimum of 2 measurements should be made at least 3 minutes apart and an average taken of the 2 readings.[67]

Home blood pressure monitoring may be appropriate in some patients and allows greater patient participation in their care. If home monitoring is introduced, it is important to provide patients with a blood pressure diary, instructions on accurate self-measurement, and criteria for blood pressure readings that should prompt them to seek attention from their oncologist or medical practitioner.[67,115]

Diagnosis of Hypertension and Targets for Treatment

A blood pressure of 140/90 mm Hg or an increase in diastolic blood pressure of 20 mm Hg from baseline are the criteria for the diagnosis of hypertension in patients receiving treatment with a VEGFI, which is based on general consensus and standard hypertension guidelines.[6,13,67,141] A lower threshold of 130/80 mm Hg should be used in patients with diabetes mellitus and/or chronic kidney disease.[6,71] VEGFI-associated hypertension is graded 1 to 5 based on severity, with increased grade mandating more intensive blood pressure–lowering therapy, often with more than one drug, as well as increased frequency of blood pressure monitoring and consideration of hospitalization in severe cases (**Table 10.2**).[142]

It is important to be aware of younger patients who are "normotensive" at baseline but who develop increases in diastolic blood pressure of greater than 20 mm Hg during treatment with absolute measurements that remain less than 140/90 mm Hg. Such patients are among those at highest risk of acute hypertensive complications, and antihypertensive therapy should be initiated even if the absolute blood pressure is less than 140/90 mm Hg.[67]

INITIATION OF ANTIHYPERTENSIVE THERAPY

It is important to adopt a robust approach to the management of elevated blood pressure before starting treatment with a VEGFI and during

TABLE 10.2
Grading of vascular endothelial growth factor inhibitor–associated hypertension by National Cancer Institute's Common Terminology Criteria for Adverse Events V. 4.0, with recommendations for blood pressure treatment and monitoring

Grade	Definition	Antihypertensive Therapy	Blood Pressure Monitoring
1	Pre-hypertension (SBP 120–139 mm Hg or DBP 80–89 mm Hg)	None or baseline therapy	Standard
2	Stage 1 hypertension (SBP 140–159 mm Hg or DBP 90–99 mm Hg); recurrent or persistent (≥24 h); symptomatic DBP increase by >20 mm Hg Monotherapy indicated	Initiate β-blocker or DHP CCB Increase doses of existing medications until BP controlled or at maximum dose	Increased frequency (weekly if asymptomatic, daily or every other day if symptomatic) Supervision by health care professional
3	Stage 2 hypertension (SBP ≥160 mm Hg or DBP ≥100 mm Hg) More than one drug or more intensive therapy than previously used indicated	Start therapy with 2-drug combination including at least a DHP CCB Increase doses until BP controlled, up to maximum dose If no or only partial BP control, add agents, up to 4 and increase dose as needed	Increased frequency (daily or every other day if symptomatic) Supervision by health care professional
4	Life-threatening consequences (eg, malignant hypertension, transient or permanent neurologic deficit, hypertensive crisis) Urgent intervention needed	Optimal management with intensive monitored support	Hospitalize
5	Death		

treatment. Antihypertensive therapy should be initiated before VEGFI treatment in patients with blood pressure measurements greater than target (Fig. 10.9, see Table 10.2). Starting treatment with the VEGFI may not need to be delayed until blood pressure is within target as long as the blood pressure is below a level likely to be associated with acute complications. An individualized approach should be taken, considering the oncologic need to start chemotherapy and relative blood pressure measurements.[67]

In patients already receiving antihypertensive therapy, it is important to ensure adherence, optimal choice of antihypertensive agent, and correct dosing. It may be necessary to switch to an alternative agent, up-titrate the current regimen, or add an additional agent (Fig. 10.10).[143] Referral to a hypertension specialist should be made if there is any difficulty in achieving blood pressure targets.[67]

It is important to consider drug pharmacokinetics and pharmacodynamics, comorbidities, and potential side effects when selecting an antihypertensive agent (Table 10.3). Particular attention should be paid to the potential for cytochrome P450 (CYP 450) inhibition by some antihypertensive drugs, because VEGFIs are metabolized through CYP 450, and therefore, inadvertently high circulating concentrations of VEGFI may be precipitated (Table 10.4).[6] ACE inhibitors/AT-II receptor antagonists tend to be the most frequently used drugs for the treatment of VEGFI-associated hypertension. Despite the lack of robust evidence for a major role of the RAAS axis in the development of VEGFI-induced hypertension, ACE inhibitors are widely used for the treatment of the condition. This approach partly reflects the widespread use of ACE inhibitors in the treatment of essential hypertension but also highlights the lack of a specific agent directed toward a clear pathophysiologic mechanism. Although the involvement of the RAAS system in VEGFI-associated hypertension is not particularly clear, the beneficial endothelial and

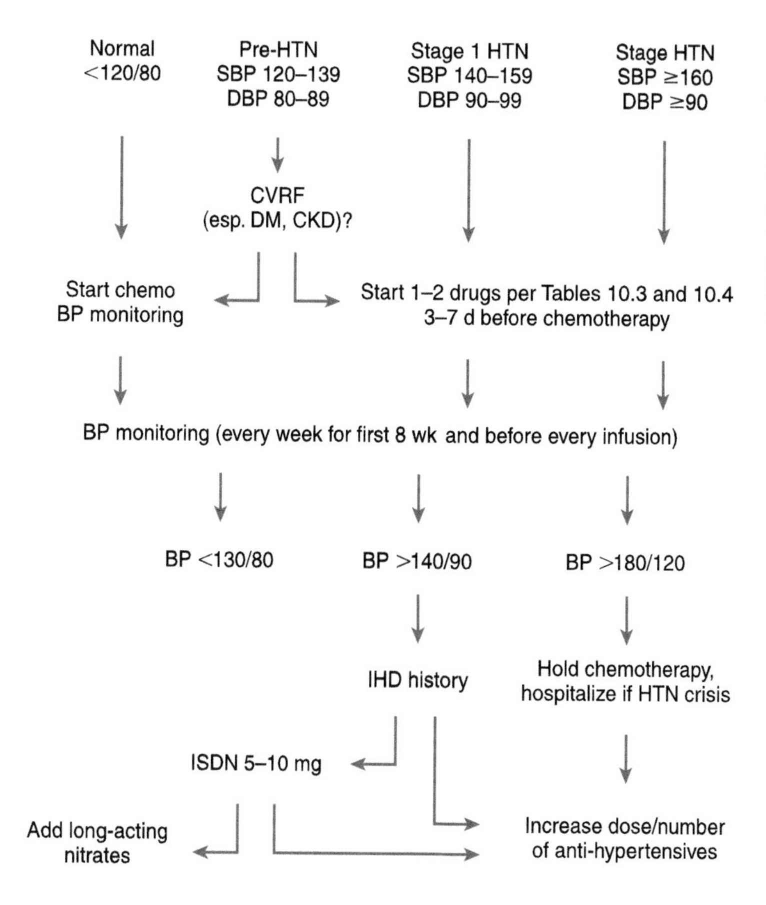

Fig. 10.9 A user-friendly algorithm for the treatment and monitoring of blood pressure in patients treated with VEGFI chemotherapy. BP, blood pressure in mm Hg; CKD, chronic kidney disease; CVRF, cardiovascular risk factor; DM, diabetes mellitus; HTN, hypertension; IHD, ischemic heart disease; ISDN, isosorbide dinitrate.

antiproteinuria effects provided by ACEi/AT-II receptor antagonists do provide some further rationale for their use.

ACE inhibitors may be particularly appropriate in patients with diabetic nephropathy, left ventricular systolic dysfunction, or situations wherein a relatively quick reduction in blood pressure is required. Ang II receptor antagonists may be considered in similar patients who develop a cough as a side effect of ACE inhibitor. ACE inhibitors and angiotensin II receptor blockers (ARBs) may not be appropriate in patients with renovascular disease, such as renal artery stenosis, patients receiving concomitant chemotherapy regimens that undergo renal clearance, and patients with a tendency toward hyperkalemia.

Dihydropyridine calcium channel antagonists are useful in elderly patients with isolated systolic hypertension, although they can predispose to ankle swelling and have a relatively slow

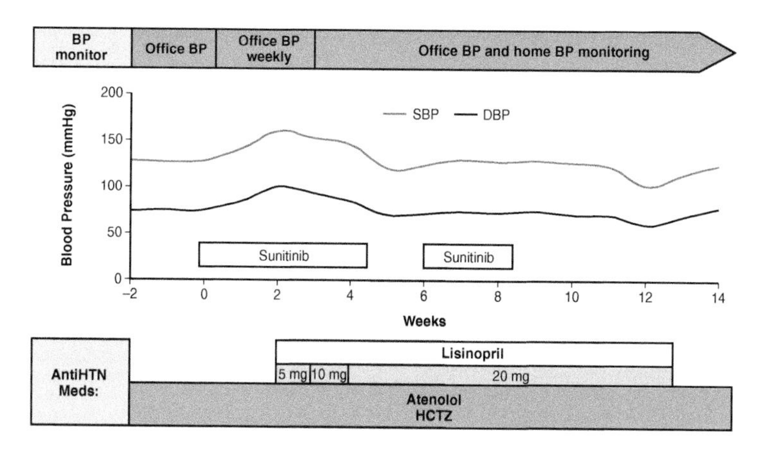

Fig. 10.10 A patient with asymptomatic, sunitinib-induced worsening hypertension on atenolol and hydrochlorothiazide, detected by weekly BP monitoring early and improved with commencement and up-titration of lisinopril. HCTZ, hydrochlorothiazide. (*From* de Jesus-Gonzalez N, Robinson E, Moslehi J, et al. Management of antiangiogenic therapy induced hypertension. Hypertension 2012;60(3):607–15; with permission.)

TABLE 10.3
Summary of antihypertensive agents used to treat vascular endothelial growth factor inhibitor–associated hypertension, their indications, benefits, and cautions/contraindications

Drug Class	Step of Therapy	Main Examples	Indications and Benefits	Cautions and Contraindications
ACE inhibitors	1st/2nd	• Captopril • Enalapril • Lisinopril • Perindopril • Ramipril	• Younger patients • Proteinuria • Diabetic nephropathy • Left ventricular dysfunction • Quick onset of action	• Renovascular disease • Peripheral vascular disease • Renal impairment • Chemotherapy with renal clearance • Hyperkalemia
Angiotensin II receptor antagonists	1st/2nd	• Candesartan • Irbesartan • Losartan • Valsartan	• Cough related to ACE inhibitor • Younger patients • Proteinuria • Diabetic nephropathy • Left ventricular dysfunction • Quick onset of action	• Renovascular disease • Peripheral vascular disease • Renal impairment • Chemotherapy with renal clearance • Hyperkalemia
Dihydropyridine calcium channel antagonists	1st/2nd	• Amlodipine • Lercanidipine	• Elderly patients • Isolated systolic hypertension	• Ankle swelling • Slow onset of action
Thiazide or loop diuretics	3rd/4th	• Bendroflumethiazide • Chlortalidone • Hydrochlorothiazide • Indapamide • Furosemide	• Elderly patients • Isolated systolic hypertension	• Gout • Hypercalcemia • Hypokalemia • QT_c prolonging drugs
β-Blockers	3rd/4th	• Atenolol • Bisoprolol • Carvedilol • Metoprolol	• Ischemic heart disease	• Bradycardia • Heart block • Asthma or chronic obstructive pulmonary disease
Mineralocorticoid receptor antagonists	3rd/4th	• Eplerenone • Spironolactone	• Resistant hypertension	• Hyperkalemia • Gynecomastia (spironolactone)

TABLE 10.4
Antihypertensive agents with the least amount of CYP 450 enzyme inhibitory potential

Class	Agent	Initial Daily Dose (mg)	Intermediate Daily Dose (mg)	Maximum Daily Dose (mg)	Hepatic Metabolism (CYP 450 Enzyme Substrate)
Calcium channel blockers	Amlodipine	2.5	5	10	CYP 3A4
	Nifedipine XL	30	60	90	CYP 3A4
β-Blockers	**Atenolol**	**25**	**50**	**100**	**None**
	Bisoprolol	2.5	5	10	CYP 3A4
	Metoprolol	50	100	200	CYP2D6
	Carvedilol	6.25	12.5	25	CYP2D6 and CYP2C9
ACE inhibitors	**Lisinopril**	**5**	**10–20**	**40**	**None**
	Enalapril	**5**	**10–20**	**40**	**None**
	Ramipril	**2.5**	**5**	**10**	**None**
	Perindopril	4	6	8	CYP 3A4
	Captopril	37.5	75	150	CYP 2D6
Angiotensin II receptor blockers	Losartan	50	75	100	CYP 2C9 and CYP 3A4
	Irbesartan	150	225	300	CYP 2C9
Diuretic	**HCTZ**	**12.5**	**25**	**50**	**None**
	Furosemide	**20**	**40**	**80**	**None**
Nitrate	Imdur	30	60	120	CYP 3A4

Note: Preferred agents are highlighted in bold.

onset of action.[67,144] It is important to avoid non-dihydropyridine calcium channel antagonists, such as verapamil and diltiazem, because these drugs inhibit CYP 3A4.[6]

Combination therapy with 2 or more antihypertensive agents may be required to achieve adequate blood pressure control in VEGFI-treated patients (see Figs. 10.9 and 10.10, Table 10.2).[115,143] A dihydropyridine calcium channel antagonist in combination with an ACE inhibitor or ARB should be used in patients who do not achieve adequate blood pressure control with monotherapy,[6,13,71] although diuretics, β-blockers, mineralocorticoid receptor antagonists, and possibly nitrates may be used if additional antihypertensive agents are required.[67,115,145]

Dose Reduction and Temporary Discontinuation of Vascular Endothelial Growth Factor Inhibitors

Reducing the dose or temporarily stopping VEGFIs may be necessary to control VEGFI-associated hypertension. Such treatment modifications are easier to achieve with tyrosine kinase inhibitors, which are given twice daily, than with bevacizumab or aflibercept, which have longer half-lives.[13,71] However, reducing the dose or temporarily stopping VEGFIs should only be considered in cases of severe or symptomatic hypertension. Clinical trials have generally used blood pressure measurements of greater than 160/90 mm Hg or symptomatic hypertension as criteria for temporary discontinuation of a VEGFI drug for at least 4 weeks until blood pressure is better controlled. It is vital to pursue aggressive blood pressure management and involve a hypertension specialist during this period to aim for the VEGFI agent to be restarted at the next scheduled cycle of chemotherapy. If blood pressure remains uncontrolled during this period, then discontinuation of the VEGFI may be considered. However, this would be a last resort, and with early involvement of a hypertension specialist, it should be able to be avoided, except in extreme cases.[67]

Additional Factors Contributing to Hypertension and Nonpharmacologic Interventions

Similar to the care of any patient with hypertension, it remains important to assess other factors that may contribute to and exacerbate VEGFI-associated hypertension, including excessive alcohol consumption, smoking, nonsteroidal anti-inflammatory drugs, adrenal steroids, erythropoietin, oral contraceptives, and sympathomimetic agents. Lifestyle interventions, including smoking cessation and reduced alcohol intake, should therefore be combined with pharmacologic interventions.[67]

Vascular Endothelial Growth Factor Inhibitor "Off Periods" and Rebound Hypotension

VEGFI regimens often have *off periods* during which patients do not receive the drug. It is important to be aware of the potential development of symptomatic rebound hypotension during this period. A particular concern during this period is for the precipitation of a "water-shed" stroke. Antihypertensive regimens may therefore need to be down-titrated during off periods.[6] Furthermore, VEGFI-induced hypertension may resolve after completing the chemotherapy regimen, and antihypertensive drugs may need to be down-titrated or stopped.[67] The intervals at which blood pressure should be monitored after completion of chemotherapy regimens remain uncertain, although a prudent approach should be taken and blood pressure measured on a relatively regular basis aiming for targets similar to those used during VEGFI therapy.

Future Directions

Clinical data have demonstrated that NO donors may have a therapeutic role in the management of elevated blood pressure associated with VEGFI agents,[77,146,147] whereas experimental data suggest a potential role for ET-1 receptor antagonists in preventing VEGFI-associated increases in blood pressure and proteinuria.[6,84,89] Although potentially promising, these strategies are in the early stages of development and require further evaluation in clinical studies.

Mineralocorticoid receptor antagonists, such as eplerenone and spironolactone, are increasingly used in the management of patients with resistant hypertension[145] and may therefore be useful in the management of VEFI-associated hypertension.

HYPERTENSION AS A SURROGATE OF ANTIVASCULAR ENDOTHELIAL GROWTH FACTOR CANCER TREATMENT

Hypertension associated with VEGFI agents occurs as a pharmacodynamic on-target toxicity, rather than a side effect, which may reflect effective inhibition of the VEGF signaling pathway.[6,8,148–150] Patients who develop VEGFI-associated hypertension have reduced tumor progression and greater overall survival compared with those who do not, and the onset of hypertension has, therefore, been proposed as an indicator of better tumor response.[4,6,67,151–153]

In a study of patients with metastatic renal cell carcinoma treated with sunitinib, those who developed hypertension had progression-free survival that was 9 months longer than those who did not become hypertensive.[154] In a further study of patients treated with sunitinib, those who developed hypertension had a 10-month longer progression-free survival and an almost 24-month greater overall survival.[152] Similar findings have been observed in patients treated with bevacizumab who developed grade 3 or 4 hypertension and had a 13-month greater overall survival.[150,155] Furthermore, in post-hoc analyses of patients treated with gemcitabine and axitinib, those who developed diastolic hypertension (>90 mm Hg) had a 7-month greater overall survival.[150]

Associations between the development of hypertension and greater progression-free and overall survival have led to suggestions that the development of hypertension could be used as an endpoint to define optimal biologically active doses of VEGFI drugs.[68] However, this suggestion should be taken with caution, and the development of hypertension should not be used as a measure to guide the maximum possible dose of VEGFI agents for individual patients.[150] The consequences of hypertension can be severe and include significant morbidity and mortality from myocardial ischemia, stroke, renal failure, and hypertensive crises in extreme cases. Furthermore, the development of VEGFI-associated hypertension is likely to involve additional host factors, such as genetic variability in the VEGF axis and pre-existing cardiovascular risk factors.[68] Thus, although associations have been observed between the development of hypertension and improved cancer-related prognosis, there is not sufficient evidence to conclude that hypertension should be used as a biomarker of favorable outcome.[4,68]

Studies that characterize the relationship between VEGFI dose, exposure, and changes in blood pressure are required to develop a better understanding of the factors contributing to VEGFI-associated hypertension.[150] In time, it may be possible to use relative changes in blood pressure rather than a binary separation of hypertensive versus normotensive patients to guide individual VEGFI doses.[150] Indeed, Keizer and colleagues[153] have proposed a detailed pharmacokinetic/pharmacodynamic model that incorporates adverse events, such as the development of hypertension, and may be effective in guiding VEGFI doses. The model would result in an overall increase in daily VEGFI dose with only marginal increases in adverse events. Although potentially promising, this approach remains experimental and is in the early phases of development.[150] VEGFI-induced hypertension can have severe and potentially devastating consequences. Vigilant detection and aggressive management of increases in blood pressure must therefore remain the focus for oncologists and cardiovascular specialists.

MAMMALIAN TARGET OF RAPAMYCIN INHIBITORS, TAXANES, AND TYROSINE KINASE INHIBITORS USED FOR HEMATOLOGIC MALIGNANCY

Other chemotherapeutic agents with a tendency to precipitate hypertension include the mTOR inhibitors, taxanes, and non-VEGF tyrosine kinase inhibitors used in the treatment of hematologic malignancies. Although these agents are associated with the development of hypertension, the incidence of this is less than that associated with VEGFIs.

Mammalian Target of Rapamycin Inhibitors

mTOR is a serine/threonine kinase involved in the regulation of cellular homeostasis that contributes to cell growth, proliferation, and angiogenesis through integration with multiple signaling pathways, including PI3K/Akt.[156–163] Activation of PI3K/Akt/mTOR contributes to tumor progression, angiogenesis, and the development of drug resistance in several malignancies and is associated with a worse prognosis.[160,164–167] mTOR inhibitors, including sirolimus, temsirolimus, everolimus, and ridaforolimus, have demonstrated antitumor activity in several malignancies, particularly advanced renal cell carcinoma and breast cancer.[160,168–171] The mTOR inhibitors sirolimus and everolimus are also used to prevent acute rejection following solid organ transplantation[168,172] and a growing body of data is derived from their use in that population.

Hypertension is a common side effect of mTOR inhibitors used in patients after transplant and is reported in up to 30% of patients treated with everolimus and almost 40% of patients treated with sirolimus.[168] The incidence of hypertension as an adverse effect of mTOR inhibitors used in the treatment of malignancy is less well described, although it could be expected to be similarly high, particularly because sirolimus, everolimus, and temsirolimus can induce or aggravate proteinuria.[173,174] A better assessment of the true incidence of hypertension in patients with cancer treated with mTOR inhibitors is overdue.[168]

Taxanes

The taxanes, including paclitaxel and docetaxel, are microtubule-targeted agents that alter the cellular microtubule mass and have profound antiangiogenic properties.[175] At low doses, they prevent cell motility and cell-cell interactions,[176,177] whereas at higher doses they cause endothelial cell detachment and apoptosis.[176] Paclitaxel attenuates vascular smooth muscle cell migration and halts endothelial cell proliferation.[176,178] Docetaxel inhibits endothelial function in vitro and angiogenesis in vivo.[176,179] Given that endothelial dysfunction is closely associated with the development of hypertension, it may be expected that the taxanes would contribute to the development of hypertension through this mechanism, although clinical data do not support this hypothesis.[180,181] In a study of patients with metastatic breast cancer, none of those treated with paclitaxel alone developed severe (grade 3 or 4) hypertension compared with 14.8% of patients treated with paclitaxel plus bevacizumab.[180] Furthermore, in a study of patients with non–small-cell lung cancer, less than 1% of patients treated with paclitaxel and carboplatin developed grade 3 or 4 hypertension compared with 7% of patients treated with paclitaxel, carboplatin, and bevacizumab.[181] Taxanes may therefore compound the development of VEGFI-associated hypertension but do not appear to cause hypertension when used in isolation.

Tyrosine Kinase Inhibitors Used for Hematologic Malignancy

Tyrosine kinase inhibitors used in the treatment of hematologic malignancy include ponatinib, nilotinib, and dasatinib.[182] These tyrosine kinase inhibitors are active against the oncogenic fusion gene, Bcr-abl, and are used in the treatment of chronic myeloid leukemia and Philadelphia chromosome positive acute lymphoblastic leukemia resistant to, or intolerant of, traditional tyrosine kinase inhibitors.[182] These agents are associated with a high incidence of acute arterial thrombotic events but are also associated with a clinically relevant incidence of systemic hypertension. In the pivotal trial of the anti-Bcr-Abl tyrosine kinase inhibitor ponatinib, 2.4% of patients developed grade 3 or 4 hypertension.[183] However, major clinical trials of nilotinib, dasatinib, and imatinib have not reported a significant incidence of hypertension.[184,185]

SUMMARY

Hypertension is a common complication of VEGFI therapy that will increase as these drugs become more frequently used for a greater number of malignancies, in older patients, and those with existing cardiovascular disease. VEGFIs have substantially improved cancer cure and survivorship for a range of previously untreatable malignancies, although patients now often survive long enough for cardiovascular complications to become the prime concern. Oncologists and cardiovascular specialists must adopt a coordinated approach to the management of VEGFI-associated hypertension to maintain improvements in cancer-related prognosis while minimizing cardiovascular morbidity and mortality.

The pathophysiology of VEGFI-associated hypertension involves a complex interplay of factors that appear primarily related to endothelial dysfunction, inhibition of NO signaling, and upregulation of the endothelin system. Blood pressure should be measured before and at regular intervals during VEGFI therapy, particularly during the first cycle of chemotherapy. Older patients, those with a history of hypertension, and smokers are at higher risk of VEGFI-associated hypertension, and extra vigilance should be adopted in these patients. Modifiable cardiovascular risk factors should be addressed and an aggressive approach taken to blood pressure management, with antihypertensive therapy commenced if blood pressure exceeds 140/90 mm Hg (130/80 mm Hg in patients with diabetes mellitus or renal impairment) or diastolic blood pressure increases by greater than 20 mm Hg.

ACE inhibitors and dihydropyridine calcium channels antagonists are first-line antihypertensive agents and prompt referral to a hypertension specialist should be made if blood pressure is difficult to manage. Novel therapeutic approaches include NO donors and ET-1 receptor antagonists, whereas mineralocorticoid receptor antagonists may also have a therapeutic role, although these strategies are in the early stages of development. Oncologists and cardiovascular specialists must adopt a collaborative approach in the management of VEGFI-associated hypertension to maintain improvements in cancer-related prognosis while minimizing cardiovascular morbidity and mortality.

ACKNOWLEDGMENTS

Work from the authors' laboratory was supported by grants from the British Heart Foundation (BHF) (RG/13/7/30099). R.M.T. is supported through a BHF Chair (CH/12/4/29762), and A.C.C. is supported through a Fellowship funded through a BHF Award of Research Excellence to the University of Glasgow.

REFERENCES

1. Suter TM, Ewer MS. Cancer drugs and the heart: importance and management. Eur Heart J 2013;34:1102–11.
2. Cameron AC, Touyz RM, Lang NN. Vascular complications of cancer chemotherapy. Can J Cardiol 2016. http://dx.doi.org/10.1016/j.cjca.2015.12.023.
3. Lankhorst S, Kappers MHW, van Esch JHM, et al. Hypertension during vascular endothelial growth factor inhibition: focus on nitric oxide, endothelin-1, and oxidative stress. Antioxid Redox Signal 2014;20(1):135–45.
4. Lankhorst S, Saleh L, Danser AJ, et al. Etiology of angiogenesis inhibition-related hypertension. Curr Opin Pharmacol 2015;21:7–13.
5. Thijs AMJ, van Herpen CML, Sweep FCGJ, et al. Role of endogenous vascular endothelial growth factor in endothelium-dependent vasodilation in humans. Hypertension 2013;61(5):1060–5.
6. Small HY, Montezano AC, Rios FJ, et al. Hypertension due to antiangiogenic cancer therapy with vascular endothelial growth factor inhibitors: understanding and managing a new syndrome. Can J Cardiol 2014;30(5):534–43.
7. Bair SM, Choueiri TK, Moslehi J. Cardiovascular complications associated with novel angiogenesis inhibitors: emerging evidence and evolving perspectives. Trends Cardiovasc Med 2013;23(4):104–13.
8. Robinson ES, Khankin EV, Karumanchi SA, et al. Hypertension induced by vascular endothelial growth factor signaling pathway inhibition: mechanisms and potential use as a biomarker. Semin Nephrol 2010;30(6):591–601.
9. Robinson ES, Matulonis UA, Ivy P, et al. Rapid development of hypertension and proteinuria with cediranib, an oral vascular endothelial growth factor receptor inhibitor. Clin J Am Soc Nephrol 2010;5(3):477–83.
10. Azizi M, Chedid A, Oudard S. Home blood-pressure monitoring in patients receiving sunitinib. N Engl J Med 2008;358(1):95–7.
11. Reimann M, Folprecht G, Haase R, et al. Anti-vascular endothelial growth factor therapy impairs endothelial function of retinal microcirculation in colon cancer patients—an observational study. Exp Transl Stroke Med 2013;5(1):7.
12. Sane DC, Anton L, Brosnihan KB. Angiogenic growth factors and hypertension. Angiogenesis 2004;7(3):193–201.
13. Abi Aad S, Pierce M, Barmaimon G, et al. Hypertension induced by chemotherapeutic and immunosuppressive agents: a new challenge. Crit Rev Oncol Hematol 2015;93(1):28–35.

14. Maitland ML, Lou XJ, Ramirez J, et al. Vascular endothelial growth factor pathway. Pharmacogenet Genomics 2010;20(5):346–9.
15. Larsen AK, Ouaret D, Ouadrani El K, et al. Targeting EGFR and VEGF(R) pathway cross-talk in tumor survival and angiogenesis. Pharmacol Ther 2011; 131(1):80–90.
16. Birk DM, Barbato J, Mureebe L, et al. Current insights on the biology and clinical aspects of VEGF regulation. Vasc Endovascular Surg 2008; 42(6):517–30.
17. Bautch VL. VEGF-directed blood vessel patterning: from cells to organism. Cold Spring Harb Perspect Med 2012;2(9):a006452.
18. Forsythe JA, Jiang BH, Iyer NV, et al. Activation of vascular endothelial growth factor gene transcription by hypoxia-inducible factor 1. Mol Cell Biol 1996;16(9):4604–13.
19. Hernandez SL, Banerjee D, Garcia A, et al. Notch and VEGF pathways play distinct but complementary roles in tumor angiogenesis. Vasc Cell 2013; 5(1):17.
20. Lee S, Chen TT, Barber CL, et al. Autocrine VEGF signaling is required for vascular homeostasis. Cell 2007;130(4):691–703.
21. Ferrara N, Gerber H-P, LeCouter J. The biology of VEGF and its receptors. Nat Med 2003;9(6):669–76.
22. Shibuya M, Claesson-Welsh L. Signal transduction by VEGF receptors in regulation of angiogenesis and lymphangiogenesis. Exp Cell Res 2006; 312(5):549–60.
23. Sawano A, Iwai S, Sakurai Y, et al. Flt-1, vascular endothelial growth factor receptor 1, is a novel cell surface marker for the lineage of monocyte-macrophages in humans. Blood 2001;97(3):785–91.
24. Clauss M, Weich H, Breier G, et al. The vascular endothelial growth factor receptor Flt-1 mediates biological activities. Implications for a functional role of placenta growth factor in monocyte activation and chemotaxis. J Biol Chem 1996;271(30): 17629–34.
25. Barleon B, Sozzani S, Zhou D, et al. Migration of human monocytes in response to vascular endothelial growth factor (VEGF) is mediated via the VEGF receptor flt-1. Blood 1996;87(8):3336–43.
26. Yogi A, O'Connor SE, Callera GE, et al. Receptor and nonreceptor tyrosine kinases in vascular biology of hypertension. Curr Opin Nephrol Hypertens 2010;19(2):169–76.
27. Terman BI, Dougher-Vermazen M, Carrion ME, et al. Identification of the KDR tyrosine kinase as a receptor for vascular endothelial cell growth factor. Biochem Biophys Res Commun 1992;187(3): 1579–86.
28. Maglione D, Guerriero V, Viglietto G, et al. Isolation of a human placenta cDNA coding for a protein related to the vascular permeability factor. Proc Natl Acad Sci U S A 1991;88(20):9267–71.
29. de Vries C, Escobedo JA, Ueno H, et al. The fms-like tyrosine kinase, a receptor for vascular endothelial growth factor. Science 1992;255(5047): 989–91.
30. Huang K, Andersson C, Roomans GM, et al. Signaling properties of VEGF receptor-1 and -2 homo- and heterodimers. Int J Biochem Cell Biol 2001;33(4):315–24.
31. Shibuya M. Vascular endothelial growth factor receptor-1 (VEGFR-1/Flt-1): a dual regulator for angiogenesis. Angiogenesis 2006;9(4):225–30.
32. Sawano A, Takahashi T, Yamaguchi S, et al. Flt-1 but not KDR/Flk-1 tyrosine kinase is a receptor for placenta growth factor, which is related to vascular endothelial growth factor. Cell Growth Differ 1996;7(2):213–21.
33. Duval M, Le Boeuf F, Huot J, et al. Src-mediated phosphorylation of Hsp90 in response to vascular endothelial growth factor (VEGF) is required for VEGF receptor-2 signaling to endothelial NO synthase. Mol Biol Cell 2007;18(11): 4659–68.
34. Neagoe P-E, Lemieux C, Sirois MG. Vascular endothelial growth factor (VEGF)-A165-induced prostacyclin synthesis requires the activation of VEGF receptor-1 and -2 heterodimer. J Biol Chem 2005;280(11):9904–12.
35. Oubaha M, Gratton J-P. Phosphorylation of endothelial nitric oxide synthase by atypical PKC zeta contributes to angiopoietin-1-dependent inhibition of VEGF-induced endothelial permeability in vitro. Blood 2009;114(15): 3343–51.
36. Dixelius J, Makinen T, Wirzenius M, et al. Ligand-induced vascular endothelial growth factor receptor-3 (VEGFR-3) heterodimerization with VEGFR-2 in primary lymphatic endothelial cells regulates tyrosine phosphorylation sites. J Biol Chem 2003;278(42):40973–9.
37. Koch S, Tugues S, Li X, et al. Signal transduction by vascular endothelial growth factor receptors. Biochem J 2011;437(2):169–83.
38. Ng YS, Krilleke D, Shima DT. VEGF function in vascular pathogenesis. Exp Cell Res 2006;312(5): 527–37.
39. Takahashi T, Yamaguchi S, Chida K, et al. A single autophosphorylation site on KDR/Flk-1 is essential for VEGF-A-dependent activation of PLC-gamma and DNA synthesis in vascular endothelial cells. EMBO J 2001;20(11):2768–78.
40. Takahashi T, Ueno H, Shibuya M. VEGF activates protein kinase C-dependent, but Ras-independent Raf-MEK-MAP kinase pathway for DNA synthesis in primary endothelial cells. Oncogene 1999;18(13):2221–30.

41. Meadows KN, Bryant P, Pumiglia K. Vascular endothelial growth factor induction of the angiogenic phenotype requires Ras activation. J Biol Chem 2001;276(52):49289–98.
42. Hood JD, Meininger CJ, Ziche M. VEGF upregulates ecNOS message, protein, and NO production in human endothelial cells. Am J Physiol 1998;274:H1054–8.
43. Wei W, Chen Z-W, Yang Q, et al. Vasorelaxation induced by vascular endothelial growth factor in the human internal mammary artery and radial artery. Vascul Pharmacol 2007;46(4):253–9.
44. Henry TD. The VIVA Trial: vascular endothelial growth factor in ischemia for vascular angiogenesis. Circulation 2003;107(10):1359–65.
45. Henry TD, Rocha-Singh K, Isner JM, et al. Intracoronary administration of recombinant human vascular endothelial growth factor to patients with coronary artery disease. Am Heart J 2001; 142(5):872–80.
46. Dvorak HF, Brown LF, Detmar M, et al. Vascular permeability factor/vascular endothelial growth factor, microvascular hyperpermeability, and angiogenesis. Am J Pathol 1995;146(5):1029–39.
47. Keck PJ, Hauser SD, Krivi G, et al. Vascular permeability factor, an endothelial cell mitogen related to PDGF. Science 1989;246(4935):1309–12.
48. Murohara T, Horowitz JR, Silver M, et al. Vascular endothelial growth factor/vascular permeability factor enhances vascular permeability via nitric oxide and prostacyclin. Circulation 1998;97(1): 99–107.
49. Senger DR, Connolly DT, Van de Water L, et al. Purification and NH2-terminal amino acid sequence of guinea pig tumor-secreted vascular permeability factor. Cancer Res 1990;50(6):1774–8.
50. Senger DR, Galli SJ, Dvorak AM, et al. Tumor cells secrete a vascular permeability factor that promotes accumulation of ascites fluid. Science 1983;219(4587):983–5.
51. Roberts WG, Palade GE. Increased microvascular permeability and endothelial fenestration induced by vascular endothelial growth factor. J Cell Sci 1995;108(Pt 6):2369–79.
52. Limaverde-Sousa G, Sternberg C, Ferreira CG. Antiangiogenesis beyond VEGF inhibition: a journey from antiangiogenic single-target to broad-spectrum agents. Cancer Treat Rev 2014; 40(4):548–57.
53. Chu TF, Rupnick MA, Kerkela R, et al. Cardiotoxicity associated with tyrosine kinase inhibitor sunitinib. Lancet 2007;370(9604):2011–9.
54. Mann DL. Targeted cancer therapeutics: the heartbreak of success. Nat Med 2006;12(8):881–2.
55. Fabian MA, Biggs WH, Treiber DK, et al. A small molecule–kinase interaction map for clinical kinase inhibitors. Nat Biotechnol 2005;23(3):329–36.
56. Force T, Krause DS, Van Etten RA. Molecular mechanisms of cardiotoxicity of tyrosine kinase inhibition. Nat Rev Cancer 2007;7(5):332–44.
57. Kerkela R, Woulfe KC, Durand J-B, et al. Sunitinib-induced cardiotoxicity is mediated by off-target inhibition of AMP-activated protein kinase. Clin Transl Sci 2009;2(1):15–25.
58. Hall PS, Harshman LC, Srinivas S, et al. The frequency and severity of cardiovascular toxicity from targeted therapy in advanced renal cell carcinoma patients. JACC Heart Fail 2013;1(1): 72–8.
59. Keefe D, Bowen J, Gibson R, et al. Noncardiac vascular toxicities of vascular endothelial growth factor inhibitors in advanced cancer: a review. Oncologist 2011;16(4):432–44.
60. Caro J, Morales E, Gutierrez E, et al. Malignant hypertension in patients treated with vascular endothelial growth factor inhibitors. J Clin Hypertens 2013;15(3):215–6.
61. Langenberg MHG, Witteveen PO, Roodhart J, et al. Phase I evaluation of telatinib, a VEGF receptor tyrosine kinase inhibitor, in combination with bevacizumab in subjects with advanced solid tumors. Ann Oncol 2011;22(11):2508–15.
62. Lazarus M, Amundson S, Belani R. An association between bevacizumab and recurrent posterior reversible encephalopathy syndrome in a patient presenting with deep vein thrombosis: a case report and review of the literature. Case Rep Oncol Med 2012;2012:819546.
63. Asaithambi G, Peters BR, Hurliman E, et al. Posterior reversible encephalopathy syndrome induced by pazopanib for renal cell carcinoma. J Clin Pharm Ther 2013;38(2):175–6.
64. Tlemsani C, Mir O, Boudou-Rouquette P, et al. Posterior reversible encephalopathy syndrome induced by anti-VEGF agents. Target Oncol 2011;6(4):253–8.
65. Nazer B, Humphreys BD, Moslehi J. Effects of novel angiogenesis inhibitors for the treatment of cancer on the cardiovascular system: focus on hypertension. Circulation 2011;124(15): 1687–91.
66. James PA, Oparil S, Carter BL, et al. 2014 evidence-based guideline for the management of high blood pressure in adults. JAMA 2014; 311(5):507–14.
67. Maitland ML, Bakris GL, Black HR, et al. Initial assessment, surveillance, and management of blood pressure in patients receiving vascular endothelial growth factor signaling pathway inhibitors. J Natl Cancer Inst 2010;102(9):596–604.
68. Horsley L, Marti K, Jayson GC. Is the toxicity of anti-angiogenic drugs predictive of outcome? A review of hypertension and proteinuria as biomarkers of response to anti-angiogenic

therapy. Expert Opin Drug Metab Toxicol 2012; 8(3):283–93.
69. Eechoute K, van der Veldt AAM, Oosting S, et al. Polymorphisms in endothelial nitric oxide synthase (eNOS) and vascular endothelial growth factor (VEGF) predict sunitinib-induced hypertension. Clin Pharmacol Ther 2012;92(4):503–10.
70. Veronese ML, Mosenkis A, Flaherty KT, et al. Mechanisms of hypertension associated with BAY 43-9006. J Clin Oncol 2006;24(9):1363–9.
71. Maitland ML, Kasza KE, Karrison T, et al. Ambulatory monitoring detects sorafenib-induced blood pressure elevations on the first day of treatment. Clin Cancer Res 2009;15(19):6250–7.
72. Robinson ES, Khankin EV, Choueiri TK, et al. Suppression of the nitric oxide pathway in metastatic renal cell carcinoma patients receiving vascular endothelial growth factor-signaling inhibitors. Hypertension 2010;56(6):1131–6.
73. Facemire CS, Nixon AB, Griffiths R, et al. Vascular endothelial growth factor receptor 2 controls blood pressure by regulating nitric oxide synthase expression. Hypertension 2009;54(3):652–8.
74. Bouloumié A. Vascular endothelial growth factor up-regulates nitric oxide synthase expression in endothelial cells. Cardiovasc Res 1999;41(3): 773–80.
75. Kappers MH, van Esch JH, Sleijfer S, et al. Cardiovascular and renal toxicity during angiogenesis inhibition: clinical and mechanistic aspects. J Hypertens 2009;27(12):2297–309.
76. Kroll J, Waltenberger J. VEGF-A induces expression of eNOS and iNOS in endothelial cells via VEGF Receptor-2 (KDR). Biochem Biophys Res Commun 1998;252(3):743–6.
77. Kruzliak P, Kovacova G, Pechanova O. Therapeutic potential of nitric oxide donors in the prevention and treatment of angiogenesis-inhibitor-induced hypertension. Angiogenesis 2012;16(2):289–95.
78. Shen BQ, Lee DY, Zioncheck TF. Vascular endothelial growth factor governs endothelial nitric-oxide synthase expression via a KDR/Flk-1 receptor and a protein kinase C signaling pathway. J Biol Chem 1999;274(46):33057–63.
79. Kappers MHW, Smedts FMM, Horn T, et al. The vascular endothelial growth factor receptor inhibitor sunitinib causes a preeclampsia-like syndrome with activation of the endothelin system. Hypertension 2011;58(2):295–302.
80. Mayer EL, Dallabrida SM, Rupnick MA, et al. Contrary effects of the receptor tyrosine kinase inhibitor vandetanib on constitutive and flow-stimulated nitric oxide elaboration in humans. Hypertension 2011;58(1):85–92.
81. Griendling KK. Oxidative stress and cardiovascular injury: part I: basic mechanisms and in vivo monitoring of ROS. Circulation 2003;108(16):1912–6.
82. Kim Y-W, Byzova TV. Oxidative stress in angiogenesis and vascular disease. Blood 2014;123(5): 625–31.
83. Schulz E, Jansen T, Wenzel P, et al. Nitric oxide, tetrahydrobiopterin, oxidative stress, and endothelial dysfunction in hypertension. Antioxid Redox Signal 2008;10(6):1115–26.
84. Kappers MHW, de Beer VJ, Zhou Z, et al. Sunitinib-induced systemic vasoconstriction in swine is endothelin mediated and does not involve nitric oxide or oxidative stress. Hypertension 2012; 59(1):151–7.
85. Attinà T, Camidge R, Newby DE, et al. Endothelin antagonism in pulmonary hypertension, heart failure, and beyond. Heart 2005;91(6):825–31.
86. Moorhouse RC, Webb DJ, Kluth DC, et al. Endothelin antagonism and its role in the treatment of hypertension. Curr Hypertens Rep 2013;15(5): 489–96.
87. Lankhorst S, Kappers MHW, van Esch JHM, et al. Mechanism of hypertension and proteinuria during angiogenesis inhibition: evolving role of endothelin-1. J Hypertens 2013;31(3):444–54.
88. Remuzzi G, Perico N, Benigni A. New therapeutics that antagonize endothelin: promises and frustrations. Nat Rev Drug Discov 2002;1(12): 986–1001.
89. Kappers MHW, van Esch JHM, Sluiter W, et al. Hypertension induced by the tyrosine kinase inhibitor sunitinib is associated with increased circulating endothelin-1 levels. Hypertension 2010; 56(4):675–81.
90. Banfor PN, Franklin PA, Segreti JA, et al. ETA receptor blockade with atrasentan prevents hypertension with the multitargeted tyrosine kinase inhibitor ABT-869 in telemetry-instrumented rats. J Cardiovasc Pharmacol 2009;53(2):173–8.
91. Cardillo C, Kilcoyne CM, Cannon RO, et al. Interactions between nitric oxide and endothelin in the regulation of vascular tone of human resistance vessels in vivo. Hypertension 2000;35(6): 1237–41.
92. Mourad JJ, Guetz des G, Debbabi H, et al. Blood pressure rise following angiogenesis inhibition by bevacizumab. A crucial role for microcirculation. Ann Oncol 2008;19(5):927–34.
93. Mitsutomi N, Akashi C, Odagiri J, et al. Effects of endogenous and exogenous nitric oxide on endothelin-1 production in cultured vascular endothelial cells. Eur J Pharmacol 1999;364(1): 65–73.
94. Dhaun N, Goddard J, Kohan DE, et al. Role of endothelin-1 in clinical hypertension: 20 years on. Hypertension 2008;52(3):452–9.
95. Te Riet L, van Esch JH, Roks AJ, et al. Hypertension: renin-angiotensin-aldosterone system alterations. Circ Res 2015;116(6):960–75.

96. Curwen JO, Musgrove HL, Kendrew J, et al. Inhibition of vascular endothelial growth factor-a signaling induces hypertension: examining the effect of cediranib (recentin; AZD2171) treatment on blood pressure in rat and the use of concomitant antihypertensive therapy. Clin Cancer Res 2008; 14(10):3124–31.
97. Belcik JT, Qi Y, Kaufmann BA, et al. Cardiovascular and systemic microvascular effects of anti-vascular endothelial growth factor therapy for cancer. J Am Coll Cardiol 2012;60(7):618–25.
98. Lankhorst S, Kappers MHW, van Esch JHM, et al. Treatment of hypertension and renal injury induced by the angiogenesis inhibitor sunitinib: preclinical study. Hypertension 2014; 64(6):1282–9.
99. Levy BI, Ambrosio G, Pries AR, et al. Microcirculation in hypertension: a new target for treatment? Circulation 2001;104(6):735–40.
100. Steeghs N, Gelderblom H, Roodt JO, et al. Hypertension and rarefaction during treatment with telatinib, a small molecule angiogenesis inhibitor. Clin Cancer Res 2008;14(11):3470–6.
101. van der Veldt AAM, de Boer MP, Boven E, et al. Reduction in skin microvascular density and changes in vessel morphology in patients treated with sunitinib. Anticancer Drugs 2010;21(4):439–46.
102. de Boer MP, van der Veldt AAM, Lankheet NA, et al. Sunitinib-induced reduction in skin microvascular density is a reversible phenomenon. Ann Oncol 2010;21(9):1923–4.
103. Kamba T, Tam BYY, Hashizume H, et al. VEGF-dependent plasticity of fenestrated capillaries in the normal adult microvasculature. Am J Physiol Heart Circ Physiol 2006;290(2):H560–76.
104. Inai T, Mancuso M, Hashizume H, et al. Inhibition of vascular endothelial growth factor (VEGF) signaling in cancer causes loss of endothelial fenestrations, regression of tumor vessels, and appearance of basement membrane ghosts. Am J Pathol 2010;165(1):35–52.
105. Baffert F, Le T, Sennino B, et al. Cellular changes in normal blood capillaries undergoing regression after inhibition of VEGF signaling. Am J Physiol Heart Circ Physiol 2006;290(2):H547–59.
106. Steeghs N, Rabelink TJ, op 't Roodt J, et al. Reversibility of capillary density after discontinuation of bevacizumab treatment. Ann Oncol 2010; 21(5):1100–5.
107. Zhu X, Wu S, Dahut WL, et al. Risks of proteinuria and hypertension with bevacizumab, an antibody against vascular endothelial growth factor: systematic review and meta-analysis. Am J Kidney Dis 2007;49(2):186–93.
108. Wu S, Kim C, Baer L, et al. Bevacizumab increases risk for severe proteinuria in cancer patients. J Am Soc Nephrol 2010;21(8):1381–9.
109. Zhang Z-F, Wang T, Liu L-H, et al. Risks of proteinuria associated with vascular endothelial growth factor receptor tyrosine kinase inhibitors in cancer patients: a systematic review and meta-analysis. Lafrenie R, ed. PLoS One 2014;9(3):e90135–10.
110. Eremina V, Jefferson JA, Kowalewska J, et al. VEGF inhibition and renal thrombotic microangiopathy. N Engl J Med 2008;358(11):1129–36.
111. Izzedine H, Rixe O, Billemont B, et al. Angiogenesis inhibitor therapies: focus on kidney toxicity and hypertension. Am J Kidney Dis 2007;50(2): 203–18.
112. Gu J-W, Manning RD, Young E, et al. Vascular endothelial growth factor receptor inhibitor enhances dietary salt-induced hypertension in Sprague-Dawley rats. Am J Physiol Regul Integr Comp Physiol 2009;297(1):R142–8.
113. Granger JP. Vascular endothelial growth factor inhibitors and hypertension: a central role for the kidney and endothelial factors? Hypertension 2009;54(3):465–7.
114. Zou AP, Cowley AW Jr. Role of nitric oxide in the control of renal function and salt sensitivity. Curr Hypertens Rep 1999;1(2):178–86.
115. Mancia G, Fagard R, Narkiewicz K, et al. 2013 ESH/ESC Guidelines for the management of arterial hypertension: the Task Force for the management of arterial hypertension of the European Society of Hypertension (ESH) and of the European Society of Cardiology (ESC). J Hypertens 2013;31(7): 1281–357.
116. Echouffo-Tcheugui JB, Batty GD, Kivimäki M, et al. Risk models to predict hypertension: a systematic review. Hernandez AV, ed. PLoS One 2013;8(7): e67370–10.
117. Greenlund KJ, Croft JB, Mensah GA. Prevalence of heart disease and stroke risk factors in persons with prehypertension in the United States, 1999-2000. Arch Intern Med 2004;164(19):2113–8.
118. Wang Y, Wang QJ. The prevalence of prehypertension and hypertension among US adults according to the new joint national committee guidelines: new challenges of the old problem. Arch Intern Med 2004;164(19):2126–34.
119. Vasan RS, Larson MG, Leip EP, et al. Assessment of frequency of progression to hypertension in non-hypertensive participants in the Framingham Heart Study: a cohort study. Lancet 2001; 358(9294):1682–6.
120. Julius S, Nesbitt SD, Egan BM, et al. Feasibility of treating prehypertension with an angiotensin-receptor blocker. N Engl J Med 2006;354(16): 1685–97.
121. Effects of weight loss and sodium reduction intervention on blood pressure and hypertension incidence in overweight people with high-normal blood pressure. The Trials of Hypertension

Prevention, phase II. The Trials of Hypertension Prevention Collaborative Research Group. Arch Intern Med 1997;157(6):657–67.
122. Wang TJ, Gona P, Larson MG, et al. Multiple biomarkers and the risk of incident hypertension. Hypertension 2007;49(3):432–8.
123. Mir O, Mouthon L, Alexandre J, et al. Bevacizumab-induced cardiovascular events: a consequence of cholesterol emboli syndrome? J Natl Cancer Inst 2007;99(1):85–6.
124. Verma S, Wang C-H, Li S-H, et al. A self-fulfilling prophecy: C-reactive protein attenuates nitric oxide production and inhibits angiogenesis. Circulation 2002;106(8):913–9.
125. Venugopal SK, Devaraj S, Yuhanna I, et al. Demonstration that C-reactive protein decreases eNOS expression and bioactivity in human aortic endothelial cells. Circulation 2002;106(12):1439–41.
126. Brasier AR, Recinos A, Eledrisi MS. Vascular inflammation and the renin-angiotensin system. Arterioscler Thromb Vasc Biol 2002;22(8):1257–66.
127. Allin KH, Nordestgaard BG. Elevated C-reactive protein in the diagnosis, prognosis, and cause of cancer. Crit Rev Clin Lab Sci 2011;48(4):155–70.
128. Miller KD, Chap LI, Holmes FA, et al. Randomized phase III trial of capecitabine compared with bevacizumab plus capecitabine in patients with previously treated metastatic breast cancer. J Clin Oncol 2005;23(4):792–9.
129. Yang JC, Haworth L, Sherry RM, et al. A randomized trial of bevacizumab, an anti-vascular endothelial growth factor antibody, for metastatic renal cancer. N Engl J Med 2003;349(5):427–34.
130. Johnson DH, Fehrenbacher L, Novotny WF, et al. Randomized phase II trial comparing bevacizumab plus carboplatin and paclitaxel with carboplatin and paclitaxel alone in previously untreated locally advanced or metastatic non-small-cell lung cancer. J Clin Oncol 2004;22(11):2184–91.
131. Motzer RJ, Hutson TE, Tomczak P, et al. Sunitinib versus interferon alfa in metastatic renal-cell carcinoma. N Engl J Med 2007;356(2):115–24.
132. Escudier B, Eisen T, Stadler WM, et al. Sorafenib in advanced clear-cell renal-cell carcinoma. N Engl J Med 2007;356(2):125–34.
133. Hurwitz H, Fehrenbacher L, Novotny W, et al. Bevacizumab plus irinotecan, fluorouracil, and leucovorin for metastatic colorectal cancer. N Engl J Med 2004;350(23):2335–42.
134. Kabbinavar FF, Schulz J, McCleod M, et al. Addition of bevacizumab to bolus fluorouracil and leucovorin in first-line metastatic colorectal cancer: results of a randomized phase II trial. J Clin Oncol 2005;23(16):3697–705.
135. Jan Danser AH. Renin and prorenin as biomarkers in hypertension. Curr Opin Nephrol Hypertens 2012;21(5):508–14.
136. Harrap SB, Dominiczak AF, Fraser R, et al. Plasma angiotensin II, predisposition to hypertension, and left ventricular size in healthy young adults. Circulation 1996;93(6):1148–54.
137. Vasan RS, Evans JC, Larson MG, et al. Serum aldosterone and the incidence of hypertension in nonhypertensive persons. N Engl J Med 2004;351(1):33–41.
138. Lewington S, Clarke R, Qizilbash N, et al. Prospective Studies Collaboration. Age-specific relevance of usual blood pressure to vascular mortality: a meta-analysis of individual data for one million adults in 61 prospective studies. Lancet 2002;360(9349):1903–13.
139. Jain RK. Lessons from multidisciplinary translational trials on anti-angiogenic therapy of cancer. Nat Rev Cancer 2008;8(4):309–16.
140. Ogden LG, He J, Lydick E, et al. Long-term absolute benefit of lowering blood pressure in hypertensive patients according to the JNC VI risk stratification. Hypertension 2000;35(2):539–43.
141. Copur MS, Obermiller A. An algorithm for the management of hypertension in the setting of vascular endothelial growth factor signaling inhibition. Clin Colorectal Cancer 2011;10(3):151–6.
142. National Cancer Institute. Common Terminology Criteria for Adverse Events (CTCAE). Washington: National Cancer Institute; 2010. p. 1–196.
143. de Jesus-Gonzalez N, Robinson E, Moslehi J, et al. Management of antiangiogenic therapy-induced hypertension. Hypertension 2012;60(3):607–15.
144. van Zwieten PA. Amlodipine: an overview of its pharmacodynamic and pharmacokinetic properties. Clin Cardiol 1994;17(9 Suppl 3):III3–6.
145. Calhoun DA, Jones D, Textor S, et al. Resistant hypertension: diagnosis, evaluation, and treatment. A scientific statement from the American Heart Association Professional Education Committee of the Council for High Blood Pressure Research. Hypertension 2008;51(6):1403–19.
146. Kruzliak P, Novák J, Novák M. Vascular endothelial growth factor inhibitor-induced hypertension: from pathophysiology to prevention and treatment based on long-acting nitric oxide donors. Am J Hypertens 2014;27(1):3–13.
147. Sunshine SB, Dallabrida SM, Durand E, et al. Endostatin lowers blood pressure via nitric oxide and prevents hypertension associated with VEGF inhibition. Proc Natl Acad Sci U S A 2012;109(28):11306–11.
148. Shah DR, Shah RR, Morganroth J. Tyrosine kinase inhibitors: their on-target toxicities as potential indicators of efficacy. Drug Saf 2013;36(6):413–26.

149. Simons M, Eichmann A. "On-target" cardiac effects of anticancer drugs: lessons from new biology. J Am Coll Cardiol 2012;60(7):626–7.
150. Snider KL, Maitland ML. Cardiovascular toxicities: clues to optimal administration of vascular endothelial growth factor signaling pathway inhibitors. Target Oncol 2009;4(2):67–76.
151. Dahlberg SE, Sandler AB, Brahmer JR, et al. Clinical course of advanced non-small-cell lung cancer patients experiencing hypertension during treatment with bevacizumab in combination with carboplatin and paclitaxel on ECOG 4599. J Clin Oncol 2010;28(6):949–54.
152. Rini BI, Cohen DP, Lu DR, et al. Hypertension as a biomarker of efficacy in patients with metastatic renal cell carcinoma treated with sunitinib. J Natl Cancer Inst 2011;103(9):763–73.
153. Keizer RJ, Gupta A, Shumaker R, et al. Model-based treatment optimization of a novel VEGFR inhibitor. Br J Clin Pharmacol 2012; 74(2):315–26.
154. Rautiola J, Donskov F, Peltola K, et al. Sunitinib-induced hypertension, neutropaenia and thrombocytopaenia as predictors of good prognosis in patients with metastatic renal cell carcinoma. BJU Int 2016;117(1):110–7.
155. Schneider BP, Wang M, Radovich M, et al. Association of vascular endothelial growth factor and vascular endothelial growth factor receptor-2 genetic polymorphisms with outcome in a trial of paclitaxel compared with paclitaxel plus bevacizumab in advanced breast cancer: ECOG 2100. J Clin Oncol 2008;26(28):4672–8.
156. Zaytseva YY, Valentino JD, Gulhati P, et al. mTOR inhibitors in cancer therapy. Cancer Lett 2012; 319(1):1–7.
157. Zoncu R, Efeyan A, Sabatini DM. mTOR: from growth signal integration to cancer, diabetes and ageing. Nat Rev Mol Cell Biol 2011;12(1):21–35.
158. Laplante M, Sabatini DM. mTOR signaling at a glance. J Cell Sci 2009;122(20):3589–94.
159. Menon S, Manning BD. Common corruption of the mTOR signaling network in human tumors. Oncogene 2008;27(S2):S43–51.
160. Yardley DA. Combining mTOR inhibitors with chemotherapy and other targeted therapies in advanced breast cancer: rationale, clinical experience, and future directions. Breast Cancer 2013;7:7–22.
161. Wullschleger S, Loewith R, Hall MN. TOR signaling in growth and metabolism. Cell 2006; 124(3):471–84.
162. Albanell J, Dalmases A, Rovira A, et al. mTOR signalling in human cancer. Clin Transl Oncol 2007; 9(8):484–93.
163. Faivre S, Kroemer G, Raymond E. Current development of mTOR inhibitors as anticancer agents. Nat Rev Drug Discov 2006;5(8):671–88.
164. Wong K-K, Engelman JA, Cantley LC. Targeting the PI3K signaling pathway in cancer. Curr Opin Genet Dev 2010;20(1):87–90.
165. Bjornsti M-A, Houghton PJ. The TOR pathway: a target for cancer therapy. Nat Rev Cancer 2004; 4(5):335–48.
166. Hay N, Sonenberg N. Upstream and downstream of mTOR. Genes Dev 2004;18(16):1926–45.
167. Bachman KE, Argani P, Samuels Y, et al. The PIK3CA gene is mutated with high frequency in human breast cancers. Cancer Biol Ther 2014;3(8): 772–5.
168. Kaplan B, Qazi Y, Wellen JR. Strategies for the management of adverse events associated with mTOR inhibitors. Transplant Rev 2014;28(3): 126–33.
169. Motzer RJ, Escudier B, Oudard S, et al. Phase 3 trial of everolimus for metastatic renal cell carcinoma : final results and analysis of prognostic factors. Cancer 2010;116(18):4256–65.
170. Hudes G, Carducci M, Tomczak P, et al. Temsirolimus, interferon alfa, or both for advanced renal-cell carcinoma. N Engl J Med 2007; 356(22):2271–81.
171. Fasolo A, Sessa C. Targeting mTOR pathways in human malignancies. Curr Pharm Des 2012; 18(19):2766–77.
172. Rostaing L, Kamar N. mTOR inhibitor/proliferation signal inhibitors: entering or leaving the field? J Nephrol 2010;23(2):133–42.
173. Pallet N, Legendre C. Adverse events associated with mTOR inhibitors. Expert Opin Drug Saf 2013;12(2):177–86.
174. Diekmann F, Andrés A, Oppenheimer F. mTOR inhibitor-associated proteinuria in kidney transplant recipients. Transplant Rev 2012;26(1):27–9.
175. Jordan MA, Wilson L. Microtubules as a target for anticancer drugs. Nat Rev Cancer 2004;4(4): 253–65.
176. Soultati A, Mountzios G, Avgerinou C, et al. Endothelial vascular toxicity from chemotherapeutic agents: preclinical evidence and clinical implications. Cancer Treat Rev 2012;38(5):473–83.
177. Schwartz EL. Antivascular actions of microtubule-binding drugs. Clin Cancer Res 2009;15(8):2594–601.
178. Belotti D, Vergani V, Drudis T, et al. The microtubule-affecting drug paclitaxel has antiangiogenic activity. Clin Cancer Res 1996;2(11):1843–9.
179. Vacca A, Ribatti D, Iurlaro M, et al. Docetaxel versus paclitaxel for antiangiogenesis. J Hematother Stem Cell Res 2002;11(1):103–18. http://dx.doi.org/10.1089/152581602753448577.
180. Miller K, Wang M, Gralow J, et al. Paclitaxel plus bevacizumab versus paclitaxel alone for metastatic breast cancer. N Engl J Med 2007;357(26): 2666–76.

181. Sandler A, Gray R, Perry MC, et al. Paclitaxel-carboplatin alone or with bevacizumab for non-small-cell lung cancer. N Engl J Med 2006; 355(24):2542–50.
182. Herrmann J, Lerman A. An update on cardio-oncology. Trends Cardiovasc Med 2014;24(7): 285–95.
183. Cortes JE, Kim DW, Pinilla-Ibarz J, et al. A Phase 2 Trial of Ponatinib in Philadelphia Chromosome–Positive Leukemias. N Engl J Med 2013;369(19): 1783–96.
184. Saglio G, Kim D-W, Issaragrisil S, et al. Nilotinib versus imatinib for newly diagnosed chronic myeloid leukemia. N Engl J Med 2010;362(24):2251–9.
185. Kantarjian H, Shah NP, Hochhaus A, et al. Dasatinib versus imatinib in newly diagnosed chronic-phase chronic myeloid leukemia. N Engl J Med 2010;362(24):2260–70.

CHAPTER 11

Thromboembolic Disease in Cancer

Ghazaleh Kazemi, MD[a,b], Oren Levine, MD[a,b], Mark N. Levine, MD, MSc[a,b,*]

INTRODUCTION

In 1865, Professor Armand Trousseau first noted that in patients with cancer "there appears in the cachexia a particular condition of the blood which predisposes it to thrombosis."[1] He also first described thrombophlebitis as the earliest manifestation of a visceral malignancy.[2] Since that time, there has been considerable research, many symposia, and hundreds of publications on the subject of the unique relationship between cancer and thrombosis. The occurrence of thrombosis complicates the management of the patient with cancer because of the need for anticoagulant therapy and the potential for bleeding. Patients with cancer with acute venous thromboembolism (VTE) are at increased risk of recurrent thrombosis compared with noncancer patients with acute VTE.[3] Thrombosis can be the first manifestation of an occult cancer.[2] Finally, patients with cancer with VTE have increased mortality compared with noncancer patients with VTE.[4] Increased mortality could be a result of fatal pulmonary embolism (PE) or that VTE is a marker of advanced cancer with a large tumor burden. It is hoped that by the end of this article, the reader will come to appreciate why this topic of cancer and thrombosis has captured the interest of so many for more than 150 years.

PATHOGENESIS

The pathogenesis of thrombosis in the patient with cancer can be considered through Virchow's triad, which includes stasis, blood components, and vessel wall damage.[5] In terms of stasis, patients with cancer are often immobile and sometimes have extrinsic compression of veins by lymph nodes or a tumor mass. Tumor cells and macrophages produce procoagulants such as tissue factor (TF) and inflammatory cytokines, which are thrombogenic (Fig. 11.1).[6,7] Finally, vessel wall damage can be caused by direct tumor invasion, indwelling catheters, chemotherapy, hematopoietic growth factors, and antiangiogenic agents.[5,6]

In addition, the hemostatic system is uniquely positioned to drive both thrombosis and tumor growth/metastases.[6,7] Thrombosis and tumor growth/metastases are very complex relationships and beyond the scope of this article. However, suffice it to say that in experimental models thrombosis can stimulate tumor growth and metastases that can be inhibited by anticoagulants.[4] These observations have been studied in clinical trials with vitamin K antagonists, unfractionated heparin, and low-molecular-weight heparin (LMWH) as anticancer agents.[4] To date, the results of these trials have not shown an improvement in survival.

EPIDEMIOLOGY

Historically, thrombosis has been most commonly observed in mucin-producing tumors, for example, pancreatic cancer and gastric cancer, and autopsy studies noted thrombosis in up to 50% of patients with metastatic cancer. However, attempting to describe the epidemiology of the condition is complex and very much depends on the question being asked. For example, one could ask, "What is the rate of thrombosis in a particular type of cancer, for example, patients with early breast cancer receiving adjuvant chemotherapy?" Rates could be obtained from prospective cohort studies, retrospective case series, or population-based studies.[8] Each type of design is associated with limitations. The thrombotic rate is also influenced by confounders such as the stage of the cancer, the performance status of the patient, and therapy (thrombotic rates with specific

[a] Department of Oncology, McMaster University, Hamilton, Ontario, Canada; [b] Hamilton Health Sciences Juravinski Cancer Centre, 711 Concession Street, Hamilton, Ontario L8V1C3, Canada
[*] Corresponding author. Room 104, G Wing, Hamilton Health Sciences, Juravinski Hospital, 711 Concession Street, Hamilton, Ontario L8C 1C3, Canada
E-mail address: mlevine@mcmaster.ca

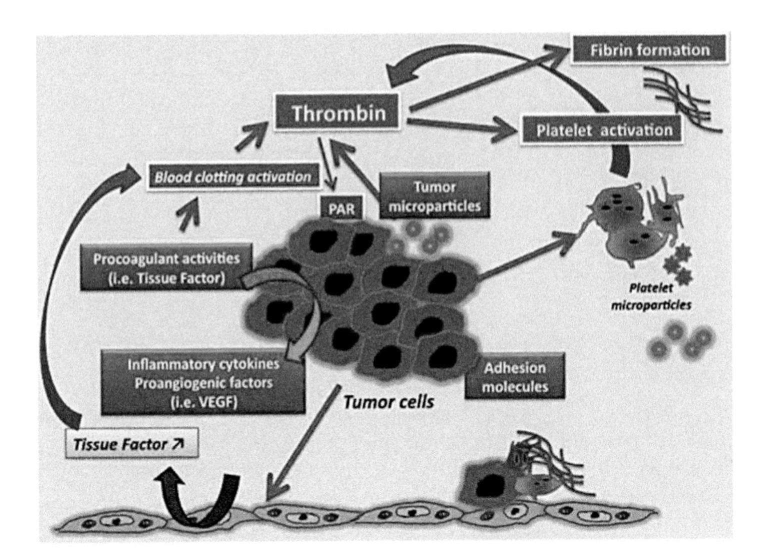

Fig. 11.1 Mechanisms involved in cancer-associated thrombosis. (*From* Falanga A. The cancer-thrombosis connection. The Hematologist: ASH News and Reports 2011:8;4; with permission.)

cancers are discussed later in the prevention section). Another question is, "in all the patients with cancer with thrombosis seen in consultation by the hematology service in the past 6 months, what is the most common cancer type?" It is important to recognize that cancer is very common, and the number of patients with cancer is increasing, so that the prevalence of patients with cancer developing thrombosis is high. About 20% of patients in trials with anticoagulants had malignant disease, and a cancer diagnosis was noted to a similar percentage in a contemporary population-based study of patients with VTE.[8,9] The frequency of the type of cancer associated with thrombosis very much depends on the frequency of the type of cancers being treated at an institution, for example, lung, colorectal, prostate in men, and breast, lung, colorectal, and ovary in women. The bottom line, however, is that thrombosis can occur with any type of cancer.

Trousseau first described the association between migratory thrombophlebitis and occult cancer. There have been several studies using different designs that have evaluated this relationship. Population-based studies using registry data showed that patients who presented with acute VTE had an increased risk of developing cancer for up to several years after diagnosis, with the highest incidence in the first year.[10] In retrospective cohort studies, the risk of cancer in the first year after the presentation of an episode of VTE was increased several fold in patients with idiopathic thrombosis versus secondary thrombosis.[10] However, many of these studies were potentially subject to bias because of the inclusion of patients who had cancer at the time of the presenting VTE. The association of acute VTE with occult cancer precipitated much discussion on whether patients presenting with idiopathic VTE should undergo screening to detect cancer.[10,11] One study suggested that screening for occult cancer, for example, computed tomographic (CT) scan thorax and abdomen in patients with idiopathic VTE, found some cancers at an early stage, but no difference in survival was detected between groups.[11] A recent Canadian trial showed that the addition of CT scan of the abdomen and pelvis to basic investigations (chest radiograph, basic laboratory tests, and screening tests for breast, prostate, and cervical cancer) for detection of occult malignancy after unprovoked VTE did not improve cancer detection or cancer-specific survival.[12] This finding is consistent with a prior *Cochrane Review* of randomized trials showing that extensive workup, including CT scans, PET scans, and endoscopy, did not improve cancer-related mortality when compared with usual care, although there was earlier detection of occult cancer in a small number of patients. In general, screening for an underlying cancer is not recommended in patients presenting with acute VTE.[13]

DIAGNOSIS OF ACUTE VENOUS THROMBOEMBOLISM

Deep Vein Thrombosis

Approximately 50% of patients with proximal deep vein thrombosis (DVT) will have asymptomatic PE. Apart from the symptoms caused by leg vein thrombosis, there is concern that calf vein thrombosis will extend into the proximal deep veins, and then the clot will fragment and travel to the pulmonary circulation. The approach to the diagnosis of DVT in patients with cancer is the same as the approach in the noncancer patient. The most common signs and symptoms for DVT are extremity swelling (80%) and pain (75%), whereas erythema is seen in only 25%.[14] Although these signs and symptoms are important for raising the suspicion of DVT, clinically they remain nonspecific for the diagnosis of DVT. The confirmation of DVT by an objective test, for example, compression ultrasound or venography, is required.

Before the turn of the century, venography was the gold standard for the diagnosis of DVT. A venogram maps the deep venous system of the calf and thigh. Proximal DVT is diagnosed when there was an intraluminal filling defect in any of the popliteal, superficial femoral, external iliac, or internal iliac veins. Over the past decade, compression ultrasound (CUS) has replaced venography for the diagnosis of DVT. Cohort studies that compared CUS with venography showed that the sensitivity and specificity of CUS for proximal DVT were 99%.[15] In fact, in many imaging departments, venography is no longer available because the radiologists lack experience with this test. The criterion required for the diagnosis of DVT with CUS is noncompressibility of either the popliteal vein or the femoral vein. As technology has improved, compression ultrasonography has been used to diagnose calf vein thrombosis, but it must be kept in mind that in calf vein thrombosis CUS ultrasound is less sensitive than venography.[15]

Because clinical symptoms are subjective, clinical risk scores for evaluating the probability of DVT have been developed. A commonly used score is the one by Wells and colleagues,[16] which quantifies the likelihood of an individual patient having DVT based on their medical history and physical examination. A score of 3 or more is considered to be associated with a high likelihood of DVT; 1 to 2 with a moderate score and 0 with a low likelihood. The parameters for the Wells score include the following: 1 point for each of active cancer, paralysis, being bedridden, localized tenderness along the distribution of the deep vein system, entire leg swelling, calf swollen by more than 3 cm when compared with the asymptomatic leg, pitting edema, collateral superficial veins; an alternative diagnosis is likely or greater than that of DVT (−2 points). Note that a patient with cancer will be assigned a score of 1, which already puts them in the moderate risk of DVT category.

D-dimer can be used to rule out DVT. D-dimer is a protein fragment produced by thrombus degradation that is formed when plasmin dissolves the fibrin strands that hold a thrombus together. A highly sensitive D-dimer test is associated with a high negative-predictive value. However, a positive D-dimer test in a patient with cancer can often be a false positive.

A clinical risk score is often used in conjunction with D-dimer and CUS to diagnose DVT. For example, in the noncancer patient with a low pretest probability and normal D-dimer, DVT is ruled out. If there is a moderate pretest probability, the patient will usually have a CUS even if the D-dimer is normal. Because there is concern that the Wells score has not been validated in patients with cancer, the patient with cancer with a suspected DVT requires a CUS, and if it is negative, the patient should have the CUS repeated in 7 days.[17] For those undergoing chemotherapy, a validated VTE risk model is available (Fig. 11.2). A more comprehensive conceptual framework toward

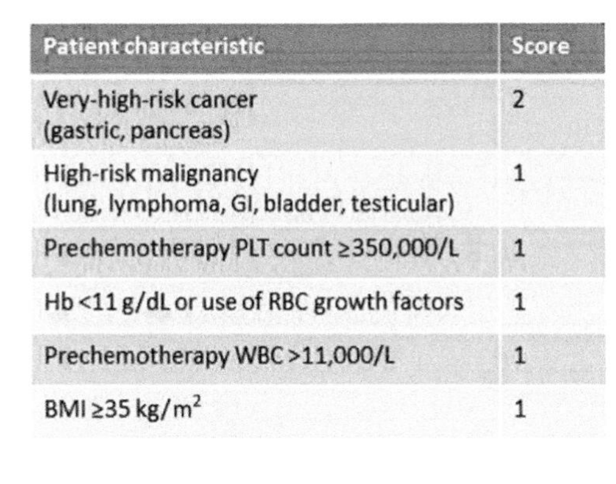

Patient characteristic	Score
Very-high-risk cancer (gastric, pancreas)	2
High-risk malignancy (lung, lymphoma, GI, bladder, testicular)	1
Prechemotherapy PLT count ≥350,000/L	1
Hb <11 g/dL or use of RBC growth factors	1
Prechemotherapy WBC >11,000/L	1
BMI ≥35 kg/m²	1

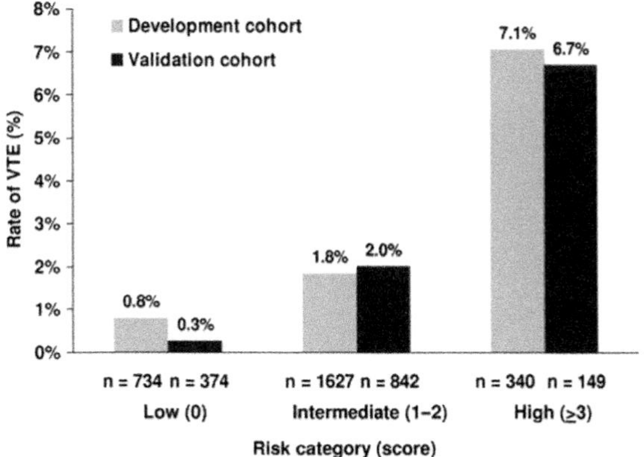

Fig. 11.2 Risk score for chemotherapy-related VTE and event rates in the derivation and validation cohorts. BMI, body mass index; GI, gastrointestinal; Hb, hemoglobulin; PAR, protease activated receptor; PLT, platelets; RBC, red blood cells; WBC, white blood cells. (*Adapted from* Khorana AA, Kuderer NM, Culakova E, et al. Development and validation of a predictive model for chemotherapy-associated thrombosis. Blood 2008;111(10):4902–7; with permission.)

the risk of VTE in patients with cancer should also be entertained (Fig. 11.3).

Pulmonary Embolism

The most common signs and symptoms of PE are dyspnea (85%), chest pain (40%), tachypnea (30%), and tachycardia (23%),[14] but again, nonspecific and objective testing is needed to diagnosis PE. Before the turn of the century, the diagnosis of PE was usually with a ventilation perfusion lung scan. A segmental mismatch, that is, a segment that was ventilated but lacked perfusion, was considered high probability for PE. Scans where the abnormalities were subsegmental or matched were considered non–high probability for PE. In such cases, the physician might go on to perform pulmonary angiography if the clinical suspicion was very high or a venogram to check for DVT. In the last decade, ventilation perfusion lung scans and pulmonary angiography have been replaced by CT angiography of the lung. Initially, spiral CT scans could reliably detect lobar and segmental thrombi. Current use of multidetector CT scanners in many centers leads to identification of arterial filling defects, presumed to represent small thrombi, in the subsegmental pulmonary arteries. These very small thrombi may have previously gone undetected, and the clinical significance is uncertain. For patients without cancer, algorithms including clinical risk score, D-dimer, and CT angiography are used to rule in or rule out PE. In patients with cancer where there is less certainty about such algorithms, CT angiography is performed.

PREVENTION OF CANCER-ASSOCIATED THROMBOSIS

Primary prevention for the patient with cancer can be considered using a framework based on the clinical setting. These settings include the patient with cancer after surgery, the patient with cancer hospitalized for a medical condition (eg, pain crisis, hypercalcemia, congestive heart failure, and septicemia), the ambulatory outpatient receiving anticancer treatment with chemotherapy, endocrine therapy, molecular targeted therapy, or radiation, and finally, the patient at the end of life.

Surgical and Medical Antithrombotic Prophylaxis

Clinical practice guidelines from several groups recommend thromboprophylaxis for patients undergoing surgery and patients hospitalized with medical conditions, for example, congestive heart failure. Patients with cancer are considered a subset of such patients. Hence, patients undergoing major cancer surgery should receive pharmacologic thromboprophylaxis with unfractionated heparin or LMWH, starting before surgery and continuing for at least 7 to 10 days after surgery.[18] Extended thromboprophylaxis up to 4 weeks should be considered in those with high-risk features. Mechanical thromboprophylaxis is often added to heparin or used alone in high-risk bleeding situations, for example, neurosurgery. The use of thromboprophylaxis at the end of life is a complex situation that weighs risks, benefits, and quality of life.

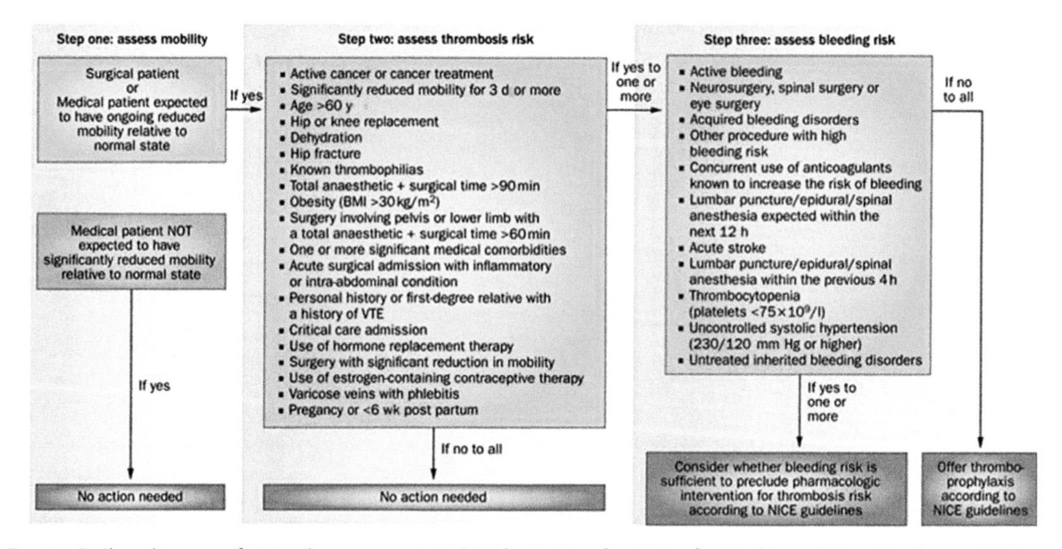

Fig. 11.3 Flow diagram of VTE risk assessment. NICE, The National Institute for Health and Care Excellence. (*Adapted from* Department of Health. Risk assessment for venous thromboembolism (VTE). 2010. Available at: http://www.dh.gov.uk/prod_consum_dh/groups/dh_digitalassets/@dh/@en/@ps/documents/digitalasset/dh_113355.pdf.)

Hospitalized medical patients with cancer are at risk for thromboembolism. They should receive the same prophylaxis as noncancer medical patients, for example, subcutaneous unfractionated heparin or LMWH, provided they are not at high risk of bleeding.[19,20]

Ambulatory Outpatients on Anticancer Treatment

There is considerable variation in the reported rates of thrombosis in patients with cancer receiving chemotherapy because of case selection and study design. Rates ranged from 1% to as high as 20%. The rate is influenced by the tumor burden, as reflected by the stage of the cancer, the treatment received, age, and the performance status of the patient. Venous thrombosis is more common than arterial thrombosis. The rate of thrombosis in patients with early breast cancer receiving adjuvant tamoxifen is ~1.5%.[21] If chemotherapy is added to the tamoxifen, the rate increases significantly; in one study, this was as high as 10%.[22] In one case series in patients with metastatic breast cancer receiving chemotherapy, the rate of thrombosis was 17.6%.[23] The gradient of thrombotic risk reflects increasing tumor burden. Thrombosis is unlikely to be specific to any specific chemotherapeutic drug per se, but is likely as a result of a general effect of this class of drug. Hematopoietic growth factors, for example, erythropoietin, are associated with thrombosis.[24] For example, in one study in women with carcinoma of the cervix receiving cisplatinum and radiotherapy, the addition of erythropoietin increased the thrombotic risk from 2.7% to 22.6%.[25] The anti–vascular endothelial growth factor agent bevacizumab is commonly used in patients with colorectal cancer. In a systematic review of trials of bevacizumab in patients with a range of malignancies, the overall increase in the rate of venous thrombosis was 1.4-fold, and renal cell carcinoma was associated with an almost 3-fold increase in venous thrombosis with bevacizumab.[26] In another analysis of trials with bevacizumab, the rate of arterial thrombosis was increased with bevacizumab compared with control from 1% to 4%.[27] In clinical studies in patients with multiple myeloma, the combination of thalidomide and dexamethasone was associated with a 19% risk of venous thrombosis compared with 6% in patients with dexamethasone alone.[28]

If primary prevention of thrombosis with an antithrombotic agent is being considered in the ambulatory patient with cancer receiving anticancer therapy, the potential magnitude of reduction in thrombosis must be weighed against the potential increase in bleeding. There have been several randomized trials of antithrombotic prophylaxis in ambulatory patients with cancer. Levine and colleagues[29] conducted a randomized trial of low-dose warfarin in 311 women with metastatic breast cancer on first- or second-line chemotherapy. Patients were randomized to 1 mg of warfarin for 6 weeks, and then the warfarin was titrated to an international normalized ratio (INR) of 1.3 to 1.9. This trial was double blinded with the placebo adjusted according to sham INRs. There were 7 events in the placebo group versus only one in the warfarin group (85% risk reduction, *P* = .03). There was no increase in major bleeding. In the PRODIGE trial by Perry and colleagues,[30] patients with newly diagnosed malignant glioma were randomized to dalteparin LMWH5000 IU subcutaneously daily versus placebo subcutaneously daily. Treatment was for at least 6 months. There were 14 events in the placebo group versus 11 in the dalteparin group; the difference was not statistically significant. However, there were 5 major bleeds in the dalteparin group compared with only one in the placebo group. In the FAMOUS trial, 385 patients with solid tumors were randomized to dalteparin or placebo. The rates of venous thrombosis were low in both groups with no statistically significant difference in bleeding.[31] In the TOPIC 1 trial, patients with stage IV breast cancer were randomized to certoparin or placebo. No difference was detected in venous thrombosis or bleeding.[32] On the other hand, in the TOPIC II trial in patients with metastatic non–small-cell lung cancer, certoparin reduced the rate of venous thrombosis from 8.3% to 4.5% (*P* = .07).[32] Finally, in the PROTECT trial, Agnelli and colleagues[33] randomized ambulatory patients with lung, gastrointestinal, pancreatic, breast, ovarian, and head and neck cancers to nadroparin LMWH (n = 779) or placebo (n = 387) for up to 4 months. The rate of VTE was 2% in the nadroparin group versus 3.9% in the placebo group (*P* = .02, one-tailed). There were 5 major bleeds in the LMWH group (0.7%) versus none in the placebo group (*P* = .09). In patients with multiple myeloma, there have been several observational studies of various prophylactic agents. There have been 2 randomized trials. In one trial, 659 patients on thalidomide were randomized to aspirin (ASA), warfarin, or LMWH.[34] The rates of thrombosis were 6.4%, 8.2%, and 5%, respectively. In the second trial, 342 patients treated with lenalidomide-based chemotherapy were randomized to low-dose ASA (100 mg) or enoxaparin LMWH.[35] The thrombosis rate was 2.3% in the ASA group versus 1.2% in the LMWH group. Finally, there has been one randomized double-blind phase II trial of apixaban, an anti-Factor Xa inhibitor, in patients with metastatic cancer on first- and second-line chemotherapy. This pilot study demonstrated that the administration of 3 months of this agent was feasible and safe.[36]

A Cochrane meta-analysis and 2 systemic reviews on the efficacy of antithrombotic agents in the prevention of thrombosis in patients with cancer on chemotherapy have shown an approximate 50% reduction in the risk of thrombosis, but the absolute benefit is modest, that is, less than 5%.[37–39] In summary, the randomized trials of various antithrombotic agents have not supported the use of such agents. Despite the at least 50% relative risk reduction demonstrated with thromboprophylaxis, the baseline rates of thrombosis were considered relatively low and the absolute benefits modest. Most oncologists think that the rates were too low to justify long-term prophylaxis. One strategy would be to identify those patients with a very high risk of thrombosis and then consider prophylaxis in these patients. There have been several studies of various biomarkers, for example, platelet count, D-dimer, p-selectin, F1+2 prothrombin fragments, and TF microparticles to identify high-risk patients. To date, the results of these studies have not been sufficient to be used in routine practice. Another approach that has been proposed to identify patients with cancer at high enough risk to justify anticoagulant prophylaxis is to use a clinical risk assessment model, such as the one developed by Khorana and McCrae.[40]

There are many questions and challenges when considering primary prophylaxis. First, one poses the question, "What is the baseline rate of thrombosis that would warrant prophylaxis?" In general, it is very difficult to predict the rate for an individual patient. Furthermore, the risk changes over time. Although there is level 1 evidence that prophylaxis can reduce the thrombosis in relative terms, the absolute reductions are relatively small. There are several disadvantages to prophylaxis, including bleeding, the necessity to monitor tests of coagulation for warfarin, and subcutaneous injections for LMWH. There is a lack of data on the new antithrombotics in terms of prevention of thrombosis in patients with cancer. Currently, the American Society of Clinical Oncology (ASCO) does not recommend routine prophylaxis for outpatients with cancer, but it may be considered for selected high-risk patients.[20] Patients with multiple myeloma receiving thalidomide- or lenalidomide-based regimens with chemotherapy and/or dexamethasone are recommended to receive prophylaxis with either ASA or LMWH.

Central Vein Catheters

In the late 1990s and early 2000s, there was much enthusiasm concerning the potential for antithrombotic prophylaxis in patients with cancer having central vein catheters. Early descriptive studies reported relatively high rates of catheter vein thrombosis. However, more contemporary randomized trials did not demonstrate the efficacy of thromboprophylaxis in patients with indwelling central vein catheters, and overall, the rates of thrombosis were very low.[41,42] Hence, in the ASCO guidelines, prophylactic use of warfarin or LMWH to prevent catheter-associated thrombosis is not recommended[43] (Case Study 1, available on Expert Consult).

TREATMENT OF VENOUS THROMBOEMBOLISM IN CANCER

Initial Treatment

Patients with proximal DVT are treated with antithrombotic therapy to improve symptoms and to prevent progression and recurrence of the thrombus, PE, and the postphlebitic syndrome. Patients with acute PE are treated with antithrombotic agents to improve symptoms, prevent pulmonary hypertension, and prevent death.

The first randomized trial of antithrombotic therapy was published by Barritt and Jordan[44] in 1960. Patients with PE diagnosed clinically were randomized to heparin 10,000 units every 6 hours for 6 doses plus concurrent nicoumalone for 14 days or no treatment. In the first 35 patients entered, none of the 16 patients on anticoagulant therapy died compared with 5 of 19 control patients ($P = .036$). Five additional control patients had recurrent PE based on clinical diagnosis. There were 3 minor bleeds on anticoagulant therapy. Randomization was discontinued at this point. Following this landmark trial, anticoagulant therapy became standard treatment for patients with acute VTE, and since then, there have been no randomized trials with a no-treatment control.

For many years, patients with acute VTE were hospitalized and received intravenous standard unfractionated heparin for approximately 7 days. This treatment was followed by oral anticoagulant therapy with a vitamin K antagonist for 3 to 6 months. LMWH appeared on the scene in the early 1990s. It had several advantages over unfractionated heparin, including binding less avidly to plasma proteins, platelets, and other cells; dose-independent renal clearance; good availability after subcutaneous injection; and less bleeding in experimental models. Several clinical trials were conducted in hospitalized patients with VTE that demonstrated no loss of efficacy with LMWH in terms of recurrent thromboembolism, and no increased bleeding risk. Hence, there was considerable uptake of LMWH for the treatment of hospitalized patients with VTE. Then, based on the properties of LMWH, a landmark trial conducted by Levine and colleagues[45] demonstrated that patients with acute VTE could be treated safely at home with subcutaneous LMWH and did not have to be admitted to hospital. These results were supported by 2 other randomized trials and subsequently patients with uncomplicated VTE were treated at home with LMWH.[46,47] Given that approximately 20% of the patients in these 3 trials had cancer, the trial results were also applied to patients with cancer with acute VTE. Thus, and consistent with the ASCO 2013 consensus guidelines, LMWH is the preferred anticoagulant as long as the estimated creatinine clearance is >30 mL/min. The alternative for those patients with a lower creatinine clearance is activated partial thromboplastin time (APTT)–adjusted infusion of unfractionated heparin. Fondaparinux remains a choice for patients with a history of heparin-induced thrombocytopenia (Table 11.1). Another important aspect is thrombocytopenia. No anticoagulation should be given if platelet counts are less than 20,000/L. For those patients with platelet counts of 20,000 to 50,000/L, a 50% dose reduction can be considered. If the platelet count is >50,000/L, full-dose anticoagulation can be considered, but other potential risk factors for bleeding need to be considered (Fig. 11.4).

Long-Term Treatment

Patients with cancer with acute VTE are a therapeutic challenge. They have a 2- to 3 fold increased risk of recurrent VTE compared with noncancer patients with VTE, but they have twice the risk of anticoagulant-associated hemorrhage compared with noncancer patients.[3] Oral warfarin therapy is complicated because it is difficult to maintain tight therapeutic control in the patient with cancer because of anorexia, vomiting, and drug interactions. There are often frequent interruptions for thrombocytopenia and procedures, for example, thoracentesis and venous access can often be difficult. Long-term therapy with LMWH does not require laboratory monitoring and can be administered with subcutaneous injections. In the landmark CLOT trial, patients with cancer with acute DVT and PE were randomized to 1 week of dalteparin LMWH followed by 6 months of LMWH compared with 1 week of dalteparin followed by 6 months of vitamin K antagonist oral anticoagulant therapy with a target INR of 2.0 to 3.0.[48] The dose of dalteparin was 200 IU/kg for 1 month, and then this was reduced by ~ 20%–25% for months 2 to 6. The risk of recurrent VTE was reduced from 16% to 8% (P = .0017) in favor of the LMWH, and the rate of major bleeding in the LMWH group was 5.6% compared with 3.6% in the oral anticoagulant group (P = .27). The ASCO 2013 clinical practice guidelines also recommend LMWH as the preferred choice for long-term treatment and for at least 6 months after the initial treatment of acute VTE (see Table 11.1).[20,49]

The results of a recent randomized trial by Lee and colleagues[50] support long-term LMWH therapy in patients with cancer with acute VTE. In the CATCH trial, 900 patients with cancer with acute symptomatic DVT and/or PE were randomized to tinzaparin LMWH (175 IU/kg) once daily for 6 months versus conventional therapy with tinzaparin (175 IU/kg) once daily for 5 to 10 days followed by warfarin at a dose adjusted to maintain the INR within the therapeutic range (2.0–3.0) for 6 months. The cumulative incidence of recurrent thrombosis at 6 months was 7.2% for tinzaparin compared with 10.5% for warfarin (hazard ratio, 0.65 [95% confidence interval, 0.41–1.03], P = .07). There was no difference in bleeding between groups.

The duration of anticoagulant therapy in patients with cancer is an important unanswered question. Clinical practice guidelines recommend continuation for as long as the cancer is active (eg, patient with symptomatic metastatic disease receiving chemotherapy and prolonged immobility; see Table 11.1).[20] However, in truth, these guidelines are based on extrapolations from patients without cancer and clinical experience. In one trial, the presence (or absence) of residual vein thrombosis after 3 months of LMWH treatment in patients with acute VTE was used as guide to continue treatment for a longer duration, but the results were inconclusive.[51,52] Tests such as D-dimer and TF microparticles have also been studied to guide the duration of anticoagulant therapy[53,54] (Case Study 2, available on Expert Consult).

Recurrent Venous Thromboembolism

Recurrent VTE is a difficult problem. There is a lack of evidence to inform what to do in such scenarios, and treatment is often based on clinical expertise and experience. If the patient has been on warfarin, they should be switched to a therapeutic dose of LMWH for a minimum of 4 weeks and then continued at a lower dose of

TABLE 11.1
Consensus guidelines for the treatment of deep venous thrombosis and pulmonary embolism in patients with cancer

	ACCP 2012[23]	NCCN 2011[15]	ASCO 2013[16]
Initial/acute treatment	Not addressed in patients with cancer	LMWH Dalteparin 200 U/kg OD Enoxaparin 1 mg/kg BID Tinzaparin 175 U/kg OD Fondaparinux 5 mg (<50 kg), 7.5 mg (50–100 kg), or 10 mg (>100 kg) OD APTT-adjusted UFH infusion	LMWH is preferred for initial 5–10 d of treatment in patients with a CrCl >30 mL/min
Long-term treatment	LMWH preferred to VKA [2B][a] In patients not treated with LMWH, VKA therapy is preferred to dabigatran or rivaroxaban [2C].[a] Patients receiving extended therapy should continue with the same agent used for the first 3 mo of treatment [2C][a]	LMWH is preferred for first 6 mo as monotherapy without warfarin in patients with proximal DVT or PE and metastatic or advanced cancer Warfarin 2.5–5 mg every day initially with subsequent dosing based on INR value targeted at 2–3	LMWH is preferred for long-term therapy VKAs (target INR, 2–3) are acceptable for long-term therapy it LMWH is not available
Duration of treatment	Extended anticoagulant therapy is preferred to 3 mo of treatment [2B][a]	Minimum 3 mo Indefinite anticoagulant if active cancer or persistent risk factors	At least 6-mo duration Extended anticoagulation with LMWH or VKA may be considered beyond 6 mo for patients with metastatic disease or patients who are receiving chemotherapy

Abbreviations: ACCP, American College of Chest Physicians; BID, twice-daily dosing; NCCN, National Comprehensive Cancer Network; OD, once-daily dosing.

[a] ACCP adaptation of the Grades of Recommendation, Assessment, Development, and Evaluation (GRADE) Working Group evidence-based recommendations: 2B, weak recommendation, moderate-quality evidence; 2C, weak recommendation, low- or very-low-quality evidence.[18]

From Lee AY, Peterson EA. Treatment of cancer-associated thrombosis. Blood 2013;122(14):2311; with permission.

LMWH. If the recurrence occurs while on LMWH, consideration should be given to raising the dose of LMWH by 25%.[55] Others have suggested to guide LMWH dosing by anti-Xa levels (Fig. 11.5), but validating trials for this strategy are missing at this point.

Direct Oral Anticoagulants

In recent years, there has been much research on the use of new direct oral thrombin inhibitors (DOACs), for example, dabigatran, and new direct oral antifactor Xa inhibitors, for example, rivaroxaban, apixaban. They have been extensively studied in patients with atrial fibrillation to prevent embolic stroke and in postoperative patients to prevent VTE. There have also been several trials evaluating DOACs for the treatment of acute VTE, which have shown that these agents are noninferior to warfarin.[56,57] However, these trials had a limited number of patients with cancer, and the patients with cancer included were often patients with a remote history of cancer and not active cancer as was in the trials of LMWH versus warfarin.[58] Furthermore, novel oral anticoagulants (NOACs) have interactions with several anticancer agents (Table 11.2). Hence, LMWH remains the standard of care for the treatment of acute VTE in the patient with cancer.[59]

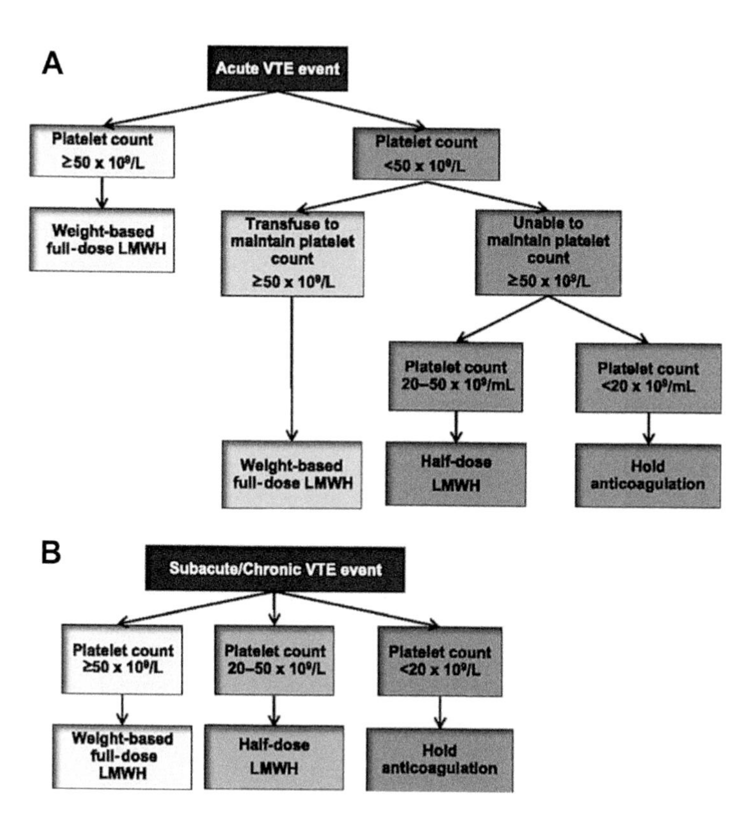

Fig. 11.4 Management algorithm of VTE in patients with cancer and thrombocytopenia (recommended). Management of acute VTE (<1 month) and subacute or chronic VTE (≥1 month) are outlined in (*A*) and (*B*), respectively. (*From* Lee AY, Peterson EA. Treatment of cancer-associated thrombosis. Blood 2013;122(14):2313; with permission.)

UNSUSPECTED (INCIDENTAL) PULMONARY EMBOLISM

Over the past decade, there has been a significant increase in the number of patients receiving chemotherapy and targeted molecular agents in part due to the aging population and the increasing number of drugs available to treat many cancers. For example, patients with non–small-cell lung cancer (one of the most common cancers) are now routinely treated with first- and second-line chemotherapy regimens, and subgroups of non–small-cell lung cancer are treated with targeted agents such as tyrosine kinase inhibitors. In parallel with the increasing use of systemic treatments for cancer, there has been the increasing use of contrast-enhanced CT imaging to stage cancer and assess its response to treatment. Contrast-enhanced CT detects incidental, or what is commonly referred to as "unsuspected" PE. The incidence of unsuspected PE is reported to be between 1% and 5% of patients with cancer.[60] The variation in the incidence is a reflection of the type and quality of CT, the tumor type, and the study design. Most studies are retrospective series that come from the radiology literature.[60] It is unclear whether unsuspected PE detected on CT scan has the same natural history as symptomatic PE. One retrospective study reported that a significant proportion of these patients in fact had symptoms compatible with PE, for example, shortness of breath and fatigue. However, this study may have suffered from bias.

There are no clinical trials evaluating anticoagulant therapy in patients with cancer with incidental PE. Hence, results of trials in patients with symptomatic PE have been extrapolated to this patient group. Accordingly, most patients are treated the same way as a patient with cancer with symptomatic PE, that is, long-term LMWH. The studies that have compared the outcome of patients with symptomatic PE with those of unsuspected PE have shown similar rates of recurrent thromboembolism and mortality.[61] Even though there are limited prospective data on this patient group, physicians are unwilling to withhold anticoagulant therapy. An area of controversy and interest is whether it is reasonable to withhold anticoagulant therapy in patients with unsuspected PE where the abnormality is in an isolated subsegmental artery, that is, a small clot in a peripheral artery. There are reports of withholding therapy in such patients, and there are reports whereby initial therapy has been withheld and the patient has developed recurrent thromboembolism. Hence, in patients with isolated subsegmental

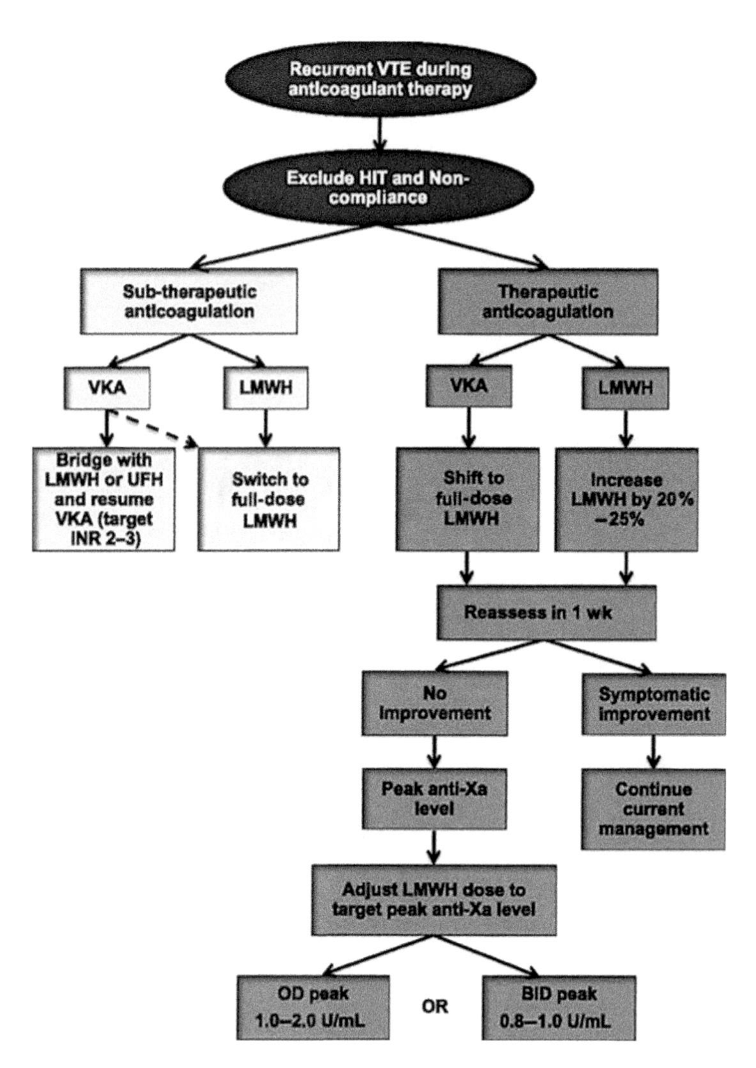

Fig. 11.5 Management algorithm of recurrent VTE in patients with cancer. BID, twice-daily dosing; HIT, heparin induced thrombocytopenia; OD, once-daily dosing; UFH, unfractionated heparin; VKA, vitamin K antagonist. (*From* Lee AY, Peterson EA. Treatment of cancer-associated thrombosis. Blood 2013;122(14):2313; with permission.)

TABLE 11.2
Interactions between antineoplastic gents and immunosuppressants with novel oral anticoagulants based on known metabolic pathway activity

Interaction Effect[a]	Dabigatran P-Glycoprotein	Rivaroxaban P-Glycoprotein CYP3A4	Apixaban P-Glycoprotein CYP3A4
Increases NOAC plasma levels[b]	Cyclosporine Tacrolimus Tamoxifen Lapatinib Nilotinib Sunitinib	Cyclosporine Tacrolimus Tamoxifen Lapatinib Nilotinib Sunitinib Imatinib	Cyclosporine Tacrolimus Tamoxifen Lapatinb Nilotinib Sunitinib Imatinib
Reduces NOAC plasma levels[c]	Dexamethasone Doxorubicin Vinblastine	Dexamethasone Doxorubicin Vinblastine	Dexamethasone Doxorubicin Vinblastine

Abbreviation: CYP3A4, cytochrome P450 3A4.

[a] Clinicians should consult with the pharmacist to determine if these and other drug interactions exist when NOACs are being considered.

[b] Drugs that inhibit P-glycoprotein transport or CYP3A4 pathway can increase NOAC levels.

[c] Drugs that induce P-glycoprotein transport or CYP3A4 pathway can lower NOAC levels.

From Lee AY, Peterson EA. Treatment of cancer-associated thrombosis. Blood 2013;122(14):2313; with permission.

PE, treatment should be individualized based on a discussion between the physician and patient (Case Study 3, available on Expert Consult).

SUMMARY

There has been much progress in the clinical management of the patient with cancer with VTE. Nonetheless, there is still much more work to be done. Despite the best treatment regimens with LMWH, still approximately 10% of patients with VTE will develop recurrence. This rate is still too high. As we look to the future with precision medicine, can the advances in molecular biology lead to the development of improved antithrombotic treatments to eliminate the risk of recurrence or can better tests be developed to better predict those patients with cancer who will develop VTE? Only time will tell.

We present one final case to illustrate the increasingly complex environment of managing VTE in patients with cancer because new therapeutic options lead to prolongation of life for many patients with advanced malignant disease (Case Study 4, available on Expert Consult).

REFERENCES

1. Trousseau A. Phlegmasia alba dolens (lecture XCV). In: Cormick JR, Bazre PV, trans. Lectures on Clinical Medicine. Philadelphia:Lindsay and Blakiston; 1873.
2. Varki A. Trousseau's syndrome: multiple definitions and multiple mechanisms. Blood 2007;110:1723–9.
3. Prandoni P, Lensing AWA, Piccioli A, et al. Recurrent venous thromboembolism and bleeding complications during anticoagulant treatment in patients with cancer and venous thrombosis. Blood 2002;100:3484–8.
4. Kuderer N, Ortel TL, Francis C. Impact of venous thromboembolism and anticoagulation on cancer and cancer survival. J Clin Oncol 2009;27:4902–11.
5. Chung I, Lip GY. Virchow's triad revisited: blood constituents. Pathophysiol Haemost Thromb 2003;33(5–6):449–54.
6. Boccacio C, Comoglio P. Genetic link between cancer and thrombosis. J Clin Oncol 2009;27:4827–33.
7. Kasthuri RS, Taubman MB, Mackman N. Role of tissue factor. J Clin Oncol 2009;27:4834–8.
8. Khorana A, Connolly GC. Assessing risk of venous thromboembolism in the patient with cancer. J Clin Oncol 2009;27:4839–47.
9. Heit JA, O'Fallon W, Petterson TM, et al. Relative impact of risk factors for deep vein thrombosis and pulmonary embolism: a population-based study. Arch Intern Med 2002;162(11):1245–8.
10. Lee AYY. Thrombosis and cancer: the role of screening for occult cancer and recognizing the underlying biological mechanisms. Hematology Am Soc Hematol Educ Program 2006;438–43.
11. Piccioli A, Lensing AW, Prins MH, et al. Extensive screening for occult malignant disease in idiopathic venous thromboembolism: a prospective randomized clinical trial. J Thromb Haemost 2004;2:884–9.
12. Carrier M, Lazo-Langner A, Shivakumar S, et al. Screening for occult cancer in unprovoked venous thromboembolism. N Engl J Med 2015;373:697–704.
13. Robertson L, Yeoh SE, Stansby G, et al. Effect of testing for cancer on cancer- and venous thromboembolism (VTE)-related mortality and morbidity in patients with unprovoked VTE. Cochrane Database Syst Rev 2015;(3):CD010837.
14. Imberti D, Agnelli G, Ageno W, et al. Characteristics and management of cancer-associated acute venous thromboembolism: findings from the MASTER Registry. Haematologica 2008;93:273–8.
15. Zierler BK. Ultrasonography and diagnosis of venous thromboembolism. Circulation 2004;109(Suppl I):I-9–14.
16. Wells PS, Anderson DR, Bormanis J, et al. Value of assessment of pretest probability of deep-vein thrombosis in clinical management. Lancet 1997;350(9094):1795–8.
17. Kearon C, Akl EA, Comerota AJ, et al, American College of Chest Physicians. Antithrombotic therapy for VTE disease: Antithrombotic Therapy and Prevention of Thrombosis, 9th ed: American College of Chest Physicians Evidence-Based Clinical Practice Guidelines. Chest 2012;141(2 Suppl):e419S–94S.
18. Kakkar AJ. Prevention of venous thromboembolism in the cancer surgical patient. J Clin Oncol 2009;27:4881–4.
19. Francis CW. Prevention of venous thromboembolism in hospitalized patients with cancer. J Clin Oncol 2009;27:4874–80.
20. Lyman GH, Bohlke K, Khorana AA, et al. Venous thromboembolism prophylaxis and treatment in patients with cancer: American Society of Clinical Oncology Clinical Practice Guideline Update 2014. J Clin Oncol 2015;33:654–6.
21. Fisher B, Costantino J, Redmond C, et al. A randomized clinical trial evaluating tamoxifen in the treatment of patients with node-negative breast cancer who have estrogen-receptor–positive tumors. N Engl J Med 1989;320:479–84.
22. Pritchard KI, Paterson AH, Paul NA, et al. Increased thromboembolic complications with concurrent tamoxifen and chemotherapy in a randomized trial of adjuvant therapy for women with breast cancer: National Cancer Institute of Canada Clinical Trials Group Breast Cancer Site Group. J Clin Oncol 1996;14:2731–7.

23. Goodnough LT, Saito H, Manni A, et al. Increased incidence of thromboembolism in stage IV breast cancer patients treated with a five-drug chemotherapy regimen. A study of 159 patients. Cancer 1984;54(7):1264–8.
24. Bohlius J, Wilson J, Seidenfeld J, et al. Recombinant human erythropoietins and cancer patients: updated meta-analysis of 57 studies including 9353 patients. J Natl Cancer Inst 2006;98:708–14.
25. Wun T, Law L, Harvey D, et al. Increased incidence of symptomatic venous thrombosis in patients with cervical carcinoma treated with concurrent chemotherapy, radiation, and erythropoietin. Cancer 2003;98:1514–20.
26. Nalluri SR, Chu D, Keresztes R, et al. Risk of venous thromboembolism with the angiogenesis inhibitor bevacizumab in cancer patients: a meta-analysis. JAMA 2008;300:2277–85.
27. Scappaticci FA, Skillings JR, Holden SN, et al. Arterial thromboembolic events in patients with metastatic carcinoma treated with chemotherapy and bevacizumab. J Natl Cancer Inst 2007;99:1232–9.
28. Cavo M, Zamagni E, Tosi P, et al. First-line therapy with thalidomide and dexamethasone in preparation for autologous stem cell transplantation for multiple myeloma. Haematologica 2004;89:826–31.
29. Levine M, Hirsh J, Gent M, et al. Double-blind randomised trial of a very-low-dose warfarin for prevention of thromboembolism in stage IV breast cancer. Lancet 1994;343:886–9.
30. Perry JR, Julian JA, Laperriere NJ, et al. PRODIGE: a randomized placebo-controlled trial of dalteparin low-molecular-weight heparin thromboprophylaxis in patients with newly diagnosed malignant glioma. J Thromb Haemost 2010;8:1959–65.
31. Kakkar AK, Levine MN, Kadziola Z, et al. Low molecular weight heparin, therapy with dalteparin, and survival in advanced cancer: the fragmin advanced malignancy outcome study (FAMOUS). J Clin Oncol 2004;22:1944–8.
32. Haas SK, Freund M, Heigener D, et al. Low molecular-weight heparin versus placebo for the prevention of venous thromboembolism in metastatic breast cancer or stage III/IV lung cancer. Clin Appl Thromb Hemost 2012;18:159–65.
33. Agnelli G, Gussoni G, Bianchini C, et al. Nadroparin for the prevention of thromboembolic events in ambulatory patients with metastatic or locally advanced solid cancer receiving chemotherapy: a randomised, placebo-controlled, double-blind study. Lancet Oncol 2009;10:943–9.
34. Palumbo A, Cavo M, Bringhen S, et al. Aspirin, warfarin, or enoxaparin thromboprophylaxis in patients with multiple myeloma treated with thalidomide: a phase III, open-label, randomized trial. J Clin Oncol 2011;29:986–93.
35. Larocca A, Cavallo F, Bringhen S, et al. Aspirin or enoxaparin thromboprophylaxis for patients with newly diagnosed multiple myeloma treated with lenalidomide. Blood 2012;119:933–9.
36. Levine MN, Gu C, Liebman HA, et al. A randomized phase II trial of apixaban for the prevention of thromboembolism in patients with metastatic cancer. J Thromb Haemost 2012;10:807–14.
37. Di Nisio M, Porreca E, Ferrante N, et al. Primary prophylaxis for venous thromboembolism in ambulatory cancer patients receiving chemotherapy. Cochrane Database Syst Rev 2012;(2):CD008500.
38. Verso M, Gussoni G, Agnelli G. Prevention of venous thromboembolism in patients with advanced lung cancer receiving chemotherapy: a combined analysis of the PROTECHT and TOPIC-2 studies. J Thromb Haemost 2010;8:1649–51.
39. Kuderer NM, Ortel TL, Khorana AA, et al. Low-molecular-weight heparin for venous thromboprophylaxis in ambulatory cancer patients: a systematic review meta-analysis of randomized controlled trials. Blood (ASH Annual Meeting Abstracts) 2009;114:490.
40. Khorana AA, McCrae KR. Risk stratification strategies for cancer-associated thrombosis: an update. Thromb Res 2014;133(Suppl 2):S35–8.
41. Verso M, Agnelli G, Bertoglio S, et al. Enoxaparin for the prevention of venous thromboembolism associated with central vein catheter: a double-blind, placebo-controlled, randomized study in cancer patients. J Clin Oncol 2005;23:4057–62.
42. Couban S, Goodyear M, Burnell M, et al. Randomized placebo-controlled study of low-dose warfarin for the prevention of central venous catheter-associated thrombosis in patients with cancer. J Clin Oncol 2005;23:4063–9.
43. Schiffer CA, Mangu PB, Wade JC, et al. Central venous catheter care for the patient with cancer: American Society of Clinical Oncology Clinical Practice Guideline. J Clin Oncol 2013;31:1357–70.
44. Barritt DW, Jordan SC. Anticoagulant drugs in the treatment of pulmonary embolism. A controlled trial. Lancet 1960;1(7138):1309–12.
45. Levine M, Gent M, Hirsh J, et al. A comparison of low-molecular-weight heparin administered primarily at home with unfractionated heparin administered in the hospital for proximal deep-vein thrombosis. N Engl J Med 1996;334:677–81.
46. Koopman MMW, Prandoni P, Piovella F, et al. Treatment of venous thrombosis with intravenous unfractionated heparin administered in the hospital as compared with subcutaneous low-molecular-weight heparin administered at home. N Engl J Med 1996;334:682–7.
47. Low-molecular-weight heparin in the treatment of patients with venous thromboembolism. The Columbus Investigators. N Engl J Med 1997;337:657–62.

48. Lee AY, Levine MN, Baker RI, et al. Low-molecular-weight heparin versus a coumarin for the prevention of recurrent venous thromboembolism in patients with cancer. N Engl J Med 2003;349:146–53.
49. Mandala M, Falanga A, Roila F, on behalf of the ESMO Guidelines Working Group. Management of venous thromboembolism (VTE) in cancer patients: ESMO Clinical Practice Guidelines. Ann Oncol 2011;22(Suppl 6):vi85–92.
50. Lee AYY, Kamphuisen PW, Meyer G, et al. Tinzaparin vs warfarin for treatment of acute venous thromboembolism in patients with active cancer. A randomized clinical trial. JAMA 2015;314(7):677–86.
51. Napolitano M, Saccullo G, Malato A, et al. Optimal duration of low molecular weight heparin for the treatment of cancer-related deep vein thrombosis: the Cancer-DACUS Study. J Clin Oncol 2014;32:3607–12.
52. Rana P, Levine MN. How long to treat acute venous thrombosis in cancer: can treatment be personalized? J Clin Oncol 2014;32:3586–7.
53. Palareti G, Cosmi B, Legnani C, et al. D-Dimer testing to determine the duration of anticoagulation therapy. N Engl J Med 2006;355:1780–9.
54. Zwicker JI, Trenor CC 3rd, Furie BC. Tissue factor–bearing microparticles and thrombus formation. Arterioscler Thromb Vasc Biol 2011;31:728–33.
55. Carrier M, Lazo–Langner A, Shivakumar S, et al. Clinical challenges in patients with cancer-associated thrombosis: Canadian expert consensus recommendations. Curr Oncol 2015;22:49–59.
56. The EINSTEIN Investigators. Oral rivaroxaban for symptomatic venous thromboembolism. N Engl J Med 2010;363:2499–510.
57. The EINSTEIN–PE Investigators. Oral rivaroxaban for the treatment of symptomatic pulmonary embolism. N Engl J Med 2012;366:1287–97.
58. Prins M, Lensing A, Brighton TA. Oral rivaroxaban versus enoxaparin with vitamin K antagonist for the treatment of symptomatic venous thromboembolism in patients with cancer (EINSTEIN-DVT and EINSTEIN-PE): a pooled subgroup analysis of two randomised controlled trials. Lancet Haematol 2014;1(1):e37–46.
59. Levine MN, Parpia S, Julian J. Treating clots in cancer: moving closer to an answer? Lancet Haematol 2014;1(1):e6–7.
60. van Esa N, Blekera SM, Di Nisio M. Cancer-associated unsuspected pulmonary embolism. Thromb Res 2014;133(Suppl 2):S172–8.
61. Den Exter PL, Hooijer J, Dekkers OM, et al. Risk of recurrent venous thromboembolism and mortality in patients with cancer incidentally diagnosed with pulmonary embolism: a comparison with symptomatic patients. J Clin Oncol 2011;29:2405–9.

CHAPTER 12

Pericardial Disease and Effusion

Dor Lotan, MD[a,*], Yishay Wasserstrum, MD[a], Massimo Imazio, MD, FESC[b], Yehuda Adler, MD, MHA[a]

PERICARDIAL DISEASE IN THE ONCOLOGIC PATIENT: AN OVERVIEW

The pericardium is a double-wall sac consisting of the outer, fibrous pericardium and the inner, serous or visceral pericardium, also known as the epicardium, which comes into contact with the myocardium. The roots of the aorta and pulmonary artery are enclosed within the pericardial sac. The pericardium encloses the pericardial cavity and prevents friction between the heart and the surrounding structures, acts as a mechanical and immunologic barrier, and limits distension of the heart, which maintains a relatively fixed maximal heart volume. In normal hearts, the pericardial space contains only a small amount of fluid, usually 20 to 50 mL, which is produced by the visceral pericardium and acts as a lubricant.

Pericardial involvement in the setting of malignancy occurs in various ways. Pericarditis and malignant pericardial effusion can be the first manifestations of cancer.[1] It can also be the consequence of radiation therapy, chemotherapy, or opportunistic infections. History, cardiac imaging, analysis of the pericardial fluid, and eventually biopsies aid in the (differential) diagnosis. The greatest functional/hemodynamic concerns relate to malignant pericardial effusions, when large in size and associated with the risk of imminent tamponade, and the development of pericardial constriction.[2,3]

Primary neoplasms of the pericardium are very rare[2,3] and are either benign (eg, lipomas, fibromas) or malignant (mainly mesothelioma, fibrosarcoma). Cardiac metastases are noted in 1.5% to 20% of autopsies in patients with cancer.[4] Most commonly, they are seen in patients with melanoma, lymphoma, and leukemia, carcinoma of the lung, breast, and esophagus. Dissemination to the heart may occur by hematologic or lymphatic pathways, transvenous extension, or direct invasion. Cardiac metastatic disease can involve all layers of the heart but most often the pericardium. Importantly, most secondary cardiac tumors do not become clinically significant, and more than 90% are discovered postmortem.[4,5] In cases of symptomatic pericardial effusion, patients are to be evaluated for the presence of tamponade and need for pericardiocentesis. The cause of the pericardial effusion needs to be defined as much as possible given the clinical implication. If, for instance, it were to be the consequence of a drug effect, stopping the offending drug would be curative. On the other hand, if it were to be malignant in nature, this would be considered a very poor prognostic sign, and palliative measures targeted at symptom reduction and prevention of recurrences would be the appropriate course of action.

PERICARDITIS AND PERICARDIAL EFFUSION

Pericarditis is the most common disease of the pericardium encountered in clinical practice, representing approximately 5% of presentations to the emergency department for nonischemic chest pain.[6] Limited epidemiologic data point out an incidence of acute pericarditis of 27.7 cases per 100,000 of the population per year in an urban area of Italy.[7] In North America and Western Europe, most cases (80%–85%) of acute pericarditis are idiopathic or presumed viral cause.[8–10] Major nonidiopathic causes include tuberculosis, neoplasia, and systemic (generally autoimmune) disease; the full list is detailed in Box 12.1.

[a] The Chaim Sheba Medical Center, Tel Hashomer, The Sackler School of Medicine, Tel Aviv University, Tel Aviv, Israel; [b] Cardiology Department, Maria Vittoria Hospital, and Department of Public Health and Pediatrics, University of Torino, Via Cibrario, 72, 10144 Torino, Italy
* Corresponding author.
E-mail address: Dor.lotan@sheba.health.gov.il

BOX 12.1
Causes of pericardial diseases

Neoplastic: Primary tumors, metastases, amyloidosis (see Box 12.2)

Infectious causes:

- Viral: Enteroviruses (coxsackieviruses, echoviruses), herpesviruses (EBV, CMV, HHV-6), adenoviruses, parvovirus B19
- Bacterial:
  - Mycobacterium tuberculosis
  - Other rare organisms: *Coxiella burnetii*, *Borrelia burgdorferi*, rarely: *Pneumococcus* spp, *Meningococcus* spp, *Gonococcus* spp, *Streptococcus* spp, *Staphylococcus* spp, *Haemophilus* spp, *Chlamydia* spp, *Mycoplasma* spp, *Legionella* spp, *Leptospira* spp, *Listeria* spp, *Providencia stuartii*
- Fungal (very rare): *Histoplasma* spp,[a] *Aspergillus* spp, *Blastomyces* spp, *Candida* spp[b]
- Parasitic (very rare): *Echinococcus* spp, *Toxoplasma* spp

Metabolic: Uremia, myxoedema, anorexia nervosa

Traumatic and iatrogenic:

- Early onset: Thoracic trauma, esophageal perforation, radiation injury
- Late-onset pericardial injury syndromes: Postmyocardial infarction syndrome, postpericardiotomy syndrome, posttraumatic

Cardiovascular: Aortic dissection, pulmonary arterial hypertension, and chronic heart failure

Rheumatic: Systemic lupus erythematosus, Sjögren syndrome, rheumatoid arthritis, scleroderma, Churg-Strauss syndrome, Horton disease, Takayasu disease, Behçet syndrome, sarcoidosis, familial Mediterranean fever, inflammatory bowel disease, adult Still disease

Drug-related:

- Antineoplastic drugs (see Box 12.2)
- Amiodarone, methysergide, mesalazine, clozapine, minoxidil, dantrolene, practolol, phenylbutazone, thiazides, streptomycin, thiouracils, streptokinase, p-aminosalicylic acid, sulfadrugs, cyclosporine, bromocriptine, several vaccines, GM-CSF, anti-TNF agents
- Lupuslike syndrome: Procainamide, hydralazine, methyldopa, isoniazid, phenytoin

[a] More likely in immunocompetent patients.
[b] More likely in immunocompromised patients.

Abbreviations: CMV, cytomegalovirus; EBV, Epstein-Barr virus; GM-CSF, granulocyte-macrophage colony-stimulating factor; HHV, human herpesvirus; spp, species; TNF, tumor necrosis factor.

From LeWinter MM, Hopkins WE. Pericardial diseases. In: Mann DL, ed. Braunwald's heart disease: a textbook of cardiovascular medicine. 10th edition. Philadelphia: Elsevier Saunders, 2015; with permission.

Acute pericarditis is an inflammatory pericardial syndrome with or without pericardial effusion. The clinical diagnosis made by 2 of 4 simple criteria: (1) typical chest pain (sharp and pleuritic in character, improved by sitting up and leaning forward); (2) pericardial friction rub (superficial scratchy or squeaking sound, best heard with the diaphragm of the stethoscope over the left sternal border); (3) widespread ST-segment elevation (J-point elevation usually >25% of the height of the T-wave peak) or PR depression in the acute phase (Fig. 12.1); and (4) pericardial effusion (Fig. 12.2). Additional signs and symptoms may be present according to the underlying cause or systemic disease.

Among patients presenting with pericarditis or a small pericardial effusion without known malignancy, the likelihood of finding previously undiagnosed cancer is between 4% and 7%.[1] A detailed evaluation for occult malignancy should generally be reserved for patients who have persistent pericarditis that is unresponsive to anti-inflammatory therapy, and for those who present with large pericardial effusion or cardiac tamponade.[11,12] When considering acute pericarditis in a patient with malignancy, it is important to investigate the underlying cause and not automatically assume its malignant nature. Because of the often immune-compromised state and recurrent hospital visits, these patients are at risk of opportunistic and nonopportunistic infections. Noninfectious pericarditis in patients with cancer can still be idiopathic, or the consequence of primary or metastatic tumors, or their

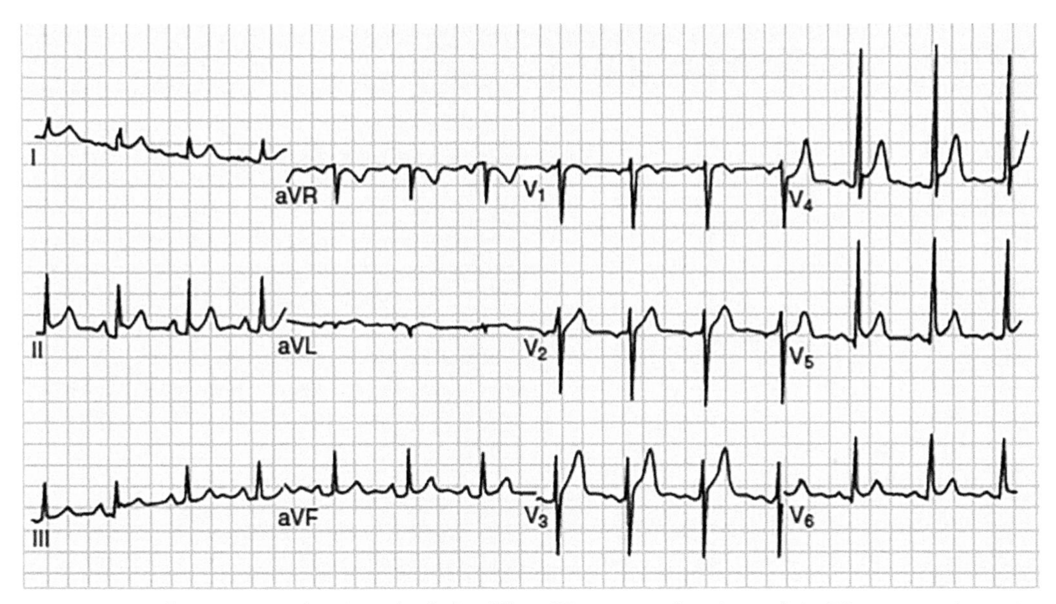

Fig. 12.1 ECG of acute pericarditis. Note both the diffuse ST-segment elevation and the PR-segment depression. (*From* LeWinter MM, Hopkins WE. Pericardial diseases. In: Mann DL, ed. Braunwald's heart disease: a textbook of cardiovascular medicine. 10th edition. Philadelphia: Elsevier Saunders, 2015; with permission.)

treatment (chemotherapy and radiation therapy) (Box 12.2).

Neoplastic pericardial disease may be considered in patients with cancer based on an incidental finding on routine chest radiograph or computed tomographic (CT) imaging. The most frequent symptoms of pleuritic chest pain, dyspnea, tachycardia are not specific in patients with cancer because they may be caused by anemia, pleural effusion, or pulmonary lymphangitis. Compared with other forms of pericarditis, a large pericardial effusion and the appearance of signs of cardiac tamponade are more frequent in neoplastic pericardial disease. This may be explained by the fact that most pericardial metastases follow a lymphatic retrograde flow, and the engorged vessels cannot drain the effusion, leading to the accumulation of a large amount of pericardial fluid in a few days, which can result in cardiac tamponade, cardiovascular collapse, and death.[13–15]

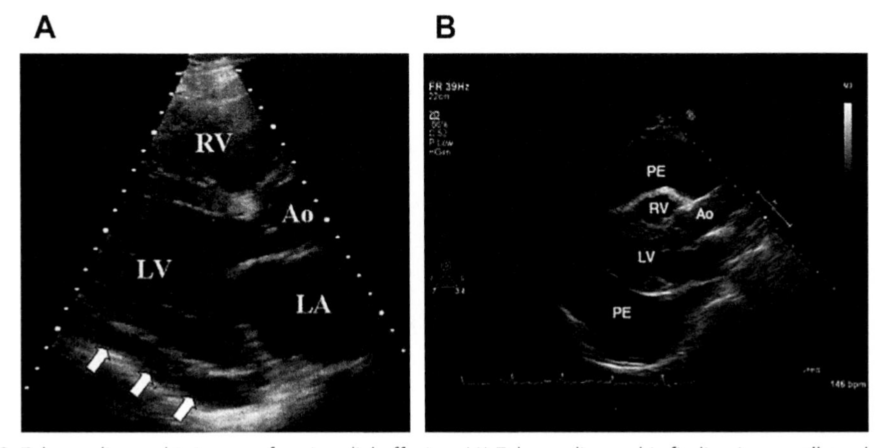

Fig. 12.2 Echocardiographic image of pericardial effusion. (*A*) Echocardiographic finding in a small moderate pericardial effusion (*white arrows*). Long-axis parasternal view. (*B*) Two-dimensional echocardiogram of a large, circumferential pericardial effusion (PE). Ao, aortic root; LA, left atrium; LV, left ventricle; RV, right ventricle. (*From* [*A*] Maisch B, Ristic AD. Pericardial diseases. In: Vincent JL, Abraham E, Moore FA. Textbook of critical care. 6th edition. Philadelphia: Elsevier Saunders, 2011; with permission; and *From* [*B*] Kabbani SS, LeWinter M. Cardiac constriction and restriction. In: Crawford MH, DiMarco JP, editors. Cardiology. St Louis (MO): CV Mosby; 2001. p. 5, 15.5; with permission.)

BOX 12.2
Causes of pericarditis in patients with cancer

- Infection
  - Nonopportunistic
  - Opportunistic
- Neoplasm
  - Primary
    - Mesothelioma
    - Synovial pericardial sarcoma
  - Metastatic
    - Melanoma
    - Lymphoma and leukemia
    - Carcinoma of lung, breast, and esophagus
  - Secondary to nonpericardial cardiac tumors
- Radiation
  - Radiation therapy early, during, or even very late after irradiation
- Systemic treatments
  - Anthracycline
    - Daunorubicin
    - Doxorubicin
  - Nonanthracycline
    - 5-Fluorouracil
    - All-*trans*-retinoic acid
    - Arsenic trioxide
    - Bleomycin
    - Busulphan
    - Cylclophosphamide
    - Cylosporine
    - Cytarabine
    - Ifosfamide
    - Fluorouracil
  - Tyrosine-kinase inhibitors
    - Bosutinib
    - Dasatinib
    - Imatinib
    - Nilotinib
- Idiopathic

From LeWinter MM, Hopkins WE. Pericardial diseases. In: Mann DL, ed. Braunwald's heart disease: a textbook of cardiovascular medicine. 10th edition. Philadelphia: Elsevier Saunders, 2015; with permission.

MALIGNANT PERICARDIAL EFFUSION

The most common malignancies associated with pericardial effusions are lung and breast cancer, adenocarcinoma, esophageal squamous cell carcinoma, melanoma, thymic carcinoma, and hematologic malignancies. Effusion can also be rarely seen in germ cell, renal, bladder malignancy, and Ewing sarcoma.[16] Primary neoplasms of the pericardium are less common. Pericardial effusion may be the first manifestation of the disease, and thus, malignancy should be excluded in every case of acute pericardial disease with rapidly increasing pericardial effusion, cardiac tamponade, or incessant or recurrent course. The rapid diagnosis and differentiation of malignant pericardial effusion are therefore of clinical relevance.

In the patient with cancer, pericardial effusion may develop through 3 main mechanisms.[17] These mechanisms are as follows:

1. Spread of the underlying malignancy,
2. Treatment complication,
3. Opportunistic infection.

With regards to the first mechanism, pericardial effusion may arise by direct extension of regional cancers (lung, breast, esophageal carcinoma) to the parietal pericardium with or without visceral involvement, lymphatic or hematogeneous spread of systemic and distant cancers (leukemia, lymphoma, Kaposi sarcoma, and melanoma), or because of obstruction to the lymphatic drainage, as seen with enlarged mediastinal lymph nodes.

Second, several drugs used in oncology patients are known to have the potential of causing cardiac adverse events. Radiation therapy, which is most commonly used in Hodgkin lymphoma as well as breast cancer, upper and lower respiratory tract cancers, thymomas, and esophageal and gastric lesions, can damage all cardiac structures (valves, myocardium, and coronary arteries). Radiation therapy most commonly causes pericardial effusion, depending on the patient's clinical condition, irradiation modality, and the dose used. Pericardial effusion related to radiation can present an acute, late, and very late consequence of irradiation from 2 months to 12 years between radiation therapies and the onset of symptoms.[18,19]

Third, in immunocompromised oncology patients, pericardial disease must be caused by a different opportunistic infection of viral (eg, CMV), bacterial (even tuberculosis), fungal (eg, Aspergillus or Candida), or autoimmune origin.[17]

Clinical Signs and Symptoms

Malignant pericardial effusion can lead to various adverse events depending on the severity of pericardial irritation and extent of fluid accumulation in the pericardial space. Pleuritic chest discomfort is the most characteristic, dyspnea the most common, and tachycardia, hypotension, and cardiogenic shock the most concerning presentations. Other symptoms include cough, fatigue, hoarseness from recurrent laryngeal nerve compression, and hiccups from phrenic nerve compression. Some patients, however, remain undiagnosed until death.

Diagnosis

The diagnosis of pericardial effusion can be challenging, especially in the asymptomatic patient, and requires a high level of suspicion. The approach to a newly discovered pericardial effusion in patients with a known malignancy should take into account the possibility of different causes even in the setting of known malignancy, as previously discussed, and management should be guided accordingly (Fig. 12.3). Establishing the cause of effusion, when possible, may be cardinal in guiding both short-term and long-term management. Current guidelines advocate for diagnostic

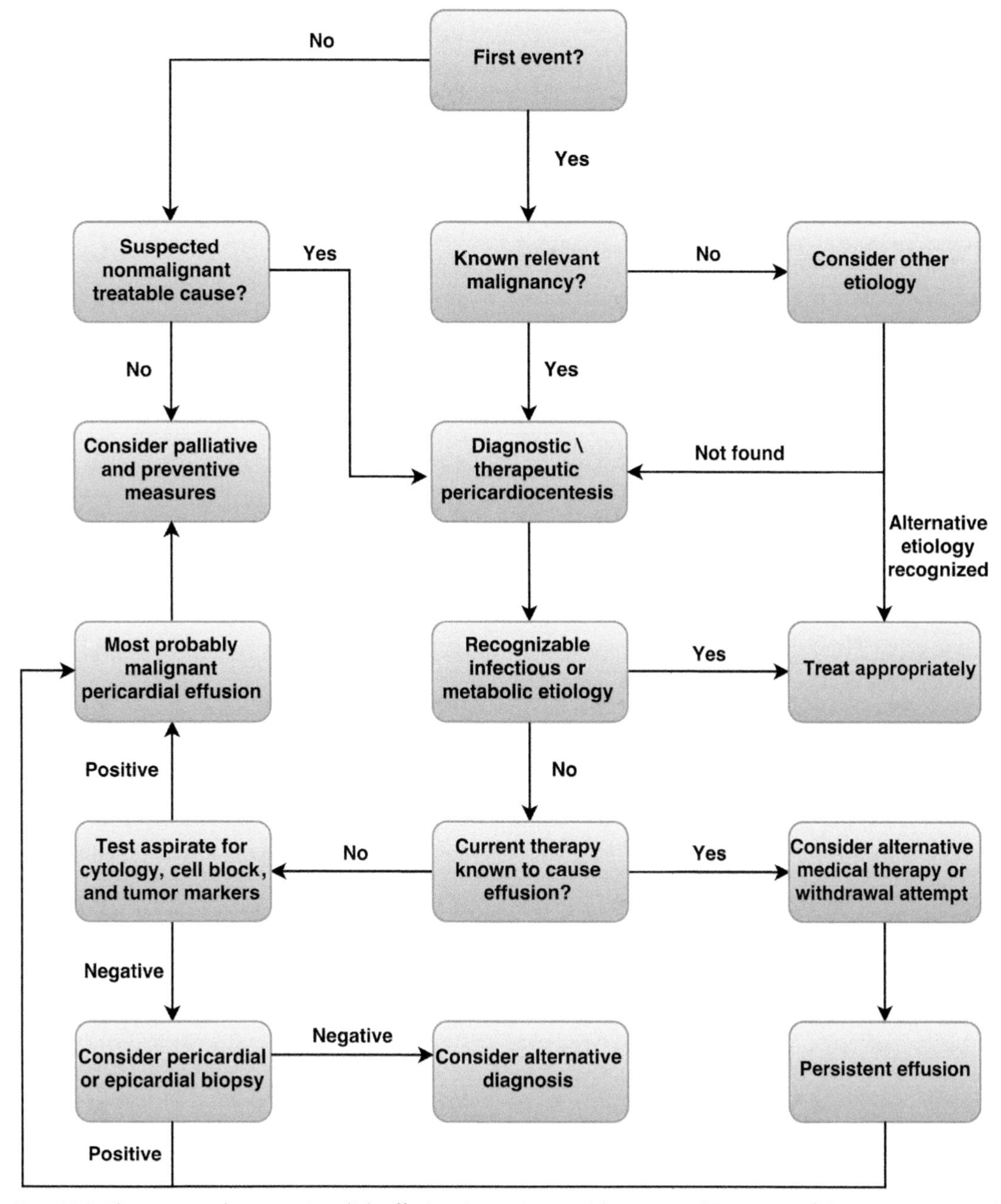

Fig. 12.3 The approach to pericardial effusion in patients with cancer. (*Courtesy of* D. Lotan, MD and Y. Wasserstrum MD; all rights reserved.)

pericardiocentesis when suspecting a neoplastic, purulent, or tuberculous underlying cause.[20–22]

Electrocardiographic Finding

A normal electrocardiography (ECG) does not exclude the presence of a pericardial effusion. The typical ECG findings are (1) sinus tachycardia, even though new-onset atrial fibrillation can be present; (2) low-voltage, defined as maximum QRS amplitude less than 0.5 mV in limb leads and less than 1 mV in the precordial leads; and (3) electrical alternans, characterized by beat-to-beat alteration in the QRS voltage. The latter represents the free motion of the entire heart within the fluid-filled pericardial cavity[17] (**Fig. 12.4**). Electrical alternans is more indicative of tamponade, but its absence does not rule out tamponade.[23]

Imaging Studies

Given that dyspnea is the most common symptom, a chest radiograph is often the first study obtained. A chest radiograph can demonstrate an enlarged cardiac silhouette, with typical "water bottle" appearance and clear lung fields (**Fig. 12.5**). "Water bottle" appearance and clear lung fields is the classic chest radiograph finding of pericardial effusion, and a concomitant left pleural effusion should only reinforce this impression. Displacement of mediastinal structures after pneumonectomy, or abnormal diaphragmatic elevation (as in the presence of large abdominal masses and/or ascites), may interfere with the diagnosis. Overall, the chest radiograph has a low sensitivity and low specificity for pericardial disease.

Echocardiography is the most widely used technique in this regard. It can provide useful information about the presence, entity, and distribution of pericardial effusion and of intrapericardial neoplastic mass. Moreover, it is very useful in assessing the hemodynamic impairment (eg, impending cardiac tamponade).[24] The size of the effusion can be determined in several ways. The fastest approach is to measure the greatest echo-free space in end-diastole on multiple views, including the parasternal axis and subcostal view. The normal pericardium is filled with 20 to 30 mL of fluid, which may be seen as systolic posterior echo-free space by M-mode recording on parasternal long-axis views. A separation of the pericardial layers throughout the whole cardiac cycle suggests pericardial effusion and can be classified as small (<10 mm, most often posterior), moderate (10–20 mm, usually circumferential), or large (>20 mm). The size of the effusion should be monitored because it can progress to cardiac tamponade.[25]

CT and cardiac magnetic resonance (CMR) are valuable imaging tools in the evaluation of pericardial disorders.[26,27] A CT may enable the initial characterization of pericardial fluid in patients first

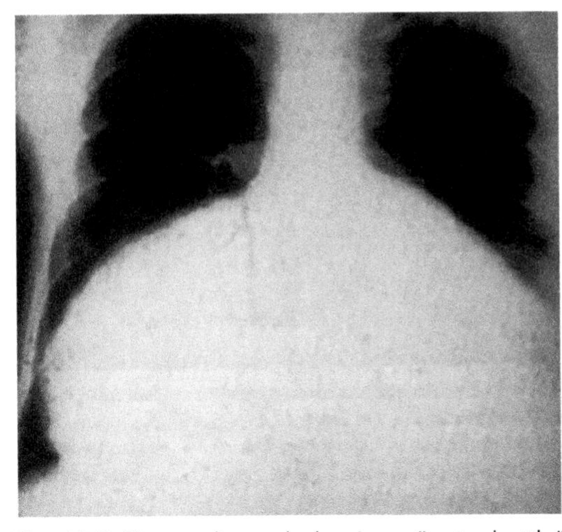

Fig. 12.5 Chest radiograph showing a "water bottle" sign. (*From* Maisch B, Ristic AD. Pericardial diseases. In: Vincent JL, Abraham E, Moore FA. Textbook of critical care. 6th edition. Philadelphia: Elsevier Saunders, 2011; with permission.)

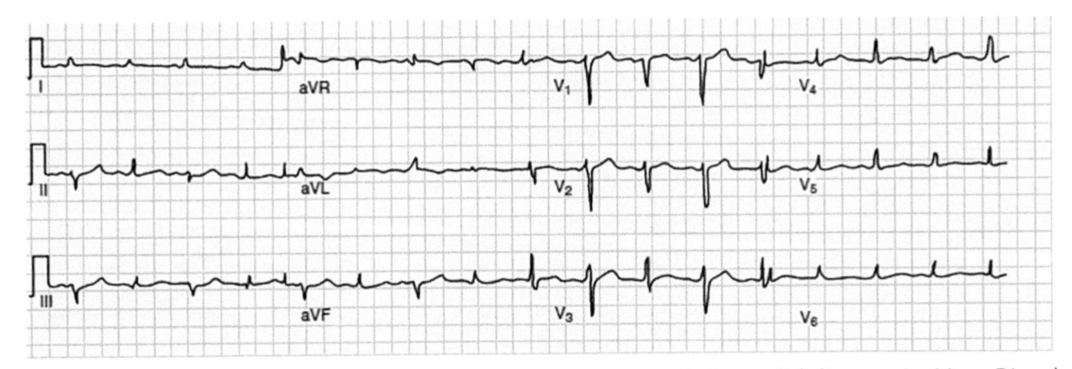

Fig. 12.4 ECG of electrical alternans. (*From* LeWinter MM, Hopkins WE. Pericardial diseases. In: Mann DL, ed. Braunwald's heart disease: a textbook of cardiovascular medicine. 10th edition. Philadelphia: Elsevier Saunders, 2015; with permission.)

presenting with pericardial effusion of unknown cause. Also, it is very useful to assess the possible presence of concomitant thoracic neoplasm. CMR has a superior ability to characterize pericardial effusion and masses. Both techniques are more reliable in the differential diagnosis between fat and tumor masses. Finally, the pericardium usually does not show any uptake on PET imaging; in the case of inflammation, however, a diffuse, low epicardial uptake may be observed, and a single mass with intense uptake is with a very high probability neoplastic.[28]

Pathology, Cytology, and Biomarkers in the Pericardial Fluid

Cytology and histology are the gold standards to define the cause of pericardial effusion when standard clinical methods remain inconclusive. False negative results, however, are still possible, for instance, when the concentration of neoplastic cells is low. Adding epicardial or pericardial biopsies to the cytologic fluid analysis reduces the rate of false negative results.[3] In this context, analyses of cytokines, inflammatory mediators, and serologic and immunologic markers may help to elucidate the underlying cause. The differentiation of malignant from benign pericardial effusion has important implications for therapy and prognosis.[29] Thus, the diagnosis should be based on pericardiocentesis followed by pericardial fluid analysis and/or epicardial and pericardial biopsies.

Cell block preparation, in addition to smears, and immunohistochemical markers are useful to yield a more accurate diagnosis and are most useful for rare tumors and lymphoproliferative disorders.[30–33] Among the immunohistochemical markers, calretinin has been used for the differential diagnosis between mesothelioma and lung carcinoma. Claudin 4 has been reported as highly sensitive and specific in recognizing neoplastic effusions due to carcinomas; it is not tumorspecific, but is useful in differentiating between mesothelioma and carcinoma.[34–36]

Tumor markers are easier than cytology and may provide positive results more rapidly and with a small amount of fluid. Carcinoembryonic antigen, α-fetoprotein, cancer antigens (CAs), CA 125, CA 72-4, CA 15-3, CA 19-9, cytokeratin 19 fragments, and adenosine deaminase, are often investigated after pericardiocentesis. However, their utility as an aid for the diagnosis of malignant pericardial effusion is not well established. Low levels of adenosine deaminase and high levels of carcinoembryonic antigen and CA 72-4 are highly suggestive of malignant cause.[19,37] In patients with lung adenocarcinoma, EGFR mutation occurred more frequently in those with malignant pericardial effusion; these patients should be managed with targeted anti-EGFR therapies. Thus, the presence of EGFR mutation should be investigated in all patients with lung carcinoma and malignant pericardial effusion.[24]

Management

Although the prognosis of patients with malignant pericardial effusion is considered to be poor, therapeutic intervention can improve quality of life and prolong survival.[38] The available treatment options vary from simple drainage to thoracic surgery. The primary aim is to relieve symptoms and improve the quality of life.

Pericardiocentesis (Figs. 12.6 and 12.7) should be performed for diagnostic purposes in cases of suspected neoplastic effusion.[20–22] In emergency cases with cardiac tamponade or significant effusion, initial relief can be obtained with percutaneous pericardiocentesis, sometimes followed by drainage with an indwelling catheter, which can, in reverse, prevent pericardial fluid accumulation. Prolonged drainage with an indwelling catheter may be required for several days, and the catheter should not be removed until drainage is less than 20 to 30 mL/24 hour. Pericardiocentesis-related major complications include chamber laceration, injury to intercostal vessels, pneumothorax, ventricular tachycardia, and bacteremia.[39] Provided that pericardiocentesis is assisted by echocardiography, such complications have been reported to be rare (1.2%), as has pericardiocentesis-related mortality (0.09%).

For decades, pericardiocentesis has been performed as a "blind" procedure, almost exclusively via a subxiphoid approach. With the wide availability of echocardiography, however, pericardiocentesis should not be attempted without echocardiographic guidance. The most useful location for pericardiocentesis is the one closest to the largest amount of the effusion, and therefore, echocardiography identifies the most suitable approach for pericardiocentesis (in most patients subxiphoid or apical).[40,41]

Without any additional treatment, the rate of recurrence of neoplastic pericarditis after drainage is high (up to 40%).[42] To prevent recurrences of symptomatic effusion in patients with an intermediate survival prognosis, 3 approaches have been used for many years: the use of extended drainage, sclerosing therapy, or the creation of a pericardial window. In patients without other metastatic sites, or in patients with cancer with an otherwise good prognosis, it is worth pursuing an attempt to cure the metastatic site and thus possibly prolong survival. This attempt can

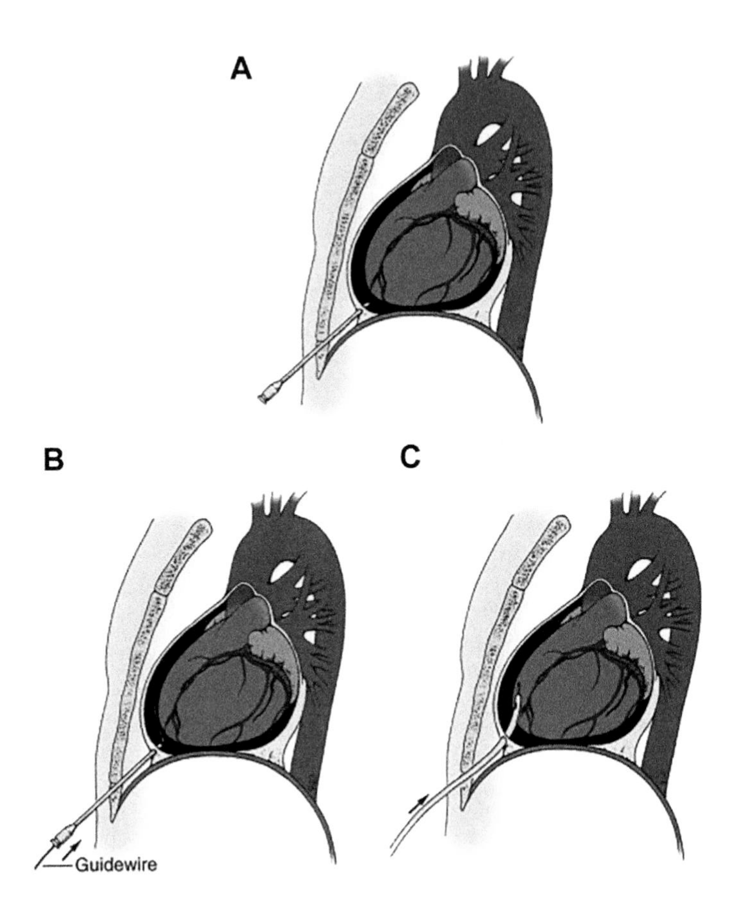

Fig. 12.6 Schematic image of pericardiocentesis. (*A*) The needle is first advanced into the pericardial space. (*B*) The syringe is then disconnected from the needle, and the flexible guidewire is advanced carefully into the pericardial space (best performed under fluoroscopic guidance). (*C*) The needle is withdrawn over the guidewire; the needle tract is dilated, and a multihole, soft pigtail catheter is advanced into the pericardial space. (*From* James D. Pericardiocentesis. In: Pfenninger JL, ed. Pfenninger and Fowler's procedures for primary care. Philadelphia: Elsevier Saunders, 2011; with permission.)

be achieved by using local and/or systemic antineoplastic treatments.[24]

- *Extended drainage:* catheter left in place, permanently or intermittently opened, until the daily drain is reduced to less than 30 mL.
- *Sclerosing therapy*: the intent is to induce irritation, inflammation, and subsequent fibrosis, thus preventing the accumulation of further effusion. The first agents used for sclerotherapy were antibiotics (tetracycline and doxycycline) with success rates of 80%, but also with high rates of adverse effects: pain, fever, atrial fibrillation, or flutter.[43,44] Bleomycin, with both antineoplastic and sclerosing effects, may be equally effective with less morbidity, but further studies need to be done. The risk of sclerosing therapy is reflected in the evolution to constrictive pericarditis and in the development of effusion-constrictive pericarditis.[45]
- *Percutanous balloon pericardiotomy:* can be performed immediately after initial pericardiocentesis or after pericardial effusion recurrences and is an alternative to a surgical creation of a pericardial window. The procedure is demanding, often painful, and involves the insertion of a deflated single catheter or double-balloon catheters into the pericardial space via a subxiphoid approach under echocardiographic or fluoroscopic guidance. Although successful (88%–100% recurrence rate prevention), it might be followed by complications, such as fever, pneumothorax, and in some cases bleeding from the pericardial blood vessels.[19,46]
- *Surgery (pericardial window):* reserved for cases of inadequate percutaneous drainage or for rapid fluid reaccumulation. No randomized trials to this date have been performed. Available reports from retrospective studies demonstrate hemodynamic benefit in most patients, minimal surgical morbidity and mortality, and a lower incidence of effusion recurrence.[8]
- *Antineoplastic treatments:* systemic chemotherapy, local chemotherapy, and external beam radiotherapy have been investigated in various studies with

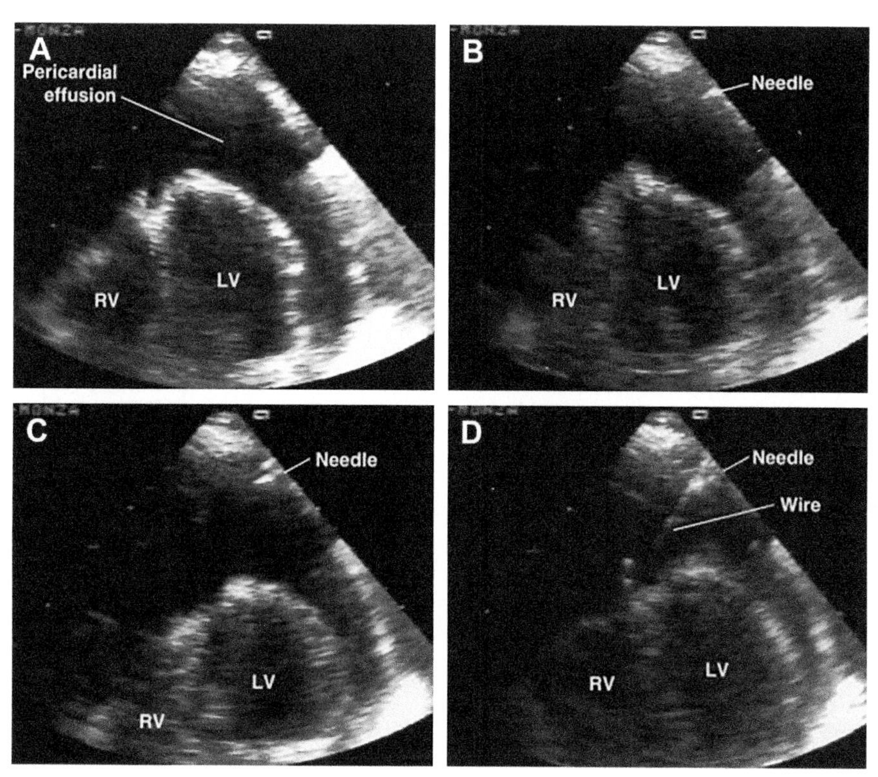

Fig. 12.7 Echocardiograph of pericardiocentesis. (*A*) Detection of pericardial effusion. (*B*) Visualization of needle tip. (*C*) Needle is advanced through tissues. (*D*) Needle enters pericardial space and guidewire is introduced. LV, left ventricle; RV, right ventricle. (*From* Maggiolini S, Bozzano A, Russo P, et al. Echocardiography-guided pericardiocentesis with probe-mounted needle: report of 53 cases. J Am Soc Echocardiogr 2001;14:821–824; with permission.)

different success rates. Systemic chemotherapy, including target therapy with monoclonal antibodies or tyrosine kinase inhibitors, has been reported to be effective for pericardial effusions because of lymphoma and breast carcinoma, but its efficacy in lung cancer is less clear.[47–49] Because the pericardium is a metastatic site, its aggressive treatment with local chemotherapy agents is a reasonable goal. Indeed, discrete pericardial implantations or infiltrations can be noted on echocardiography in many patients with lung cancer, and in some even diffuse neoplastic deposits. Thus, the rationale of local chemotherapy is to control not only the pericardial fluid reaccumulation but also the neoplastic process as well. The injection of a chemotherapeutic agent into the pericardial space, layering on the pericardial surface, and slow reabsorption through the lymphatic vessels (which are the main means of metastasization to the pericardium in lung and other cancer) has several advantages in pursuing the goal of cancer control, namely high intrapericardial concentration (and few systemic side effects) and beneficial effects on lymphatic system obstructions.[15,19,45] Several chemotherapeutic and radioactive agents have been investigated depending on the origin of the malignancy, for example, thiotepa, carboplatin, cisplatin, mitoxantrone, colloidal 32P, aclarubicin, and cytokines, such as interferon-α2b and interleukin-2.[19] Colloidal 32P and cytokines also have sclerosing effects, whereas platins and thiotepa are mainly antineoplastic agents and reduce the neoplastic burden rather than induce adherence between the pericardial layers. External beam radiation was used in the 1970s, delivering 25 to 30 Gy to the pericardium. Intracardial radiotherapy may be obtained by the instillation of radioactive compounds (such as colloid 32P) within the pericardial space. It has been proven to be very effective and well tolerated in some studies.[50] However, radiation therapy is not routinely used, due to concerns regarding the risks associated with radiation and the availability and cost of the radioactive compound for the intrapericardial instillation.[24] External beam radiotherapy may have a role in very selected cases, for instance, tumor encasement of the heart or extensive pericardial infiltration by nonresectable tumors. Modern techniques, such as intensity-modulated radiation therapy or proton beam therapy, allow focusing the irradiation treatment on the neoplastic mass more than ever before, thereby reducing the exposure and injury of cardiovascular structures. Surgery in these cases has a very high perioperative mortality and morbidity.[51]

Prognosis

In terms of relapse and overall survival, the prognosis of malignant pericardial involvement and effusion depends mostly on the type of primary tumor, the grade of metastatic involvement, and its chemosensitivity. In lung cancer and mesothelioma, the recurrence rates are higher and survival times are shorter than in other tumors. Neoplastic pericardial disease due to breast cancer has a better prognosis, and even large effusions in lymphoma patients may be easily and definitively cured by systemic chemotherapy. The exception is primary effusive lymphoma, which has a poor prognosis.

CARDIAC TAMPONADE

Cardiac tamponade is defined as a pericardial effusion resulting in restriction of chamber filling and hemodynamic collapse. This process is more commonly associated with acute accumulation of fluid in the pericardium (eg, after trauma or open heart surgery), but may also occur when slow accumulating effusions reach a critical volume. Malignant pericardial effusions may account for 9% to 39% of moderate- to larger-sized pericardial effusions.[11,12,52–54] They usually develop slowly and allow the pressure within the pericardial cavity to increase gradually as large volumes of fluid are accumulating, some of which may even surpass 1000 mL and reach up to 3000 mL.

The relationship between intrapericardial pressure and the hemodynamic effect of the accumulating fluid is exponential, and the critical clinical presentation correlates with the rapid incline phase of the curve, the so-called last-drop phenomenon.[55,56] In clinical practice, this translates into the rapid correction of the hemodynamics with removal of only a small volume of fluid. One caveat, however, is hemorrhagic pericardial effusion, for example, with aortic or coronary dissection, which requires surgical treatment (see later discussion).

The clinical presentation can be acute (sudden onset of chest pain and dyspnea) or subacute (nonspecific fatigue and exertional intolerance). Tachycardia, hypotension, specifically with low pulse pressure, elevated jugular venous pressure, and pulsus paradoxus are the classical clinical signs on examination. Although in practice it is not often used in the establishment of the diagnosis of cardiac tamponade, right heart catheterization remains the reference standard because it provides confirmation of elevated filling pressures and even equalization of right- and left-sided end-diastolic pressures.[17,19]

Current guidelines advocate rapid echocardiographic evaluation and urgent drainage. Sonographically guided pericardiocentesis has been shown to have higher recurrence rates, but also better safety outcomes, than an open surgical approach.[57] This represents a challenge in patients who are fragile and at a higher surgical risk while at the same time more prone toward recurrences. Prolonged pericardial drainage may significantly reduce recurrence rates. In general, acute drainage should be limited to 1000 mL. If a larger volume removal is needed, prolonged drainage should be considered.[58,59]

Several indications for urgent surgical intervention in cardiac tamponade are recommended. Among these, a purulent effusion in unstable septic patients and loculated effusions that cannot be managed percutaneously are the most relevant in the setting of malignancy. Other generally accepted indications include cases of type A aortic dissection, ventricular free wall rupture, and trauma. In selected cases, intervention may be postponed for up to 48 hours (Fig. 12.8).[59]

CONSTRICTIVE PERICARDITIS

Constrictive pericardial disease, shown in Fig. 12.9, occurs when fibrosis and/or calcification leads to an increase in pericardial stiffness and alteration of filling dynamics. Common histopathologic findings include mild and focal fibrosis, inflammation, calcification, fibrin deposition, and focal noncaseating granulomas. Incidence rate varies among the different causes, but in general, it remains a rare complication of pericardial disease. Malignancy-associated constrictive pericarditis is seen in 2% to 5% of patients with neoplastic pericardial manifestations.[60] In patients with cancer, this can arise directly from pericardial involvement of the underlying disease, or as a complication of radiotherapy. Constrictive pericarditis usually presents as a chronic disorder,

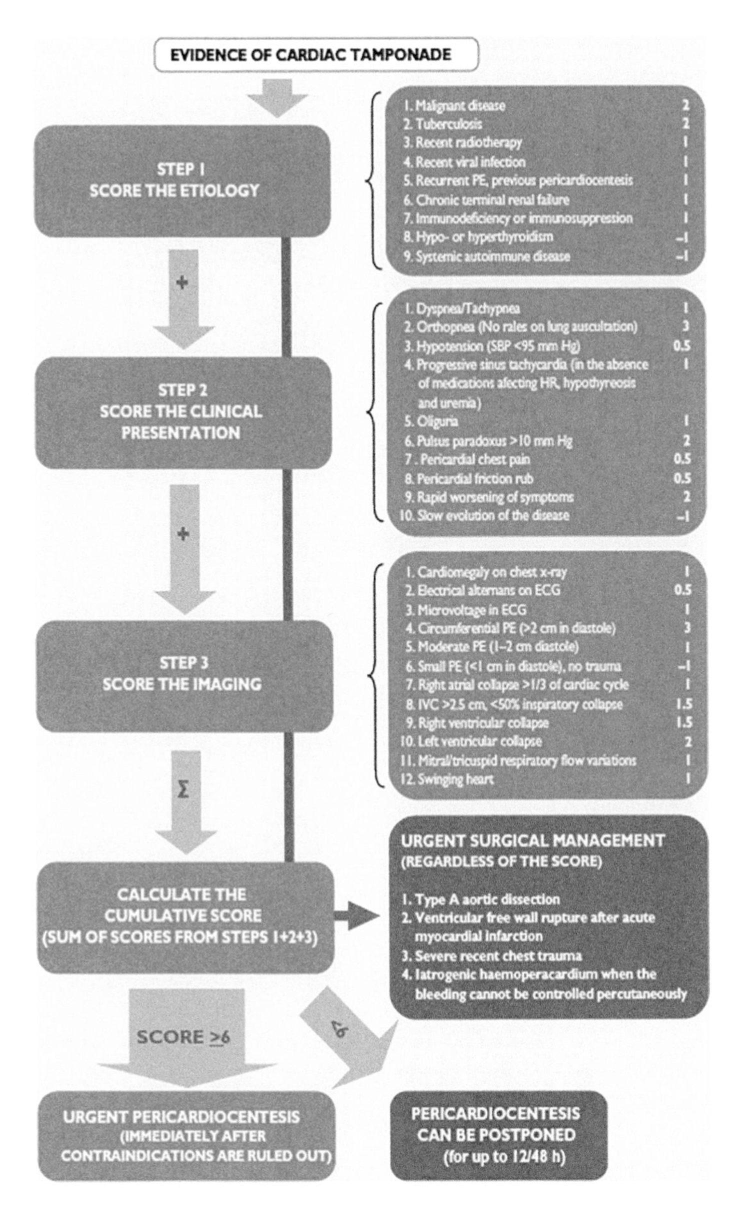

Fig. 12.8 Cardiac tamponade triage. IVC, inferior vena cava; SBP, systolic blood pressure. (*From* Adler Y, Charron P, Imazio M, et al; European Society of Cardiology (ESC). 2015 ESC Guidelines for the diagnosis and management of pericardial diseases: the Task Force for the Diagnosis and Management of Pericardial Diseases of the European Society of Cardiology (ESC) Endorsed by: the European Association for Cardio-Thoracic Surgery (EACTS). Eur Heart J 2015;36(42):2936; with permission.)

but in practice, more subacute and transient presentations are also seen.

When there is clinical suspicion for constrictive pericarditis with or without effusion, the systolic area index (ratio of right ventricle to left ventricle systolic area during 2 cycles of respiration) can be determined, with a nearly absolute positive predictive value.[61]

Preferred management of constrictive pericarditis is surgical, with pericardiectomy being the treatment of choice. Interestingly, up to 20% of patients do not have increased pericardial thickness, although this has not been shown to have significant effects on the outcome of surgical management.[62]

PERICARDIAL MASSES

Autopsy studies show that metastatic involvement of the pericardium is 20 times more common than primary lesions.[63] These tumors may involve all components of the pericardial sac and cavity, as shown in Fig. 12.10, but most of these remain limited to the pericardium, thus not invading the myocardium.

The overall incidence of both malignant and benign pericardial tumors is 0.02% to 1.28%. Benign primary tumors of the pericardium are mainly lipomas and sarcomas; the main malignant tumors are mesotheliomas and synovial sarcomas.[13,64] Pericardial neoplasms, both primary and secondary, may present as a

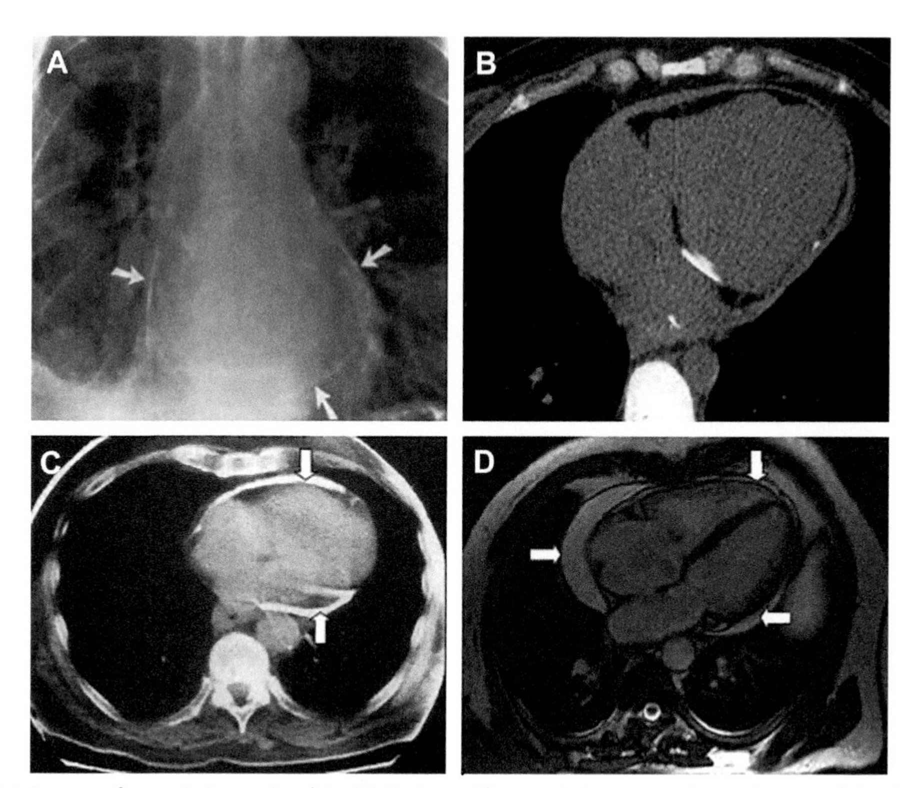

Fig. 12.9 Images of constrictive pericarditis. (*A*) Patient with constrictive pericarditis and pericardial calcifications (*arrows*). (*B*) CT scan showing increased pericardial thickness and mild calcifications in a patient with constrictive pericarditis. (*C, D*) CT finding in constrictive pericarditis (*C*). White vertical arrows depict thickened pericardium and pericardial calcification. MRI of a patient with effusive-constrictive pericarditis (*D*). Horizontal arrows show loculated pericardial effusion, and the vertical arrow shows thickened pericardium. ([*A, D*] *From* Maisch B, Ristic AD. Pericardial diseases. In: Vincent JL, Abraham E, Moore FA. Textbook of critical care. 6th edition. Philadelphia: Elsevier Saunders, 2011; with permission and [*B, C*] *From* LeWinter MM, Hopkins WE. Pericardial diseases. In: Mann DL, ed. Braunwald's heart disease: a textbook of cardiovascular medicine. 10th edition. Philadelphia: Elsevier Saunders, 2015; with permission.)

pericardial effusion, cardiac tamponade, or constrictive pericardial disease. The clinical presentation depends mainly on the lesion size and location as well as myocardial invasion. The histopathological classification plays a lesser role in this context.

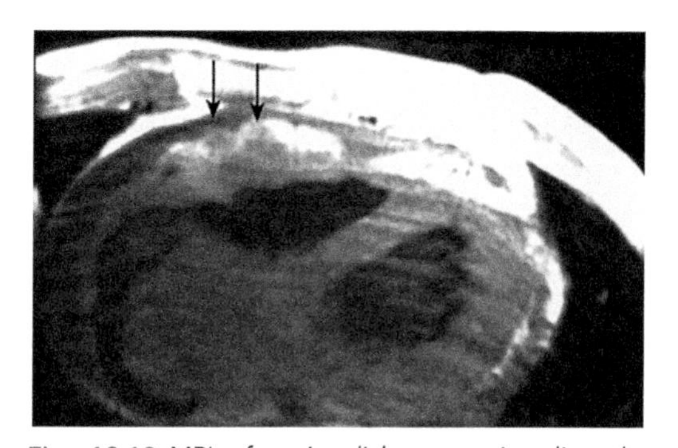

Fig. 12.10 MRI of pericardial masses invading the epicardial fat. Axial spin-echo black-blood gated MRI demonstrates a pericardial effusion and pericardial metastasis invading the epicardial fat (*arrows*). (*From* Malguria N, Miller SW, Abbara S. Myocardium, pericardium, and cardiac tumor. In: Boxt LM, Abbara S, eds. Cardiac imaging: the requisites. Philadelphia: Elsevier, 2016; with permission.)

The diagnosis is based on cytology studies of pericardial aspirate. The role of biomarker detection in pericardial remains controversial yet may still be of some benefit.[20] A biopsy may be considered when there are suspicious findings on imaging studies and negative cytology tests, or when a nonneoplastic cause (eg, tuberculosis) is suspected in the setting of a known malignancy. Although it is advisable to perform a pericardial or epicardial biopsy in order to confirm the diagnosis, in practice, if the primary source of malignancy is found to be extrapericardial, it is advisable to reconsider this approach.

Mesothelioma

Benign cardiac mesotheliomas are extremely rare tumors that arise from the atrioventricular (AV) node and may cause subsequent AV block.

Malignant mesotheliomas (Fig. 12.11), on the other hand, are neoplasms that can arise from

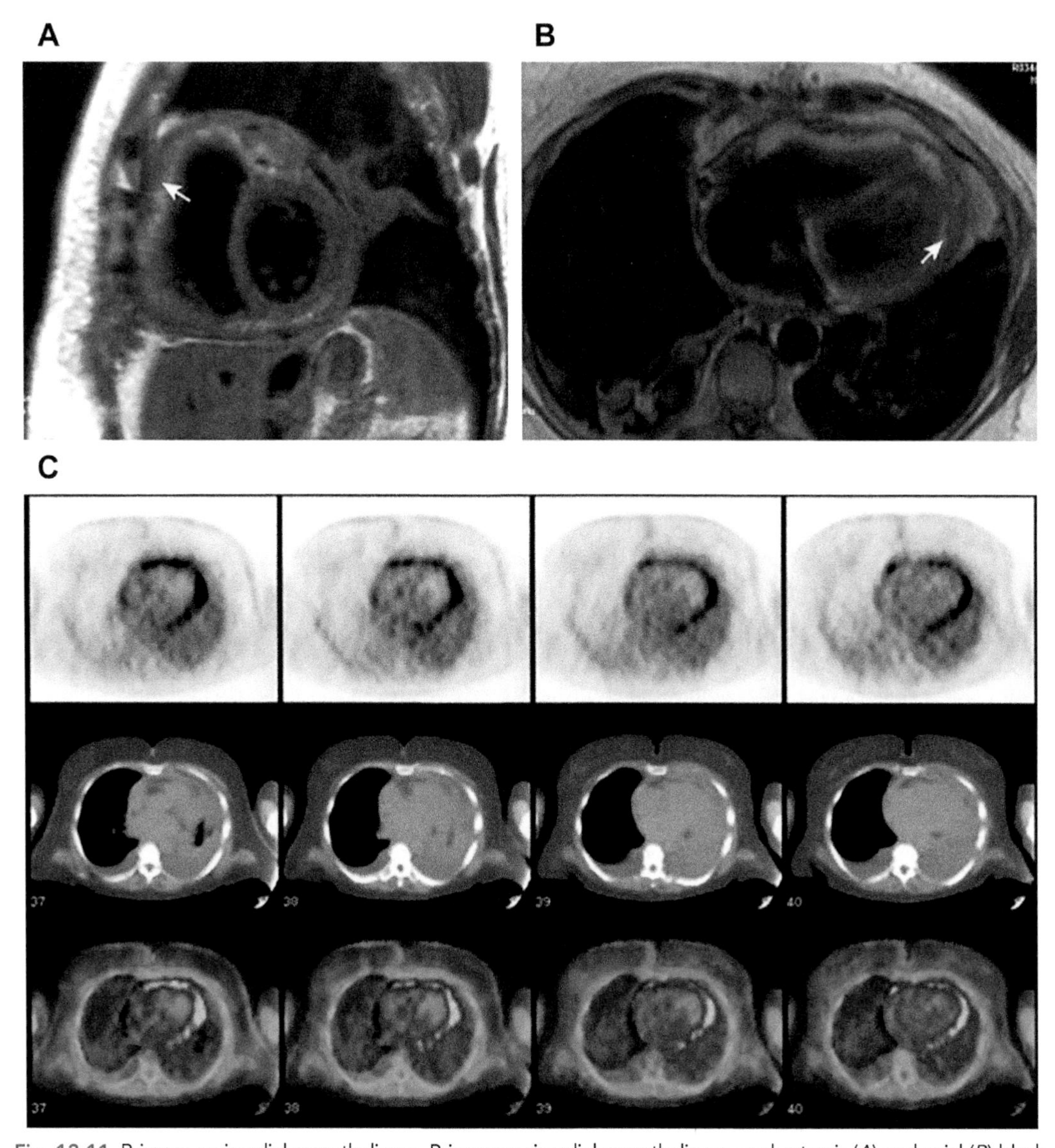

Fig. 12.11 Primary pericardial mesothelioma. Primary pericardial mesothelioma on short-axis (*A*) and axial (*B*) black-blood T1-weighted MRI through the heart. There is diffuse nodularity of the pericardium infiltrating the epicardial fat (*arrow*). On imaging alone, this would be difficult to distinguish from pericardial metastasis. (*C*) Axial images from PET-CT. There is diffuse uptake in the pericardium along the tumor. Top row, axial PET images; middle row, axial CT; bottom row, fused PET-CT images. There are bilateral pleural effusions. (*From* Malguria N, Miller SW, Abbara S. Myocardium, pericardium, and cardiac tumor. In: Boxt LM, Abbara S, eds. Cardiac imaging: the requisites. Philadelphia: Elsevier, 2016; with permission.)

the pericardial mesothelial cell layer and account for 50% of primary pericardial tumors. Patients range in age from 2 to 78 years with a mean age of 46 years, and the male-to-female ratio is 2:1.[65] Most of the pericardial mesotheliomas are diffuse, cover visceral and parietal surfaces, and grow by direct extension into surrounding surfaces. The epicardial myocardium may be focally invaded, but the tumor does not extend to the endocardial surface.

Clinical symptoms include chest pain, cough, dyspnea, and palpitations. Patients with diffuse pericardial involvement may present with signs and symptoms that mimic pericarditis or cardiac tamponade. These patients seldom have evidence of widespread metastatic disease but nevertheless face a poor prognosis.

Although there appears to be some causal effect of asbestos exposure, a definite association has not been established because of the rare nature of pericardial mesothelioma. Most of the literature discussing the subject is descriptive and is mainly in the form of individual case reports or small case series. More recently published reports are mostly on patients with no known exposure.[66]

Multidetector computed tomography (MDCT) is the superior imaging technique, and pericardial mesotheliomas appear as multiple enhancing and coalescing pericardial masses that envelope the pericardial space.[67] The diagnosis is usually confirmed by cytology studies of the pericardial aspirate. Currently, there is no immunohistochemical marker that distinguishes pericardial mesothelioma from other sources of mesothelioma that may metastasize to the pericardium; thus, these should be excluded in order to define the diagnosis of primary pericardial mesothelioma.[66]

Surgery combined with radiation therapy may be palliative, but the prognosis of all patients, even those who are treated, is extremely poor, with survival of 6 months to 1 year after diagnosis.[65]

Pericardial Synovial Sarcomas

Synovial sarcomas are more commonly associated with joint capsules and other components of the musculoskeletal system, although rare cases of primary head, neck, and thoracic tumors have also been reported.

Primary pericardial sarcomas are very rare aggressive tumors that are composed of spindle and epithelioid cells. The diagnosis is established via biopsy, although detection of the SYT/SSX1 or SYT/SSX2 genes (seen in the t(X;18)(p11; q11) translocation) may be useful, as found in most synovial sarcomas.[68]

Imaging characteristics may overlap with cardiac angiosarcoma, and MDCT has been suggested as a means to establish the diagnosis. The typical finding is that of a heterogeneously enhancing, multilobulated mass with extensive pericardial infiltration and deep invasion.[69]

Management is mainly by broad resection, limited only by surgical considerations. Adjuvant systemic therapy with combinations of ifosfamide and doxorubicin may be considered. Even with optimal management, local and metastatic recurrences are common and prognosis is poor with 5-year survival estimates of 35% to 50%.[70]

Pericardial Metastases

Most commonly associated with hematologic malignancies, melanoma and lung, breast, or esophageal malignancies, metastases develop by either local invasion or distal dissemination via the bloodstream or the lymphatic system. Lung metastases are the most common of those listed. Kaposi sarcoma has also been associated with pericardial metastases.[63]

A high index of suspicion for pericardial involvement should arise whenever a patient with cancer presents with a new pericardial effusion, although other possible causes as outlined above (eg, cancer therapy, infections) should not be overlooked.

The optimal treatment varies according to the tumor type. For leukemia or lymphoma, steroids and chemotherapy are the first choice of treatment. In solid tumors, a combination of local chemotherapy or a pericardial window together with systemic chemotherapy provides a significantly better chance of long-term disease control.[71] With regards to intrapericardial chemotherapy, platinum seems to be the drug of choice in lung cancer, whereas in breast cancer, both thiotepa and platinum are effective. Intrapericardial chemotherapy is usually well tolerated without any significant systemic side effects. In patients with solid tumor who are in poor general condition, local chemotherapy alone is recommended, which is well tolerated and is at least as effective as systemic chemotherapy alone for the local disease process.[24]

SUMMARY, PERSPECTIVE, AND UNMET NEEDS

Pericardial disease in the patient with cancer is not rare and may manifest either as a mass, pericarditis, or pericardial effusion. The underlying mechanisms of these processes are diverse and may be either directly related to the patient's malignancy, its treatments, or infectious complications.

Cytology and pathology studies play a key role in the assessment of pericardial involvement in malignancy. For patients with a new pericardial effusion, pericardiocentesis is advised, regardless of the presence of tamponade. Establishing the nature of the patient's pericardial syndrome may have a significant effect on both short- and long-term management. Examples of this include the recognition of a treatable infectious cause, discovering a surgically resectable lesion, avoiding cessation of systemic treatment by recognizing a specific cause, and so forth. An increase in neoplastic markers in the pericardial fluid may orient toward a diagnosis of malignant pericardial effusion. However, the usefulness of tumor marker concentrations in pericardial fluid remains controversial.

Pericardial tumors are generally associated with a poor prognosis. It will be interesting to see future studies describing the effect of novel antineoplastic systemic therapies on the clinical course of this subset of patients. At least in the case of metastatic pericardial involvement, the prospect seems positive. The lack of population studies is still a setback in the quest to better define the epidemiologic, genetic, and biologic nature of primary pericardial malignancies as well as their susceptibility to novel systemic therapies. Common knowledge is still that the management of these tumors is surgical, because they are relatively resistant to radiotherapy and systemic antineoplastic therapy.

REFERENCES

1. Imazio M, Demichelis B, Parrini I, et al. Relation of acute pericardial disease to malignancy. Am J Cardiol 2005;95(11):1393–4.
2. Vaitkus PT, Herrmann HC, LeWinter MM. Treatment of malignant pericardial effusion. JAMA 1994; 272(1):59–64.
3. Maisch B, Ristic A, Pankuweit S. Evaluation and management of pericardial effusion in patients with neoplastic disease. Prog Cardiovasc Dis 2010; 53(2):157–63.
4. Al-Mamgani A, Baartman L, Baaijens M, et al. Cardiac metastases. Int J Clin Oncol 2008;13(4):369–72.
5. Rafajlovski S, Tatić V, Ilić S, et al. Frequency of metastatic tumors in the heart. Vojnosanit Pregl 2005; 62(12):915–20 [in Serbian].
6. Troughton RW, Asher CR, Klein AL. Pericarditis. Lancet 2004;363(9410):717–27.
7. Imazio M, Cecchi E, Demichelis B, et al. Myopericarditis versus viral or idiopathic acute pericarditis. Heart 2008;94(4):498–501.
8. Imazio M, Cecchi E, Demichelis B, et al. Indicators of poor prognosis of acute pericarditis. Circulation 2007;115(21):2739–44.
9. Permanyer-Miralda G, Sagrista-Sauleda J, Soler-Soler J. Primary acute pericardial disease: a prospective series of 231 consecutive patients. Am J Cardiol 1985;56(10):623–30.
10. Zayas R, Anguita M, Torres F, et al. Incidence of specific etiology and role of methods for specific etiologic diagnosis of primary acute pericarditis. Am J Cardiol 1995;75(5):378–82.
11. Corey GR, Campbell PT, Van Trigt P, et al. Etiology of large pericardial effusions. Am J Med 1993;95(2): 209–13.
12. Sagrista-Sauleda J, Mercé J, Permanyer-Miralda G, et al. Clinical clues to the causes of large pericardial effusions. Am J Med 2000;109(2):95–101.
13. Abraham KP, Reddy V, Gattuso P. Neoplasms metastatic to the heart: review of 3314 consecutive autopsies. Am J Cardiovasc Pathol 1990;3(3):195–8.
14. Kim Y, Park CJ, Roh J, et al. Current concepts in primary effusion lymphoma and other effusion-based lymphomas. Korean J Pathol 2014;48(2):81–90.
15. Burazor I, Imazio M, Markel G, et al. Malignant pericardial effusion. Cardiology 2013;124(4):224–32.
16. Jeong TD, Jang S, Park CJ, et al. Prognostic relevance of pericardial effusion in patients with malignant diseases. Korean J Hematol 2012;47(3):237–8.
17. Refaat MM, Katz WE. Neoplastic pericardial effusion. Clin Cardiol 2011;34(10):593–8.
18. Perrault DJ, Levy M, Herman JD, et al. Echocardiographic abnormalities following cardiac radiation. J Clin Oncol 1985;3(4):546–51.
19. Pohjola-Sintonen S, Tötterman KJ, Salmo M, et al. Late cardiac effects of mediastinal radiotherapy in patients with Hodgkin's disease. Cancer 1987; 60(1):31–7.
20. Adler Y, Charron P, Imazio M, et al, European Society of Cardiology (ESC). 2015 ESC Guidelines for the diagnosis and management of pericardial diseases: the Task Force for the Diagnosis and Management of Pericardial Diseases of the European Society of Cardiology (ESC) Endorsed by: The European Association for Cardio-Thoracic Surgery (EACTS). Eur Heart J 2015;36(42):2921–64.
21. Imazio M, Brucato A, Trinchero R, et al. Diagnosis and management of pericardial diseases. Nat Rev Cardiol 2009;6(12):743–51.
22. Maisch B, Rupp H, Ristic A, et al. Pericardioscopy and epi- and pericardial biopsy—a new window to the heart improving etiological diagnoses and permitting targeted intrapericardial therapy. Heart Fail Rev 2013;18(3):317–28.
23. Seferovic PM, Ristić AD, Maksimović R, et al. Pericardial syndromes: an update after the ESC guidelines 2004. Heart Fail Rev 2013;18(3):255–66.
24. Lestuzzi C, Berretta M, Tomkowski W. 2015 update on the diagnosis and management of neoplastic pericardial disease. Expert Rev Cardiovasc Ther 2015;13(4):377–89.
25. Imazio M, Mayosi BM, Brucato A, et al. Triage and management of pericardial effusion. J Cardiovasc Med (Hagerstown) 2010;11(12):928–35.
26. Verhaert D, Gabriel RS, Johnston D, et al. The role of multimodality imaging in the management of pericardial disease. Circ Cardiovasc Imaging 2010; 3(3):333–43.
27. Rajiah P. Cardiac MRI: part 2, pericardial diseases. AJR Am J Roentgenol 2011;197(4):W621–34.
28. Korn RL, Coates A, Millstine J. The role of glucose and FDG metabolism in the interpretation of PET studies. In: Lin EC, Alavi A, editors. PET and PET/CT. A clinical guide. 2nd edition. New York: Thieme; 2009. p. 22–30.
29. Kraft A, Weindel K, Ochs A, et al. Vascular endothelial growth factor in the sera and effusions of patients with malignant and nonmalignant disease. Cancer 1999;85(1):178–87.
30. Nathan NA, Narayan E, Smith MM, et al. Cell block cytology. Improved preparation and its efficacy in diagnostic cytology. Am J Clin Pathol 2000;114(4): 599–606.

31. Chute DJ, Kong CS, Stelow EB. Immunohistochemistry for the detection of renal cell carcinoma in effusion cytology. Diagn Cytopathol 2011;39(2):118–23.
32. Su XY, Huang J, Jiang Y, et al. Serous effusion cytology of extranodal natural killer/T-cell lymphoma. Cytopathology 2012;23(2):96–102.
33. Shield PW, Papadimos DJ, Walsh MD. GATA3: a promising marker for metastatic breast carcinoma in serous effusion specimens. Cancer Cytopathol 2014;122(4):307–12.
34. Shield PW, Koivurinne K. The value of calretinin and cytokeratin 5/6 as markers for mesothelioma in cell block preparations of serous effusions. Cytopathology 2008;19(4):218–23.
35. Lonardi S, Manera C, Marucci R, et al. Usefulness of Claudin 4 in the cytological diagnosis of serosal effusions. Diagn Cytopathol 2011;39(5):313–7.
36. Jo VY, Cibas ES, Pinkus GS. Claudin-4 immunohistochemistry is highly effective in distinguishing adenocarcinoma from malignant mesothelioma in effusion cytology. Cancer Cytopathol 2014;122(4):299–306.
37. Karatolios K, Maisch B, Pankuweit S. Tumor markers in the assessment of malignant and benign pericardial effusion. Herz 2011;36(4):290–5 [in German].
38. Jama GM, Scarci M, Bowden J, et al. Palliative treatment for symptomatic malignant pericardial effusion†. Interact Cardiovasc Thorac Surg 2014;19(6):1019–26.
39. Tsang TS, Enriquez-Sarano M, Freeman WK, et al. Consecutive 1127 therapeutic echocardiographically guided pericardiocenteses: clinical profile, practice patterns, and outcomes spanning 21 years. Mayo Clin Proc 2002;77(5):429–36.
40. Maisch B, Ristic AD, Seferovic PM, et al. Interventional pericardiology. Berlin: Springer; 2011.
41. Silvestry FE, Kerber RE, Brook MM, et al. Echocardiography-guided interventions. J Am Soc Echocardiogr 2009;22(3):213–31 [quiz: 316–7].
42. Tsang TS, Seward JB, Barnes ME, et al. Outcomes of primary and secondary treatment of pericardial effusion in patients with malignancy. Mayo Clin Proc 2000;75(3):248–53.
43. Liu G, Crump M, Goss PE, et al. Prospective comparison of the sclerosing agents doxycycline and bleomycin for the primary management of malignant pericardial effusion and cardiac tamponade. J Clin Oncol 1996;14(12):3141–7.
44. Maher EA, Shepherd FA, Todd TJ. Pericardial sclerosis as the primary management of malignant pericardial effusion and cardiac tamponade. J Thorac Cardiovasc Surg 1996;112(3):637–43.
45. Lestuzzi C, Lafaras C, Bearz A, et al. Malignant pericardial effusion: sclerotherapy or local chemotherapy? Br J Cancer 2009;101(4):734–5 [author reply: 736–7].
46. Imazio M, Brucato A, Cumetti D, et al. Corticosteroids for recurrent pericarditis: high versus low doses: a nonrandomized observation. Circulation 2008;118(6):667–71.
47. Zaharia L, Gill PS. Primary cardiac lymphoma. Am J Clin Oncol 1991;14(2):142–5.
48. Reynolds PM, Byrne MJ. The treatment of malignant pericardial effusion in carcinoma of the breast. Aust N Z J Med 1977;7(2):169–71.
49. Primrose WR, Clee MD, Johnston RN. Malignant pericardial effusion managed with Vinblastine. Clin Oncol 1983;9(1):67–70.
50. Dempke W, Firusian N. Treatment of malignant pericardial effusion with 32P-colloid. Br J Cancer 1999;80(12):1955–7.
51. Buyukbayrak F, Aksoy E, Dedemoglu M, et al. Pericardiectomy for treatment of neoplastic constrictive pericarditis. Asian Cardiovasc Thorac Ann 2014;22(3):296–300.
52. Levy PY, Corey R, Berger P, et al. Etiologic diagnosis of 204 pericardial effusions. Medicine (Baltimore) 2003;82(6):385–91.
53. Ma W, Liu J, Zeng Y, et al. Causes of moderate to large pericardial effusion requiring pericardiocentesis in 140 Han Chinese patients. Herz 2012;37(2):183–7.
54. Reuter H, Burgess LJ, Doubell AF. Epidemiology of pericardial effusions at a large academic hospital in South Africa. Epidemiol Infect 2005;133(3):393–9.
55. Spodick DH. Acute cardiac tamponade. N Engl J Med 2003;349(7):684–90.
56. Shabetai R. Pericardial effusion: haemodynamic spectrum. Heart 2004;90(3):255–6.
57. Gumrukcuoglu HA, Odabasi D, Akdag S, et al. Management of cardiac tamponade: a comperative study between echo-guided pericardiocentesis and surgery-a report of 100 patients. Cardiol Res Pract 2011;2011:197838.
58. Rafique AM, Patel N, Biner S, et al. Frequency of recurrence of pericardial tamponade in patients with extended versus nonextended pericardial catheter drainage. Am J Cardiol 2011;108(12):1820–5.
59. Ristic AD, Imazio M, Adler Y, et al. Triage strategy for urgent management of cardiac tamponade: a position statement of the European Society of Cardiology Working Group on Myocardial and Pericardial Diseases. Eur Heart J 2014;35(34):2279–84.
60. Imazio M, Brucato A, Maestroni S, et al. Risk of constrictive pericarditis after acute pericarditis. Circulation 2011;124(11):1270–5.
61. Talreja DR, Nishimura RA, Oh JK, et al. Constrictive pericarditis in the modern era: novel criteria for diagnosis in the cardiac catheterization laboratory. J Am Coll Cardiol 2008;51(3):315–9.

62. Talreja DR, Edwards WD, Danielson GK, et al. Constrictive pericarditis in 26 patients with histologically normal pericardial thickness. Circulation 2003;108(15):1852–7.
63. Lam KY, Dickens P, Chan AC. Tumors of the heart. A 20-year experience with a review of 12,485 consecutive autopsies. Arch Pathol Lab Med 1993;117(10):1027–31.
64. Butany J, Leong SW, Carmichael K, et al. A 30-year analysis of cardiac neoplasms at autopsy. Can J Cardiol 2005;21(8):675–80.
65. Grebenc ML, Rosado de Christenson ML, Burke AP, et al. Primary cardiac and pericardial neoplasms: radiologic-pathologic correlation. Radiographics 2000;20(4):1073–103 [quiz: 1110–1, 1112].
66. Kerger BD, James RC, Galbraith DA. Tumors that mimic asbestos-related mesothelioma: time to consider a genetics-based tumor registry? Front Genet 2014;5:151.
67. Burazor I, Aviel-Ronen S, Imazio M, et al. Primary malignancies of the heart and pericardium. Clin Cardiol 2014;37(9):582–8.
68. Kawai A, Woodruff J, Healey JH, et al. SYT-SSX gene fusion as a determinant of morphology and prognosis in synovial sarcoma. N Engl J Med 1998;338(3):153–60.
69. Hoey E, Ganeshan A, Nader K, et al. Cardiac neoplasms and pseudotumors: imaging findings on multidetector CT angiography. Diagn Interv Radiol 2012;18(1):67–77.
70. Spillane AJ, A'Hern R, Judson IR, et al. Synovial sarcoma: a clinicopathologic, staging, and prognostic assessment. J Clin Oncol 2000;18(22):3794–803.
71. Lestuzzi C, Bearz A, Lafaras C, et al. Neoplastic pericardial disease in lung cancer: impact on outcomes of different treatment strategies. A multicenter study. Lung Cancer 2011;72(3):340–7.

CHAPTER 13

Arrhythmias and QTc Prolongations

Marzia Locatelli, MD, Giuseppe Curigliano, MD, PhD*

INTRODUCTION

Torsades de pointes (TdP) was first described in 1966 by the French cardiologist Dessertenne. Until 1989, TdP was known to occur fairly frequently during the initiation of antiarrhythmic drugs with class III effect (so that patients were placed on telemetry to initiate such drugs), fairly rarely in patients receiving psychiatric drugs (so that nothing systematic was done for these patients), and occasionally in very sick hospitalized patients receiving intravenous erythromycin.

In the fall of 1989, the first recognized case of QT prolongation and TdP associated with terfenadine was described by physicians at the National Naval Medical Center in Bethesda, Maryland. This case of drug reaction was a landmark adverse drug reaction that triggered the awareness that many apparently benign noncardiovascular drugs could rarely have the unwanted ability to prolong cardiac repolarization and thus cause TdP in susceptible patients. In the process of elucidating the mechanism of terfenadine-associated QT prolongation and TdP, it was demonstrated that terfenadine, but not its active metabolite fexofenadine, had the unanticipated property of blocking the rapid component of the delayed rectifier potassium current (IK_r) and thus prolonging the QT interval.

The first regulatory document addressing the evaluation of noncardiovascular drugs to alter cardiac repolarization in humans was published in 1997.[1] Subsequently, the US Food and Drug Administration (FDA) and the International Conference on Harmonization (ICH) adopted a tripartite harmonized guidance (ICH E14) document entitled, "The Clinical Evaluation of QT/QTc Interval Prolongation and Proarrhythmic Potential for Non-Antiarrhythmic Drugs," that was accepted by the regulatory authorities in the United States, the European Union, and Japan in 2005.[2] ICH E14 focuses on a more systematic clinical evaluation of a drug for its effect on QT_c interval in humans. According to ICH E14, drugs are expected to receive a clinical electrocardiographic evaluation, beginning early in clinical development, typically including a single trial dedicated to evaluating their effect on cardiac repolarization (thorough QT/QT_c study or TQTS). Indeed, the TQT is an in vivo bioassay designed to evaluate the propensity of a drug to prolong the QT interval in humans. Normal volunteers receive in a randomized crossover sequence, or in parallel groups, a placebo, a positive control that slightly prolongs the QT interval, the study drug at therapeutic dose, and the study drug at a supratherapeutic dose. A thorough QT study is described as negative when the upper bound of the 95% one-sided confidence interval for the largest time-matched mean effect of the drug on the QT interval excludes 10 milliseconds. A TQT is required for most new drugs and is typically performed after in vitro testing, and pilot data have suggested that the drug is unlikely to affect cardiac repolarization. If a drug is known to prolong the QT interval or is unsuitable for administration to normal volunteers, then precise QT data must be generated from clinical trials in patients performed "in the spirit of a TQT" as is the case for oncology products. Traditionally, TQT studies are performed in normal volunteers, except in oncology phase 1 trials where patients with incurable cancer often serve as subjects in early trials. This situation makes electrocardiogram (ECG) evaluation more complex in the sense that pre-existing cardiac disease and concomitant medications may complicate the precise assessment of the effect of study drug on the ECG. Thoughtful review of a potential participant's medical history, ECG, and concomitant medications is sufficient screening; however, more aggressive testing is rarely being justified.

Division of Development of New Drugs, European Institute of Oncology, Via Ripamonti, 435, 20141 Milano, Italy
* Corresponding author.
E-mail address: giuseppe.curigliano@ieo.it

RHYTHM DISTURBANCES: "WHAT IS QT INTERVAL"?

The development of new drugs in the past decade has revealed a new spectrum of proarrythmogenic effects of anticancer drugs, the most important one consisting of QT interval prolongation. In the ECG, the QT interval is measured from the beginning of the QRS complex to the end of the T wave (Fig. 13.1). Although prolongation of the QT interval is not the best predictor of this proarrhythmic risk, it represents the principal clinical surrogate marker by which to evaluate the torsadogenic risk of a drug, and it has been a common cause of withdrawal from the market for several drugs.[3,4]

The assessment of cardiac safety and risk/benefit of a drug is more complicated in the field of oncology. The decision of a regulatory agency to approve a promising anticancer agent, and the physician to administer it, is based on the assumption that the benefits of therapy outweigh the risks. Thus, although clinicians, regulatory bodies, and drug developers may be able to predict that a given drug may carry some risks due to QT_c prolongation, precise determination of the risk/benefit remains difficult if not elusive for the development and clinical use of many anticancer agents.

QT interval is a measure of the total duration of ventricular activation and recovery (depolarization and repolarization). These electrical processes in cardiac myocytes are mediated through channels, complex molecular structures within the myocardial cell membrane that regulate the flow of ions in and out of cardiac cells in a well-synchronized sequence. The ventricular action potential proceeds through 5 phases (0 through 4) (Fig. 13.2):

- Phase 0 (action potential upstroke)
- Phase 1 (notch or rapid repolarization phase)
- Phase 2 (plateau phase)
- Phase 3 (period of rapid repolarization)
- Phase 4 (diastolic period).

The initial upstroke (phase 0, depolarization) occurs through the opening and closing of Na^+ channels. The repolarization process begins with the rapid transient outflow of K^+ ions (phase 1). Phase 1 is followed by a relatively more sustained flow of outward current through 2 components of delayed rectifier K^+ channels (the slow component or IK_s and IK_r) and of inward current through Ca^{++} channels, constituting phase 2 or the plateau phase of repolarization (phase 3). Phase 4 represents a return of the action potential to baseline. The rapid inflow of positively charged ions (sodium and calcium) results in normal myocardial depolarization. When this inflow is exceeded by outflow of potassium ions, myocardial repolarization occurs. Malfunction of ion channels that lead to sustained inward flow of positively charged sodium ions or to impaired outward flow of potassium ions results in prolongation of QT interval. QT interval prolongation can result from drugs, electrolyte abnormalities, or other factors. Almost all drugs that prolong the QT interval have been shown to impair the function of IK_r channel. At a submolecular level, the effect of a drug on IK_r current is recapitulated by its effect on human ether-a-go-go (HERG) subunit that is encoded by the KCNH2 gene. Table 13.1 summarizes the risk factors that could provoke TdP.

Cancer patients may be at risk of QT prolongation because many of them have electrolyte disturbance, have baseline ECG abnormalities, or take concomitant medications that could enlarge QT interval, listed in Table 13.2.

MEASUREMENT AND INTERPRETATION OF THE QT INTERVAL

The duration of QT interval varies with the heart rate (HR). Therefore, a drug can influence the duration of QT interval not only by an inhibitory effect on IK_r but also indirectly by an effect on HR. Given the QT interval prolonging at slower

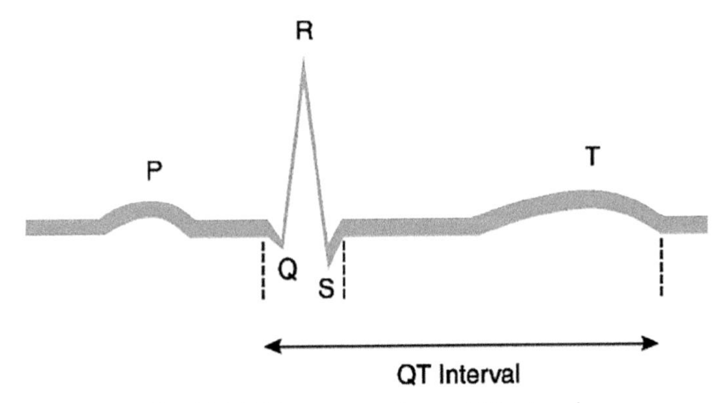

Fig. 13.1 ECG representation and QT interval.

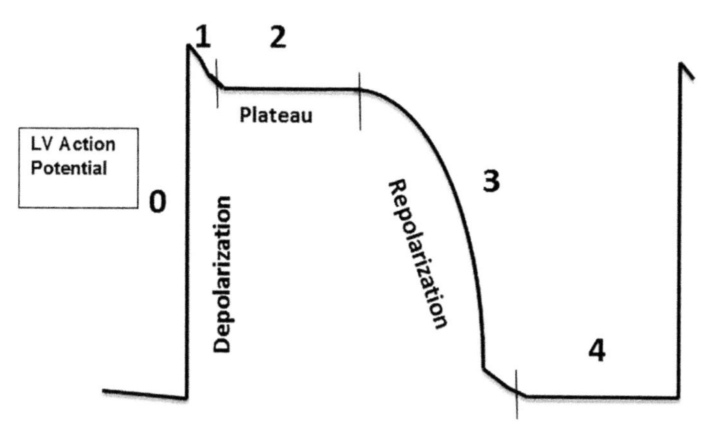

Fig. 13.2 Ventricular action potential process.

HRs and shortening at faster HRs, the measured QT interval requires a correction for HR to standardize it to HR. Table 13.3 shows the principal formulae proposed to correct QT for HR variation. None of these corrections has been thoroughly evaluated and compared with each other in patients to determine the most effective formula in predicting which patients are at the greatest risk of the actual clinical risk, namely, TdP. For evaluation of drug effects, however, analyses of drug effect using the Fridericia correction (QT_cF interval) have been considered generally satisfactory in studies that are conducted in patients. Although the QTc has been the standard measurement of ventricular repolarization, it includes both depolarization and repolarization and may not always be a sensitive indicator of the type of repolarization abnormalities seen in bundle branch block or in patients with pacemaker activity or with the hereditary long QT syndrome (LQTS) (Case Study, available on Expert Consult). Intraventricular conduction abnormalities complicate evaluation of the QTc interval. The rate-corrected JT interval (JTc) is a more accurate measurement of

TABLE 13.1
Risk factors for torsades de pointes in case of QT_c prolongation

Gender	Female sex
Age	>65 y
Cardiovascular disease	Bradycardia (especially recent heart-rate slowing), mitral valve prolapse, congestive HF or cardiac hypertrophy, myocarditis, atrioventricular block
Endocrine disorders	Hypothyroidism, hyperparathyroidism, hyperaldosteronism
Clinical or subclinical congenital LQTS	
Ion-channel polymorphisms	
Baseline ECG alteration	Prolongation QT or T-wave liability
Postexposure ECG that shows	QT prolongation, pathologic TU morphology, and marked post-extrasystolic QTU changes
Drugs	Diuretic use (independent of electrolyte serum concentration), drugs-induced proarrhythmic effects
Electrolyte disturbance	Hypokalemia, hypomagnesemia, hypocalcemia
Other disease	Anorexia nervosa, liquid proteins diets, major gastrointestinal bypass, diabetes, cirrhosis, AIDS
Nervous system injuries	Subarachnoid hemorrhage, stroke, intracranial trauma, pheochromocytoma
Related to drug administration	High drug concentration, rapid rate of intravenous infusion with a QT prolonging drug

TABLE 13.2
Drugs producing prolonged QT interval

Class of Drugs	Drugs
Antidepressants	Amitriptyline, imipramine, desipramine, clomipramine
Antipsychotics	Phenothiazine, droperidol, haloperidol
Serotonin agonist/ antagonist	Cisapride, zimeldine
Antiarrhythmic drugs	IA: quinidine, amaline, disopyramide, procainamide IB: flecaine, propafenone II: amiodarone, sotalol, dofetilide, ibutilide
Vasodilators	Bepridil, perhexiline
Antibiotics	Clarithromycin, sparfloxacin, pentamide, erythromycin
Antifungals	Miconazole, itraconazole, ketokonazole
Other	Methadone

ventricular repolarization, and therefore, may be a more sensitive means of assessing abnormalities. The JTc is a more specific measurement of ventricular repolarization than the QTc by eliminating QRS duration variability. It appears to be a more sensitive predictor of repolarization abnormalities and may be helpful in identifying patients with LQTS who have borderline or normal QTc measurements on resting ECGs.

QT_C INTERVAL PROLONGATION AND NEW DRUGS

New drugs present a special problem, because clinical experience with each drug is limited at the time of their evaluation by regulatory authorities, such as the FDA or the European Medicines Agency. Until the effects of the drug on the QT/QT_c interval have been characterized, the following exclusion criteria are suggested:

- A marked baseline prolongation of QT/QT_c interval (eg, repeated demonstration of a QT_c interval of >450 milliseconds)
- A history of additional risk factors for TdP (eg, heart failure [HF], hypokalemia, and family history of LQTS)
- The use of concomitant medications that prolong the QT/QT_c interval

For the development of cytotoxic oncology products, discussions continue between regulators and other stakeholders about the most optimal methods for gathering data on their QT liability.

There are several other concerns that need to be highlighted when designing phase 1 trials in oncology. Patient capabilities and compliance in tolerating trial demands must be considered. The timing of ECG collection is usually concomitant with pharmacokinetic blood sampling and requires an outstanding level of compliance from patients enrolled into the study. Because of concomitant medications, rapid assessment and decision making during administration of the drug with a significant risk of QT_c prolongation can induce psychological distress that needs to be mitigated through education and preparation, including the informed consent process.

Another level of concerns is related to protocol issues. Oncology trial issues can be divided into design issues and technical ECG issues. The trial design issues originate from defining the purpose of the study and how the potential QT evaluation will affect the trial. Definition of clinical trial inclusion criteria is an important consideration. The definition of QT_c prolongation varies in the literature, but most investigators consider normal QT_c of $\leq$400 milliseconds and prolonged QT_c of greater than 450 milliseconds in men and greater than 470 milliseconds in women. Ventricular arrhythmias, particularly TdP, are correlated with QT_c of $\geq$500 milliseconds, but there is no threshold below which prolongation QT interval is considered free of proarrhythmic risk.[5,6] In view of the major difficulties encountered in conducting a formal TQTS for a cytotoxic oncology product, it is not appropriate or ethical to exclude all patients with prolonged QT_c at baseline. Such exclusions also raise significant clinical dilemmas for investigators, patients, and caregivers alike because phase 1 studies offer access to new agents that can provide perhaps the only opportunity for disease control. In addition, and perhaps more importantly, the risk and the frequency of QT_c prolongation do not correlate well with the risk and the frequency of significant arrhythmia or other adverse clinical outcomes. There is also a need to make many protocol decisions related to the technical aspects of capturing ECGs. Although these issues can be approached

TABLE 13.3
QT correction formulae

Reference	Formula	Advantages	Disadvantages
Nonlinear formulae			
Bazett	$QT_cB = (HR/60)^{1/2} = QT\ (RR)^{-1/2}$	The most used; simple, limited number of ECG records; more corrections at HR <60 bpm	Nonsubjective variable; less correction with long QT
Fridericia	$QT_cFri = (HR/60)^{1/3} = QT\ (RR)^{-1/3}$	More correction at HR <100 bpm	Nonsubjective variable; less correction with short QT
Malik	$QTij = QTij\ 1000^{\beta\hat{J}}/RR^{\beta\hat{J}}$	Subjective variable	Require high ECG records
Linear formulae			
Framingham	$QT_cFr = QT + 154\ (1 - HR/60) = QT + 0.154\ (1000 - RR)$	Expresses in milliseconds; more correction with long QT; adaptable for men and women	Less correction with short QT
Hodges	$QT_cH = QT + 1.75\ (HR - 60) = QT + 105\ (1/RR - 1)$	Expresses in seconds; fits globally the ECGs database; works well with wide populations	Less correction with HR <60 bpm

Abbreviations: β, treatment variable; B, Bazett; Fr, Framingham; Fri, Fridericia; H, Hodges; i, subject variable; QT, QT interval; QT_c, corrected QT interval; RR, RR interval.

essentially in the same manner in oncology trials as in trials in any other therapeutic area, the special needs of oncology patients must be recognized. These special needs are related to the performance status of the patients: a rapid disease progression or a symptomatic disease could affect compliance of the patient with an "intensive" cardiac monitoring protocol.

INTERNATIONAL CONFERENCE ON HARMONIZATION S7B GUIDELINE AND NEW DRUGS: NONCLINICAL ASSESSMENT QT_C INTERVAL PROLONGATION

S7B is an ICH guideline that deals with nonclinical evaluation of the potential for delayed ventricular repolarization by human pharmaceuticals. It promotes a concept of integrated risk assessment, based on the chemical and pharmacologic class of the drug, together with data from 2 core tests—in vitro IK_r or HERG assay and in vivo studies in a suitable species. Although great progress has been made over the last 10 years or so, no single nonclinical assay has an absolute positive and/or negative predictive value or can be considered a gold standard.[7]

The sensitivity of nonclinical tests (ie, their ability to label as positive those drugs with a real risk of inducing QT prolongation in humans) is sufficiently good, but their specificity (ie, their ability to label as negative those drugs carrying no risk) has been challenged. Although S7B does not refer to it, transmural dispersion of repolarization seems to be another marker of the torsadogenic potential of a compound.[8] This parameter is a measure of the radial dispersion of repolarization across the ventricular wall and is the interval from the first repolarization of the specialized M cells located in the midmyocardial layer to the epicardial cells.[9] This radial dispersion of repolarization generates local electrical gradients and appears to provide the electrophysiological substrate necessary for induction of TdP. Consequently, transmural dispersion of repolarization, rather than QT_c interval prolongation, is thought to be more predictive of the potential risk of developing TdP.

CURRENT GUIDELINES FOR CLINICAL ASSESSMENT OF QT INTERVAL

The ICH E14 guideline was not specifically developed for cancer clinical trials. Although the ICH E14 does review different HR correction formulas to determine QT, it does not explicitly state which formula should be used. ICH E14 recommends that data from uncorrected QT and QT_c (via Bazett, Fridericia, or another formula), as well HR data, be recorded and monitored. This ambiguity limits the applicability of the guideline's recommendations for baseline QT_c and drug-related QT prolongation. Thus, for feasibility and convenience, multiple early-phase oncology trials have adapted alternative protocol designs other than the TQTS to address the question of drug-induced QT prolongation. A revision of current standards for QT interval assessment, such that they are more applicable and specific to oncology drug development, is required.

Table 13.4 presents the National Cancer Institute's (Bethesda, MD) toxicity criteria for QT_c[10] interval prolongation.

These criteria are practically limited, because no parameters for QT_c measurement or correction are outlined, and the distinction between different grades of QT_c toxicity may be arbitrary (ie, QT of >500 milliseconds without serious cardiovascular symptoms is grade 3, whereas the same QT interval in the presence of symptoms is grade 4). Definition of these terms that are validated by clinical relevance would be useful for oncology drug developers. For current practice, the QTc interval should not exceed 470 milliseconds before the start of a drug with QTc prolonging properties. During therapy, the QTc interval should not be longer than 500 milliseconds. If this cutoff is exceeded, therapy is to be held but may be resumed at a reduced dose after normalization unless the patient developed symptoms in which case it is to be stopped permanently. In order to detect these changes, ECGs should be obtained at baseline, at 2 to 4 weeks, at 8 to 12 weeks, and every 3 months thereafter. The same ECG frequency is required after dose reductions or therapy interruptions over 2 weeks.

TABLE 13.4
National Cancer Institute prolonged QT_c clinical terminology criteria for adverse events

QTc Prolongation Grade	Definition
I	QT_c >450–470 ms
II	QT_c >470–500 ms or >60 ms above baseline
III	QT_c >500 ms
IV	QT_c >500 ms; life-threatening signs or symptoms (ie, arrhythmia, shock, syncope, hypotension), TdP
V	Death

Abbreviations: CHF, congestive heart failure; QT_c, corrected QT interval.

QT PROLONGATION AND TARGETED DRUGS

QT prolongation has been associated with several classes of targeted agents, including the histone deacetylase (HDAC) inhibitors, multitargeted tyrosine kinase inhibitors (TKIs), vascular disruption agents (VDAs), farnesyl protein transferase (FPTase) inhibitors, Src/Abl kinase inhibitors, and protein kinase C (PKC) inhibitors.

Histone Deacetylase Inhibitors

The HDAC inhibitors (HDIs) target an epigenetic mechanism of acetylation that modulates transcription, resulting in accumulation of hyperacetylated histone proteins, which causes cell cycle arrest in G1 and G2.[10,11] Because of asymptomatic ECG changes noted in early trials, patients receiving these agents have been closely monitored; however, HDIs do not appear to be associated with a greater incidence of cardiac adverse events than other chemotherapeutic agents. Vorinostat and romidepsin have been the most studied, followed by entinostat and belinostat.

Depsipeptide (FK228, romidepsin)

Depsipeptide is a cyclic peptide HDI that has been variably associated with QT prolongation, and rarely, sudden cardiac death.[12,13] Neither ECG abnormalities nor cardiac hemorrhage was observed when depsipeptide was infused over 4 hours. With QT interval prolongation and ST segment abnormalities observed in preclinical and phase 1 studies, intensive cardiac monitoring was incorporated into the phase 2 trials of depsipeptide. The effect of romidepsin on cardiac function was evaluated in 42 patients with T-cell lymphoma, who received a total of 736 doses in 282 cycles of romidepsin with intensive cardiac monitoring that included more than 2000 ECGs and 161 left ventricular ejection fraction (LVEF) evaluations.[14] Grade I (T-wave flattening) and grade II (ST segment depression) ECG changes occurred in more than half of the ECGs obtained after treatment; however, these changes were reversible and of short duration, with no elevation in cardiac enzymes and no significant changes in LVEF. Overall, after-treatment ECGs had a mean Bazett HR corrected QT_c interval prolongation of 14 milliseconds compared with baseline. Although cardiac dysrhythmias (supraventricular and ventricular tachycardia [VT]) were observed in a small number of patients, most of these patients had pretreatment-documented dysrhythmias, and some cases had abnormal electrolyte levels, which prompted the recommendation to maintain potassium and magnesium levels in the high-normal reference range, particularly at the time of infusion. Similar ECG changes and QT interval prolongation have been reported in other phase 1/2 romidepsin studies.[15–20] There have been reports of sudden death in a few romidepsin studies; however, the relationship to the drug remains unclear. In a phase 2 study of 15 patients with metastatic neuroendocrine tumors, using romidepsin at a standard dose of 14 mg/m^2 intravenous infusion over 4 hours, one sudden death was reported in a 48-year-old patient 20 hours after completion of the fifth dose of romidepsin.[20] However, this patient had a history of hypertension, and post-mortem examination revealed biventricular hypertrophy, both of which are known risk factors for sudden death. In addition, the patient had chronic hypokalemia and received concomitant ondansetron and octreotide therapy (both of which are known to cause QT interval prolongation).

Another case of sudden death was reported in 1 of 29 patients with refractory renal cell cancer (RCC) in a phase 2 romidepsin study; once again, this patient had multiple risk factors for sudden death, including hypertension, chronic obstructive airway disease, and a history of heavy smoking.[21] In a retrospective analysis of 500 patients who received Fk228, 5 sudden deaths were reported. All of these patients had risk factors, such as electrolyte abnormalities, concomitant medications with a QT_c-prolonging agent, or hypertrophic cardiomyopathy. Documentation of enlarged QT was not observed before sudden death.

Vorinostat

Vorinostat is a small-molecule inhibitor of class I and II HDAC enzymes,[22] which binds directly to the catalytic pocket of HDAC enzymes and is orally bioavailable. Clinical activity has been shown in patients with a variety of malignancies, including cutaneous T-cell lymphoma (CTCL). Currently, vorinostat is marketed with an indication for the treatment of patients with CTCL who have progressive, persistent, or recurrent disease on or following 2 systemic therapies at a daily dose of 400 mg.[23] Cardiac-associated adverse experiences have not been reported commonly.

Cardiac rhythm and ECG alterations have been suggested to be a class effect with HDIs.[13,14] However, a specific hypothesis explaining the underlying mechanism or mechanisms has yet to be determined. A dedicated QT_c assessment study was conducted in patients with cancer to provide a more rigorous assessment of the potential for vorinostat to prolong ventricular repolarization. In 24 patients with advanced cancer, a single supratherapeutic 800-mg dose of vorinostat did not prolong the QT_c interval (monitored over 24 hours). Results indicate that a supratherapeutic single dose of vorinostat is not associated with significant prolongation of ventricular repolarization. This study was designed using many of the recommendations in the ICH E14 QT/QT_c guidance and could be a more general approach for QT_c evaluation of cancer drugs.

Oral panobinostat (LBH589)

Oral panobinostat is a novel cinnamic acid hydroxamate that inhibits HDAC and hinders HERG K^+ in preclinical studies, currently being investigated in several human malignancies.

When 2 phase 1 studies of LBH589 were compared for cardiac effects, a dose-related increase in Fridericia QT of at most 20 milliseconds was observed on day 3 of drug delivery. In a phase 2 nonrandomized single-arm trial, LBH589 was tested in patients with low/intermediate-1-risk myelodisplastic syndrome. No major adverse events were documented except for one patient that developed significant QT_c prolongation. QT_c interval increased from a baseline of 409 to 556 milliseconds. The patient was asymptomatic, and the event did not result in cardiac arrhythmia. At the time of the event, the patient also had severe anemia (hemoglobin 6 g/dL). QT_c normalized with drug cessation and correction of anemia. The patient was discontinued from study drug.

Table 13.5 shows incidence and severity of suspected drug-related QT_c prolongation of any grade in panobinostat clinical trials.[24]

Similarly, LAQ824, another cinnamic acid hydroxamate inhibitor of HDAC that blocks the HERG K^+, also increases QT_c in phase 1 studies. Nonspecific, asymptomatic, and reversible ST-T wave changes were also observed. LAQ824 did not affect cardiac function in serial assessments of cardiac function by acquisition scans.

Other members of the HDIs, including CI-994 and MS275, have been also tested in early-phase clinical trials, without documentation of QT effects.

Table 13.6 shows a summary of preclinical cardiac markers and clinical effects of HDIs.

In summary, the ECG changes observed to date with HDI treatment appear to be clinically insignificant; however, additional studies may be needed to rule out any long-term cardiac effects.

TABLE 13.5
Incidence and severity of suspected drug-related QT_c prolongation of any grade in panobinostat clinical trials

Route of Administration	Giles et al, 2006[94] Intravenous	Sharma et al, 2007[95] Intravenous	Prince et al, 2007[96] Oral
Dose	4.8, 7.2, 9.0, 11.5, or 14.0 mg/m^2	10, 15, or 20 mg/m^2	15, 20, or 30 mg
Schedule	Days 1–7 of 21-d cycle	Days 1, 8, and 15 of 28-d cycle	Days 1, 3, and 5 every week on 28-d cycle
Patient population	Refractory hematologic malignancies	Advanced solid tumors or non-Hodgkin lymphoma (NHL) with/without prior systemic therapy	Advanced solid tumors or NHL with/without prior systemic therapy
Cardiovascular exclusion criteria	Impaired cardiac function, clinically significant cardiac disease, congenital LQTS	Impaired cardiac function, clinically significant cardiac disease, or congenital prolonged QT syndrome	Impaired cardiac function, clinically significant cardiac disease, or congenital prolonged QT syndrome
Overall incidence of grade ≥2 QT_cF prolongation (regardless of dose)	5/15 (33.3%) patients	3/44 (6.8%) patients	2/32 (6.3%) patients
Severity of QT_cF prolongation	Grade 3; 14 mg/m^2 dose; 3 patients[a] Grade 3; 11.5 mg/m^2 dose; 1 patient Grade 2; 9.0 mg/m^2 dose; 1 patient[b]	Grade 3; 20 mg/m^2 dose; 1 patient[c] Grade 2; 20 mg/m^2 dose; 2 patients	Grade 3; 20 mg dose; 1 patient Grade 2; 30 mg dose; 1 patient[d]

[a] Grade 3 QT_cF prolongation defined as greater than 500 ms.
[b] Grade 2 QT_cF prolongation defined as change from baseline of greater than 60 ms.
[c] This patient entered the study with left bundle branch block.
[d] Isolated event after first dose, which did not recur with continued therapy at same daily dose.

Multitarget Tyrosine Kinase Inhibitors

TKIs are effective in the targeted treatment of various malignancies. Imatinib was the first to be introduced into clinical oncology, and drugs such as gefitinib, erlotinib, sorafenib, sunitinib, and dasatinib followed it. Almost 30 TKIs have been approved for use in oncology with more in development or under regulatory review. Although they share the same mechanism of action, namely, competitive ATP inhibition at the catalytic binding site of tyrosine kinase, they differ from each other in the spectrum of targeted kinases and their pharmacokinetics as well as substance-specific adverse effects. Their use has been found to be associated with serious toxicities, including cardiac toxicity. The QT effect of most QT-prolonging TKIs (except lapatinib, nilotinib, sunitinib, and vandetanib) is relatively mild at clinical doses and has not led to appreciable morbidity clinically.

Lu and colleagues[25] exposed canine heart muscle cells to TKIs and other drugs known to prolong the QT interval and reported that TKI-induced QT prolongation was actually due to inhibition of the phosphoinositide 3-kinase (PI3K) signaling pathway, which affects multiple ion channels, not just the potassium channels. Drug-induced PI3K inhibition resulted in prolongation of action potential duration (APD), and the addition of a second messenger produced by the PI3K pathway normalized the APD. For 3 of 16 TKIs (erlotinib, imatinib, and regorafenib), there are no significant data concerning their QT liability. Nine of the other 13 TKIs carry a standard set of warnings and cautions with respect to their potential to prolong the QT_c interval and recommendations or restrictions during their clinical use. Prescribing information for the remaining 4 TKIs is either cautiously noncommittal (axitinib and gefitinib) or simply describes the results of a negative study (bosutinib and ruxolitinib).

In a review article, Rashmi and colleagues[26] evaluated the QT-related preclinical and

TABLE 13.6
Selected histone deacetylase inhibitors in clinical use or development and summary of drug effect in preclinical cardiac markers and clinical cardiac effects

Compound by Class	Manufacturer	HDAC Class Specificity	Preclinical Effects	Clinical Cardiac Effects
Hydroxamic acid				
Vorinostat	Merck	I, II, IV	Unknown	Nonspecific ECG changes
Trichostatin A	Merck	I, II, IV	Unknown	Nonspecific ECG changes
LAQ824 (dacinostat)	Novartis	I, II, IV	HERG K+ interaction	Dose-related increase QT_c
Panobinostat (LBH589)	Novartis	I, II, IV	HERG K+ interaction	Dose-related increase QT_c
Belinostat (PXD101)	CuraGen	I, II, IV	Significant effect on plasma PlGF and b-FGF	QT_c prolongation was the reason for dose reduction in 3 patients, but this was not symptomatic and did not require treatment
ITF2357 (givinostat)	Italfarmaco	I, II, IV	Unknown	Not significant cardiac side effects
Cyclic tetrapeptide				
Depsipeptide (romidepsin, FK228)	Gloucester Pharmaceuticals	I (particularly HDAC1, HDAC2)	Canine/murine models, cardiac enzyme elevation, myocardium inflammation, QT/QT_c prolongation	QT_c prolongation (mean, 14 ms), 3-s sinus pause VT, 6 sudden deaths
Benzamide				
Entinostat (SNDX-275/MS-275)	Syndax Pharmaceuticals	I (particularly HDAC1, HDAC2, HDAC3)	Unknown	Not significant cardiac side effects
MGCD0103 (Mocetinostat)	Celgene	I	Unknown	Not significant cardiac side effects
Short-chain aliphatic acids				
Valproic acid	—	I, IIa	NA	NA
Phenyl butyrate	—	I, IIa	NA	NA
AN-9, pivanex	Titan Pharmaceutical	NA	NA	NA

Abbreviation: NA, not available.

clinical data (summarized in Table 13.7) from the regulatory reviews of TKIs, especially the pharmacology, medical, and QT-IRT reviews of the data submitted to the FDA, and the prescribing information. Inevitably, a question arises as to whether the QT liability of TKIs may be a pharmacologic effect linked to inhibition of one or more tyrosine kinases, which may regulate HERG function (on-target effect) or an effect related to a particular chemical class (off-target effect). Mechanisms that modulate HERG channel activity are now known, in particular, its regulation by serine/threonine phosphorylation.[27–29]

TABLE 13.7
Preclinical and clinical data on cardiac repolarization effects of approved tyrosine kinase inhibitors

TKI	Preclinical Data In Vitro (HERG IC50, APD Study)	Preclinical Data In Vivo	Author's Assessment of Overall Preclinical Evidence for an Effect on QT_c Interval	Clinical Data (Clinical Trials, QT Study, TQT Study)	Author's Assessment of Overall Preclinical Evidence for an Effect on QT_c Interval
Axitinib	Not done APD study	No effect on QT_c in dogs	Negative	TQT study, no data	Possible negative
Bosutinib	Not done APD study	Slight, dose-independent QT_c prolongation observed at high doses	Questionable	QT study, no data	Negative
Crizotinib	Antagonism of calcium and sodium channels in dogs	QT_c prolonged at high doses in dogs	Positive	No QT and TQT study	Positive
Dasatinib	Slight APD 90 prolongation at 30 μM in rabbit	No effects on QT_c interval in monkeys	Negative	No QT and TQT study	Equivocal
Erlotinib	No effects on APD 90 at 3 μM in rabbit	No ECG effects in dogs	Negative	No QT and TQT study	Negative
Gefitinib	ADP 90 increased at ≥2.5 μM in dogs	Mild QT_c prolongation in dogs at 5 and 50 mg/kg doses	Positive	No QT and TQT study	Equivocal
Imatinib	No data, APD not done	No ECG effects in rats and dogs	Data not adequate	No data on QT interval	Questionable
Lapatinib	No effects on APD 90 in dogs	No effects on QT_c interval in rats and dogs	Negative	No QT and TQT study	Positive

Nilotinib	In isolate rabbits hearts, APD 90 increased	No effects on QT_c in dogs at doses up to 300 mg/kg	Positive	QT study no data	Positive
Pazopanib	No effects on APD 90 in dogs	No QT_c effects in monkeys	Negative	QT study no data	Minimal
Regorafenib	No effect of the parent drug in rabbits	No effect from the parent drug and metabolites in dogs	Negative	TQT study no data	Negative
Ruxolitinib	APD 90 not done	Slight increase in QT_c in dogs at high doses	Negative	Only TQT study	Negative
Sorafenib	In rabbit APD 90 increased (? calcium channel block)	No QT_c effect in dogs	Positive	No QT and TQT study	Possible positive
Sunitinib	? Calcium channel block	QT_c prolonged at high doses in excess of 50 mg/kg in monkeys	Positive	No QT study	Positive
Vandetanib	In dogs APD 90 prolonged	Dose-dependent increase in QT_c and changes in T-wave morphology in dogs	Positive	No QT and TQT study	Positive
Vemurafenib	Interpretation difficult, but APD 90 seemed prolonged in dogs	No effect on QT_c but AV block detected in dogs	Positive	No QT and TQT study	Positive

Rashmi and colleagues[26] summarize some key observations:

- Cyclic adenosine 5′-monophosphate (cAMP)-dependent protein kinase A (PKA) is a serine/threonine kinase that can be stimulated by extracellular signals that elevate intracellular cAMP concentrations.[28]
- HERG channels can be subject to acute regulation by changes in cAMP and cAMP-dependent PKA.
- Normal HERG function in HEK293 cells requires basal activity of AKT, another serine/threonine protein kinase.[30] Activation of AKT occurs downstream of PI3K (the PI3K/AKT/mammalian target of rapamycin pathway and other signaling pathways).
- HERG is modulated also by the EGF family of receptor tyrosine kinase.[31] Regulation of HERG channels by tyrosine kinases modifies the channel activity and thus likely alters the electrophysiological properties, including APD and cell excitability in the human heart.

Although these interactions may suggest a class-related effect of TKIs that acts on certain kinases linked to a specific ligand and inhibition of PI3K, there is no indication at the moment of a consistent predictable link. In fact, TKIs with and TKIs without a QT liability inhibit tyrosine kinases that are frequently linked to the same ligand or set of ligands. The authors focused on sunitinib, vandetanib, nilotinib, and dasatinib because of their QT effects that led to appreciable clinically morbidity.

Sunitinib malate

Sunitinib malate is a small molecule TKI used in the treatment of RCC and gastrointestinal stromal tumors. It has also demonstrated efficacy in treating pancreatic neuroendocrine tumors and is being evaluated for the treatment of other cancers. In preclinical studies, sunitinib malate and its active metabolite SU012662 interact with HERG K^+. In addition, sunitinib mesylate induced in vitro APD prolongation in Purkinje fibers and in vivo QT prolongation in monkey studies. Initially developed for its inhibition of the vascular endothelial growth factor (VEGF) signaling pathway, sunitinib has been associated with hypertension and HF. A study of 75 patients found an 8% incidence of HF and a 28% incidence of LVEF decrease of greater than 10%.[32] A multicenter analysis has also confirmed cardiac events following sunitinib treatment.[33] The molecular mechanism for cardiotoxicity is unknown. Myocardial biopsy in patients who developed sunitinib-related left ventricular (LV) dysfunction demonstrated hypertrophy and structural abnormalities of the mitochondria, but no necrosis or fibrosis was seen, and sarcomere structure was preserved.[32] These pathologic findings were confirmed in mice.[33] In both of the above studies, significant improvement in LV dysfunction was seen after stopping sunitinib (83% and 58% of patients, respectively), and no cumulative dose relationship was present. TdP has been observed in less than 0.1% of patients receiving sunitinib.[32] Sunitinib, however, is associated with hypertension, which probably contributes to the pathogenesis of HF in this group. Mechanistic insights suggest that an attentive clinical strategy for hypertension could prevent severe cardiotoxicity. Indeed, the sunitinib scenario is similar in that the hearts of older patients stressed with increased afterload and who experience detectable declines in cardiac reserve as a consequence have persistent vulnerability of their myocytes. Although the final explanation will have to take other possible mechanisms into account as well, sequential stress associated with hypertension is probably part of the involved mechanism. Cardiac monitoring during treatment is appropriate.

Vandetanib (Zactima, ZD 6474)

Vandetanib is a once-daily potent inhibitor of rearranged during transfection receptor tyrosine kinase activity and of VEGFR-2 and epidermal growth factor receptor (EGFR) tyrosine kinase activity. Preclinical studies showed an interaction on vandetanib with cardiac ion channels, in particular HERG K^+, leading to repolarization abnormalities and QT_c prolongation.[34] In a phase 1 trial of vandetanib in solid tumors, 9% of patients developed asymptomatic QT_c prolongation, whereas in a Japanese phase 1 trial, the incidence increased to 61%.[5,35] Hammett and colleagues[36] carried out a study of ZD6474 pharmacodynamic effect on cardiac repolarization in combination with ondansetron in 28 healthy male volunteers. The combination of vandetanib with ondansetron demonstrated a direct additive effect on the increase of QT interval. In another phase 1 trial, 2 of 7 patients experienced QT_c prolongation.[37] In phase 2 trials, the incidence of asymptomatic QT prolongation was 15%; all events were of grade 1 to 2.[6] In a phase 2 trial,[38] assessing vandetanib in combination with docetaxel for patients with platinum refractory non–small-cell lung cancer (NSCLC), no clinically symptomatic changes in ECG was observed between treatment groups. All episodes of QT_c prolongation were asymptomatic and manageable with dose interruption and/or reduction. One patient in the run-in phase experienced asymptomatic, no sustained VT in the setting of electrolyte abnormalities and QT_c prolongation, both of which normalized following electrolyte repletion.[38] In a phase 2 trial evaluating this drug among patients suffering from relapsed multiple myeloma, no ECG QT prolongation was found.[39] In a phase 2 trial conducted in patients with previously treated metastatic breast cancer (BC), the mean QT_c increased. Seven patients in the 300-mg cohort had asymptomatic grade 1 prolongation of the QT_c interval. No patient developed symptomatic arrhythmia. Although QT_c prolongation was reported at a variety of dose levels, repolarization abnormalities, including changes in T-wave morphology as well as QT and QT_c prolongation, were more frequent with doses of greater than 500 mg daily.[35] Vandetanib was evaluated also in patients with small-cell lung cancer. Asymptomatic QT_c prolongation was observed in 8 patients on vandetanib. All grade QT prolongation was found in 15% of patients on vandetanib versus 0 in control patients. No grade 3 or 4 QT_c prolongation was observed.[40] Vandetanib is now being tested in phase 3 trials. In a phase 3 study assessing the efficacy of vandetanib versus erlotinib in unselected patients with advanced NSCLC after treatment failure with 1 to 2 prior cytotoxic chemotherapy regimens, a protocol defined QT_c prolongation occurred in 32 patients (5.1%) receiving vandetanib and in 1 patient (0.2%) receiving erlotinib. These events were asymptomatic and resolved after dose interruption/reduction with the exception of 2 patients for whom this event led to the discontinuation of vandetanib; these events resolved after study treatment was stopped. TdP occurred in one patient, who recovered without sequelae after vandetanib was discontinued.[41] In a randomized, placebo-controlled phase 3 study assessing the efficacy of vandetanib plus pemetrexed as second-line therapy in advanced NSCLC, elevated blood pressure (>160 mm Hg systolic; <100 mm Hg or change from baseline >20 mm Hg diastolic) was more common in the vandetanib arm (29 vs 13%). Most hypertension adverse events were of grade 1 to 2, with grade 3 to 4 events reported in 2% of the patients in the vandetanib arm and in 1% in the placebo arm. One patient in the vandetanib arm experienced protocol-defined QT_c prolongation, which was asymptomatic and resolved without dose interruption or reduction.[42] Finally, in a randomized, double-blind phase 3 trial, in patients with locally advanced or metastatic medullary thyroid cancer, more patients required dose reduction of vandetanib compared with placebo for adverse events or QT_c prolongation (35 vs 3%). Nineteen patients (8%) developed protocol-defined QT_c prolongation, but there were no reports of TdP.[43]

Vandetanib has obtained approval for the treatment of symptomatic or progressive medullary thyroid cancer in patients with unresectable locally advanced or metastatic disease. Monitoring ECGs and levels of serum potassium, calcium, magnesium, and TSH at baseline, 2 to 4 weeks, and 8 to 12 weeks after starting treatment with vandetanib, and every 3 months thereafter and following adjustments may be mandatory. Vandetanib should not be used in patients with hypocalcemia, hypokalemia, hypomagnesemia, or LQTS.

Nilotinib

A decade ago, the introduction of imatinib was a key advance in molecularly targeted treatment of cancer. Imatinib greatly improved the outcome of patients with chronic-phase chronic myeloid leukemia (CML), with event-free survival greater than 80% after 6 years.[44,45] However, intolerance, resistance, and disease progression all limit success of imatinib therapy. Several second-generation TKIs, including nilotinib and dasatinib, have been developed. Nilotinib is a multiprotein kinase inhibitor, targeting the BCRABL fusion protein, c-Kit, and platelet-derived growth factor receptor a (PDGFRa), and PDGFRh. Nilotinib received fast-track approval by the FDA for the treatment of chronic phase and accelerated phase Ph+CML in adults resistant or intolerant to at least one prior therapy that included imatinib. Nilotinib, like imatinib, binds to the inactive conformation of BCR-ABL, but is 30 times more potent at inhibiting BCR-ABL activity. Results from the ENESTnd study showed superiority of nilotinib over imatinib as first-line therapy for chronic-phase CML after 12 months of follow-up.[46]

In healthy volunteers, the maximum mean QT_c prolongation change from baseline was 18 milliseconds.[47] In the phase 1 and 2 studies, QT_cF (Fredericia's method) prolongation superior to 60 milliseconds was reported in 1.9% of CML-chronic phase and 2.5% of CML accelerated phase patients. Grade 3/4 drug-related QT prolongation was reported in less than 3% of cases.[48] Five sudden deaths (0.6%) were reported in patients receiving nilotinib in a phase 1/2 study considered probably or potentially related to nilotinib use. Their occurrence suggests that ventricular repolarization abnormalities may have contributed to their occurrence.[48]

Dasatinib

Dasatinib is an oral, dual Src/Abl kinase inhibitor, which has been designed to target populations with BCR-ABL point mutations that interfere with imatinib binding. In vitro analysis of dasatinib demonstrated its interaction with HERG K+ and Purkinje assays. In collected analysis of 467 patients with cancer on phase 2 studies with the drug, the mean change in Fridericia QT_c was 3 to 6 milliseconds, with only 3 patients experiencing QT_c of more than 500 milliseconds, and 14 patients with QT_c that increased for more than 60 milliseconds from baseline.[47] Dasatinib has obtained FDA approval for imatinib-resistant chronic myelogenous leukemia and Philadelphia chromosome–positive acute lymphoblastic leukemia, without specification of QT-monitoring precautions.

As summarized in Table 13.8, TKIs are also associated with several other serious cardiovascular adverse effects unrelated to QT interval.

Ceritinib

ALK is a receptor tyrosine kinase of the insulin receptor superfamily that plays a role in neural development and function. It is translocated, mutated, or amplified in several tumor types, including NSCLC, neuroblastoma, and anaplastic large cell lymphoma, and these alterations play a key role in the pathogenesis of these tumors. Other fusion partners of ALK have been described (eg, KIF5B, TFG, KLC1, and PTPN3), but these are less common than EML4. Preclinical experiments have shown that the various ALK fusion partners mediate ligand-independent dimerization/oligomerization of ALK resulting in constitutive kinase activity and in potent oncogenic activity both in vitro and in vivo. This activity can be effectively blocked by small-molecule inhibitors that target ALK. The first evidence that ALK-positive NSCLC responds to ALK inhibitors was seen with crizotinib, an ALK and MET inhibitor, which in single-arm trials was shown to induce durable responses in 50% to 61% of patients. Although crizotinib has impressive activity in patients with ALK-rearranged NSCLC, these cancers invariably progress, typically in less than 1 year, because of the development of resistance to crizotinib. Therefore, the development of ALK TKIs with clinical activity against ALK-positive NSCLC resistant to crizotinib is crucial. Ceritinib is an orally available ALK inhibitor, approximately a 20-fold more potent ALK inhibitor than crizotinib and more selective for ALK. Ceritinib does not inhibit MET. Ceritinib has potent activity on the hERG channel with an IC50 (half maximal inhibitory concentration) of 0.4 μM. However, there were no ceritinib-related effects in vivo in monkeys at doses as high as 100 mg/kg (human equivalent dose of 1950 mg). In Fase 1 study, Shaw and colleagues[49] administered oral ceritinib in doses of 50 to 750 mg once daily to patients with advanced cancers harboring genetic alterations in ALK. Patients were assessed to determine the safety, pharmacokinetic properties, and antitumor activity of ceritinib. They observed one case of asymptomatic grade 3 prolongation of the corrected QT interval that was possibly related to ceritinib. Overall, 8 patients experimented asymptomatic QT_c prolongation in phase escalation (2/10 [20%] at the dose level of 600 mg, 1/5 [20%] at the dose level of 700 mg, and 5/81 [6%] at the dose level of 750 mg).

Fibroblast Growth Factor Receptors Inhibitors

Recently, the field of fibroblast growth factor receptors (FGFRs) targeting has exponentially progressed thanks to the development of novel agents inhibiting the fibroblast growth factor (FGF) or its receptors (FGFRs), including nonselective and selective TKIs, FGF ligand traps, and monoclonal antibodies (mAbs) (Table 13.9).

Lucitanib

Lucitanib is an oral, potent, selective inhibitor of the tyrosine kinase activity of FGFR1-3, VEGFR1–3, and PDGFRα/β. Fifty-nine patients were treated in the expansion phase I study.[50] Arterial hypertension grade 3 and proteinuria grade 3, qualifying for dose-limiting toxicity (DLT), were the most frequent cardiotoxicities observed. Based on the clinical experience with lucitanib to date, 15 mg on a continuous daily schedule has been identified as the dose that provides meaningful clinical activity with a manageable toxicity profile. The observed toxicity profile is consistent with the mechanism of action and in line with the preclinical safety findings.

BGJ398

BGJ398 is an orally bio-available, selective, and ATP-competitive pan FGFR kinase inhibitor. In vivo safety pharmacology studies in rats and dogs did not reveal any effects on electrocardiographic parameters.

Monoclonal antibodies and fibroblast growth factor ligand traps

mAbs targeting fibroblast growth factors (FGFs) or FGRs can block FGFR signaling by interfering with ligand binding or receptor dimerization.

MFGR1877S is a human anti-FGFR3 mAb that showed antitumor activity in preclinical models

TABLE 13.8
Cardiovascular toxicity of approved tyrosine kinase inhibitors

TKI	Effusion Edema	Hypertension	Pulmonary Hypertension	Pulmonary Embolism	CHF/LV Dysfunction	QT Liability	Bleeding	Venous Thrombosis	Arterial Thrombosis
Crizotinib	X	—	—	X	—	X	—	—	—
Dasatinib	X	—	X	X	X	—	X	X	X
Erlotinib	—	—	—	—	—	—	—	X	X
Gefitinib	—	—	—	—	—	?	—	—	—
Imatinib	X	—	—	—	—	—	X	—	X
Lapatinib	—	—	—	—	X	X	—	—	—
Sunitinib	X	X	—	X	X	X	X	X	X
Sorafenib	—	X	—	—	X	X	X	X	X
Pazopanib	—	X	—	X	X	X	X	X	X
Regorafenib	—	X	—	—	—	—	X	—	X
Vandetanib	—	X	—	—	X	X	X	—	X
Axitinib	—	X	—	—	—	—	X	X	X
Nilotinib	X	—	—	—	X	X	—	—	—
Vemurafenib	X	—	—	—	—	X	—	—	—
Bosutinib	X	—	—	—	—	X	—	—	—
Ruxolitinib	—	—	—	—	—	—	—	—	—

TABLE 13.9
Clinical trials evaluating fibroblast growth factor receptor signaling-targeted therapies currently under development

Type of Cancer	Phase I	Phase II	Phase III
Lung cancer	—	Nindetanib[a] Lenvatinib[a] Lucitanib[a] Ponatinib[a] Brivanib[a] AZD4547[c]	—
Breast cancer	BGJ398[c] AZD4547[c]	Lucitanib[a] Dovitinib[a]	—
All other solid tumors	BGJ398[c] AZD4547[c] ARQ087[d] JNJ-42756493[d] TAS-120[d] Debio 1347[d] LY287445[d] Orantinib[a] GSK3052230[b] MGFR1877S[b]	Ponatinib[a] Nindetanib[a] Lucitanib[a] Lenvatinib[a]	Dovitinib[a] Brivanib[a]

[a] Nonselective FGFR TKIs.
[b] MAbs and FGF-ligand traps.
[c] Selective FGFR TKIs (genomic enrichment).
[d] Selective FGFR TKIs.

of bladder cancer with FGFR3 overexpression. Two phase I studies of MFGR1877S in patients with advanced solid tumors or myeloma have been completed. No significant cardiotoxicity was reported.

Given the multiple physiologic function of FGFR signaling, the feasibility of long-term FGFR signaling inhibition is uncertain. Although nonselective FGFR inhibitors have toxicity profiles close to those for VEGFR TKIs, selective FGFR TKIs display their own class-specific toxicity related to a potent and specific FGFR signaling inhibition. The main specific drug-related adverse events observed to date are all mild and manageable.

Vascular Disrupting Agents

VDAs such as combretastatin A4 phosphate (CA4P) and plinabulin are a rapidly advancing class of oncology therapeutics that elicit antitumor activity by causing a rapid and selective vascular shutdown in tumors to produce extensive secondary neoplastic cell death due to ischemia. The differences between tumor neovasculature and normal vasculature have been recognized for more than 20 years, and several drugs targeting the growth of the tumor vasculature (eg, sunitinib and bevacizumab) have become standard of care validating this approach. These agents principally target the VEGF pathway to inhibit tumor angiogenesis. Because VDAs target the existing tumor vasculature through a different set of molecular targets, preclinical and clinical data showed that the efficacy and toxicity profiles of VDAs may be different from, and complementary to, the VEGF-targeted agents and standard cytotoxic agents.[51–54]

Combretastatin

Zybrestat, otherwise known as fosbretabulin or CA4P, is a target natural tubulin inhibitor that acts as a VDA. The mechanism responsible for the selective vascular damage has not been completely understood.[54,55]

The adverse event profile of CA4P, along with that of other VDAs, includes events of hypertension and cardiac ischemia.[56] In rodents, hypertension after CA4P administration has been linked to mild smooth muscle contraction, which causes an increase in peripheral vascular resistance.[57] In vivo testing resulted in dog bradycardia.[57,58]

In a phase 1 trial, Dowlati and colleagues[58] documented 7 asymptomatic episodes of grade 1 Bazett QT_c prolongation with CA4P 60 mg/m^2 (peak 550 milliseconds, occurring 44 hours after infusion). The mean prolongation in QT_c in the study population of 25 patients was 30.8 milliseconds, 4 hours after drug administration. Two patients developed cardiac ischemia in the trial.[58,59]

Another phase 1 study in 20 patients testing CA4P at a dose of 50 mg/m^2 combined with radiotherapy documented a mean asymptomatic increase in Bazett QT_c of 13 milliseconds, 4 hours after infusion; all QT_c were less than 480 milliseconds. One patient experienced postural syncope after his first dose of CA4P without documentation of prolonged QT_c.[60]

Other clinical trials with CA4P have showed tachycardia or bradycardia, but no further QT-prolonging effects or ventricular arrhythmias have been reported.[61–63] A review of serious adverse events in the greater than 350 patients treated to date with CA4P revealed 2 instances of myocardial infarction and 2 instances of symptomatic ischemia with ECG changes, suggesting an event rate of around 1% to 2%. This event rate is comparable to that reported for antiangiogenic agents.[64] Myocardial ischemia and ECG changes occur in temporal association with after-infusion hypertension. CA4P-related hypertension tends to peak by 1 to 2 hours after infusion and resolves by around 2 to 6 hours.[60,65] Subjects with symptomatic cardiac ischemia have been in this subset with a large increase in systolic blood pressure. Transient asymptomatic ECG changes such as T-wave inversion or ST-segment depression have been reported in some additional patients. Myocardial infarction has been excluded by lack of elevation in cardiac enzymes, such as troponin. Specific guidelines for management of hypertension or cardiac ischemia are included in all ongoing clinical trials. By an unrelated and less well-characterized mechanism, CA4P causes mild-to-moderate asymptomatic QT_c prolongation. Also, the most common arrhythmias observed after CA4P are sinus bradycardia and sinus tachycardia, which may be secondary to changes in peripheral resistance. Meticulous attention to electrolyte management, particularly potassium and magnesium levels, also is critical for minimization of QT changes.

Plinabulin

Plinabulin (NPI-2358) is a VDA showing to produce antitumor activity in animal models alone and synergistically with chemotherapy agents including taxanes.[66,67] Overall, preclinical studies indicated that plinabulin had a favorable safety and activity profile leading to the initiation of this single-agent phase 1 first-in-human trial. Consistent with what was predicted by preclinical toxicologic assessment, plinabulin did not appear to induce QT_c prolongation or impair LVEF, and the incidence of cardiac and neurologic events was not notably different than what would be expected in a phase 1 oncology population. As reported with CA4P administration,[57] these may represent a reactive decrease in HR from the transient increases in blood pressure. Of particular interest, only one significant cardiac adverse event was reported, myocardial infarction remote from plinabulin administration, which differs from multiple occurrences of acute after-infusion ischemia reported in studies with several other VDA. Furthermore, intensive cardiac monitoring did not show that plinabulin affects cardiac function, other than the transient changes in blood pressure and HR described. Therefore, QT_c prolongation has been associated with some VDA but not others and thus may be related to the structure of the individual drug (ie, "off-target" effects, differential interactions with the same target, or differences in pharmacokinetics, metabolism, or distribution).

Farnesyl Protein Transferase Inhibitors

Farnesyltransferase (FT) itself is a heterodimeric enzyme consisting of a 49-kDa subunit, which houses the catalytic site of the enzyme, and a 46-kDa subunit, which is responsible for binding farnesyl pyrophosphate and a protein or peptide substrate. Protein substrates that depend on FT for their activity include Ras, a G protein that governs cell proliferation and survival. Ras is mutated in 30% or less of all human cancers, and its role in carcinogenesis is well established.

FTPase inhibitors selectively inhibit posttranslational farnesylation of Ras and other proteins from other signaling pathways. Therefore, they have antiproliferative, antiangiogenic, and proapoptotic effects.[68] Several farnesyltransferase inhibitors (FTIs) have progressed into clinical trials due to encouraging preclinical and clinical results.

L-778123

Merck developed L-778123. In a phase 1 study of 25 patients, L-778123 has been administered as 7 days continuous. Five patients experienced an asymptomatic increase in QT_c of up to 563 milliseconds. The sixth patient developed syncope on day 2 of drug administration, which was associated with atrial fibrillation. QT prolongation was not documented.[69] Another phase 1 study with L-778123 using a 2-week continuous dosing regimen reported asymptomatic QT_c prolongation of more than 490 milliseconds.[70] In a phase 1 trial, L-778123 was combined with radiotherapy in patients with NSCLC and head and neck cancer (HNC).[71] L-778123 was given by 3 days continuous intravenous infusion in conjunction with standard radiotherapy. Nine patients (6 NSCLC patients and 3 HNC patients) were enrolled. Two episodes of QT_c prolongation were observed. One patient treated on dose level 1 had a prolonged QT_c in the setting of grade III hypokalemia and grade I hypomagnesemia. The electrolyte abnormalities were related to the effects of prior chemotherapy. FTI treatment was continued, and the patient was monitored overnight in the hospital. After electrolyte repletion, the QT_c returned to baseline. A second patient treated on dose level 2 developed QT prolongation, and L-778123 was discontinued. After review by the attending cardiologist, the QT_c prolongation was thought to be an artifact. On rechallenge with L-778123, no QT prolongation was observed. These episodes of QT_c prolongation were not thought to represent DLTs. No patient was removed from the study because of QT prolongation.

In combination with the radiotherapy, L-778123 was studied also in locally advanced patients with pancreatic cancer. L-778123 was given by continuous intravenous infusion with concomitant radiotherapy. One patient on dose level 1 experienced mild QT_c prolongation, toxicity thought to be unique among FTIs to L-778123.[72]

Lonafarnib

In a phase 2 trial of lonafarnib (SCH66336) in patients with refractory HNC, 1 of 15 patients developed grade 3 QT_c prolongation, and another patient presented syncope without previously documented QT_c prolongation.[5] Other phase 2 trials with lonafarnib have not reported this toxicity. In any case, among the various FTIs in clinical evaluation, QT prolongation is toxic unique to L-778123.[70]

Protein Kinase C Inhibitors

The PKC family of isoenzymes, which belongs to the widely expressed group of serine/threonine kinases and is involved in key cellular processes,[73,74] is a possible target for antitumor therapy.[75–77] Activation of PKC is implicated in tumor-induced angiogenesis and the regulation of key processes that lead to tumor growth and survival.[78] PKC overexpression and increased activity have been linked to many cancers, including colon, RCC, hepatocellular cancer, prostate cancers, and NSCLC. In patients with fatal/refractory diffuse large B-cell lymphoma, PKCβ is one of the most prominently overexpressed genes and is linked to poor prognosis. PKC is also involved in the PI3K/AKT pathway, responsible for apoptosis regulation.[79,80]

Enzastaurin

Enzastaurin HCl (LY317615), an acyclic bisindolylmaleimide, is a potent selective serine/threonine kinase inhibitor.

Enzastaurin induced apoptosis and decreased proliferation of various cancer cell lines[81] and decreased VEGF expression and microvessel density in human tumor xenografts.[82] In a phase 1 dose escalation and pharmacokinetic study of enzastaurin, 47 patients with advanced cancer were enrolled. Three DLTs (QT_c changes) occurred. One patient at the 700-mg dose level was initially diagnosed with a DLT of QT_c interval prolongation by more than 50 milliseconds (later amended to ST-T wave changes), and 2 patients in the expansion cohort at the 525-mg dose level had QT_c interval prolongation by more than 50 milliseconds over baseline (which did not require treatment or discontinuation). Both reports of QT_c prolongation in the expansion cohort were transient, with no clinical consequence, and did not result in treatment discontinuation.

The event of ST-T wave change was reported as drug related, although confounding factors such as a previous history of nonspecific ST-T wave changes and concomitant medications were present. Two deaths were reported: one patient died as a result of disease progression and one patient died of myocardial infarction. At the time of autopsy, it was revealed that the latter patient had severe underlying coronary artery disease.[83] A combination phase 1 study with enzastaurin, gemcitabine, and cisplatin in advanced, refractory, solid tumors also demonstrated one event of grade 2 QT_c interval prolongation of 33 patients.[84] In a phase 2 study, enzastaurin was tested in patients with relapsed or refractory diffuse large B-cell lymphoma. Fifty-five patients were enrolled. There were no treatment-related deaths. No cardiac toxicity was reported.[85]

Novel Targeted Therapeutics: Inhibitors of MDM2 and PARP

MDM2, also known as HDM2 in human, is a key regulator of p53 inducing the proteosomal degradation and the inhibition of transcriptional activity of p53.[86] HDM2 is overexpressed in a wide variety of tumor types, including melanoma, NSCLC, BC, esophageal cancer, leukemia, non-Hodgkin lymphoma, and sarcoma. Inhibition of MDM2 can restore p53 activity in cancers containing wild-type p53, leading to antitumor effects with apoptosis and growth inhibition.[87–89] There are 3 main categories of MDM2 inhibitors: inhibitors of MDM2-p53 interaction by targeting to MDM2, inhibitor of MDM2-p53 interaction by targeting top 53, and inhibitors of MDM2 E3 ubiquitin ligase.

JNJ-26854165 (serdemetan) is an oral MDM2 inhibitor. Results for phase 1 study using continuously daily oral dosing in patients with advanced solid tumors were presented in the 2009 annual meeting of American Society of Clinical Oncology.[90] Forty-seven patients were treated at 11 dose levels. One patient at the 300-mg dose level experienced DLT with grade 3 asymptomatic QT_c prolongation, which resolved after discontinuation of treatment. Dose escalation was stopped at the 400-mg dose level because of 2 of 3 patients having DLT, including one grade 3 skin rash and one grade 3 QT_c prolongation. Dose level of 350 mg was used on an expanded cohort of patients to confirm maximum tolerated dose, and trial with alternate dosing schedule to minimize QT_c prolongation was started with 150 mg 2 times a day. In light of the observed QT_c prolongation in the daily dosing schedule, a twice-daily dosing escalation was also done in the expectation that a lowered C_{max} might mitigate the risk of this toxicity. Two cohorts were treated on a twice-daily dosing schedule (150 and 200 mg), with the resulting observation of QT_c prolongation as a DLT at both doses. The MTD for this dosing schedule was determined to be 150 mg twice daily. The most frequently occurring grade 3 treatment-emergent adverse events (TEAEs) reported as possibly related to the study drug were as follows: QT_c prolongation (N = 6 [8.5%]); asthenia/fatigue (N = 9 [12.7%]); and diarrhea, decreased appetite, and abnormal hepatic function (each in 2 [2.8%] patients). Twelve (16.9%) patients discontinued the study due to TEAEs, of which 6 discontinued because of TEAEs considered related to study drug (QT_c prolongation [N = 4]). Ten (14.1%) patients experienced QT_cF increases of more than 60 milliseconds from baseline, of which 5 patients showed QT_cF of more than 500 milliseconds. The relatively frequent observation of QT_c prolongation prompted a more thorough examination of this toxicity. QT_c prolongation was directly correlated with serdemetan plasma concentration.[91] Therefore, although serdemetan showed evidence of clinical efficacy in this patient population with limited treatment options, the identification of exposure-related QT_c toxicity is of concern.

Preliminary data of RO5045337 (RG7112), another MDM2 inhibitor, has shown acceptable safety profiles.

PARPs are a family of nuclear enzymes that regulates the repair of DNA single-strand breaks through the base excision repair pathway. Targeting the PARP-mediated DNA repair pathway is a promising therapeutic approach for potentiating the effects of chemotherapy and radiation therapy and overcoming drug resistance.[92] No significant cardiotoxicity was seen from PARP inhibitors, such as BSI-201-iniparib, AZD2281 (olaparib), AG-014699 (PF-01367338), ABT-888 (veliparib), MK-4827, CEP-9722, and E7016.[93]

ARRHYTHMIAS IN PATIENTS WITH CANCER

Obviously, QTc prolongation is a setup for the development of polymorphic VT and ventricular fibrillation. Even so, the reported incidence of malignant tachyarrhythmias is not high. One may argue that this is an area not well studied, and thus, the true incidence remains unknown. Such cases have essentially only been described with 5-fluorouracil (5-FU) and its derivate capecitabine alone or in combination with cisplatin. Given the vascular toxicity spectrum of these drugs, one may speculate on an additional acute ischemic component. Nonsustained VT may occur in 5% to 10% of patients during the acute exposure phase to doxorubicin and in less than 1% of patients undergoing taxane therapy. The risk resolves once therapy is discontinued. An implantable cardioverter defibrillator is rarely indicated in this setting unless for secondary prevention with a presumed irreversible cause. Primary prevention defibrillator therapy, however, may become a consideration for patients with persistently reduced cardiac function as generally indicated.

Taxanes are more notorious for bradycardia and first-degree atrioventricular (AV) block (30% and 25%, respectively, with paclitaxel) occurring within the first day of therapy in most cases and resolving in 2.5 hours to 6 days after discontinuation. The combination with other bradycardia-prone cancer and negative chronotropic and dromotropic CV drugs increases the risk as does a history of bradycardia, AV block, bundle branch block, myocardial infarction, HF, and electrolyte imbalances. These risk factors may also be considered for tachyarrhythmias and bradycardia-induced tachyarrhythmias. Cardiac monitoring is not recommended for patients without history, risk factors, and symptoms. Antihistamine and steroid pretreatment intriguingly reduces the risk of taxane-induced bradycardia. Thalidomide is the other chemotherapeutic notoriously associated with bradycardia. Mild forms may occur in more than half of the patients, but in severe degrees only in 1% to 3%. The indication for pacemaker implantation is in keeping with current guidelines but often becomes a requirement with the need for continuation of chemotherapy.

The prevalence of atrial fibrillation among patients with newly diagnosed cancer seems to be similar to the general population, that is, around

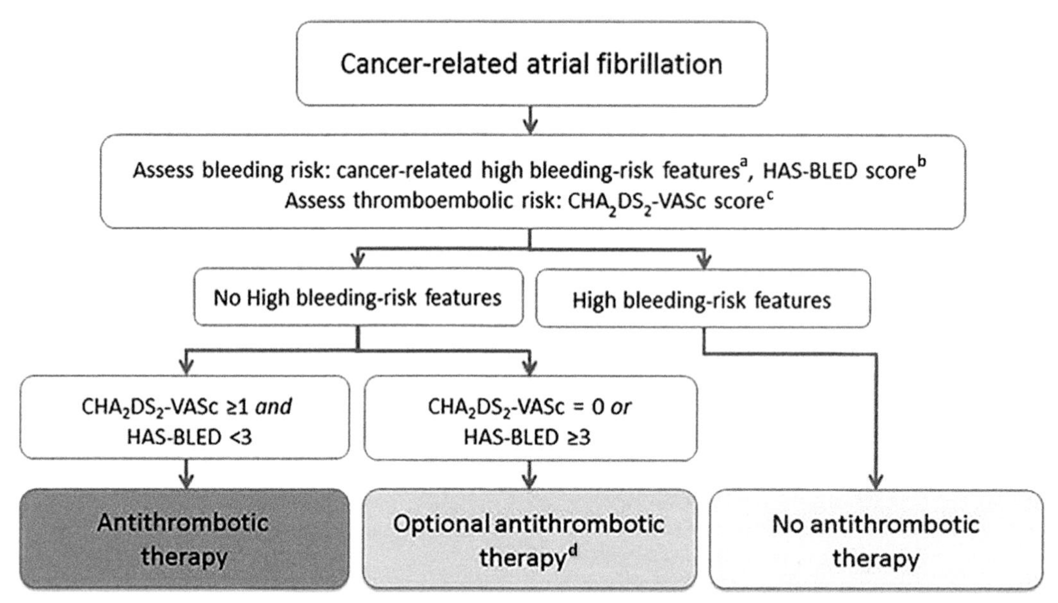

Fig. 13.3 A practical algorithm for antithrombotic therapy in cancer-related atrial fibrillation. [a] Intracranial tumor, hematologic malignancies with coagulation defects, cancer therapy-induced thrombocytopenia, severe metastatic hepatic disease, and so forth. [b] HAS-BLED, Hypertension, Abnormal renal/liver function, Stroke, Bleeding history or predisposition, Labile INR, Elderly, Drugs/alcohol concomitantly [c] CHA2DS2-VASc, Congestive heart failure or left ventricular dysfunction Hypertension, Age ≥75 (doubled), Diabetes, Stroke (doubled)-Vascular disease, Age 65 to 74, Sex (female). [d] Antithrombotic therapy may be considered in high thromboembolic risk associated with certain cancers (eg, pancreatic, ovarian, lung, primary hepatic) or cancer therapies (eg, cisplatin, gemcitabine, 5-FU, erythropoietin, granulocyte colony stimulating factors). (*From* Farmakis D, Parissis J, Filippatos G. Insights into onco-cardiology: atrial fibrillation in cancer. J Am Coll Cardiol 2014;63(10):947; with permission.)

2%. A similar percentage will develop atrial fibrillation subsequently in association with a 2-fold increased risk of thromboembolism and 6-fold increased risk of HF. Most of these occurrences are at the time of or after surgery, especially lung surgery, overall in the order of 4% to 30%. Beyond the standard risk factors, paraneoplastic phenomena such as hyperparathyroidism and autoimmunity against atrial structures may be factors unique to patients with cancer. Furthermore, it can be a reflection of atrial masses and the cancer treatment. The chemotherapeutics most commonly associated with atrial fibrillation include doxorubicin, 5-FU, cisplatin, taxanes, ifosfamide, gemcitabine, mitoxantrone, high-dose dexamethasone corticosteroids, and melphalan. For the perioperative setting, amiodarone is an effective preventive strategy, and there might be some merit to β-blocker. The long-term use of amiodarone and other antiarrhythmics can be complicated in patients with cancer because of the issues of QTc prolongation as discussed above. Similarly, anticoagulation may prove difficult in the patient with cancer for reasons of drug-drug interactions, thrombocytopenia, anemia, coagulopathy, and bleeding risk. Both the risk of thromboembolism and the bleeding must be addressed in patients with cancer and treatment must be adjusted accordingly (Fig. 13.3). Left atrial appendix closure devices may be an option for the patient with cancer who is not a candidate for anticoagulation but has a high thromboembolic risk and a relatively favorable long-term survival prognosis.

SUMMARY

Clinicians are increasingly faced with both old and new anticancer agents that have the potential to prolong the QT interval, a laboratory finding that is associated with the risk of significant arrhythmia. As more sensitive methods for electrocardiographic testing are applied, an increasing number of anticancer agents or treatments for supportive care will likely be described with some risk for QT_c prolongation. For many agents, the frequency of QT_c prolongation may be common, whereas the risk of clinical arrhythmia (TdP) may be very rare.

To enable the development and application of future treatments, detailed analyses and publication about TdP events, observed in cancer treatment settings, should continue to support rational strategies for risk management with broad relevance. Oncologists have demonstrated their ability to identify and manage complicated cardiac risks in clinical investigations and general practice. Across multiple geographic regions, successful risk management is exemplified by the published experiences with arsenic trioxide, highlighting the value of systematic ECG testing and attention to concomitant medications, electrolyte abnormalities, and comorbidities, all likely contributing to the low frequency of clinical cardiac toxicities reported after approval. Given the growing introduction of promising agents, designed to address unmet medical needs, efforts are needed to promote strategies for risk management, avoiding unintended consequences that can impede development, regulatory approval, and patient access. More research is needed to assess and manage cardiovascular safety of patients treated with anticancer agents, building from organized collaborations between oncologists and cardiologists, and these efforts should have broad relevance to therapeutics designed for treatment or supportive care.

Risk-benefit assessments might be relatively straightforward in nononcologic studies and are provided in the ICH E14 document. In principle, risk-benefit must be interpreted in the context of the nature and severity of the disease, and conservative approaches will delay or prevent patient access to innovative treatment. Currently, different criteria are used in defining which prolongation of the QT-QT_c time or change over baseline is feasible. The use of uniform thresholds to describe changes of concern for all protocol applications can simplify study conduct and subsequent data collection.

Grading according to the Common Toxicities Adverse Events version 3 might be considered a uniform guideline in which grade 3 QT-QT_c prolongation is defined as a value exceeding 500 milliseconds. In oncology trials, treatment-related events of grade 3 or higher are often considered for decision making and dosing decisions. Asymptomatic prolongation of the QT-QT_c time exceeding 60 milliseconds over baseline may be too sensitive to guide dosing in oncologic studies, because these changes can already be observed as a diurnal variation, even in healthy volunteers, and might even be larger in oncologic patients. Of utmost importance is that the data generated in oncologic studies are pooled to provide additional information on the QT/QT_c interval in patients with cancer and to guide us in broadening the eligibility criteria of studies in the oncologic setting, to implement the concomitant use of oncology-relevant medication, to standardize dose modification and discontinuation criteria, and to search for alternatives in study design, resulting in timely approval of drugs by the regulatory authorities providing access for patients to promising new anticancer agents.

Various arrhythmias have been reported with the administration of antineoplastic drugs. Indeed, transient electrocardiographic changes and arrhythmias are known to be acute manifestations of cardiotoxicity secondary to cancer therapy with anthracycline, alkylating agents, antimetabolites, taxanes, interferon, and interleukin-2. Paclitaxel most commonly has caused transient, asymptomatic bradyarrhythmias. Higher-grade bradyarrhythmias, including complete heart block, have been reported, but the incidence is small. VTs also have been described with paclitaxel. Arrhythmias also have been reported with anthracyclines (eg, doxorubicin), ifosfamide, and 5-FU, but the toxicity of these drugs is mainly myocardial or ischemic. Treatment with interferon is associated with a variety of cardiac toxicities, including cardiomyopathy, ischemia, myocardial infarction, and sudden death, but the most common cardiac toxicity is supraventricular and ventricular arrhythmias.

No treatment is required for asymptomatic changes, but progressive/symptomatic disturbances may require dose reduction, treatment discontinuation, or pacemaker placement. In any case, before the patient starts the chemotherapy, proper treatment of coexisting cardiovascular disease and careful monitoring of cardiac function are necessary, although uniform recommendations regarding cardiac monitoring in adult patients undergoing anticancer treatment are lacking. Cardiotoxicity related to anticancer treatment is important to recognize because it may have a significant impact on the overall prognosis and survival of patients with cancer, and it is likely to remain a significant challenge for both cardiologists and oncologists in the future because of an increasing aging population of patients with cancer and the introduction of many new cancer therapies.

REFERENCES

1. The clinical evaluation of QT/QT_c interval prolongation and proarrhythmic potential for non antiarrhythmic drugs. Available at: http://www.fda.gov/cder/calendar/meeting/qt4jam.pdf. Accessed March 25, 1997.

2. Food and Drug Administration, HHS. International Conference on Harmonisation; guidance on E14 clinical evaluation of QT/QTc interval prolongation and proarrhythmic potential for non-antiarrhythmic drugs; availability. Notice. Fed Regist 2005;70:61134–5.
3. Shah RR. Can pharmacogenetics help rescue drugs withdrawn from the market? Pharmacogenomics 2006;7(6):889–908.
4. Roden DM. Drug-induced prolongation of the QT interval. N Engl J Med 2004;350:1013–22.
5. Strevel EL, Ing DJ, Siu LL. Molecularly targeted oncology therapeutics and prolongation of the QT interval. J Clin Oncol 2007;25:3362–71.
6. Ederhy S, Cohen A, Dufaitre G, et al. QT interval prolongation among patients treated with angiogenesis inhibitors. Target Oncol 2009;4:89–97.
7. Gintant GA, Limberis JT, McDermott JS, et al. The canine Purkinje fiber: an in vitro model system for acquired long QT syndrome and drug-induced arrhythmogenesis. J Cardiovasc Pharmacol 2001; 37:607–18.
8. Weissenburger J, Nesterenko VV, Antzelevitch C. Transmural heterogeneity of ventricular repolarisation under baseline and long QT conditions in the canine heart in vivo: torsades de pointes develops with halothane but not pentobarbital anesthesia. J Cardiovasc Electrophysiol 2000;11:290–304.
9. Antzelevitch A. Role of transmural dispersion of repolarization in the genesis of drug-induced torsade de pointes. Heart Rhythm 2005;2(11):S9–15.
10. National Cancer Institute: Cancer therapy evaluation program, Common terminology for adverse events, version 3.0, DCTD, NCI, NIH, DHHS. 2006. Available at: https://ctep.cancer.gov/protocolDevelopment/electronic_applications/docs/ctcaev3.pdf.
11. Johnstone RW. Histone-deacetylase inhibitors: novel drugs for the treatment of cancer. Nat Rev Drug Discov 2002;1:287–99.
12. Ueda H, Manda T, Matsumoto S, et al. FR901228, a novel antitumor bicyclic depsipeptide produced by Chromobacterium violaceum No. 968. III. Antitumor activities in experimental mice. J Antibiot (Tokyo) 1994;47:315–23.
13. Bates SE, Rosing DR, Fojo T, et al. Challenges of evaluating the cardiac effects of anticancer agents. Clin Cancer Res 2006;12:3871–4.
14. Pickarz RL, Frye AR, Wright JJ, et al. Cardiac studies in patients treated with depsipeptide, FK228, in a phase II trial for T-cell lymphoma. Clin Cancer Res 2006;12:3762–73.
15. Sandor V, Bakke S, Robey RW, et al. Phase I trial of the histone deacetylase inhibitor, depsipeptide (FR901228, NSC 630176) in patients with refractory neoplasms. Clin Cancer Res 2002;8(3):718–28.
16. Marshall JL, Rizvi N, Kauh J, et al. A phase I trial of depsipeptide (FR901228) in patients with advanced cancer. J Exp Ther Oncol 2002;2(6):325–32.
17. Whittaker S, Mcculloch W, Robak T, et al. International multicenter Phase II study of the HDCA inhibitor (HDACi) depipeptide (FK228) in cutaneous T-cell lymphoma (CTCL): interim report. J Clin Oncol 2006;24(Suppl 18) [abstract 3063].
18. Parker C, Molife R, Karavasilis V, et al. Romidepsin (FK228), a hystone deacetylase inhibitor: final results of a phase II study in metastatic refractory prostate cancer (HRPC). 2007 ASCO Annual Meeting Proceedings (Post-Meeting Edition). J Clin Oncol 2007;25(Suppl 18) [abstract 15507].
19. Niesvizky R, Ely S, Diliberto M, et al. Multicenter phase II trial of the histone deacetylase inhibitor depsipeptide (FK228) for the treatment of relapsed or refractory multiple myeloma (MM). Blood 2005; 106:2574.
20. Shah MH, Binkley P, Chan K, et al. Cardiotoxicity of histone deacetylase inhibitor depsipeptide in patients with metastatic neuroendocrine tumors. Clin Cancer Res 2006;12(13):3997–4003.
21. Stadler WM, Margolin K, Ferber S, et al. A Phase II study of depsipeptide in refractory metastatic renal cell cancer. Clin Genitourin Cancer 2006;5(1):57–60.
22. Marks PA, Rifkind RA, Richon VM, et al. Histone deacetylases and cancer: causes and therapies. Nat Rev Cancer 2001;1:194–202, 1.
23. Zolinza [package insert]. Whitehouse Station, NJ: Merck&Co; 2006.
24. Zhang L, Lebwohl D, Masson E, et al. Clinically relevant QTc prolongation is not associated with current dose schedules of LBH589 (panobinostat). J Clin Oncol 2008;26(2):332–9.
25. Lu Z, Wu CY, Jiang YP, et al. Suppression of phosphoinositide-3-kinase signalling and alteration of multiple ion currents in drug induced long QT syndrome. Sci Transl Med 2012;4:131–50.
26. Rashmi RS, Morganroth J, Devron RS. Cardiovascular safety of tyrosine kinase inhibitors: with a special focus on cardiac repolarisation (QT interval). Drug Saf 2013;36:295–316.
27. Barros F, Gomez-Varela D, Viloria CG, et al. Modulation of human erg K+ channel gating by activation of a G protein coupled receptor and protein kinase C. J Physiol 1998;511(Pt 2):333–46.
28. Thomas D, Zhang W, Karle CA, et al. Deletion of protein kinase. a phosphorylation sites in the HERG potassium channel inhibits activation shift by protein kinase A. J Biol Chem 1999;274:27457–62.
29. Davis MJ, Wu X, Nurkiewicz TR, et al. Regulation of ion channels by protein tyrosine phosphorylation. Am J Physiol Heart Circ Physiol 2001;281:H1835–62.
30. Zhang Y, Wang H, Wang J, et al. Normal function of HERG K? channels expressed in HEK293 cells requires basal protein kinase B activity. FEBS Lett 2003;534:125–32.
31. Zhang DY, Wang Y, Lau CP, et al. Both EGFR kinase and Src related tyrosine kinases regulate human

ether-a-go-go-related gene potassium channels. Cell Signal 2008;20:1815–21.
32. Chu TF, Rupnick MA, Kerkela R, et al. Cardiotoxicity associated with tyrosine kinase inhibitor sunitinib. Lancet 2007;370:2011–9.
33. Di Lorenzo G, Autorino L, Bruni G, et al. Cardiovascular toxicity following sunitinib therapy in metastatic renal cell carcinoma: a multicenter analysis. Ann Oncol 2009;20:1535–42.
34. Miller KD, Trigo JM, Wheeler C, et al. Multicenter phase II trial of ZD6474, a vascular endothelial growth factor receptor-2 and epidermal growth factor receptor tyrosine kinase inhibitor, in patients with previously treated metastatic breast cancer. Clin Cancer Res 2005;11(9):3369–76.
35. Tamura T, Minami H, Yamada Y, et al. A phase I dose escalation study of ZD6474 in Japanese patients with solid malignant tumors. J Thorac Oncol 2006;1(9):1002–9.
36. Hammett T, Oliver S, Ghahramani P, et al. The pharmacodynamics effect on cardiac repolarization of combination single dose ZD6474 and ondansetron in healthy subjects. J Clin Oncol 2005;23:16S [abstract: 3197].
37. Holden SN, Eckhardt SG, Basser R, et al. Clinical evaluation of ZD6474, an orally active inhibitor of VEGF and EGF receptor signaling, in patients with solid, malignant tumors. Ann Oncol 2005;16:1391–7.
38. Heymach JV, Johnson BE, Prager D, et al. Randomized, placebo-controlled phase II study of vandetanib plus docetaxel in previously treated non small-cell lung cancer. J Clin Oncol 2007;25(27):4270–7.
39. Kovacs MJ, Reece DE, Marcellus D, et al. A phase II study of ZD6474 (Zactima, a selective inhibitor of VEGFR and EGFR tyrosine kinase in patients with relapsed multiple myeloma—NCIC CTG IND.145. Invest New Drugs 2006;24(6):529–35.
40. Kiura K, Nakagawa K, Shinkai T, et al. A randomized, double blind, phase IIa dose-finding study of Vandetanib (ZD6474) in Japanese patients with non-small cell lung cancer. J Thorac Oncol 2008;3(4): 386–93.
41. Natale RB, Thongprasert S, Greco FA, et al. Phase III trial of vandetanib compared with erlotinib in patients with previously treated advanced non–small-cell lung cancer. J Clin Oncol 2011;29:1059–66.
42. De Boer RH, Arrieta O, Yang CH, et al. Vandetanib plus pemetrexed for the second-line treatment of advanced non–small-cell lung cancer: a randomized, double-blind phase III trial. J Clin Oncol 2011;29:1067–74.
43. Wells SA Jr, Robinson BG, Gagel RF, et al. Vandetanib in patients with locally advanced or metastatic medullary thyroid cancer: a randomized, double-blind phase III trial. J Clin Oncol 2011;30:134–41.
44. Hochhaus A, O'Brien SG, Guilhot F, et al. Six-year follow-up of patients receiving imatinib for the first-line treatment of chronic myeloid leukemia. Leukemia 2009;23:1054–61.
45. Davies J. First-line therapy for CML: nilotinib comes of age [comment]. Lancet Oncol 2011;12:826–7.
46. Saglio G, Kim DW, Issaragrisil S, et al. Nilotinib versus imatinib for newly diagnosed chronic myeloid leukemia. N Engl J Med 2010;362:2251–9.
47. US Food and Drug Administration (FDA). Dasatinib (BMS-35825) Oncologic drug advisory committee briefing document NDA 21–96. Washington, DC: US Food and Drug Administration (FDA); 2006. p. 52.
48. Tam CS, Kantarjian H, Garcia-Manero G, et al. Failure to achieve a major cytogenetic response by 12 months defines inadequate response in patients receiving nilotinib or dasatinib as second or subsequent line therapy for chronic myeloid leukemia. Blood 2008;112(3):516–8.
49. Shawn AT, Dong-Wan K, Ranee M, et al. Ceritinib in ALK-rearranged non–small-cell lung cancer. N Engl J Med 2014;370(13):1189–97.
50. Dienstmann R, Andre F, Soria JC, et al. Significant antitumour activity of E-3810, a novel FGFR and VEGF inhibitor, in patients with FGFR1 amplified breast cancer. Ann Oncol, Proceeding ESMO Congress 2012. Abstract 2115.
51. Denekamp J. Endothelial cell proliferation as a novel approach to targeting tumour therapy. Br J Cancer 1982;45:136–9.
52. Denekamp J. The current status of targeting tumour vasculature as a means of cancer therapy: an overview. Int J Radiat Biol 1991;60:401–8.
53. Shi W, Siemann DW. Targeting the tumor vasculature: enhancing antitumor efficacy through combination treatment with ZD6126 and ZD6474. In Vivo 2005;19:1045–50.
54. Nathan PD, Judson I, Padhani A, et al. A phase I study of combretastatin A4 phosphate (CA4P) and bevacizumab in subjects with advanced solid tumors. J Clin Oncol 2008;26(Suppl):3550.
55. Siemann DW, Bibby MC, Dark GG, et al. Differentiation and definition of vascular-targeted therapies. Clin Cancer Res 2005;11:416–20.
56. Siemann DW, Chaplin DJ. An update on the clinical development of drugs to disable tumor vasculature. Expert Opin Drug Discov 2007;2:1–11.
57. Haverkamp W, Breithardt G, Camm AJ, et al. The potential for QT prolongation and proarrhythmia by non-antiarrhythmic drugs: clinical and regulatory implications. Report on a policy conference of the European Society of Cardiology. Cardiovasc Res 2000;47:219–33.
58. Dowlati A, Robertson K, Cooney M, et al. A phase I pharmacokinetic and translational study of the novel vascular targeting agent combretastatin a-4 phosphate on a single-dose intravenous schedule in patients with advanced cancer. Cancer Res 2002;62:3408–16.

59. Cooney MM, Radivoyevitch T, Dowlati A, et al. Cardiovascular safety profile of combretastatin a4 phosphate in a single-dose phase I study in patients with advanced cancer. Clin Cancer Res 2004;10:96–100.
60. Ng QS, Carnell D, Milner J, et al. Phase Ib trial of combrestastatin A4 phosphate in combination with radiotherapy: initial clinical results. J Clin Oncol 2005;23:16S [abstract: 3117].
61. Rustin GJ, Galbraith SM, Anderson H, et al. Phase I clinical trial of weekly combretastatin A4 phosphate: clinical and pharmacokinetic results. J Clin Oncol 2003;21:2815–22.
62. Stevenson JP, Rosen M, Sun W, et al. Phase I trial of the antivascular agent combretastatin A4 phosphate on a 5-day schedule to patients with cancer: magnetic resonance imaging evidence for altered tumor blood flow. J Clin Oncol 2003;21: 4428–38.
63. Bilenker JH, Flaherty KT, Rosen M, et al. Phase I trial of combretastatin a-4 phosphate with carboplatin. Clin Cancer Res 2005;11:1527–33.
64. Jones R, Ewer M. Cardiac and cardiovascular toxicity of non anthracycline anticancer drugs. Expert Rev Anticancer Ther 2006;6:1249–69.
65. Rustin GJ, Nathan PD, Boxhall J, et al. A phase Ib trial of combretastatin A-4 phosphate (CA4P) in combination with carboplatin or paclitaxel chemotherapy in patients with advanced cancer [abstract]. J Clin Oncol 2005;23:3013.
66. Lloyd GK, Nicholson B, Neuteboom STC, et al. NPI-2358: a new vascular/tubulin modifying agent greatly potentiates standard chemotherapy in xenograft models. EORTC-NCI-AACR Molecular Targets and Therapeutics Meeting. Boston, 2003.
67. Neuteboom STC, Medina E, Palladino MA, et al. NPI-2358, a novel tumor vascular disrupting agent potentiates the anti-tumor activity of docetaxel in the non small cell lung cancer model MV522 [abstract]. Eur J Cancer 2008;6(Suppl):141.
68. End DW, Smets G, Todd AV, et al. Characterization of the antitumor effects of the selective farnesyl protein transferase inhibitor R115777 in vivo and in vitro. Cancer Res 2001;61:131–7.
69. Britten CD, Rowinsky EK, Soignet S, et al. A phase I and pharmacological study of the farnesyl protein transferase inhibitor L-778123 in patients with solid malignancies. Clin Cancer Res 2001;7:3894–903.
70. Rubin E, Abbruzzese J, Morrison B, et al. Phase I trial of farnesyl protein transferase inhibitor (FPTase) L778123 on a 14- or 28-day dosing schedule. Proc Am Soc Clin Oncol 2000;19(abstract 689):178a.
71. Hahn SM, Bernhard EJ, Regine W, et al. A phase I trial of the farnesyltransferase inhibitor L-778,123 and radiotherapy for locally advanced lung and head and neck cancer. Clin Cancer Res 2002;8: 1065–72.
72. Martin NE, Brunner TB, Kiel KD, et al. A phase I trial of the dual farnesyltransferase and geranylgeranyltransferase inhibitor L-778,123 and radiotherapy for locally advanced pancreatic cancer. Clin Cancer Res 2004;10:5447–54.
73. Livneh E, Fishman DD. Linking protein kinase C to cell-cycle control. Eur J Biochem 1997;248:1–9.
74. Nishizuka Y. Intracellular signaling by hydrolysis of phospholipids and activation of protein kinase C. Science 1992;258:607–14.
75. Da Rocha AB, Mans DR, Regner A, et al. Targeting protein kinase C: new therapeutic opportunities against high-grade gliomas? Oncologist 2002;7: 17–33.
76. Gescher A. Analogs of staurosporine: potential anticancer drugs? Gen Pharmacol 1998;31:721–8.
77. Goekjian PG, Jirousek MR. Protein kinase C inhibitors as novel anticancer drugs. Expert Opin Investig Drugs 2001;10:2117–40.
78. Blobe GC, Obeid LM, Hannun YA. Regulation of protein kinase C and role in cancer biology. Cancer Metastasis Rev 1994;13:411–31.
79. Balendran A, Hare GR, Kieloch A, et al. Further evidence that 3-phosphoinositide-dependent protein kinase-1 (PDK1) is required for the stability and phosphorylation of protein kinase C (PKC) isoforms. FEBS Lett 2000;484:217–23.
80. Partovian C, Simons M. Regulation of protein kinase B/Akt activity and Ser473 phosphorylation by protein kinase C alpha in endothelial cells. Cell Signal 2004;16:951–7.
81. Graff JR, McNulty AM, Hanna KR, et al. The protein kinase C beta–selective inhibitor, enzastaurin (LY317615.HCl), suppresses signaling through the AKT pathway, induces apoptosis, and suppresses growth of human colon cancer and glioblastoma xenografts. Cancer Res 2005; 65:7462–9.
82. Keyes KA, Mann L, Sherman M, et al. LY317615 decreases plasma VEGF levels in human tumor xenograft-bearing mice. Cancer Chemother Pharmacol 2004;53:133–40.
83. Carducci MA, Musib L, Kies MS, et al. Phase I dose escalation and pharmacokinetic study of Enzastaurin, an oral protein kinase C beta inhibitor, in patients with advanced cancer. J Clin Oncol 2006;24: 4092–9.
84. Beerepoot L, Rademaker-Lakhai J, Witteveen E, et al. Phase I and pharmacokinetic evaluation of enzastaurin combined with gemcitabine and cisplatin in advanced cancer. J Clin Oncol 2006;24: 18S [abstract: 2046].
85. Robertson MJ, Kahl BS, Vose JM, et al. Phase II study of enzastaurin, a protein kinase C beta inhibitor, in patients with relapsed or refractory diffuse large B-cell lymphoma. J Clin Oncol 2007; 25:1741–6.

86. Chen J, Marechal V, Levine AJ. Mapping of the p53 and MDM-2 interaction domains. Mol Cell Biol 1993;13:4107–14.
87. Wasylyk C, Salvi R, Argentini M, et al. p53 mediated death of cells overexpressing MDM2 by an inhibitor of MDM2 interaction with p53. Oncogene 1999; 18(11):1921–34.
88. Chene P, Fuchs J, Bohn J, et al. A small synthetic peptide, which inhibits the p53-hdm2 interaction, stimulates the p53 pathway in tumour cell lines. J Mol Biol 2000;299(1):245–53.
89. Wang H, Nan L, Yu D, et al. Anti-tumor efficacy of a novel antisense anti-MDM2 mixed-backbone oligonucleotide in human colon cancer models: p53-dependent and p53-independent mechanisms. Mol Med 2002;8(4):185–99.
90. Tabernero J, Dirix L, Schoffski P, et al. Phase I pharmacokinetic (PK) and pharmacodynamic (PD) study of HDM-2 antagonist JNJ-26854165 in patients with advanced refractory solid tumors. J Clin Oncol 2009;27(15S):3514 [meeting abstracts].
91. Tabernero J, Dirix L, Schoffski P, et al. A phase I first-inhuman pharmacokinetic and pharmacodynamic study of serdemetan in patients with advanced solid tumors. Clin Cancer Res 2011;17:6313–21.
92. Ratnam K, Low JA. Current development of clinical inhibitors of poly (ADP-ribose) polymerase in oncology. Clin Cancer Res 2007;3(5): 1383–8.
93. Yuan Y, Liao YM, Chung TH, et al. Novel targeted therapeutics: inhibitors of MDM2, ALK and PARP. J Hematol Oncol 2011;4:16.
94. Giles F, Fischer T, Cortes J, et al. A phase I study of intravenous LBH589, a novel cinnamic hydroxamic acid analogue histone deacetylase inhibitor, in patients with refractory hematologic malignancies. Clin Cancer Res 2006;12:4628–35.
95. Sharma S, Vogelzang N, Beck J, et al. Phase I pharmacokinetic and pharmacodynamic study of once-weekly i.v. panobinostat (LBH589). ECCO 2007, Poster presented. Barcelona, Spain, September 23–27, 2007 [abstract: 702].
96. Prince HM, George D, Patnaik A, et al. Phase I study of oral panobinostat (LBH589) in advanced solid tumors and non-Hodgkin's lymphoma. ECCO 2007, Poster presented. Barcelona, Spain, September 23–27, 2007 [abstract: 701].

CHAPTER 14

Radiation-Induced Heart Disease

Long-Term Manifestations, Diagnosis, and Management

William Finch, MD*, Michael S. Lee, MD, Eric H. Yang, MD

INTRODUCTION

Radiation therapy (RT) is an important cause of cardiovascular disease in patients treated for cancer, especially in those receiving chest radiotherapy for Hodgkin disease or breast cancer (Table 14.1) as well as after total body irradiation for bone marrow transplantation.[1] Factors that influence the development of cardiotoxicity include the total radiation dose and the dose fractionation. Radiation damage may involve the pericardium, myocardium, valves, coronary arteries, and the conduction system (Box 14.1, Fig. 14.1).[2,3] Injury to the endothelial cells in these compartments, inflammation, and fibrosis are key elements. Diagnosis and treatment do not differ from conventional heart disease; however, screening for radiation-induced heart disease (RIHD) should be pursued even in asymptomatic patients in an effort to ameliorate at least some of the disease manifestations.

RT is commonly used as an adjuvant treatment modality in patients with breast cancer (nearly 40% in the Surveillance Epidemiology, and End Results registry).[4] Randomized trials and meta-analyses confirm that radiation exposure, especially of the left chest, is associated with an increased cardiovascular mortality, attributed mainly to ischemic heart disease and acute myocardial infarction.[4–6]

In patients who received mediastinal RT for Hodgkin disease, cardiovascular mortality becomes a leading cause of death over time.[7,8] Extending prior studies,[9–11] the most recent and comprehensive analysis of more than 2500 patients who underwent mediastinal RT between 1965 and 1995 and had survived more than 5 years reported a cumulative incidence of any cardiovascular disease of 54.6% after 40 years.[12]

Mediastinal RT increased the hazard for any type of cardiovascular disease by a factor of 3.6 (95% confidence interval [CI] 2.8–4.6). The highest risk was found for valvular heart disease (hazard ratio [HR] 6.6, 95% CI 4.0–10.8), followed by an equivalent risk of coronary heart disease or CHF. At 20 years out from RT, childhood cancer survivors develop clinically relevant valvular heart disease at a cumulative incidence rate of 6% versus 3% for other RIHD manifestations (Fig. 14.2).

There is little discussion in the literature on the impact of radiation from diagnostic imaging studies on the heart.[13,14] However, doses of RT are frequently greater than 10 Gy, compared with the radiation dose of a computed tomography (CT) scan of around 0.01 Gy. Therefore, it is unlikely that the radiation from diagnostic CT is cardiotoxic.

RELATION OF RADIATION FIELD, DOSE, AND FRACTIONATION TO RADIATION-INDUCED HEART DISEASE

Both the cumulative radiation dose and the dose fractionation (the division of the total dose into smaller fractions separated by time) are factors in the development of radiation cardiotoxicity. In animal studies, single (unfractionated) radiograph doses of 35 to 40 Gy caused severe heart failure (HF) after several months, whereas 10 to 15 Gy caused only minor HF after 1 year.[15] Cardiotoxicity likely develops with single doses of less than 10 Gy, whereas cumulative doses of 50 to 70 Gy (in fractions of 2, 3, or 4 Gy) cause myocardial

Division of Cardiology, Department of Medicine, University of California, Los Angeles, Los Angeles, CA, USA
* Corresponding author. UCLA Cardiovascular Center, 100 Medical Plaza, Suite 630, Los Angeles, CA 90095
E-mail address: ehyang@mednet.ucla.edu

TABLE 14.1
Malignancies whose treatment may include radiation therapy at the outlined doses and generation of a radiation risk to the heart

Malignancy	Dose (Gy)
Hodgkin lymphoma	30–36
Breast cancer	45–50
Gastric carcinoma	45–50
Esophageal carcinoma	45–50
Lung cancer	50–60
Thymoma	60

cytolysis.[16] Pericardial fibrosis and HF occurred earlier when larger fractions were used. In a human autopsy study, significant myocardial fibrosis was observed only in patients that received greater than 30 Gy.[3] This being said, in recent years there has been a shift from an exponential model with a "safe" threshold value for radiation dose to a more linear model.

BREAST CANCER

The radiation dose that the heart receives varies depending on the type and location of tumor being treated. As described above, there is a higher risk for cardiac disease after RT for cancer of the left breast when compared with irradiation of the right breast.[4] This finding is not surprising given the radiation dose the heart receives for left-sided tumors is more than double that received for right-sided tumors.[17] With irradiation of the left breast, the left anterior descending artery (LAD) is the structure that receives the highest radiation dose.

Changes to contemporary RT regimens for breast cancer have improved cardiac outcomes. Tangential radiation fields rather than anterior fields result in lower cardiac doses,[18] and CT radiation planning can exclude the heart from the treatment field.[19] These changes have produced a steady decline in the laterality of coronary artery disease (CAD) observed with left-sided versus right-sided irradiation since 1979, and laterality was no more seen in a modern cohort study.[20,21] Although early randomized controlled trials of RT for breast cancer found a higher risk of ischemic heart disease in the RT than in the surgery-only arm, the Danish Breast Cancer Cooperative Group 82b and 82c trials randomized patients to surgery with or without RT and found no increased risk of ischemic heart disease.[18,21–23] In these trials, cardiac radiation protection blocks, lower volume of heart irradiated, and RT treatment planning using ultrasound measurement of chest wall thickness were contributing factors to reduced cardiotoxicity. However, a more recent retrospective analysis of women who underwent RT for breast cancer in Sweden and Denmark between 1958 and 2001 revealed a linear relationship between major coronary events and radiation dose (7.4% risk increase per gray) with no obvious threshold. This increase started within the first 5 years after radiotherapy and continued into the third decade. In addition, patients with pre-existing cardiovascular risk factors had a greater absolute risk of death from ischemic heart disease and/or coronary events compared with patients who did not have risk factors.[24] Avoidance of internal mammary lymph node irradiation reduces cardiac radiation dose; however, recent trials of internal mammary node irradiation for breast cancer have shown benefits in terms of disease-free survival.[25,26] At a follow-up time of 10 years, there were no significant increases in cardiac disease; however, longer-term follow-up of these patients is warranted.

BOX 14.1
Cardiac disease associated with radiation exposure

- Pericardial disease
  - Pericardial effusion
  - Acute pericarditis
  - Constrictive pericarditis
- Cardiomyopathy
- Vascular disease
  - Coronary artery disease
- Microvascular coronary disease
- Carotid artery disease
- Valvular disease
- Conduction abnormalities
  - Bundle branch blocks
  - Atrioventricular block

HODGKIN DISEASE

Historically, mantle field irradiation (lymph nodes in the neck, mediastinum, and axillae) with 35 to 45 Gy was used for Hodgkin disease (HD).[27] The whole heart receives a dose of 27.5 Gy with mantle field RT, and some parts receive greater than 35 Gy.[28,29] Most cardiovascular deaths in patients

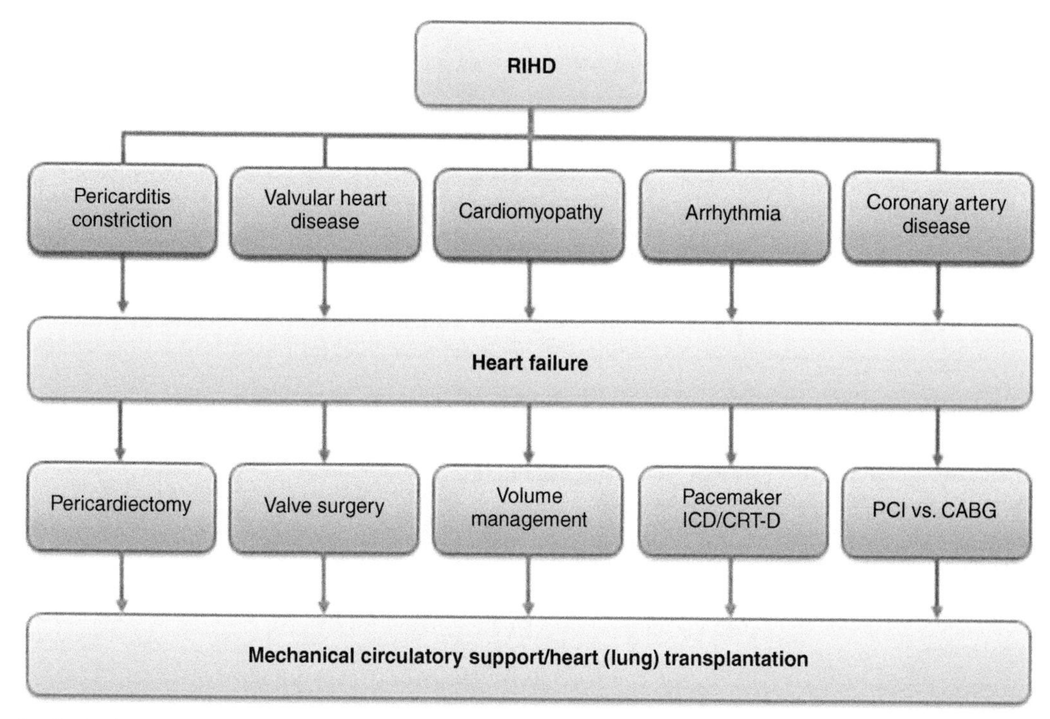

Fig. 14.1 The spectrum of RIHD, common final pathway of presentation with HF, and treatment modalities directed toward the disease aspects. ICD, implantable cardioverter defibrillator.

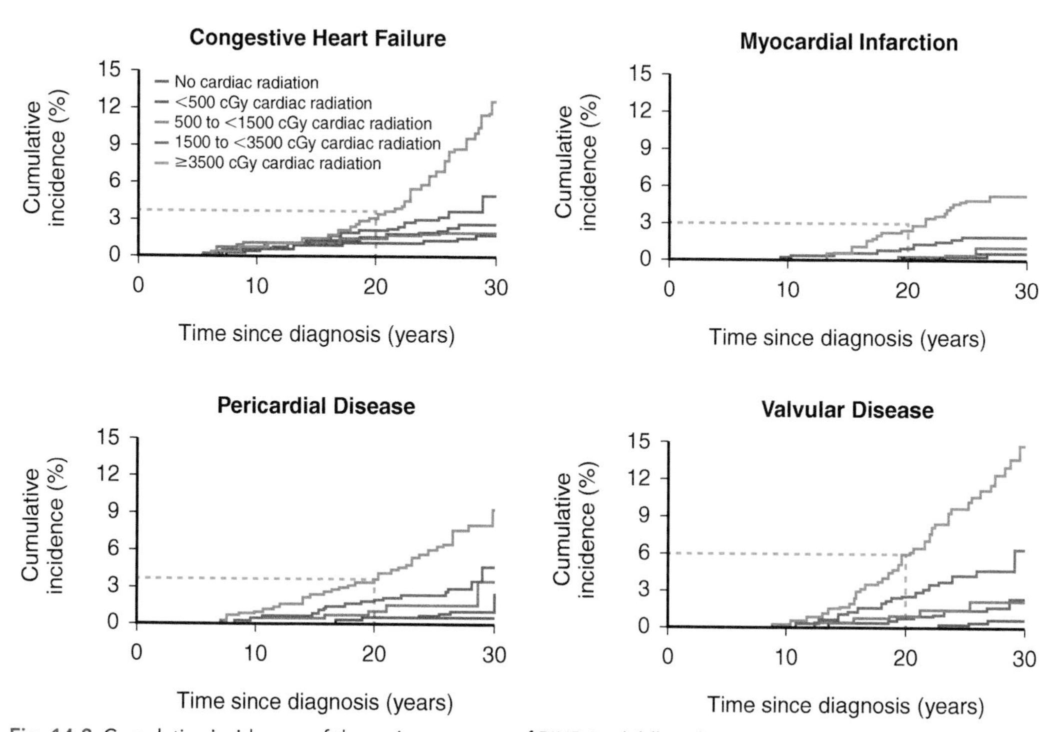

Fig. 14.2 Cumulative incidences of the various aspects of RIHD in childhood cancer survivors. Notice the dose dependency and the timeline of 15 years from diagnosis for clinical appearance. (*From* Mulrooney DA, Yeazel MW, Kawashima T, et al. Cardiac outcomes in a cohort of adult survivors of childhood and adolescent cancer: retrospective analysis of the Childhood Cancer Survivor Study cohort. BMJ 2009;339:b4606; with permission.)

with heart disease occur in those that received greater than 30 Gy.[7] Acute pericardial effusion following RT occurred in patients who received an average pericardial dose of 53.25 Gy.[30] A dose of 2.8 Gy was the lowest dose that has been shown to increase the rate of CAD.[31]

RT for HD has been refined since the 1970s. Radiation protection blocks covering the left ventricle limit the total cardiac dose to 15 Gy, and modern-era regimens have used a reduced fraction size.[7,32,33] With these interventions, the relative risk for non-acute myocardial infarction-related cardiac death was reduced from 5.3 to 1.4. Involved-node RT and involved-field RT include the involved nodes and their surrounding regions, respectively.[27,28] These regimens have resulted in further reductions in cardiac radiation dose when compared with extended-field (mantle) radiation.

DOSE FRACTIONATION

Fractionation of total radiation dose is another factor in the development of RIHD, and it is thought that risk of RIHD is higher with a lower number of fractions.[31–34] Indeed, twice weekly fractionation compared with 5 times weekly increases the risk of complications in noncardiac tissues such as pulmonary fibrosis and pathologic fractures.[35,36] Dose plan analysis of hypofractionated RT (larger dose fractions given in fewer treatments) furthermore confirms a lower cardiac radiation dose compared with normofractionated RT.[35] However, hypofractionated RT of 42.5 Gy in 16 fractions versus 50 Gy in 25 fractions, which is commonly used for breast cancer, resulted in no differences in cardiovascular mortality after 10 years.[37,38] Thus, the value of this strategy has yet to be fully defined.

PATHOPHYSIOLOGY OF RADIATION-INDUCED HEART DISEASE

Human autopsy studies have characterized the pathologic findings of RIHD, and pathophysiologic concepts have been described (Fig. 14.3).[2,3] It is unlikely that age-related CAD or degenerative changes are responsible for the

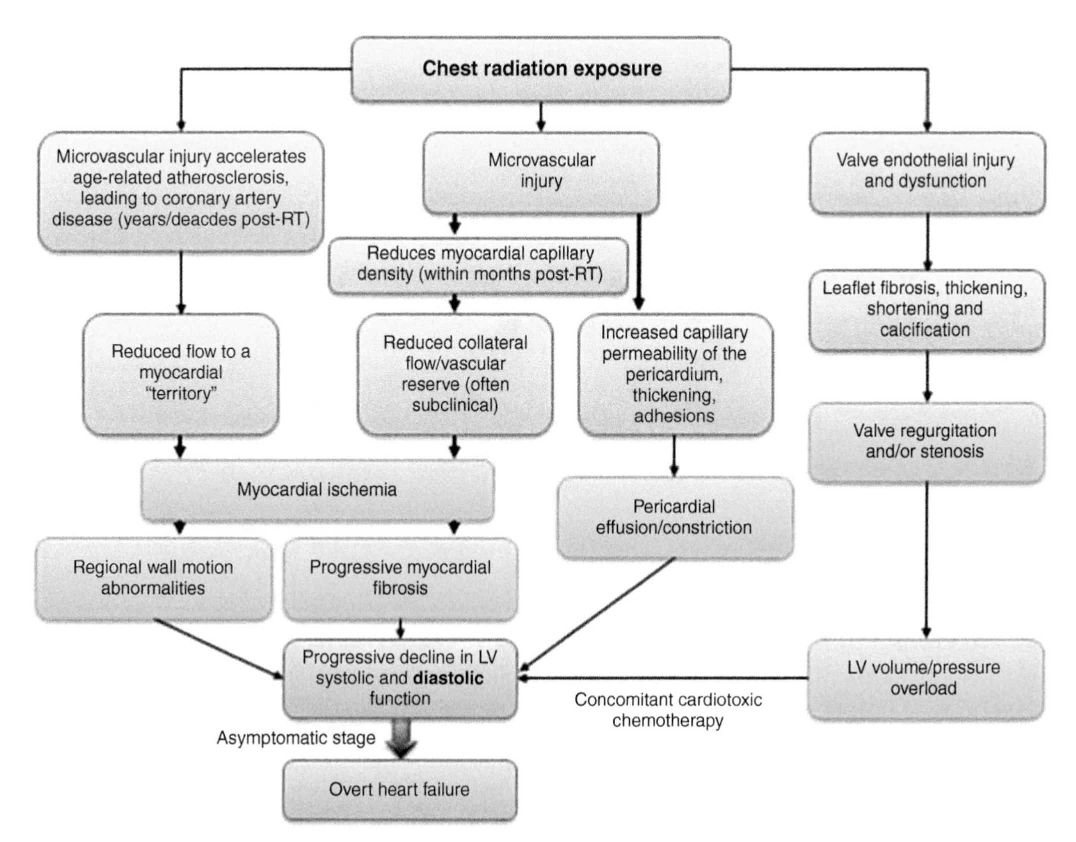

Fig. 14.3 Outline of the pathophysiology of RIHD. (*From* Lancellotti P, Nkomo VT, Badano LP, et al. Expert consensus for multi-modality imaging evaluation of cardiovascular complications of radiotherapy in adults: a report from the European Association of Cardiovascular Imaging and the American Society of Echocardiography. Eur Heart J Cardiovasc Imaging 2013;14(8):723; with permission.)

lesions observed given the young age of many of these patients. Pericardial disease was the most common finding, with 70% to 100% of patients having an abnormal pericardium. Some of the lesions observed include constrictive pericarditis, fibrinous pericardial adhesions, and pericardial fibrosis. Pericardial effusions and thickening with fibrous tissue were seen in most patients. Diffuse fibrosis and calcification were found in each of the 4 valves, and some surgically removed specimens were severely fibrosed and stenotic. Myocardial interstitial fibrosis was also found in most patients, although necrosis of myocardial cells was not observed. Up to a third of autopsies revealed severe CAD (>75% stenosis) attributable to radiation. Although conventional atherosclerosis was often present, fibrous tissue was a dominating feature in essentially all 3 layers of the arterial wall.

Fibrosis becomes the dominant pathologic feature 1 year after radiation, whereas inflammation is the dominant finding early on.[15,16,39] This also has been attributed to injury of the endothelial layer with subsequent activation and release of cytokines as well as loosening of tight junction and increased permeability. This process is pertinent to the process of acute and constrictive pericarditis but also affects the valves and the capillaries in the myocardium. Cytokines such as tumor necrosis factor-α and transforming growth factor-β have been implicated in increased type I and III collagen deposition and thus fibrosis.[40–43]

However, because interstitial fibrosis is often perivascular, some investigators have hypothesized that tissue hypoxia from capillary damage may be the primary insult causing radiation-induced tissue fibrosis.[15,16,37,42–45] Endothelial damage exposes von Willebrand factor, which stimulates thrombus formation and can occlude myocardial capillaries.[46,47] The theory that ischemia is a key factor in RIHD is supported by the observation that histopathological changes are most evident in the subendocardium. However, direct radiation injury appears to affect the intercalated discs and mitochondria of myocytes.[48–52] Reactive oxygen species are produced by inhibition of mitochondrial respiration, which is associated with radiation-induced myocardial dysfunction.[41,48–54] The renin-angiotensin-aldosterone system is also activated by this oxidative stress, and angiotensin II is another profibrotic mediator.[55,56] In addition, studies have suggested that angiotensin-receptor blockers and angiotensin-converting enzyme (ACE) inhibitors can potentially inhibit the development of radiation-induced fibrosis.[55–59] Finally, there is also the potential for direct injury of the cardiomyocytes (myocytolysis).[16]

Radiation exposure accelerates atherosclerosis by causing direct endothelial injury. Intimal cholesterol plaques may occur rapidly when lysosomal enzymes are activated and endothelial permeability is increased following coronary irradiation.[60–65] Furthermore, there is endothelial activation with expression of adhesion molecules and release of von Willebrand factor.[46,66–69] These processes favor inflammation, plaque progression, and vulnerability as well as thrombosis.[70,71] A unique observation is the presence of fibrotic changes of all 3 layers of the epicardial coronary arteries.[2,3] However, changes of the microvasculature are also observed after chest irradiation.[72,73]

Structural alterations of the valves seem to be stimulated by conversion of interstitial cells into an osteoblast-like cell.[74,75] In addition, multiple osteogenic proteins, including osteopontin and bone morphogenetic protein 2, are upregulated and likely play a role in the development of calcific aortic stenosis following cardiac irradiation.

PERICARDIAL DISEASE

Radiation-induced pericardial disease ranges from acute pericarditis and pericardial effusions to constrictive pericarditis. Historically, with older, more radiation-intense protocols, pericardial disease was one of the most frequent cardiac complications of RT.[76,77] Pericardial effusions with cardiac tamponade were among the first case reports of RIHD following thoracic radiation. Acute pericarditis presenting with chest pain and friction rubs was also reported.[77,78] Management of these cases does not differ from management of acute pericarditis and includes nonsteroidal anti-inflammatory drugs.

Although pericardial disease-related sequelae is less frequently encountered nowadays due to changes in radiation exposure and techniques, patients may also develop chronic pericardial effusions and/or constrictive pericarditis due to evolving adhesions and fibrosis anywhere from 1 to 20 years following irradiation.[3,77–85] Patients may complain of shortness of breath, increased girth size, lower extremity swelling, and lightheadedness to the point of presyncope and syncope. The physical examination findings include jugular venous distention, Kussmaul sign, ascites, and peripheral edema. Electrocardiogram findings are nonspecific but include low-voltage and T-wave changes. Although echocardiography, CT, or MRI scans may reveal pericardial thickening, these findings can be nonspecific, and cardiac catheterization to evaluate for ventricular discordance and interdependence may aid in the diagnosis.[86]

Pericardiocentesis is sometimes needed for large effusions and pericardial stripping (pericardectomy) for hemodynamically and clinically relevant constriction.[77,86,87] Mortality following pericardial stripping is significantly higher in radiation-induced constrictive pericarditis compared with pericardiectomy performed for other causes (5-year mortality 89.0% vs 35.7%, $P<.001$; Fig. 14.4).[86,87] The likely reason for higher mortality rates in this population is due to more extensive pericardial and mediastinal fibrosis as well as fibrosis of the myocardium, and concomitant valvular and ischemic heart disease. Once diagnosed, pericardiectomy should be done sooner rather than later but may only expose the presence of restrictive cardiomyopathy.[86] A thorough preoperative evaluation is therefore needed to determine the value of surgery as is experience with managing these cases in general for best overall outcomes.

CARDIOMYOPATHY

The clinical presentation of radiation-induced myocardial disease is similar to HF of other causes.[88] MRI may show diffuse and patchy fibrosis that does not correspond to a coronary artery perfusion territory. Left ventricular ejection fraction (LVEF), on average, may still be within the normal range but lower than expected in comparison with healthy controls (62%, $P<.05$).[89] The impairment in cardiac function can be more profoundly impaired in patients who also received anthracycline treatment, even when there is temporal separation between these treatment modalities (Fig. 14.5).[90–92] The most distinctive feature is the development of restrictive cardiomyopathy as a consequence of endocardial and myocardial fibrosis.[93,94]

As with HF not caused by radiation exposure, ACE inhibitors and β-blockers are the mainstays of therapy.[95] Orthotopic heart transplantation (OHT) is the last resort in cases that are refractory to medical therapy. It may also be preferred to pericardiectomy given the technical difficulties of pericardial stripping in the presence of severe mediastinal fibrosis.[96,97] OHT may also be the only remaining option in the case of diffuse CAD not amendable to coronary artery bypass surgery (CABG), which can similarly be challenged in its technical aspects by mediastinal fibrosis. In the RIHD population, OHT may also carry a significant perioperative risk, although at least one center has reported excellent short- and intermediate-term results in a small cohort of patients.[96,97] Patients should be carefully selected for OHT given the significant perioperative risk.

VALVULAR DISEASE

Most patients develop clinically relevant valvular disease 20 years or more after mediastinal radiation (on average 22 years to symptom development).[98] A cardiac radiation dose of greater than 25 Gy carries the highest risk for radiation-induced valvular disease,[99–102] and in general, the aortic and mitral valves are the most commonly affected valves. Regurgitation is more common than stenosis (aortic regurgitation in 60%, mitral regurgitation in 52%, and aortic stenosis in 16% in one series).[3,11,98,103,104]

Surgical management is the standard of care for radiation-induced valvular disease.[103] The 30-day mortality after valvular surgery for radiation-induced valvular disease (including aortic, mitral, and tricuspid valves) is 12%, whereas the 5-year survival is 66%.[105,106] Constrictive pericarditis significantly raises the 30-day mortality to 40%.[102,105–107] It might be because of a direct role, or more likely, constrictive pericarditis serves as an indicator of higher

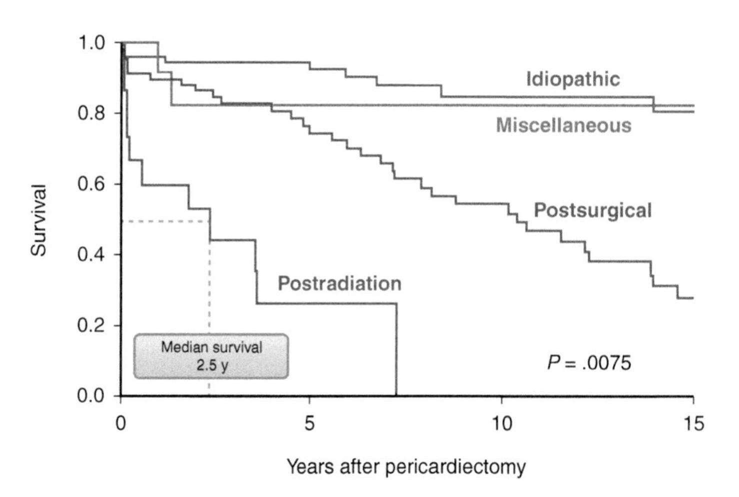

Fig. 14.4 Survival after pericardiectomy by type of pericardial disease. (*Adapted from* Bertog SC, Thambidorai SK, Parakh K, et al. Constrictive pericarditis: etiology and cause-specific survival after pericardiectomy. J Am Coll Cardiol 2004;43(8):1448; with permission.)

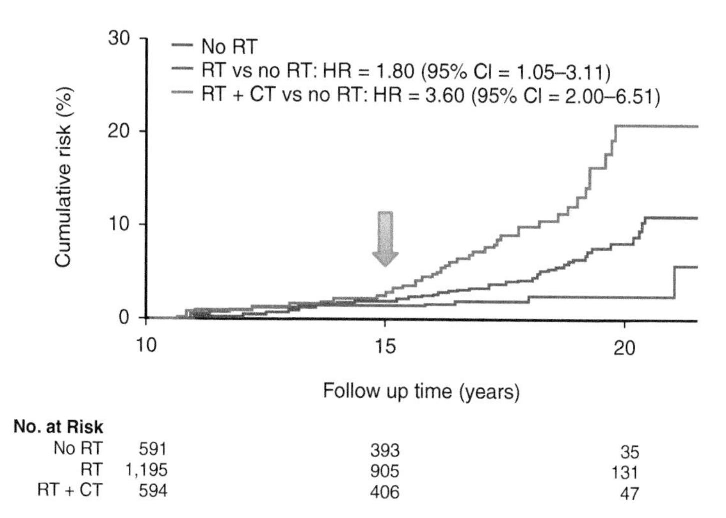

Fig. 14.5 Cumulative incidences of HF in patients with breast cancer. Notice the more than synergistic impact of chemotherapy (mainly anthracyclines) and the emergence of differences after 15 years. (*From* Hooning MJ, Botma A, Aleman BM, et al. Long-term risk of cardiovascular disease in 10-year survivors of breast cancer. J Natl Cancer Inst 2007;99(5):370; with permission.)

radiation dose exposure and greater burden of cardiac and mediastinal disease. In patients with advanced aortic stenosis who are poor surgical candidates due to comorbidities such as radiation pulmonary fibrosis and severe aortic calcifications (ie, porcelain aorta), transcatheter aortic valve replacement (TAVR) may be a less invasive option.[108] Intervention for radiation-induced valvular disease should be individually tailored to the valve involved and the patient's other comorbidities.

CORONARY ARTERY DISEASE

Irradiation of the coronary arteries rapidly accelerates atherosclerosis. CAD is the most common clinically significant manifestation of RIHD, with acute myocardial infarctions occurring even in young patients without traditional cardiac risk factors (see **Fig. 14.3**).[11,77,109] The distribution of CAD reflects the radiation field.[110] Accordingly, the mid to distal segments of the LAD are the most likely areas to be involved with left-breast irradiation.[111] On the contrary, ostial right and left main lesions have classically been reported with mediastinal, mantle, or involved field radiation. A third of patients screened with coronary angiography will also have 2- or 3-vessel disease with stenoses 70% or greater.[112–114] Concerns for aggravation of in-stent restenoses after thoracic radiotherapy have been raised but not always confirmed.[115–117]

Radiation-induced CAD typically presents clinically with angina or myocardial infarction, just like conventional CAD.[113,118] The diagnostic workup is in keeping with published guidelines, and coronary angiography remains the reference standard.[109,113] Consideration has to be given to the presence of microvascular disease, ideally assessed by regional myocardial perfusion imaging with PET or invasive measures of coronary flow reserve and vasoreactivity. Under these circumstances, technetium-99m tetrofosmin perfusion may show reversible perfusion defects that do not correspond to coronary artery distribution territories but microvascular dysfunction.[119,120] Stress echocardiography is generally not as sensitive but more specific for regional perfusion defects, which may not be present with microvascular disease. Computed tomography angiography (CTA) with or without coronary artery calcium (CAC) scoring is an alternative imaging technique. The prevalence of coronary calcium in patients who received RT for Hodgkin disease is overall higher, and the overall plaque burden is more quantifiable; however, no systematic studies have yet been performed.[121–123] In one of the most comprehensive studies thus far, conventional functional stress testing underestimated the burden of CAD in these patients (**Fig. 14.6**).

Guidelines for management of stable CAD and acute coronary syndromes do not specifically address RIHD; however, it is reasonable to follow the existing recommendations for conventional CAD.[124,125] Either percutaneous coronary intervention (PCI) or CABG may be considered for complex, multivessel CAD, although if valve surgery or pericardiectomy is needed, then CABG may be done concurrently to avoid reoperation.[126,127] The internal mammary artery (IMA) is in the radiation field of some RT regimens, and there have been concerns that it may be potentially a dysfunctional conduit.[128] The IMA, however, was found to be free of radiation-induced injury in one study of

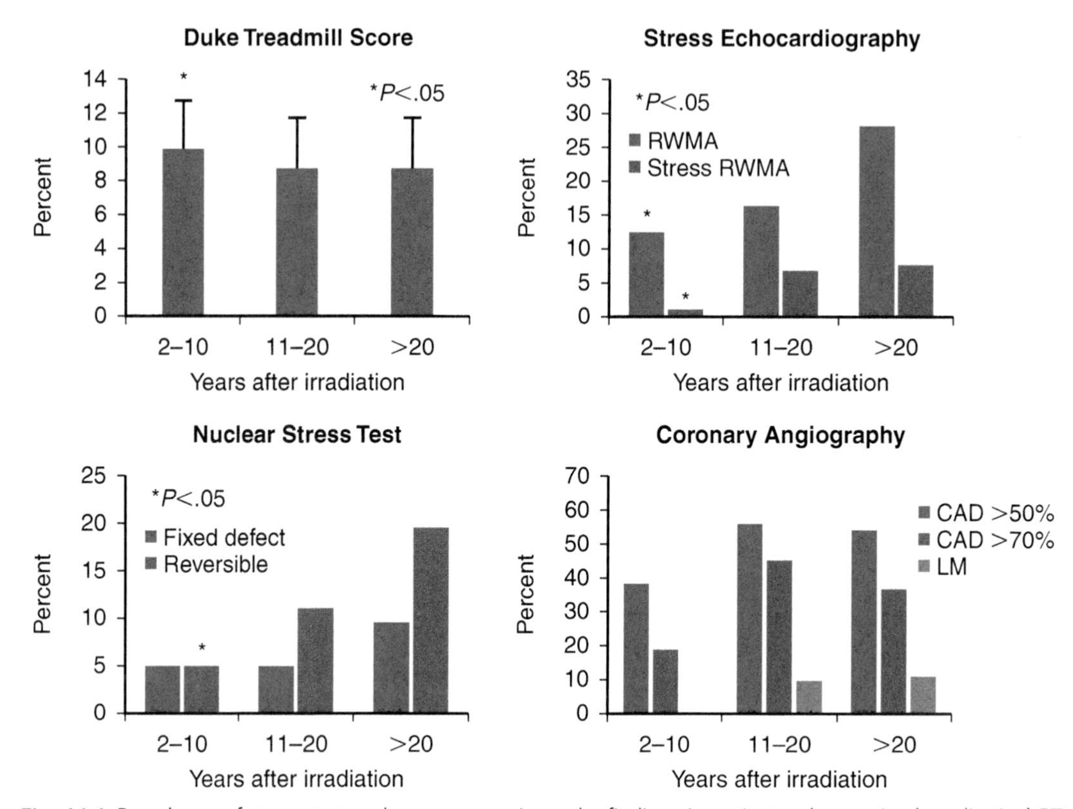

Fig. 14.6 Prevalence of stress test and coronary angiography findings in patients who received mediastinal RT (≥35 Gy) for Hodgkin lymphoma. LM, left main coronary artery; RWMA, regional wall motion abnormalities. (*Data from* Heidenreich PA, Schnittger I, Strauss W, et al. Screening for coronary artery disease after mediastinal irradiation. J Clin Oncol 2007;25:43–9.)

125 patients who had received thoracic RT[129]; thus, no definitive conclusions can be made about IMA graft patency in the setting of mediastinal radiation. It may, however, be prudent to perform angiography on any potential mammary grafts to exclude pre-existing disease before surgery. In general, PCI and CABG are both reasonable options for the management of severe radiation-induced CAD, but the final decision is case based.[130,131]

NONCORONARY ATHEROSCLEROTIC DISEASE

In addition to CAD, atherosclerosis affects the carotid and subclavian arteries following thoracic radiation as well.[11] Stenosis of 40% or greater of the carotid or subclavian artery was observed in 7.4% of patients with prior RT for Hodgkin disease at a median of 17 years after treatment. The median age of patients at the time of radiotherapy was 34 years, and the median time from treatment to diagnosis of carotid or subclavian arterial disease was 17 years. Patients who developed subclavian stenosis were exposed to a higher median low-cervical radiation dose than those who did not (44 vs 36 Gy, $P = .002$).

RT for head and neck tumors also increases the risk of carotid artery stenosis. Patients who had received a mean radiation dose of 56.4 Gy to the neck for nasopharyngeal carcinoma had a prevalence of carotid stenosis of 79% compared with 21% in controls.[132] Ten years after RT to the neck, the relative risk of stroke was 10.1 (95% CI 4.4–20.0).

Carotid endarterectomy and carotid artery stenting are options for severe carotid artery stenosis, and stenting of the subclavian artery or bypass subclavian artery bypass grafting are options for subclavian artery stenosis.

ELECTROPHYSIOLOGIC ABNORMALITIES

Cardiac irradiation may cause damage to the conduction system, such as atrioventricular (AV) block and bundle branch blocks.[98,133] Although most patients are asymptomatic, the most common clinical presentation reported in the literature is syncope. In one study of patients who presented with complete heart block, the average latency period from irradiation to clinical presentation was 12 years. Ostial stenosis of the right coronary artery (RCA) from radiation exposure has been reported to cause AV block from exercise-induced AV nodal ischemia.[134,135] Radiation-induced fibrosis may also disrupt the conduction system.[136,137] Calcifications of the mitral-aortic junction are a peculiar sign to note on imaging studies as associated with complete heart block in these patients (Fig. 14.7). Patients with high-degree AV blocks may require pacemakers.[133,134] Treatment with anthracyclines in addition to RT may increase the risk of developing supraventricular tachycardia and ventricular tachycardia.[138]

AUTONOMIC DYSFUNCTION

Patients treated with thoracic RT may also develop autonomic dysfunction, likely due to the disruption in the parasympathetic and sympathetic regulatory mechanisms. In fact, in Hodgkin lymphoma survivors after mediastinal RT, autonomic dysfunction ranks second after electrocardiogram (ECG) abnormalities as one of the most common abnormalities (Fig. 14.8). A more recent retrospective study of 263 patients with Hodgkin lymphoma evaluated the resting heart rates and heart rate recovery before and during exercise treadmill testing. Compared with control patients, patients that had received RT a median of 19 years prior (median radiation dose 38 Gy) had an elevated resting heart rate.[139] In addition, after 1 minute of recovery from Bruce protocol, a significantly greater percentage of RT patients had an abnormal heart rate recovery (31.9% vs 9.3%, *P*<.0001). An abnormal heart rate recovery was associated with higher all-cause mortality (HR 4.6, 95% CI 1.6–13.0), as has previously been described in patients without radiation history or known heart disease.[140] The authors of this study hypothesized that radiation injury to the autonomic nervous system is disruptive of the sympathovagal balance.

SCREENING AND PREVENTION

Although modern RT has become more sophisticated and results in lower radiation doses, patients are also living longer after treatment of cancer, increasing the likelihood of developing clinically significant RIHD. Prevention of radiation exposure by excluding the heart from the radiation field with radiation planning or use of radiation protection blocks (shielding) is the primary method of preventing RIHD.

There is a dearth of literature regarding prevention of RIHD during or after radiation exposure. Animal studies have demonstrated a cardioprotective effect of ACE inhibitors and angiotensin-receptor blockers after irradiation,

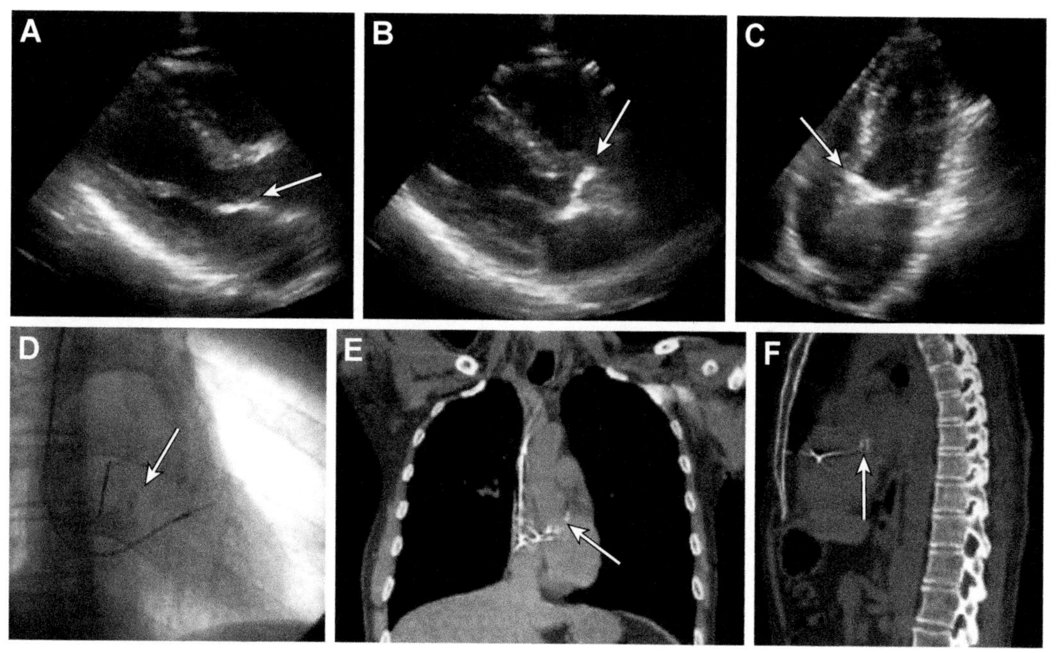

Fig. 14.7 Calcification of mitral-aortic junction. (*From* Santoro F, Ieva R, Lupo P, et al. Late calcification of the mitral-aortic junction (*arrows*) causing transient complete atrio-ventricular block after mediastinal radiation of Hodgkin lymphoma: multimodal visualization. Int J Cardiol 2012;155:e50; with permission.)

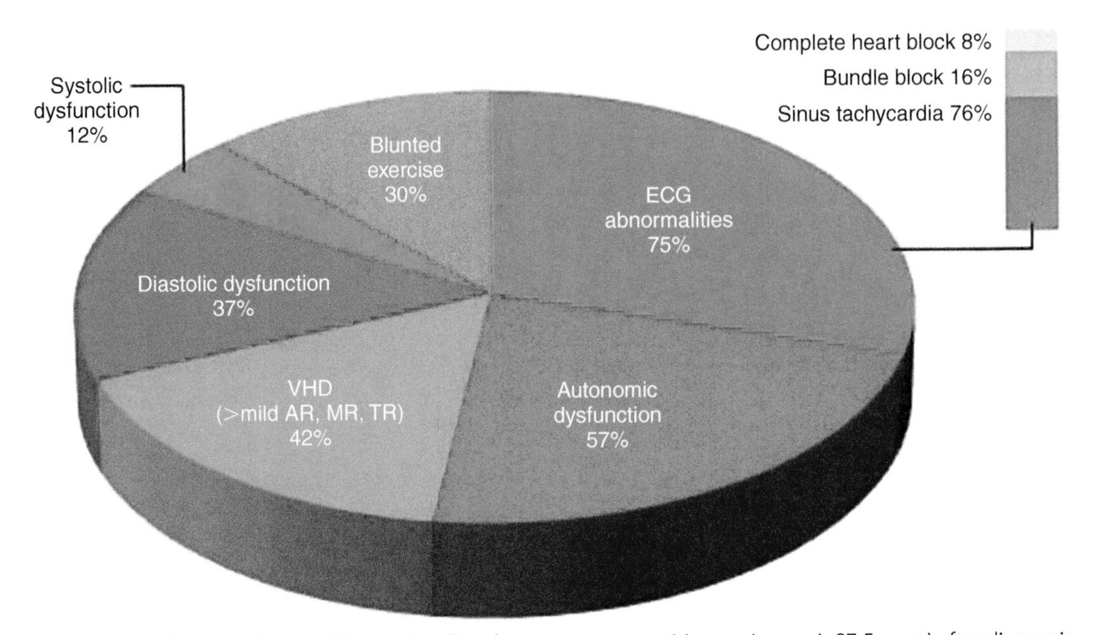

Fig. 14.8 Prevalence of abnormalities and cardiac disease on average 14 years (range 6–27.5 years) after diagnosis in survivors of Hodgkin lymphoma who underwent mediastinal radiation. AR, aortic regurgitation; MR, mitral regurgitation; TR, tricuspid regurgitation; VHD, valvular heart disease. (*Data from* Adams MJ, Lipsitz SR, Colan SD, et al. Cardiovascular status in long-term survivors of Hodgkin's disease treated with chest radiotherapy. J Clin Oncol 2004;22(15):3139–48.)

and patients who are on ACE-inhibitors are at lower risk of radiation pneumonitis.[141–144] HMG-CoA reductase inhibitors (statin drugs) also decrease the degree of cardiac fibrosis due to radiation exposure.[145] Statin therapy should be considered in patients undergoing thoracic RT. Similarly, if patients undergoing RT require antihypertensive treatment, ACE inhibitors or angiotensin receptor blockers (ARBs) should be considered the initial agents. Prospective studies in humans though are needed to confirm the benefits of statins and ACE inhibitors/ARBs in patients with possible cardiac radiation exposure.

Patients with a history of thoracic radiation treatment should be followed by a cardiologist lifelong. This includes asymptomatic patients given that even those without symptoms may have significant cardiovascular disease. The value of brain natriuretic peptide and troponin I is unknown,[146] and the emphasis has been on imaging studies, as endorsed in the European Association of Cardiovascular Imaging and American Society of Echocardiography 2013 consensus statement on follow-up screening after RT.[147] Screening echocardiography is recommended starting 10 years after radiation exposure, or 5 years after RT in higher-risk patients (Box 14.2).[98,147,148] Echocardiograms are then to be repeated be every 5 years. Likewise, functional stress tests are recommended 5 to 10 years after RT in high-risk patients to screen for CAD.[148] Other investigators recommend CAD screening following mediastinal RT >35 Gy.[147] The Society for Cardiac Angiography and Intervention (SCAI) recently further refined screening recommendations after RT as summarized in Fig. 14.9 (see Box 14.2).[149] The SCAI consensus document specifically mentions the use of computerized tomography coronary angiography (CCTA) with CAC scoring and exercise oxygen consumption stress testing with echocardiographic imaging as additional screening techniques. Although CCTA outlines the anatomic burden of CAD more than any other technique, exercise oxygen consumption stress testing evaluates both the cardiac and the pulmonary reserve, which may also be impaired because of concomitant lung fibrosis in these patients. If abnormalities are found on CT or functional stress testing, coronary angiography may be considered. Screening for and treatment of traditional CAD risk factors, including hypertension, dyslipidemia, diabetes, and smoking, are imperative.[91,150] Indeed, RT may be considered as yet another potent cardiovascular risk factor (Fig. 14.10), and for instance, the risk of acute coronary events is higher and emerges earlier (<10 years, and even <5 years) in those with other cardiovascular risk factors[24] (Fig. 14.11). These observations provide another strong impetus for screening efforts. Even though intuitive and extrapolated from studies on conventional atherosclerotic cardiovascular disease, evidence

BOX 14.2
Screening recommendations for asymptomatic patients with cardiac radiation exposure

Screening for CAD

van Leeuwen-Segarceanu et al

- CT angiography/coronary artery calcium scoring
- Screening recommended for patients receiving ≥35 Gy to the mediastinum (or those who received older RT techniques that do not minimize cardiac irradiation)
- Starting 5 years after radiation exposure for patients 45 or older
- Starting 10 years after radiation exposure for patients less than 45
- Reassess every 5 years
- Lipid panel every 3 years
- Blood pressure and fasting blood glucose screening annually

European Association of Cardiovascular Imaging and the American Society of Echocardiography (EACVI/ASE) consensus statement

- Functional noninvasive stress test
- Screening recommended in high-risk patients[a]
- Starting 5 to 10 years after radiation exposure
- Reassess every 5 years

Screening for valvular disease

van Leeuwen-Segarceanu et al

- Echocardiogram
- Screening recommended for patients receiving 35 Gy or greater to the mediastinum (or those who received older RT techniques that do not minimize cardiac irradiation)
- Starting 10 years after radiation
- Reassess every 5 years

EACVI/ASE consensus statement

- Echocardiogram
- Starting 5 years after radiation in high-risk patients[a]
- Starting 10 years after radiation in all others
- Reassess every 5 years

Screening for noncoronary atherosclerotic disease

Both van Leeuwen-Segarceanu et al and the EACVI/ASE consensus statement do not recommend screening for noncoronary atherosclerotic disease in asymptomatic patients, but recommend carotid artery ultrasonography in patients with carotid bruits or neurologic symptoms. However, given the significant elevation in risk of stroke related to carotid stenosis in patients who have received head and neck radiotherapy, screening with ultrasonography in select asymptomatic patients is reasonable.

[a] High-risk patients were defined as having had anterior or left chest irradiation as well as one of the following risk factors: dose greater than 30 Gy, dose fraction greater than 2 Gy, age less than 50 years, lack of shielding, concomitant anthracyclines, cardiovascular risk factors, or known cardiac disease.

Data from Nellessen U, Zingel M, Hecker H, et al. Effects of radiation therapy on myocardial cell integrity and pump function: which role for cardiac biomarkers? Chemotherapy 2010;56:147–52; and Lancellotti P, Nkomo VT, Badano LP, et al. Expert consensus for multi-modality imaging evaluation of cardiovascular complications of radiotherapy in adults: a report from the European Association of Cardiovascular Imaging and the American Society of Echocardiography. J Am Soc Echocardiogr 2013;26:1013–32.

is yet to be provided that this knowledge and reaction to this knowledge yield improved cardiovascular outcomes in patients who underwent RT. Until this proof is provided, all patients may be considered to be at higher risk in the respective radiation territories than captured by conventional risk calculators and should be proactively managed with aspirin and statins. Experimental studies indicate that these medications may not be as efficacious for radiation-induced

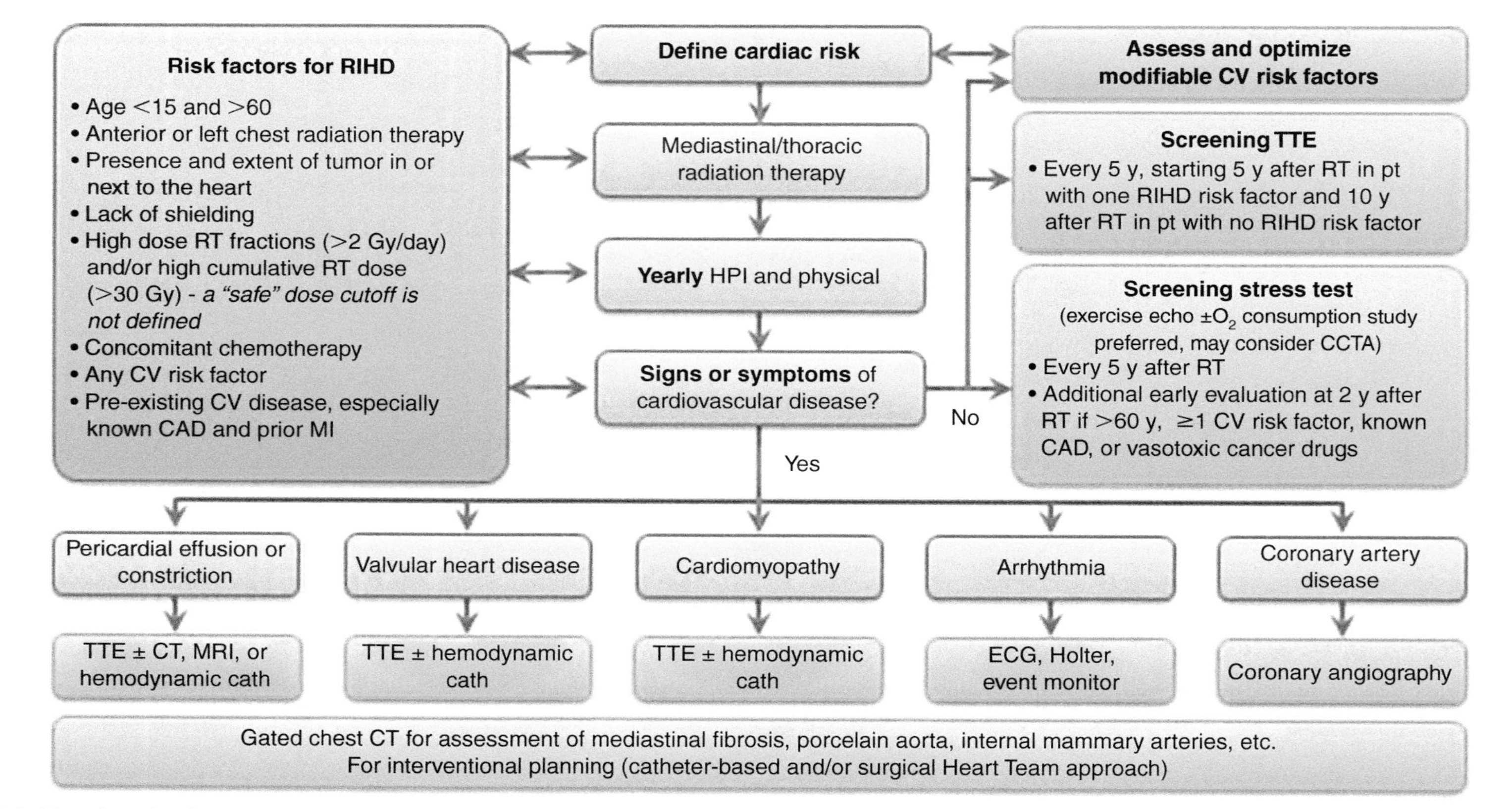

Fig. 14.9 SCAI algorithm for the management of patients undergoing chest RT. (*From* Iliescu CA, Grines CL, Herrmann J, et al. SCAI expert consensus statement: evaluation, management, and special considerations of cardio-oncology patients in the cardiac catheterization laboratory (endorsed by the Cardiological Society of India, and Sociedad Latino Americana de Cardiologıa Intervencionista). Catheter Cardiovasc Interv 2016;87(5):E206; with permission.)

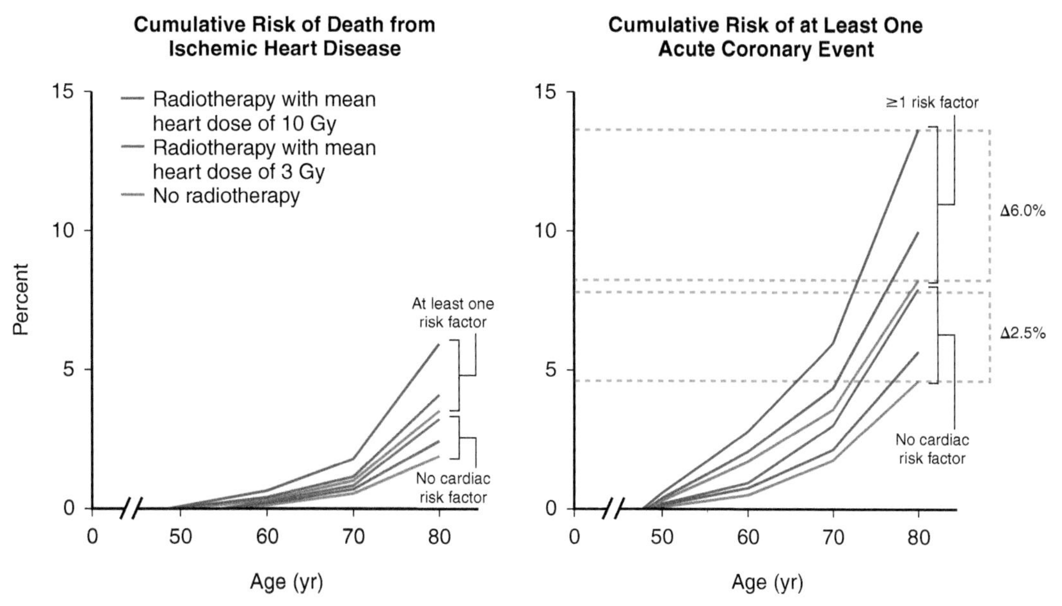

Fig. 14.10 Cumulative risk of death from ischemic heart disease (*left*) and of an acute coronary event (*right*) in patients after chest radiation for breast cancer. (*From* Darby SC, Ewertz M, McGale P, et al. Risk of ischemic heart disease in women after radiotherapy for breast cancer. N Engl J Med 2013;368:997; with permission.)

vascular injury, but there is no substance to these concerns in patients yet.

With regards to the other manifestations for RIHD, there are currently no known strategies that would prevent their development or progression after radiation-induced injury.

SUMMARY

RT is a highly prevalent cause of cardiovascular disease in survivors of breast cancer and Hodgkin disease. CAD, cardiomyopathy, and valvular disease have a high prevalence, so it is recommended that patients with significant prior radiation

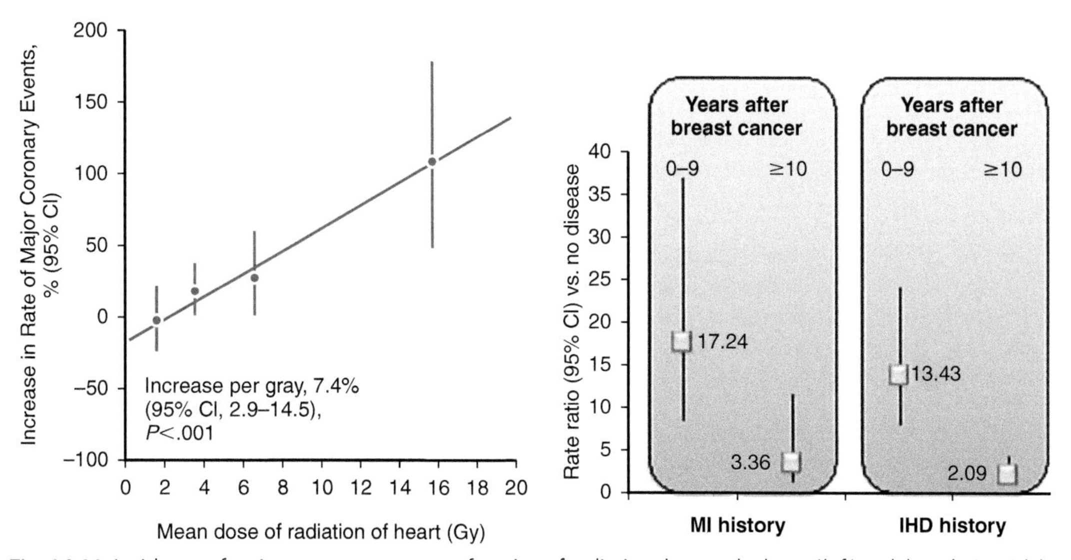

Fig. 14.11 Incidence of major coronary event as a function of radiation dose to the heart (*left*) and the relative risk by time from chest radiation for breast cancer (*right*). MI, myocardial infarction. (*From* Darby SC, Ewertz M, McGale P, et al. Risk of ischemic heart disease in women after radiotherapy for breast cancer. N Engl J Med 2013;368:993; with permission.)

TABLE 14.2
Commonly used units of radiation exposure

Unit	Type of Unit	Conversion Factor
Rad[a]	Absorbed radiation dose	1 rad = 0.01 Gy
Gray (Gy)[a]	Absorbed radiation dose; SI unit	1 J/kg = 1 Gy = 100 rad
Rem[b]	Dose equivalent	1 rem = 0.01 Sv; 1 rem = 1 rad[c]
Sievert (Sv)[b]	Dose equivalent; SI unit	1 Sv = 100 rem; 1 Sv = 1 Gy[c]

[a] Rad and grays are units of energy per mass.
[b] Rem and sieverts are units of energy per mass adjusted by a dimensionless factor to account for potential for biological damage.
[c] Rem and rad are equivalent and sieverts and grays are equivalent for radiograph and gamma radiation.
Data from Topolnjak R, Borst GR, Nijkamp J, et al. Image-guided radiotherapy for left-sided breast cancer patients: geometrical uncertainty of the heart. Int J Radiat Oncol Biol Phys 2012;82:e647–55.

exposure be followed by a cardiologist lifelong (Case Studies 1-4, available on Expert Consult, Table 14.2). Screening for RIHD with echocardiograms and for accelerated CAD with either functional stress testing or CT coronary angiography is warranted. Advances continue to be made in reducing cardiac radiation exposure with RT, and with these refinements the incidence of RIHD may decline.

SUPPLEMENTARY MATERIAL

Go to ExpertConsult.com to listen to an interview with the authors.

REFERENCES

1. Finch W, Shamsa K, Lee MS. Cardiovascular complications of radiation exposure. Rev Cardiovasc Med 2014;15:232–44.
2. Brosius FC, Waller BF, Roberts WC. Radiation heart disease: analysis of 16 young (aged 15 to 33 years) necropsy patients who received over 3,500 rads to the heart. Am J Med 1981;70:519–30.
3. Veinot JP, Edwards WD. Pathology of radiation-induced heart disease: a surgical and autopsy study of 27 cases. Hum Pathol 1996;27:766–73.
4. Darby SC, McGale P, Taylor CW, et al. Long-term mortality from heart disease and lung cancer after radiotherapy for early breast cancer: prospective cohort study of about 300,000 women in US SEER cancer registries. Lancet Oncol 2005;6:557–65.
5. Favourable and unfavourable effects on long-term survival of radiotherapy for early breast cancer: an overview of the randomised trials. Early Breast Cancer Trialists' Collaborative Group. Lancet 2000;355:1757–70.
6. Cuzick J, Stewart H, Rutqvist L, et al. Cause-specific mortality in long-term survivors of breast cancer who participated in trials of radiotherapy. J Clin Oncol 1994;12:447–53.
7. Hoppe RT. Hodgkin's disease: complications of therapy and excess mortality. Ann Oncol 1997;8:S115–8.
8. Mauch PM, Kalish LA, Marcus KC, et al. Long-term survival in Hodgkin's disease relative impact of mortality, second tumors, infection, and cardiovascular disease. Cancer J Sci Am 1995;1:33–42.
9. Piovaccari G, Ferretti RM, Prati F, et al. Cardiac disease after irradiation for Hodgkin's disease: incidence in 108 patients with long follow-up. Int J Cardiol 1995;49:39–43.
10. Applefeld MM, Wiernik PH. Cardiac disease after radiation therapy for Hodgkin's disease: analysis of 48 patients. Am J Cardiol 1983;51:1679–81.
11. Hull MC, Morris CG, Pepine CJ, et al. Valvular dysfunction and carotid, subclavian, and coronary artery disease in survivors of Hodgkin lymphoma treated with radiation therapy. JAMA 2003;290:2831–7.
12. Van Nimwegen FA, Schaapveld M, Janus CP, et al. Cardiovascular disease after Hodgkin lymphoma treatment. JAMA Intern Med 2015;75:1007–17.
13. Davies HE, Wathen CG, Gleeson FV. Risks of exposure to radiological imaging and how to minimise them. BMJ 2011;342:589–93.
14. Brenner DJ, Hall EJ. Computed tomography—an increasing source of radiation exposure. N Engl J Med 2007;357:2277–84.
15. Lauk S, Kiszel Z, Buschmann J, et al. Radiation-induced heart disease in rats. Int J Radiat Oncol Biol Phys 1985;11:801–8.
16. Gillette SM, Gillette EL, Shida T, et al. Late radiation response of canine mediastinal tissues. Radiother Oncol 1992;23:41–52.
17. Taylor CW, Nisbet A, McGale P, et al. Cardiac exposures in breast cancer radiotherapy: 1950s-1990s. Int J Radiat Oncol Biol Phys 2007;69:1484–95.

18. Rutqvist LE, Lax I, Fornander T, et al. Cardiovascular mortality in a randomized trial of adjuvant radiation therapy versus surgery alone in primary breast cancer. Int J Radiat Oncol Biol Phys 1992;22:887–96.
19. Buchholz TA. Radiation therapy for early-stage breast cancer after breast-conserving surgery. N Engl J Med 2009;360:63–70.
20. Giordano SH, Kuo YF, Freeman JL, et al. Risk of cardiac death after adjuvant radiotherapy for breast cancer. J Natl Cancer Inst 2005;97:419–24.
21. Host H, Brennhovd IO, Loeb M. Postoperative radiotherapy in breast cancer—long-term results from the Oslo study. Int J Radiat Oncol Biol Phys 1986;12:727–32.
22. Overgaard M, Hansen PS, Overgaard J, et al. Postoperative radiotherapy in high-risk premenopausal women with breast cancer who receive adjuvant chemotherapy. N Engl J Med 1997;337:949–55.
23. Hojris I, Overgaard M, Christensen JJ, et al. Morbidity and mortality of ischaemic heart disease in high-risk breast-cancer patients after adjuvant postmastectomy systemic treatment with or without radiotherapy: analysis of DBCG 82b and 82c randomised trials. Lancet 1999;354:1425–30.
24. Darby SC, Ewertz M, McGale P, et al. Risk of ischemic heart disease in women after radiotherapy for breast cancer. N Engl J Med 2013;368:987–98.
25. Poortmans PM, Collette S, Kirkove C, et al. Internal mammary and medial supraclavicular irradiation in breast cancer. N Engl J Med 2015;373:317–27.
26. Whelan TJ, Olivotto IA, Parulekar WP, et al. Regional nodal irradiation in early-stage breast cancer. N Engl J Med 2015;373:307–16.
27. Hodgson DC. Late effects in the era of modern therapy for Hodgkin lymphoma. Hematology Am Soc Hematol Educ Program 2011;2011:323–9.
28. Maraldo MV, Brodin NP, Vogelius IR, et al. Risk of developing cardiovascular disease after involved node radiotherapy versus mantle field for Hodgkin lymphoma. Int J Radiat Oncol Biol Phys 2012;83:1232–7.
29. Glanzmann C, Huguenin P, Lutolf UM, et al. Cardiac lesions after mediastinal irradiation for Hodgkin's disease. Radiother Oncol 1994;30:43–54.
30. Byhardt R, Brace K, Ruckdeschel J, et al. Dose and treatment factors in radiation-related pericardial effusion associated with the mantle technique for Hodgkin's disease. Cancer 1975;35:795–802.
31. Carr ZA, Land CE, Kleinerman RA, et al. Coronary heart disease after radiotherapy for peptic ulcer disease. Int J Radiat Oncol Biol Phys 2005;61:842–50.
32. Hancock SL, Tucker MA, Hoppe RT. Factors affecting late mortality from heart disease after treatment of Hodgkin's disease. JAMA 1993;270:1949–55.
33. Lauk S, Ruth S, Trott KR. The effects of dose-fractionation on radiation-induced heart disease in rats. Radiother Oncol 1987;8:363–7.
34. Schultz-Hector S, Sund M, Thames HD. Fractionation response and repair kinetics of radiation-induced heart failure in the rat. Radiother Oncol 1992;23:33–40.
35. Cosset JM, Henry-Amar M, Girinski T, et al. Late toxicity of radiotherapy in Hodgkin's disease: the role of fraction size. Acta Oncol 1988;27:123–9.
36. Overgaard M, Bentzen SM, Christensen JJ, et al. The value of the NSD formula in equation of acute and late radiation complications in normal tissue following 2 and 5 fractions per week in breast cancer patients treated with postmastectomy irradiation. Radiother Oncol 1987;9:1–11.
37. Appelt AL, Vogelius IR, Bentzen SM. Modern hypofractionation schedules for tangential whole breast irradiation decrease the fraction size-corrected dose to the heart. Clin Oncol 2012. http://dx.doi.org/10.1016/j.clon.2012.07.012.
38. Whelan TJ, Pignol JP, Levine MN, et al. Long-term results of hypofractionated radiation therapy for breast cancer. N Engl J Med 2010;362:513–20.
39. McChesney SL, Gillette EL, Powers BE. Radiation-induced cardiomyopathy in the dog. Radiat Res 1988;113:120–32.
40. Chello M, Mastroroberto P, Romano R, et al. Changes in the proportion of types I and III collagen in the left ventricular wall of patients with post-irradiative pericarditis. Cardiovasc Surg 1996;4:222–6.
41. Kruse J, Zurcher C, Strootman EG, et al. Structural changes in the auricles of the rat heart after local ionizing irradiation. Radiother Oncol 2001;58:303–11.
42. Rodemann HP, Bamberg M. Cellular basis of radiation-induced fibrosis. Radiother Oncol 1995;35:83–90.
43. Boerma M, Bart CI, Wondergem J. Effects of ionizing radiation on gene expression in cultured rat heart cells. Int J Radiat Biol 2002;78:219–25.
44. Fajardo LF, Stewart JR. Capillary injury preceding radiation-induced myocardial fibrosis. Radiology 1971;101:429–33.
45. Paris F, Fuks Z, Kang A, et al. Endothelial apoptosis as the primary lesion initiating intestinal radiation damage in mice. Science 2001;293:293–7.
46. Boerma M, Kruse J, van Loenen MM, et al. Increased deposition of von Willebrand factor in the rat heart after local ionizing irradiation. Strahlenther Onkol 2004;180:109–16.
47. Verheij M, Dewit LGH, Boomgaard MN, et al. Ionizing radiation enhances platelet adhesion to

the extracellular matrix of human endothelial cells by an increase in the release of von Willebrand factor. Radiat Res 1994;137:202–7.
48. Cilliers GD, Harper IS, Lochner A. Radiation-induced changes in the ultrastructure and mechanical function of the rat heart. Radiother Oncol 1989;16:311–26.
49. Yang VV, Stearner SP, Tyler SA. Radiation induced changes in the fine structure of the heart: comparison of fission neutrons and 60Co gamma rays in the mouse. Radiat Res 1976;67:344–60.
50. Kahn MY. Radiation induced cardiomyopathy. I. An electron microscopic study of cardiac muscle cells. Am J Pathol 1973;73:131–46.
51. Maeda S. Pathology of experimental radiation pancarditis. II. Correlation between ultrastructural changes of the myocardial mitochondria and succinic dehydrogenase activity in rabbit heart receiving a single dose of X-ray irradiation. Acta Pathol Jpn 1982;32:199–218.
52. Barcellos-Hoff MH. How do tissues respond to damage at the cellular level? The role of cytokines in irradiated tissues. Radiat Res 1998;150:S109–20.
53. Barjaktarovic Z, Schmaltz D, Shyla A, et al. Radiation–induced signaling results in mitochondrial impairment in mouse heart at 4 weeks after exposure to X-rays. PLoS One 2011;6(12):e27811.
54. Schultz-Hector S, Bohm M, Blochel A, et al. Radiation-induced heart disease: morphology, changes in catecholamine synthesis and content, β-adrenoceptor density, and hemodynamic function in an experimental model. Radiat Res 1992;129:281–9.
55. Robbins ME, Diz DI. Pathogenic role of the renin-angiotensin system in modulating radiation-induced late effects. Int J Radiat Oncol Biol Phys 2006;64:6–12.
56. Wu R, Zeng Y. Does angiotensin II–aldosterone have a role in radiation-induced heart disease? Med Hypotheses 2009;72:263–6.
57. Yarom R, Harper IS, Wynchank S, et al. Effect of captopril on changes in rats' hearts induced by long-term irradiation. Radiat Res 1993;133:187–97.
58. Sridharan V, Tripathi P, Sharma SK. Cardiac inflammation after local irradiation is influenced by the kallikrein-kinin system. Cancer Res 2012;72:4984–92.
59. Boerma M, Wang J, Wondergem J, et al. Influence of mast cells on structural and functional manifestations of radiation-induced heart disease. Cancer Res 2005;65:3100–7.
60. Amromin GD, Gildenhorn HL, Solomon RD, et al. The synergism of X-irradiation and cholesterol-fat feeding on the development of coronary artery lesions. J Atheroscler Res 1964;4:325–34.
61. Konings AW, Hardonk MJ, Wieringa RA, et al. Initial events in radiation-induced atheromatosis I. Activation of lysosomal enzymes. Strahlentherapie 1975;150:444–8.
62. Konings AW, Smit Sibinga CT, Aarnoudse MW, et al. Initial events in radiation-induced atheromatosis. II. Damage to intimal cells. Strahlentherapie 1978;154:795–800.
63. Konings AW, Smit Sibinga CT, Lamberts HB. Initial events in radiation-induced atheromatosis. IV. Lipid composition of radiation-induced plaques. Strahlentherapie 1980;156:134–8.
64. Konings AW, de Wit SS, Lamberts HB. Initial events in radiation-induced atheromatosis. III. Effect on lipase activity. Strahlentherapie 1979;155:655–7.
65. Evans ML, Graham MM, Mahler PA, et al. Changes in vascular permeability following thorax irradiation in the rat. Radiat Res 1986;107:262–71.
66. Zhou Q, Zhao Y, Li P, et al. Thrombomodulin as a marker of radiation-induced endothelial cell injury. Radiat Res 1992;131:285–9.
67. Stewart FA, Hoving S, Russell NS. Vascular damage as an underlying mechanism of cardiac and cerebral toxicity in irradiated cancer patients. Radiat Res 2010;174:865–9.
68. Khaled S, Gupta KB, Kucik DF. Ionizing radiation increases adhesiveness of human aortic endothelial cells via a chemokine-dependent mechanism. Radiat Res 2012;177:594–601.
69. Beckman JA, Thakore A, Kalinowski BH, et al. Radiation therapy impairs endothelium-dependent vasodilation in humans. J Am Coll Cardiol 2001;37:761–5.
70. Stewart FA, Heeneman S, Te Poele J, et al. Ionizing radiation accelerates the development of atherosclerotic lesions in ApoE-/- mice and predisposes to an inflammatory plaque phenotype prone to hemorrhage. Am J Pathol 2006;168:649–58.
71. Hoving S, Heeneman S, Gijbels MJ, et al. Single-dose and fractionated irradiation promote initiation and progression of atherosclerosis and induce an inflammatory plaque phenotype in ApoE(-/-) mice. Int J Radiat Oncol Biol Phys 2008;71:848–57.
72. Gabriels K, Hoving S, Seemann I, et al. Local heart irradiation of ApoE(-/-) mice induces microvascular and endocardial damage and accelerates coronary atherosclerosis. Radiother Oncol 2012. http://dx.doi.org/10.1016/j.radonc.2012.08.002.
73. Tribble DL, Barcellos-Hoff MH, Chu BM, et al. Ionizing radiation accelerates aortic lesion formation in fat-fed mice via SOD-inhibitable processes. Arterioscler Thromb Vasc Biol 1999;19:1387–92.
74. Stewart FA. Mechanisms and dose–response relationships for radiation-induced cardiovascular disease. Ann ICRP 2012. http://dx.doi.org/10.1016/j.icrp.2012.06.031.
75. Nadlonek NA, Weyant MJ, Yu JA, et al. Radiation induces osteogenesis in human aortic valve

interstitial cells. J Thorac Cardiovasc Surg 2012; 144:1466–70.
76. Hurst DW. Radiation fibrosis of pericardium, with cardiac tamponade. Can Med Assoc J 1959;81: 377–80.
77. Cohn KE, Stewart JR, Fajardo LF, et al. Heart disease following radiation. Medicine 1967;46: 281–98.
78. Ruckdeschel JC, Chang P, Martin RG, et al. Radiation-related pericardial effusions in patients with Hodgkin's disease. Medicine 1975;54:245–59.
79. Kumar PP. Pericardial injury from mediastinal irradiation. J Natl Med Assoc 1980;72:591–4.
80. Cameron J, Oesterle SN, Baldwin JC, et al. The etiologic spectrum of constrictive pericarditis. Am Heart J 1987;113:354–60.
81. Ling LH, Oh JK, Schaff HV, et al. Constrictive pericarditis in the modern era: evolving clinical spectrum and impact on outcome after pericardiectomy. Circulation 1999;100:1380–6.
82. Talreja DR, Edwards WD, Danielson GK, et al. Constrictive pericarditis in 26 patients with histologically normal pericardial thickness. Circulation 2003;108:1852–7.
83. Greenwood RD, Rosenthal A, Cassady R, et al. Constrictive pericarditis in childhood due to mediastinal irradiation. Circulation 1974;50:1033–9.
84. Applefeld MM, Cole JF, Pollock SH, et al. The late appearance of chronic pericardial disease in patients treated by radiotherapy for Hodgkin's disease. Ann Intern Med 1981;94:338–41.
85. Kane GC, Edie RN, Mannion JD. Delayed appearance of effusive-constrictive pericarditis after radiation for Hodgkin lymphoma. Ann Intern Med 1996;124:534–5.
86. Barbetakis N, Xenikakis T, Paliouras D, et al. Pericardiectomy for radiation-induced constrictive pericarditis. Hellenic J Cardiol 2010;51:214–8.
87. George TJ, Arnaoutakis GJ, Beaty CA, et al. Contemporary etiologies, risk factors, and outcomes after pericardiectomy. Ann Thorac Surg 2012;94:445–51.
88. H-Ici DO, Garot J. Radiation-induced heart disease. Circ Heart Fail 2011;4:e1–2.
89. Tsai HR, Gjesdal O, Wethal T, et al. Left ventricular function assessed by two-dimensional speckle tracking echocardiography in long-term survivors of Hodgkin's lymphoma treated by mediastinal radiotherapy with or without anthracycline therapy. Am J Cardiol 2011;107:472–7.
90. Billingham ME, Bristow MR, Glatstein E, et al. Adriamycin cardiotoxicity: endomyocardial biopsy evidence of enhancement by irradiation. Am J Surg Pathol 1977;1:17–23.
91. Aleman BM, van den Belt-Dusebout AW, De Bruin ML, et al. Late cardiotoxicity after treatment for Hodgkin lymphoma. Blood 2007;109:1878–86.
92. Shapiro CL, Hardenbergh PH, Gelman R, et al. Cardiac effects of adjuvant doxorubicin and radiation therapy in breast cancer patients. J Clin Oncol 1998;16:3493–501.
93. Kushwaha SS, Fallon JT, Fuster V. Restrictive cardiomyopathy. N Engl J Med 1997;336:267–76.
94. Heidenreich PA, Hancock SL, Vagelos RH, et al. Diastolic dysfunction after mediastinal irradiation. Am Heart J 2005;150:977–82.
95. Hunt SA, Abraham WT, Chin MH, et al, American College of Cardiology Foundation, American Heart Association. 2009 focused update incorporated into the ACC/AHA 2005 Guidelines for the Diagnosis and Management of Heart Failure in Adults: a report of the American College of Cardiology Foundation/American Heart Association Task Force on Practice Guidelines: developed in collaboration with the International Society for Heart and Lung Transplantation. J Am Coll Cardiol 2009;53:e1–90.
96. Uriel N, Vainrib A, Jorde UP, et al. Mediastinal radiation and adverse outcomes after heart transplantation. J Heart Lung Transplant 2010; 29:378–81.
97. Handa N, McGregor CG, Daly RC, et al. Heart transplantation for radiation-associated end-stage heart failure. Transpl Int 2000;13:162–5.
98. Heidenreich PA, Hancock SL, Lee BK, et al. Asymptomatic cardiac disease following mediastinal irradiation. J Am Coll Cardiol 2003;42:743–9.
99. Cella L, Liuzzi R, Conson M, et al. Dosimetric predictors of asymptomatic heart valvular dysfunction following mediastinal irradiation for Hodgkin's lymphoma. Radiother Oncol 2011; 101:316–21.
100. Bose AS, Shetty V, Sadiq A, et al. Radiation induced cardiac valve disease in a man from Chernobyl. J Am Soc Echocardiogr 2009;22:973.e1-3.
101. Bruhl SR, Sheikh M, Adlakha S, et al. Endovascular therapy for radiation-induced pulmonary artery stenosis: a case report and review of the literature. Heart Lung 2012;41:87–9.
102. Janelle GM, Mnookin SC, Thomas JJ, et al. Surgical approach for a patient with aortic stenosis and a frozen mediastinum. J Cardiothorac Vasc Anesth 2003;17:770–2.
103. Adabag AS, Dykoski R, Ward H, et al. Critical stenosis of aortic and mitral valves after mediastinal irradiation. Catheter Cardiovasc Interv 2004;63: 247–50.
104. Carlson RG, Mayfield WR, Normann S, et al. Radiation-induced valvular disease. Chest 1991;99: 538–45.
105. Handa N, McGregor CG, Danielson GK, et al. Valvular heart operation in patients with previous mediastinal radiation therapy. Ann Thorac Surg 2001;71:1880–4.

106. Crestanello JA, McGregor CG, Danielson GK, et al. Mitral and tricuspid valve repair in patients with previous mediastinal radiation therapy. Ann Thorac Surg 2004;78:826–31.
107. Veeragandham RS, Goldin MD. Surgical management of radiation-induced heart disease. Ann Thorac Surg 1998;65:1014–9.
108. Latib A, Montorfano M, Figini F, et al. Percutaneous valve replacement in a young adult for radiation-induced aortic stenosis. J Cardiovasc Med 2012;13:397–8.
109. Letsas KP, Korantzopoulos P, Evangelou D, et al. Acute myocardial infarction with normal coronary arteries in a patient with Hodgkin's disease: a late complication of irradiation and chemotherapy. Tex Heart Inst J 2006;33:512–4.
110. Annest LS, Anderson RP, Li W, et al. Coronary artery disease following mediastinal radiation therapy. J Thorac Cardiovasc Surg 1983;85:257–63.
111. Nilsson G, Holmberg L, Garmo H, et al. Distribution of coronary artery stenosis after radiation for breast cancer. J Clin Oncol 2012;30:380–6.
112. Heidenreich PA, Schnittger I, Strauss HW, et al. Screening for coronary artery disease after mediastinal irradiation for Hodgkin's disease. J Clin Oncol 2007;25:43–9.
113. Santoro F, Ferraretti A, Centola A, et al. Early clinical presentation of diffuse, severe, multi-district atherosclerosis after radiation therapy for Hodgkin lymphoma. Int J Cardiol 2012. http://dx.doi.org/10.1016/j.ijcard.2012.08.027.
114. Orzan F, Brusca A, Conte MR, et al. Severe coronary artery disease after radiation therapy of the chest and mediastinum: clinical presentation and treatment. Br Heart J 1993;69:496–500.
115. Schomig K, Ndrepepa G, Mehilli J, et al. Thoracic radiotherapy in patients with lymphoma and restenosis after coronary stent placement. Catheter Cardiovasc Interv 2007;70:359–65.
116. Waksman R, Ajani AE, White RL, et al. Five-year follow-up after intracoronary gamma radiation therapy for in-stent restenosis. Circulation 2004;109:340–4.
117. Wiedermann JG, Marboe C, Amols H, et al. Intracoronary irradiation markedly reduces restenosis after balloon angioplasty in a porcine model. J Am Coll Cardiol 1994;23:1491–8.
118. Ellis GR, Penny WJ. Hibernating myocardium caused by isolated, radiation induced left main stem coronary artery stenosis. Heart 1997;78:419–20.
119. Seddon B, Cook A, Gothard L, et al. Detection of defects in myocardial perfusion imaging in patients with early breast cancer treated with radiotherapy. Radiother Oncol 2002;64:53–63.
120. Marks LB, Yu X, Prosnitz RG, et al. The incidence and functional consequences of RT-associated cardiac perfusion defects. Int J Radiat Oncol Biol Phys 2005;63:214–23.
121. Andersen R, Wethal T, Günther A, et al. Relation of coronary artery calcium score to premature coronary artery disease in survivors >15 years of Hodgkin's lymphoma. Am J Cardiol 2010;105:149–52.
122. Kupeli S, Hazirolan T, Varan A, et al. Evaluation of coronary artery disease by computed tomography angiography in patients treated for childhood Hodgkin's lymphoma. J Clin Oncol 2010;28:1025–30.
123. Rademaker J, Schoder H, Ariaratnam NS, et al. Coronary artery disease after radiation therapy for Hodgkin's lymphoma: coronary CT angiography findings and calcium scores in nine asymptomatic patients. Am J Roentgenol 2008;191:32–7.
124. Wright RS, Anderson JL, Adams CD, et al, American College of Cardiology Foundation/American Heart Association Task Force on Practice Guidelines. 2011 ACCF/AHA focused update incorporated into the ACC/AHA 2007 Guidelines for the Management of Patients with Unstable Angina/Non-ST-Elevation Myocardial Infarction: a report of the American College of Cardiology Foundation/American Heart Association Task Force on Practice Guidelines developed in collaboration with the American Academy of Family Physicians, Society for Cardiovascular Angiography and Interventions, and the Society of Thoracic Surgeons. J Am Coll Cardiol 2011;57:e215–367.
125. Gibbons RJ, Abrams J, Chatterjee K, et al, American College of Cardiology, American Heart Association Task Force on practice guidelines (Committee on the Management of Patients With Chronic Stable Angina). ACC/AHA 2002 guideline update for the management of patients with chronic stable angina–summary article: a report of the American College of Cardiology/American Heart Association Task Force on practice guidelines (Committee on the Management of Patients With Chronic Stable Angina). J Am Coll Cardiol 2003;41:159–68.
126. Salemi VM, Dabarian AL, Nastari L, et al. Treatment of left main coronary artery lesion after late thoracic radiotherapy. Arq Bras Cardiol 2011;97:e53–55.
127. Aqel RA, Lloyd SG, Gupta H, et al. Three-vessel coronary artery disease, aortic stenosis, and constrictive pericarditis 27 years after chest radiation therapy: a case report. Heart Surg Forum 2006;9:E728–30.
128. Khan MH, Ettinger SM. Post mediastinal radiation coronary artery disease and its effects on arterial conduits. Catheter Cardiovasc Interv 2001;52:242–8.
129. Gansera B, Schmidtler F, Angelis I, et al. Quality of internal thoracic artery grafts after mediastinal irradiation. Ann Thorac Surg 2007;84:1479–84.

130. Handler CE, Livesey S, Lawton PA. Coronary ostial stenosis after radiotherapy: angioplasty or coronary artery surgery? Br Heart J 1989;61:208–11.
131. Patel MR, Dehmer GJ, Hirshfeld JW, et al. ACCF/SCAI/STS/AATS/AHA/ASNC/HFSA/SCCT 2012 Appropriate use criteria for coronary revascularization focused update: a report of the American College of Cardiology Foundation Appropriate Use Criteria Task Force, Society for Cardiovascular Angiography and Interventions, Society of Thoracic Surgeons, American Association for Thoracic Surgery, American Heart Association, American Society of Nuclear Cardiology, and the Society of Cardiovascular Computed Tomography. J Am Coll Cardiol 2012;59:857–81.
132. Dorresteijn LD, Kappelle AC, Boogrd W, et al. Increased risk of ischemic stroke after radiotherapy on the neck in patients younger than 60 years. J Clin Oncol 2001;20:282–8.
133. Slama MS, Le Guludec D, Sebag C, et al. Complete atrioventricular block following mediastinal irradiation: a report of six cases. Pacing Clin Electrophysiol 1991;14:1112–8.
134. de Waard DE, Verhorst PM, Visser CA. Exercise-induced syncope as late consequence of radiotherapy. Int J Cardiol 1996;57:289–91.
135. Orzan F, Brusca A, Gaita F, et al. Associated cardiac lesions in patients with radiation-induced complete heart block. Int J Cardiol 1993;39:151–6.
136. Cohen SI, Bharati S, Glass J, et al. Radiotherapy as a cause of complete atrioventricular block in Hodgkin's disease. An electrophysiological-pathological correlation. Arch Intern Med 1981;141:676–9.
137. Santoro F, Ieva R, Lupo P, et al. Late calcification of the mitral-aortic junction causing transient complete atrio-ventricular block after mediastinal radiation of Hodgkin lymphoma: multimodal visualization. Int J Cardiol 2012;155:e49–50.
138. Larsen RL, Jakacki RI, Vetter VL, et al. Electrocardiographic changes and arrhythmias after cancer therapy in children and young adults. Am J Cardiol 1992;70:73–7.
139. Groarke JD, Tanguturi VK, Hainer J, et al. Abnormal exercise response in long-term survivors of Hodgkin lymphoma treated with thoracic irradiation. J Am Coll Cardiol 2015;65:573–83.
140. Cole CR, Blackstone EH, Pashkow FJ, et al. Heart-rate recovery immediately after exercise as a predictor of mortality. N Engl J Med 1999;341:1351–7.
141. Moulder JE, Fish BL, Cohen EP. Radiation nephropathy is treatable with an angiotensin converting enzyme inhibitor or an angiotensin II type-1 (AT1) receptor antagonist. Radiother Oncol 1998;46:307–15.
142. Kohl RR, Kolozsvary A, Brown SL, et al. Differential radiation effect in tumor and normal tissue after treatment with ramipril, an angiotensin-converting enzyme inhibitor. Radiat Res 2007;168:440–5.
143. van der Veen SJ, Ghobadi G, de Boer RA, et al. ACE inhibition attenuates radiation-induced cardiopulmonary damage. Radiother Oncol 2015;114:96–103.
144. Kharofa J, Cohen EP, Tomic R, et al. Decreased risk of radiation pneumonitis with incidental concurrent use of angiotensin-converting enzyme inhibitors and thoracic radiation therapy. Int J Radiat Oncol Biol Phys 2012;84:238–43.
145. Lenarczyk M, Su J, Haworth ST, et al. Simvastatin mitigates increases in risk factors for and the occurrence of cardiac disease following 10 Gy total body irradiation. Pharmacol Res Perspect 2015;3:e00145.
146. Nellessen U, Zingel M, Hecker H, et al. Effects of radiation therapy on myocardial cell integrity and pump function: which role for cardiac biomarkers? Chemotherapy 2010;56:147–52.
147. Lancellotti P, Nkomo VT, Badano LP, et al. Expert consensus for multi-modality imaging evaluation of cardiovascular complications of radiotherapy in adults: a report from the European Association of Cardiovascular Imaging and the American Society of Echocardiography. J Am Soc Echocardiogr 2013;26:1013–32.
148. van Leeuwen-Segarceanu EM, Bos WJ, Dorresteijn LD, et al. Screening Hodgkin lymphoma survivors for radiotherapy induced cardiovascular disease. Cancer Treat Rev 2011;37:391–403.
149. Iliescu CA, Grines CL, Herrmann J, et al. SCAI Expert consensus statement: evaluation, management, and special considerations of cardio-oncology patients in the cardiac catheterization laboratory (endorsed by the Cardiological Society of India, and Sociedad Latino Americana de Cardiologıa Intervencionista). Catheter Cardiovasc Interv 2016. http://dx.doi.org/10.1002/ccd.26379.
150. Wethal T, Lund MB, Edvardsen T, et al. Valvular dysfunction and left ventricular changes in Hodgkin's lymphoma survivors. A longitudinal study. Br J Cancer 2009;101:575–81.

CHAPTER 15

Miscellaneous Syndromes (Takotsubo's, Orthostasis, and Differentiation Syndrome)

Ezequiel Munoz, MD[a], Gloria Iliescu, MD[a],
Konstantinos Marmadgkiolis, MD, MBA, FSCAI[b,c],
Cezar Iliescu, MD, FSCAI[a,*]

INTRODUCTION

Takotsubo cardiomyopathy was named after the shape of an ancient Japanese octopus trap, but is also known as stress or stress-induced cardiomyopathy (SC), (transient) apical ballooning syndrome or cardiomyopathy.[1] The abnormality results from a dysfunctional left ventricle during systole, causing wall motion abnormalities. The characteristic octopus trap and apical ballooning appearance is evident on a left ventriculogram as a consequence of extensive apical dyskinesia and preserved or even increased basal contractility.[2] Interestingly, this "typical" form is seen in only two-thirds of Takotsubo patients. Variant forms constitute the remaining one-third and include isolated basal, midventricular (mid cavitary akinesis and basal as well as apical hyperkinesis),[3] or apical segment involvement.[1] In the general population, SC is mainly seen in postmenopausal women, but there also appears to be a higher prevalence of SC in patients with cancer.[4]

CLINICAL SUBTYPES

SC can be classified as either primary or secondary[5]:

- *Primary SC* is caused by a stressor, many times nonidentifiable; the cardiac symptoms are the primary reason for seeking care, and the clinical management depends on the specific complications.[5]
- *Secondary SC* is caused by sudden activation of the adrenergic system, while the patient is already hospitalized, for example, for cancer therapy (medical, radiation, or surgical). The treatment should focus not only on SC and its cardiac complications but also on the conditions that triggered the syndrome.[5]

PATHOPHYSIOLOGY

The exact pathophysiologic mechanisms are not known, but existing evidence shows that the main physiologic pathway is physical or psychological stress precipitating adrenaline release by the adrenal glands. This evidence is supported by the observation that levels of catecholamines 1 or 2 days after the clinical presentation are significantly higher than in patients with acute coronary syndrome (ACS).[6] In addition, catecholamine storm associated predominantly with epinephrine-secreting pheochromocytomas and less with norepinephrine and dopamine secreting pheochromocytomas can also precipitate SC.[7]

To understand the development of this pathophysiologic event, one needs to consider the gradient of β-adrenergic receptor (βAR) density that exists on the level of the left ventricle, with the apex having the highest βAR and lowest sympathetic nerve density.[8] This intends to ensure optimal ventricular ejection fraction during fight-or-flight responses

[a] The University of Texas MD Anderson Cancer Center, 1515 Holcombe Boulevard, Houston, TX 77030, USA; [b] University of Missouri, Columbia, MO 65211, USA; [c] Pepin Heart Institute, Florida Hospital, 3100 E Fletcher Avenue, Tampa, FL 33613, USA
* Corresponding author.
E-mail address: CIliescu@mdanderson.org

(Fig. 15.1). In normal physiologic situations, norepinephrine released by the sympathetic nervous system acts on β_1-adrenergic receptors (AR) to increase contractility through the cyclic adenosine monophosphate (cAMP)–protein kinase A (PKA) signaling pathway.

Epinephrine also binds to β_1AR, but has higher affinity for β_2AR. These subtypes of βAR have pleiotropic effects, being able to couple through G_s (like β_1AR), but also through G_i and non–G-protein pathways.[9] At physiologic range, epinephrine coupling to β_2AR subsequently increases cAMP–PKA levels to further increase myocardial contractility.

At supraphysiologic levels, epinephrine has a negative inotropic effect via ligand-mediated trafficking of the β_2AR from G_s protein to G_i protein subcellular signaling pathways, a process known as biased agonism. This event is dependent on β_2AR phosphorylation by PKA and G protein receptor coupled kinases (Fig. 15.2). The understanding of this process is essential considering the evidence of L41Q GRK5 polymorphism found in patients with SC. This polymorphism enhances desensitization and impairs βAR response.[10]

The G_i negative inotropic effect results from inhibition of G_s-cAMP production and through other pathways, such as p38 mitogen-activated protein kinase (MAPK) alteration of myofilament sensitivity.[11,12] This negative inotropic effect affects predominantly the apex, developing the characteristic wall motion abnormality seen in patients with SC.[13] Although this is detrimental from a mechanical perspective, it represents a cardioprotective mechanism against βAR: catecholamine toxicity.[14]

This pathophysiologic model helps us understand the reversibility of SC. As levels of epinephrine decrease, β_2AR dephosphorylation or internalization, and replacement with de novo unphosphorylated β_2ARs, reduces the β_2AR-G_i stimulus trafficking and restores normal contractile function in the surviving cardiomyocytes.[15]

CLINICAL PRESENTATION

SC mimics the clinical presentation of acute myocardial infarction. In patients undergoing cardiac catheterization for acute coronary syndrome, there is an approximately 1% incidence of this disorder[16] in the general population. In cancer

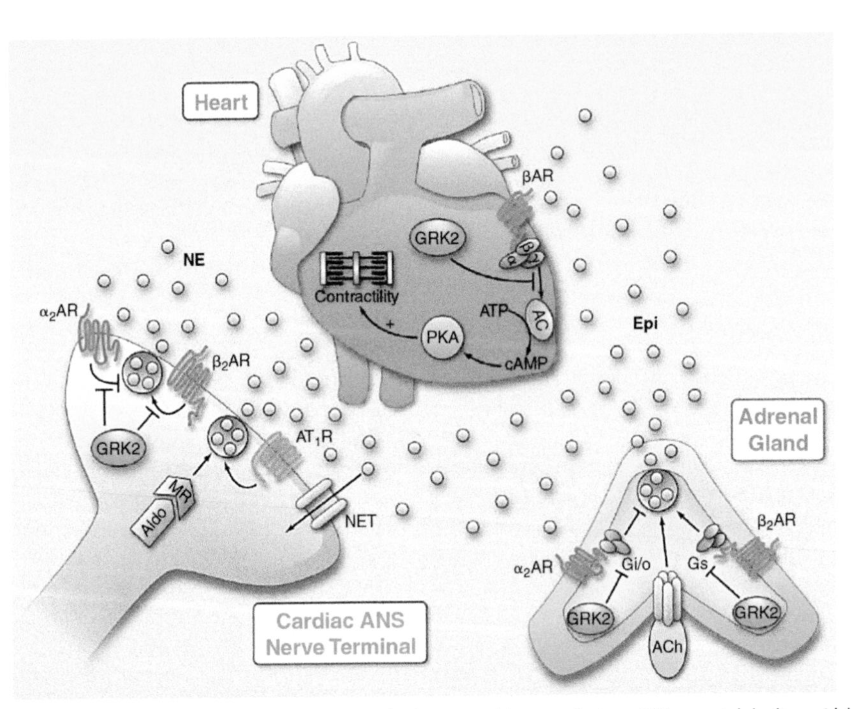

Fig. 15.1 Adrenergic nervous system (ANS) input to the heart and its regulation. ACh, acetylcholine; Aldo, aldosterone; Epi, epinephrine; Gi/o, inhibitory or other G protein; Gs, stimulatory G protein; MR, mineralocorticoid receptor; NE, norepinephrine; NET, norepinephrine transporter. (*From* Lymperopoulos A, Rengo G, Koch WJ. Adrenergic nervous system in heart failure: pathophysiology and therapy. Circ Res 2013;113(6):741; with permission.)

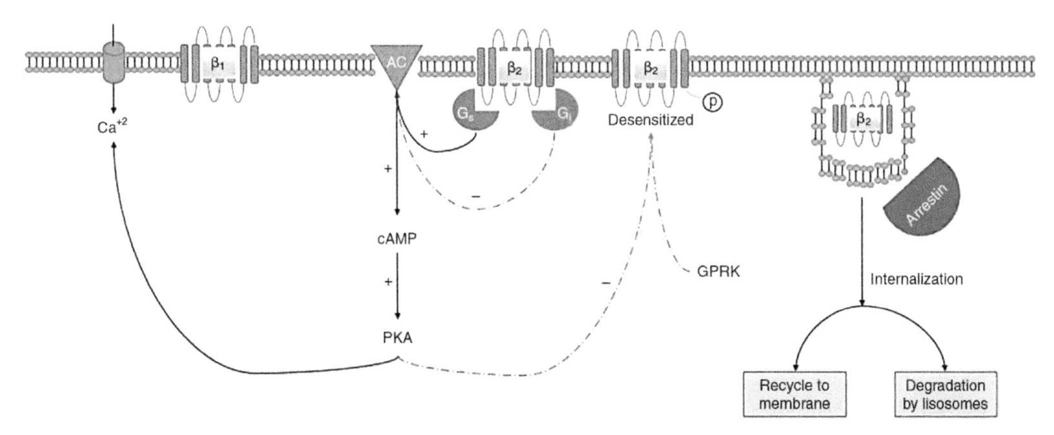

Fig. 15.2 Molecular mechanisms of B2 AR signaling pathway. GPRK, G protein receptor coupled kinase.

patients, the incidence seems to be 10 to 20 times compared to general population.[17]

The predominant clinical presentation in patients with cancer is chest pain, followed by shortness of breath/dyspnea on exertion. Nonspecific symptoms including failure to thrive or hypotension account for 33% of the cases. Hypertension and dyslipidemia are considered the most common cardiovascular risk factors. Intensive care unit patients are likely to present with pulmonary edema, ischemic changes on the electrocardiogram (ECG), or elevated cardiac biomarkers. In general, hemodynamic compromise is unusual, but mild to moderate congestive heart failure is frequent. Hypotension may occur because of the reduction in stroke volume and, occasionally, because of dynamic left ventricular (LV) outflow tract obstruction. Cardiogenic shock has been reported as a rare complication.

TRIGGERS AND RISK FACTORS IN A PATIENT WITH CANCER POPULATION

Patients with cancer seem to be unique in that the usual triggering event for SC in the form of extreme physical, emotional, or psychological stress is seen only in a minority of patients with cancer with SC. Other triggers are therefore to be considered.

Procedural/Surgery Related

SC is a rare postoperative cardiac complication in the general population. However, surgical procedures, such as tumor resection, endoscopic procedure, or pericardiocentesis, are the most common triggers for SC in patients with cancer.[17] Surgeons should consider this condition in their patients who manifest with cardiac symptoms suggestive of myocardial infarction, particularly postmenopausal women.[18]

Chemotherapy-Induced Stress-Induced Cardiomyopathy

Chemotherapy also has been linked with SC (Box 15.1). It is predominantly seen in patients who are being treated with 5-fluorouracil (5-FU), a widely used chemotherapeutic for solid tumors, but there are also case reports on SC with cytarabine, daunorubicin, bevacizumab, sunitinib, and ibrutinib.

Chemotherapy induces increased sympathetic tone with resulting elevation of cytokine, free radical, prostaglandin, catecholamine, and growth factor levels. The excess of these modulators can potentiate worsening adrenoceptor sensitivity and can contribute to the clinical

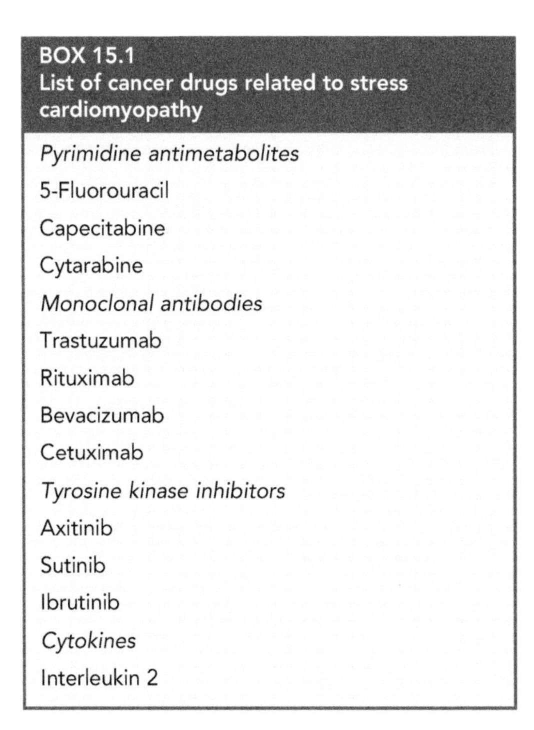
BOX 15.1
List of cancer drugs related to stress cardiomyopathy

Pyrimidine antimetabolites
5-Fluorouracil
Capecitabine
Cytarabine
Monoclonal antibodies
Trastuzumab
Rituximab
Bevacizumab
Cetuximab
Tyrosine kinase inhibitors
Axitinib
Sutinib
Ibrutinib
Cytokines
Interleukin 2

presentation.[19] It is presumed that the method of chemotherapy delivery affects the incidence of cardiotoxicity. Continuous infusion is more likely to cause SC compared with a bolus or an oral route.[20]

Emotional and physical stress

SC is described in association with sudden and severe emotional stressors (unexpected loss, frightening situation, among others).[21,22] Moreover, Singh and Harle[23] presented a case of cancer-related pain crisis as a contributory precipitating cause for the development of SC. It is important to consider, however, that although frequently seen as a trigger of SC, emotional or physical stress is not universally documented preceding the acute event.[24]

Neurologic triggers

Cerebrovascular accidents, which are known to produce LV dysfunction because of excess catecholamine production, are associated with 10-fold higher odds of SC.[25]

Cathecholamine-excreting tumors

Many SC cases in patients with cancer are associated with catecholamine-excreting neoplasms (eg, a pheochromocytoma).[24] It has not been proven that cancer leads to SC (although an association cannot be excluded); thus, patients presenting with cardiac stunning may be considered for prompt screening for cancer. It is possible that patients with cancer present with higher circulating catecholamine levels, making them more susceptible for the development of this cardiomyopathy with additional stress. The presence of paraneoplastic syndrome can alter the cardiac adrenoceptors and favor the development of SC.[26]

DIAGNOSTIC CRITERIA

To standardize all the information related to SC diagnosis, the European Society of Cardiology proposed the following diagnostic criteria[5]:

1. Transient regional wall motion abnormalities of the left ventricle or right ventricular myocardium, which are frequently but not always preceded by a stressful trigger (emotional or physical).
2. The regional wall motion abnormalities usually extend beyond a single vascular distribution and often result in circumferential dysfunction of the ventricular segment involved.
3. The absence of culprit atherosclerotic coronary artery disease, including acute plaque rupture, thrombus formation, and coronary dissection or other pathologic conditions that could explain the pattern of temporary LV dysfunction observed (eg, hypertrophic cardiomyopathy, viral myocarditis).
4. New and reversible ECG abnormalities (ST-segment elevation, ST depression, left bundle branch clock, T-wave inversion, and/or QTc prolongation) during acute phase (3 months).
5. Significantly elevated serum natriuretic peptide (brain natriuretic peptide [BNP] or NT-proBNP) during the acute phase.
6. Positive but relatively small elevation in cardiac troponin measured with a conventional assay (ie, disparity between the troponin level and the amount of dysfunctional myocardium present).
7. Recovery of ventricular dysfunction on cardiac imaging at follow-up (3–6 months).

ELECTROCARDIOGRAM AND CARDIAC BIOMARKERS

The most common ECG abnormalities in patients with cancer with SC at the time of admission are the extensive T-wave inversions followed by ST-segment elevation.[17] These changes are slightly different from those typically seen in SC in the general population, which include ST-segment elevation, mimicking ST-elevation myocardial infarction (STEMI), as well as nonspecific T-wave abnormalities or new bundle-branch block. The 12-lead ECG itself is insufficient for differentiating SC from STEMI.[27] Characteristic and common evolutionary changes that may occur over 2 to 3 days include resolution of the ST-segment elevation, development of diffuse and often deep T-wave inversion that involves most leads, and prolongation of the corrected QT interval.[28]

Cardiac biomarkers are moderately elevated. Cardiac troponin T peaks within 24 hours, but levels are less that those observed with an STEMI.[29] Circulating BNP is elevated and correlates with LV end-diastolic pressure.[30] Nguyen and colleagues[30] revealed that BNP and NT-proBNP were substantially elevated and significantly increased during the first 24 hours after onset of SC, with slow and incomplete resolution over the course of 3 months thereafter. They showed that peak NT-proBNP levels correlate with the severity of regional wall motion abnormality or systolic dysfunction assessed by echocardiography and could predict complications during hospitalization.

MULTIMODALITY IMAGING

Echocardiography

Echocardiography is essential in the diagnosis of SC because it is the ideal imaging modality for early evaluation of LV segmental systolic function in the acute setting as well as for monitoring of myocardial function recovery during the relatively quick follow-up.[31] Regional wall motion abnormalities are seen, namely, apical hypokinesis, akinesis, or dyskinesis and compensatory hypercontractility found on the basal segment. Other patterns include regional wall motion abnormality with apical sparring (apical-sparring variant) or right ventricular involvement.

Global longitudinal strain has proven so far to be the most sensitive and reproducible of the various strain measurements performed with speckle tracking when suspecting SC. Using speckle tracking echocardiography, the specific deformation values for the apex have been described to be of higher value than that of the midcavity and base segments in groups describing normal populations.[32,33] A characteristic pattern (not typical of any specific coronary distribution) is seen, affecting only the apical/tip segments and being known as the "evil-eye" pattern.[34] Sosa and Banchs[34] stated that this pattern is helpful in increasing recognition for this process, at the very least being able to expand the differential diagnosis. Echocardiography is also useful in detecting acute complications such as cardiogenic shock, left ventricular outflow tract obstruction (LVOTO), apical thrombus, or cardiac rupture.[1]

Coronary Angiography and Invasive Left Ventriculography

Although a variety of clinical examination tools are available, cardiac catheterization is still the gold standard for definitive differentiation between SC and ACS due to complicated coronary artery disease.[35] The most frequent finding on coronary angiography (CA) in patients with SC is "normal coronary arteries."[36] Invasive evaluation of SC patients should include left ventriculography (if not contraindicated) to confirm the regional wall motion abnormality pattern.[35]

Cardiac Computed Tomography

In patients with acute chest pain, cardiac computed tomography can rule out high-grade coronary stenosis[37] and also exclude pulmonary embolism and acute aortic disease.[38] However, this must be weighed against delays to immediate invasive CA as the more definitive test.[35]

Cardiac Magnetic Resonance

Cardiac magnetic resonance (CMR) provides accurate assessment of global ventricular function, defines regional wall motion abnormalities, shows the presence or absence of myocardial edema, and detects common complications associated with SC.[39] Cine CMR sequences demonstrate a circumferential LV regional wall motion abnormality (hypokinesia or, more typically, akinesia) involving the mid- and apical myocardial segments with normal or hyperdynamic contraction of the base as well as a circumferential transmural increase in T2 signal intensity.[39]

Late gadolinium enhancement (LGE) sequences are important in differentiating SC from acute myocardial infarction and acute myocarditis.[40] In SC, LGE is frequently less bright ("low-intensity LGE") than the LGE usually associated with myocardial infarction[41]; the distribution of LGE typically matches the sites of wall motion abnormality, in contrast with myocarditis, where wall motion abnormalities are typically global.[41]

MANAGEMENT

The key elements in the treatment of SC are restoration of normal cardiac function, provision of supportive care, and minimization of complications.

The European Society of Cardiology proposes that the first step in management should be assessment of the in-hospital mortality risk, even though not validated in clinical trials and not to replace clinical judgment.

Individuals at higher risk are those who have at least one of the following major risk factors: greater than 75 years old, levels of systolic blood pressure (SBP) less than 110, signs of pulmonary edema, unexplained syncope, ventricular arrhythmias, mitral regurgitation, apical thrombus, ejection fraction less than 35%, and LVOTO; or 2 of the following minor risk factors: age 70 to 75, QTc greater than 500 ms, pathologic Q waves, persistent ST elevation, left ventricular ejection fraction (LVEF) 35% to 45%, BNP greater than 600 pg/mL, NT-proBNP $\geq$ 2000 pg/mL, biventricular involvement, and coronary artery disease.[5]

Patients considered at higher risk of in-hospital mortality should be monitored in a critical care unit (CCU or medical intensive care unit) or at least with continuous ECG monitoring and access to resuscitation equipment for at least 72 hours after the presentation. In cases of low cardiac output (CO), serial limited echocardiographic studies should be performed to monitor evolution if the patient does not improve clinically. When excessive atrial or ventricular tachyarrhythmias are present, β-blockers should be considered. The use of inotropes (eg, dobutamine, norepinephrine, epinephrine, dopamine, milrinone, and isoproterenol) is generally contraindicated in SC[42] because further activation of catecholamine receptors or their downstream molecular pathways might worsen the clinical status and prognosis of patients with SC cardiomyopathy and cardiogenic shock.[9]

Patients at lower risk may be transferred to wards with lower levels of monitoring and potentially discharged early. They should be followed 3 to 6 months after the discharge with a review of medications and cardiac imaging to confirm that cardiac function has fully recovered.

The use of specific β_2AR antagonists or p38 MAPK inhibitors has been associated with an increase in mortality and represents a counterproductive strategy, exacerbating the epinephrine-induced negative inotropic effect. Levosimendan increases myofilament calcium sensitivity, and study results were favorable, preventing further decline in cardiac function in patients with SC.[43]

COMPLICATIONS

SC is generally a relatively benign disease with rapid recovery of LV function. However, it can be associated with acute high-risk complications.[44]

Acute Heart Failure

Acutely decompensated heart failure is the most common complication, occurring in approximately 20% of patients.[45] Standard therapies such as diuretics or nitroglycerin are effective in most cases. Inotropes such as dobutamine and pressors with β-agonist activity typically worsen the scenario, thus vasopressin and mechanical circulatory support might be preferred options. When patients have severe congestive heart failure or significant hypotension, it is important to assess whether LVOTO or mitral regurgitation is associated with their condition.[45]

Cardiogenic Shock

Cardiogenic shock is primarily caused by LV dysfunction, but LVOTO due to basal hypercontractility might have a contributing role. LVOTO may be associated with systolic anterior movement of the mitral valve anterior leaflet and mitral regurgitation.[46] When LVOTO is identified, nitroglycerin or inotropic agents should be immediately discontinued to avoid further obstruction.[46] Cardiogenic shock because of acute pump failure represents a challenging scenario, and mechanical support in the form of an Impella device or extracorporeal membrane oxygenation device may become necessary. As alluded to above, inotropic agents and intra-aortic balloon pump may induce LVOTO through basal hypercontractility and reduced afterload, respectively.[47] In those cases, serial echocardiography is useful in detecting and monitoring such adverse effects.

Thrombus Formation

Thrombus is observed in 2% to 8% in the akinetic apex, occasionally resulting in stroke or arterial embolism. Most develop 2 to 5 days after symptoms onset, when LV function is still depressed. They are best visualized by CMR in early postcontrast acquisition sequences.[48] Prophylactic anticoagulation in higher-risk SC cases has an undetermined role, but may be considered.

Arrhythmias

Madias and colleagues[49] reported that life-threatening ventricular arrhythmias such as torsades de pointes (TdP) and ventricular fibrillation occurred in 8.6% of patients with SC. Patients with a QTc interval greater than 500 ms were at higher risk.

Presumed new onset of atrioventricular (AV) block has also been described,[50] but it remains unclear if it requires pacemaker implantation or when it should be considered. However, when AV block results in hemodynamic instability or marked QTc interval prolongation, temporary ventricular pacing should be considered at least.[51]

Ventricular Rupture

Ventricular rupture is a rare life-threatening complication (<1%) that occurs 2 to 8 days after symptom onset, often with persistent ST segment elevation.

Cardiac rupture is associated with higher LV intramural pressure and wall stress.[48]

Pericardial Effusion

Pericardial effusion has been observed in some patients during recovery phase that present with recurrent chest pain and reappearance of ST segment elevation.[52] CMR imaging early after admission has detected small pericardial effusion in 43% of patients. However, pericardial tamponade is rare.[53]

PROGNOSIS AND CLINICAL IMPLICATIONS

The main causes of death in SC are cardiogenic shock and ventricular fibrillation. The mortality in hospitalized patients is 2% to 5%. Experience at MD Anderson Cancer Center shows that 95% of the patients who required further oncologic treatment were able to continue it without recurrent SC. The mean time to restart therapy was 21 days.[17] The risk of recurrence may be estimated on an individual according to the triggering event and coexisting medical conditions (in the patient with cancer the most important factors for recurrence might be).

Five-year recurrence rates are in the order of 5% to 22%, with the second episode occurring 3 months to 10 years after the first.[54] For this reason, β-blockers and angiotensin-converting enzyme inhibitors (when not contraindicated) should be continued indefinitely for potential prevention of future recurrences as well as general cardioprotection during cancer therapy. In the authors' experience, patients have complete recovery of LV function, and resumption of cancer therapy did not cause adverse cardiovascular events when patients were on cardioprotective therapy.[17] In the general population, long-term prognosis is favorable, with a high index of recovery.

SUMMARY

Stress cardiomyopathy is an important disease that has to be differentiated from AMI promptly for appropriate management.[55] Diagnosis is critical because anticoagulant/antiplatelet therapy is different. Furthermore, because of the different pathophysiology and different prognosis, physicians involved in the cardiovascular care of patients with cancer should pursue the diagnosis with the additional tests required. The key is to include SC in the differential of the presenting patient. The new oncologic therapies with their targeted design might provide newer insight in SC as well. The potential for early identification of high-risk patient groups may lead to a decrease in both morbidity and mortality.[56] Resumption of cancer therapy should be encouraged after recovery from an SC event (Fig. 15.3–15.7).

ORTHOSTATIC HYPOTENSION

Definition and Epidemiology

Orthostatic hypotension (OH) is defined as a sustained reduction of SBP of at least 20 mm Hg and/or diastolic blood pressure of at least 10 mm Hg, or an SBP decrease greater than 30 mm Hg in hypertensive patients with supine SBP >160 mm Hg,

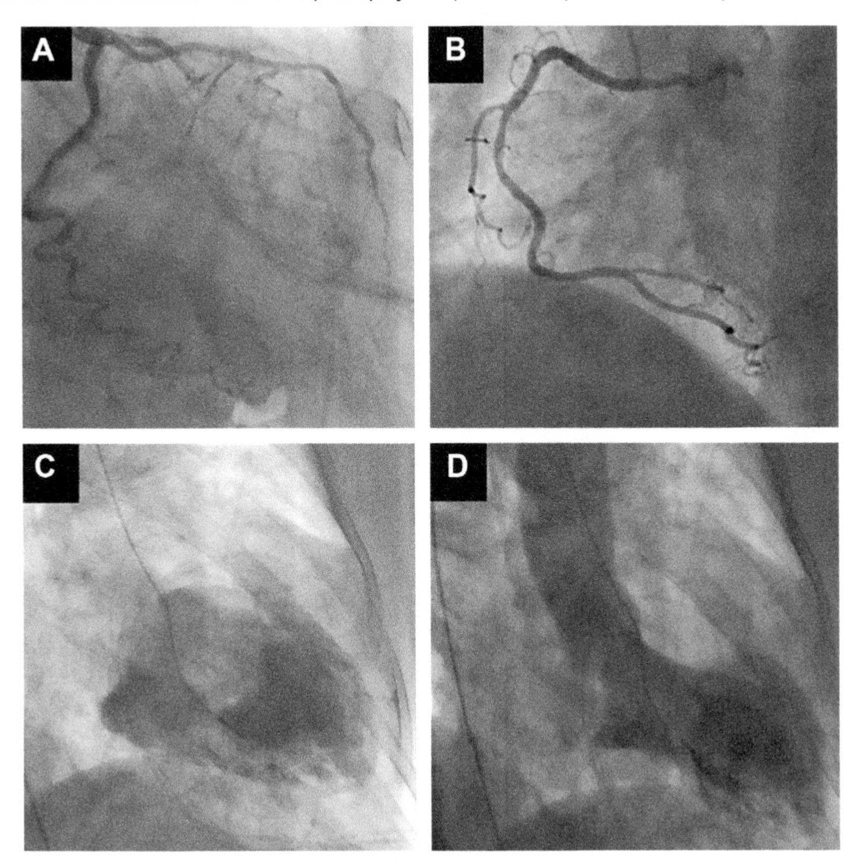

Fig. 15.3 A 75-year-old woman diagnosed with multiple myeloma presented with angina pectoris. (*A*) Coronary angiography of left coronary tree showed no obstructive disease. (*B*) Coronary angiography of right coronary artery with no angiographic evidence of obstructive disease. (*C*) Left diastolic ventriculogram. (*D*) Left systolic ventriculogram showing apical dyskinesis with sparing of the base.

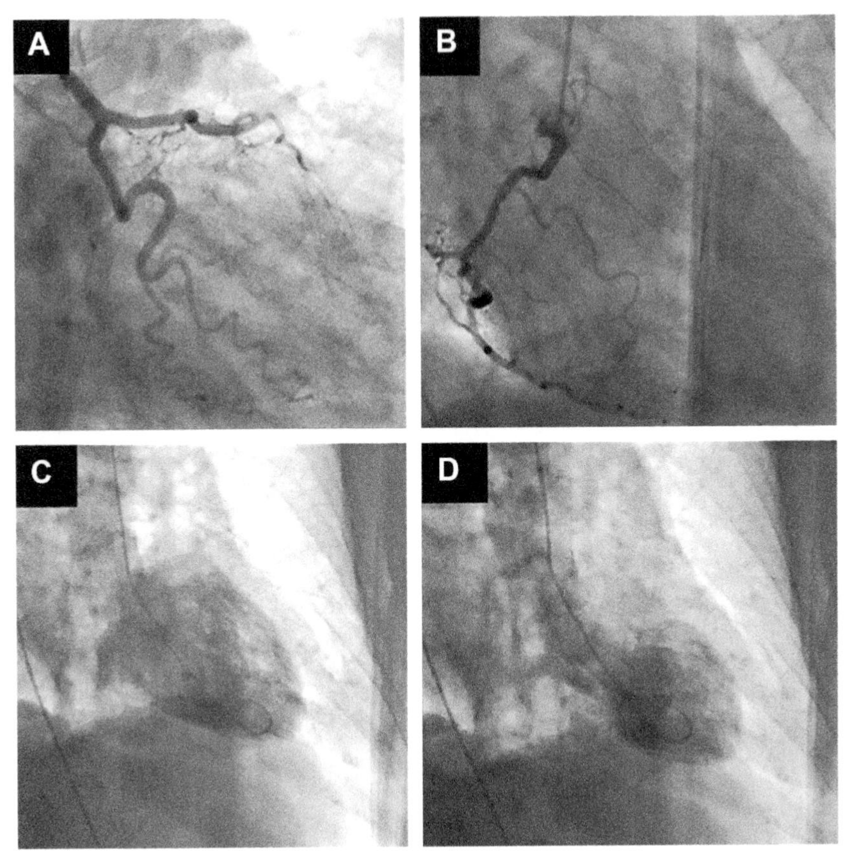

Fig. 15.4 A 77-year-old woman diagnosed with non–small-cell lung carcinoma presented to the Emergency Room with chest tightness radiating to her shoulder associated with dyspnea and nausea. (*A*) Coronary angiography of left coronary tree with no angiographic evidence of obstructive disease. (*B*) Coronary angiography of right coronary artery with no angiographic evidence of obstructive disease. (*C*) Left diastolic ventriculogram. (*D*). Left systolic ventriculogram showing apical dyskinesis with sparing of the base.

when assuming a standing position or during a head-up tilt test of at least 60°[57] (Fig. 15.8).

The prevalence of this condition increases with age, ranging from 5% in patients less than 50 years to 30% in those greater than 70 years.[58] Several contributing factors have been implied including medications (α-blockers, diuretics, tricyclic antidepressants), systemic diseases involving peripheral autonomic nerves (diabetes mellitus, amyloidosis), and in rare cases, primary neurodegenerative disorders (Parkinson disease, pure autonomic failure, multiple systems atrophy).[59] It is also relatively common among hospitalized elderly in the United States with an overall annual rate of 36 per 100,000 adults and is consistently higher in male patients.[59] Patients with OH have increased risk of death (relative risk [RR] 1.50; 95% confidence interval [CI] 1.24–1.81) and heart failure events (RR 2.25; 95% CI 1.52–3.33).[60]

Mechanisms Involved in Blood Pressure Regulation

The control of blood pressure is essentially the control of blood flow to a given tissue in proportion to its metabolic needs. It is a complex physiologic function that depends on a continuum of actions of the cardiovascular, neural, renal, and endocrine systems.[61]

The mechanisms by which blood flow is controlled can be divided into intrinsic and extrinsic factors (Fig. 15.9). The intrinsic factors are important for local blood flow regulation, whereas extrinsic mechanisms are involved in arterial blood pressure regulation and systemic vascular resistance.

Contribution of Autonomic Nervous System to Blood Pressure Regulation

Mean arterial pressure (mAP) is expressed by the relationship between CO and total peripheral

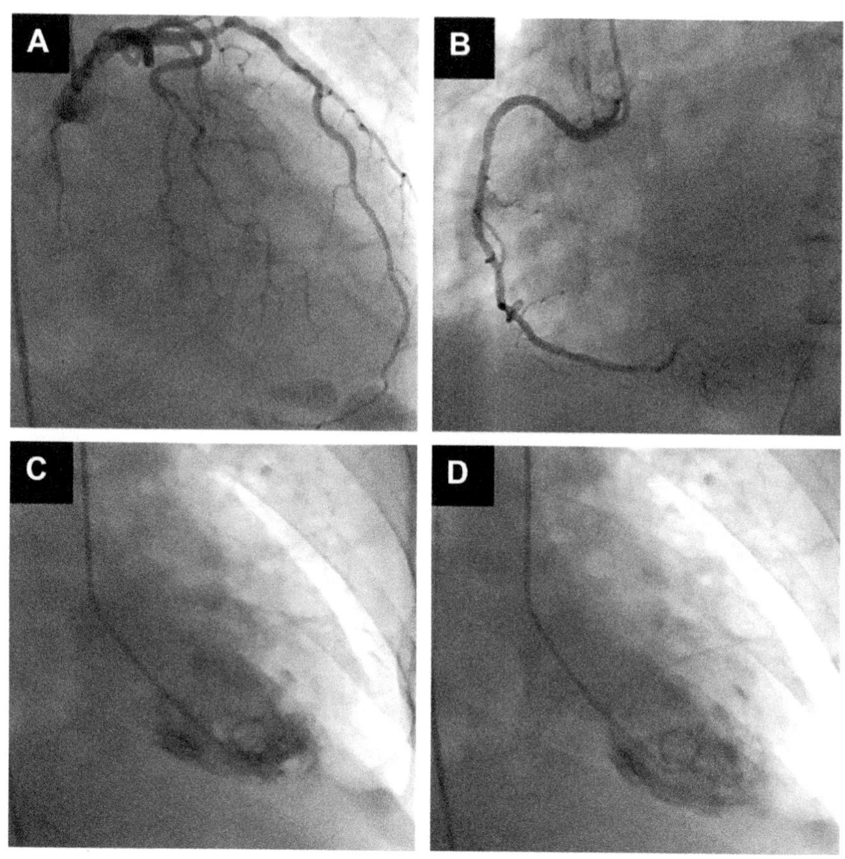

Fig. 15.5 A 78-year-old woman diagnosed with low-grade ovarian cancer admitted for a small bowel obstruction and a recent fall. Laboratory workup showed abnormal troponins. (*A*) Coronary angiography of left coronary tree with no angiographic evidence of obstructive disease. (*B*) Coronary angiography of the right coronary artery with no angiographic evidence of obstructive disease. (*C*) Left diastolic ventriculogram. (*D*) Left systolic ventriculogram showing apical dyskinesis with sparing of the base.

vascular resistance, and changes in any of these 2 modify in direct proportion the value of the mAP. Global neural control is essentially through the sympathetic nervous system, releasing norepinephrine and making its effect either on B1 receptors located in the heart (increasing heart rate and contractility) or on $\alpha1$ receptors located on the membrane of the vascular smooth muscle (producing vasoconstriction).

Changes in blood pressure due to neuronal effect can be divided by its duration in short-term response and long-term response.

Short-term regulation of blood pressure and baroreceptor reflex

High-pressure baroreceptors in the carotid sinus and aortic arch respond to acute elevations in systemic BP by causing a reflex vagal bradycardia that is mediated through the parasympathetic systems and inhibition of sympathetic output from the central nervous system.

Standing produces pooling of approximately 700 mL of blood in the lower extremities, in pulmonary and splanchnic circulations, as well as translocation of fluid from intravascular to interstitial spaces. This shift in blood compartmentalization attenuates venous return to the heart and ventricular filling, to transiently reduce stroke volume. As a result, there is unloading of the arterial baroreceptors to enhance sympathetic outflow and subsequently increase systemic vascular resistance, venous return, and CO[62] (**Fig. 15.10**). Sympathetic effects also take action in long-term BP regulation, as the most important stimulus to renin release in the juxtaglomerular apparatus is through renal sympathetic nerves.[63]

Renal-endocrine mechanism

Renin is synthesized in the juxtaglomerular cells (surrounding the renal afferent arteriole) and is released in response of B1-adrenergic stimulation, decrease of NaCl reabsorption by the

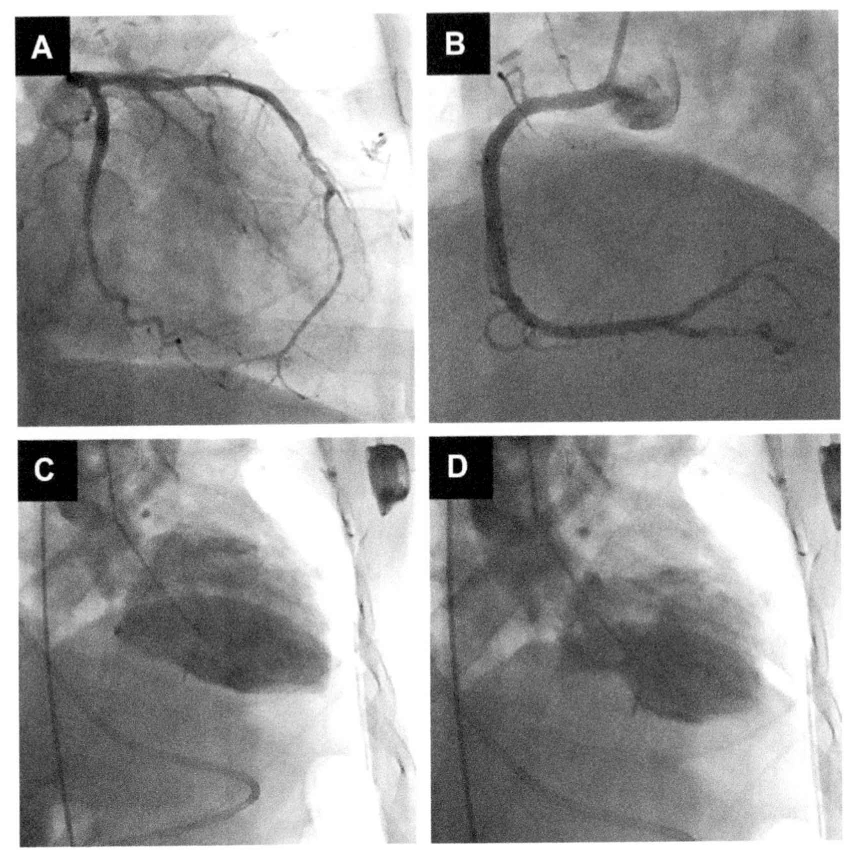

Fig. 15.6 A 65-year-old woman diagnosed with stage IV breast cancer admitted for respiratory distress and stridor. ECG: T-wave abnormality in lead I, aVL, V5, and V6. Abnormal troponins. (*A*) Coronary angiography of left coronary tree with no angiographic evidence of obstructive disease. (*B*) Coronary angiography of right coronary artery with no angiographic evidence of obstructive disease. (*C*) Left diastolic ventriculogram. (*D*) Left systolic ventriculogram showing apical and basal hyperkinesis and midcavitary akinesis.

macula densa, or decreases in blood pressure in the preglomerular vessels. It acts on circulating angiotensinogen to form angiotensin I that becomes angiotensin II by the effect of the angiotensin converting enzyme. Angiotensin II acts as a vasoconstrictor of the vessel as well as a stimulus for aldosterone release, the main effect of which is going to be the increase in sodium and water reabsorption on the distal nephron (see Fig. 15.3).

It is very important to take into consideration all of these aspects related to blood pressure physiology to understand and properly evaluate OH. Any abnormality that compromises the

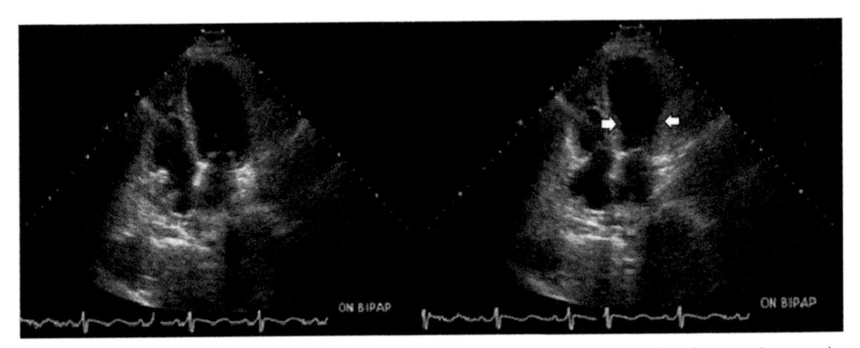

Fig. 15.7 A 77-year-old woman diagnosed with marginal cell lymphoma. During her hospital stay, she developed acute systolic heart failure, ST segment elevation in ECG, and abnormal troponins. Two-dimensional transthoracic echocardiogram shows regional wall motion abnormalities in left ventricle of anterior wall hypokinesis.

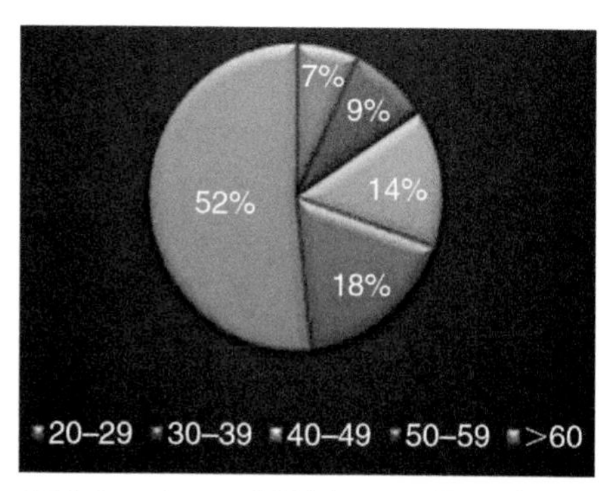

Fig. 15.8 Prevalence of OH by age. (*Data from* Wu J, Yang Y, Lu F, et al. Population-based study on the prevalence and correlates of orthostatic hypotension/hypertension and orthostatic dizziness. Hypertens Res 2008;31(5):897–904.)

systems mentioned above is going to promote the development of OH. Some of the causes in general population related to this abnormality are mentioned in Table 15.1.

Cancer survivors may be at risk for orthostatic intolerance because of the known autonomic effects of chemotherapy and radiation therapy,[38] together with the relative hypovolemia that would be expected to accompany nausea, dehydration, and prolonged bed rest during cancer treatment.[64]

Anatomic lesions of the baroreflex loop may lead to baroreflex failure, producing severe, labile hypertension, headache, diaphoresis, and emotional instability. These lesions have been described after neck surgery and/or radiation therapy for familiar paraganglioma and pharyngeal carcinoma.[65] Damage to carotid artery baroreceptors, glossopharyngeal or vagal nerves, or these pathways in the brainstem can result in blood pressure and heart rate volatility.[66] Radiation-induced cardiovascular autonomic impairment is a dynamic and progressive process long after irradiation, and chronic inflammation plays a major role.[67]

Mechanisms proposed for radiation-induced baroreceptor failure include the following.[68]

Carotid artery stenosis

Neck radiotherapy results in chronic inflammation of carotid arterial walls causing carotid artery stenosis secondary to intimal fibrosis and also leads to disruption of carotid sinus baroreceptors and atherosclerosis. Elerding and colleagues[69] published a study among 5-year survivors of head and neck squamous cell carcinoma, where approximately 17% developed clinically significant carotid artery stenosis. Increased intima media thickness in the carotid bulb has been shown to correlate with reduced baroreceptor sensitivity.[70] Atherosclerosis and fibrosis may result in a decreased distensibility of the carotid sinus and thereby may reduce stretch-induced afferent carotid sinus nerve activity.[71] In line with these observations, removal of an atherosclerotic plaque from the carotid artery in some patients enhances baroreflex function.[72]

Vascular ischemia

Irradiation injury to the vasa vasorum of the carotid artery and the consequent ischemic lesions of the arterial wall may induce necrotizing vasculitis and occlusive thrombosis,[73] causing baroreceptor failure.

Cranial neuropathy

Damage to the glossopharyngeal and vagus nerves is likely the predominant reason for baroreflex failure in these patients.[66] Development of cranial neuropathy has a mean latent period of 7.6 years and is both dose and fractionation dependent.[74]

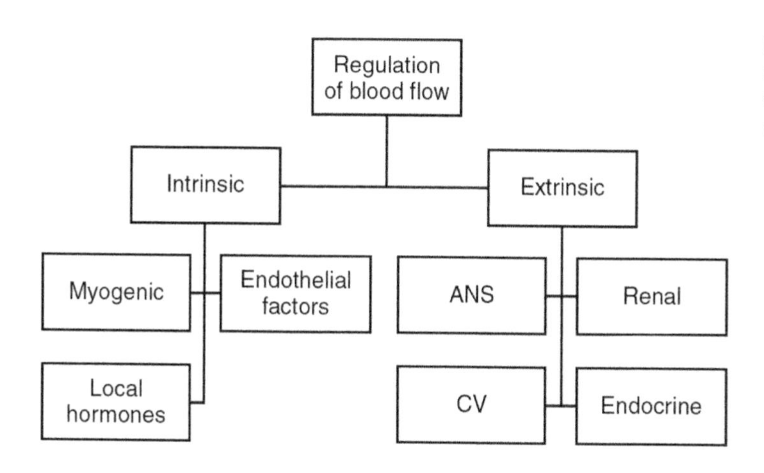

Fig. 15.9 Intrinsic and extrinsic mechanisms involved in the regulation of blood flow. CV, cardiovascular.

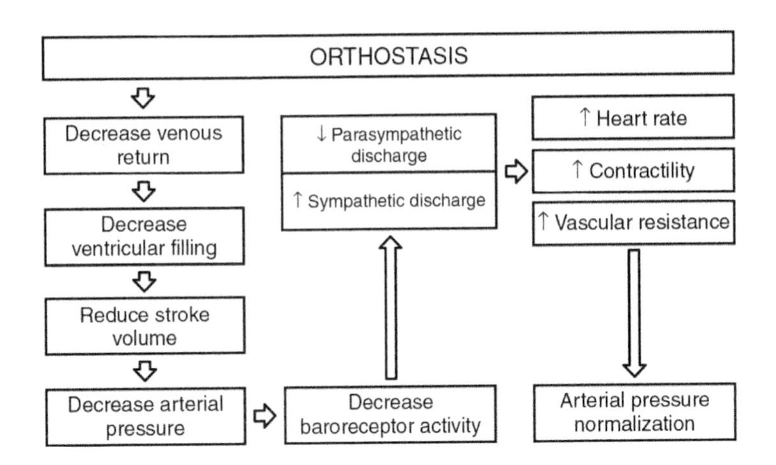

Fig. 15.10 Baroreceptor reflex.

Radiation doses after which cranial nerve palsies occur are relatively high, mostly greater than an equivalence of 70 Gy with conventional fractionation.[75]

Chemotherapy has also been involved in baroreflex dysfunction. Studies have shown that oxaliplatin in combination with 5-FU or capecitabine affects significantly the adrenergic cardiovascular reaction and the parasympathetic heart innervation.[76]

Autonomic nervous system effects of paraneoplastic origin are associated with the presence of anti-Hu antibodies in the context of small-cell lung cancer.[77]

Classification of Othrostatic Hypotension

According to the 2011 updated consensus statement endorsed by major international autonomic nervous system and neurologic societies and in agreement with the European Society of Cardiology, OH is included in the classification of orthostatic intolerance syndromes (accompanied with neutrally mediated syncope and postural tachycardia syndrome).[78]

On a pathophysiologic basis, OH may be divided into 2 broad categories dealing with structural (neurogenic) or functional (or nonneurogenic) causes of autonomic nervous system failure (see earlier discussion).

More clinically relevant is to classify OH based on temporal changes in orthostatic BP. Three different clinical variants of OH have been proposed: classic, delayed, and initial OH[79] (Fig. 15.11):

- *Classic:* a sustained reduction in SBP of at least 20 mm Hg and/or diastolic BP of at least 10 mm Hg, within 30 to 180 seconds of active standing or during a head-up tilt test of at least 60°. In patients with supine hypertension, a reduction in systolic BP of at least 30 mm Hg is considered to be a

TABLE 15.1
Neurogenic, nonneurogenic, and pharmacologic causes of orthostatic hypotension

Neurogenic	Nonneurogenic	Pharmacologic
Autonomic neuropathy	Cardiac pump failure:	Alcohol
Dementia with Lewy body	• Aortic stenosis	Antidepressant drugs
Multiple system atrophy	• Bradyarrhythmia/tachyarrhythmia	Antihypertensive drugs
Amyloidosis	• Constrictive pericarditis	Antiparkinsonism drugs
Diabetes mellitus	• Myocardial infarction	β-Blockers
Familial dysautonomia	• Myocarditis	Antipsychotic drugs
Paraneoplastic syndromes	Venous pooling:	Diuretics
Stroke	• Alcohol	Vaccines: gardasil
Pure autonomic failure	• Postprandial splanchnic expansion	Hypoglycemic drugs: insulin
Pernicious anemia	• Sepsis	Narcotics
Porphyria	• Vigorous exercise	Sedatives
Transverse myelitis	• Deficient blood volume	Calcium channel blockers
	• Adrenal insufficiency	
	• Burns	

From Perlmuter LC, Sarda G, Casavant V, et al. A review of the etiology, associated comorbidities, and treatment of orthostatic hypotension. Am J Ther 2013;20(3):280–81; with permission.

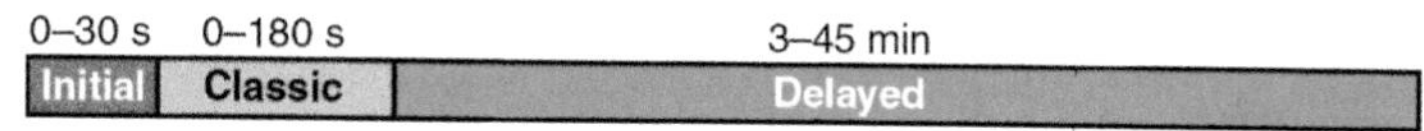

Fig. 15.11 OH timeline classification.

more appropriate criterion for OH because the magnitude of the BP decrease is proportional to baseline values.[80]

- *Delayed:* caused by a gradual impairment of adaptive mechanisms during orthostasis, resulting in a slow progressive drop in arterial pressure (BP decrease ≥20/10 mm Hg or ≥30/15 mm Hg in patients with hypertension) between 3 and 45 minutes. It has been associated with milder abnormalities of sympathetic adrenergic function, suggesting that this disorder may be a less severe or an early form of autonomic failure, along with age-related impairment of compensatory reflexes and with a stiffer, more preload-dependent heart in older patients.[80]
- *Initial:* a transient BP decrease (SBP decrease >40 mm Hg and/or diastolic BP decrease >20 mm Hg) within 30 seconds of standing. The mechanism of initial OH involves a short-lasting mismatch between a sudden decrease in venous return and neurally mediated compensatory vasoconstriction. The diagnosis of initial OH is quite challenging and can only be confirmed by an active standing test with continuous BP monitoring.[79]

Diagnosis

At present, there is no active surveillance for those at risk. Further assessment is made as patients present with signs and symptoms suggestive of OH.

OH is diagnosed on the basis of a simple principle: to demonstrate a significant persistent BP decrease during orthostasis, either by the bedside active-standing test or by using a more sophisticated head-up tilting test.

Typical symptoms of cerebral hypoperfusion include lightheadedness, dizziness, blurred vision, fatigue, headache, and cognitive impairment, among others. It should be noted that similar symptoms may be induced by postural change, but without a decrease in blood pressure, and be caused by a panic attack, occult hyperventilation, cerebrovascular disease, or postural tachycardia syndrome.[81]

Orthostatic Stress Tests

The lying-to-standing orthostatic test

A frequently used protocol is the short, bedside orthostatic test: the patient's blood pressure is measured after 5 to 10 minutes of rest in the supine position; the patient arises and the measurements are then repeated while he stands motionless for 3 to 5 minutes with the cuffed arm supported at heart level. On standing, the patient is asked to report dizziness, faintness, or lightheadedness. The procedure is aborted for safety reasons if blood pressure drops precipitously or presyncope ensues.[82]

It is important to highlight that orthostatic symptoms are often worse in the morning, suggesting diurnal variability. Therefore, it is essential to instruct patients to keep a blood pressure diary with orthostatic blood pressure measurements taken over several days and at various different time points to increase the sensitivity for detection of OH.[83]

The head-up tilt test

In patients unable to tolerate standing or in those with suspicion of OH despite normal vital signs, head-up tilt table testing to an angle at least 60° should be considered.[83] The test comprises 2 phases: supine pretilt phase, and the passive head-up tilt.[79] According to recommendations of the European Society of Cardiology, the supine pretilt phase should last at least 5 minutes, when no venous cannulation is performed, and at least 20 minutes, when venous blood sampling is part of the study. The tilt angle recommended is 60°–70°; the duration of passive tilt should be a minimum of 20 minutes and maximum of 45 minutes.[84] Repeated measurements are taken at 30-second intervals when self-reported dizziness or faintness occurs. The test is discontinued in the event of loss of consciousness. Continuous blood pressure and heart rate monitoring with finger plethysmography are preferable to discontinuous measurement.[83]

The accuracy of postural tests has not been well studied. Different results can be found because of diurnal variability, day-to-day variability, and seasonal variability.[83] A single orthostatic test demonstrating the presence of OH is sufficient for diagnosis. As OH is poorly reproducible, it has been shown that several measurements may be required to detect the abnormality.

Management of Orthostatic Hypotension

The first steps in the management are correcting reversible causes (eg, anemia, hypovolemia), initiating no pharmacologic measures, and removing or reducing high-risk medications when possible.

If these measures fail, pharmacologic management of OH should be considered.

Nonpharmacologic measures

Elastic stockings and abdominal binding. Limb and abdomen compression improves orthostatic tolerance in up to 40% of symptomatic patients. The recommended compression pressure is 30 to 50 mm Hg for leg compression and 20 to 30 mm Hg for the abdomen. However, leg compression alone is not as effective as compression of the abdomen because the venous compartment of the lower limbs is smaller than that of the splanchnic region. The main disadvantage of this method is that compression garments are inconvenient to put on and wear, particularly for older and disabled patients.[85]

Bolus of water and elevating head of bed. Water-bolus treatment consists of the patient drinking two 8-ounce glasses of cold water in rapid succession. This treatment results in the abrupt increase in standing SBP by about 20 mm Hg for 1 to 2 hours.

Pharmacologic treatment. There are several drugs that can be used when treating OH. Table 15.2 shows the mechanism of action, dosage, and contraindications of each drug.[86]

The efficacy of such pharmacologic therapy has been repeatedly questioned, and very few substances, including droxidopa and midodrine, have shown positive results in randomized trials.[88] At present, droxidopa and midodrine are preferred and administered during the daytime to avoid nocturnal (supine) hypertension because both substances have favorable half-lives of approximately 3 hours. A volume expander, preferably fludrocortisone, may complement vasoactive treatment. The use of fludrocortisone in patients with heart failure, kidney failure, or hypertension is relatively contraindicated.[87]

Because several drugs used for the treatment of ischemic heart disease, heart failure, cardiac arrhythmias, and hypertension may have a negative impact on postural homeostasis, tailored therapy is needed to avoid worsening of orthostatic symptoms.

Pyridostigmine, a cholinesterase inhibitor, will improve standing BP in patients with OH without aggravating supine hypertension.

SUMMARY

OH is a frequent condition in the general population, with a prevalence close to 6%, and the frequency increases with age and the presence of comorbidities.[58] In patients with cancer, OH has

TABLE 15.2
Pharmacologic treatment of orthostatic hypotension

Drug	Mechanism of Action	Dosage	Side Effects
Midodrine	Peripheral selective α-1-adrenergic agonist	Starting dosage of 2.5 mg 3 times per day, titrate by 2.5-mg increments weekly until maximum dosage of 10 mg 3 times per day[86]	Hypertension reflex, bradycardia, dry mouth, sedation, rebound hypertension upon abrupt withdrawal
Fludrocortisone	Synthetic mineralocorticoid	Starting dosage of 0.1 mg per day, titrate in increments of 0.1 mg per week, maximum dosage of 1 mg per day	Hypokalemia, headache, supine hypertension, congestive heart failure, edema
Pyridostigmine	Cholinesterase inhibitor that improves neurotransmission at acetylcholine-mediated neurons of the autonomic nervous system	Starting dosage of 30 mg 2 to 3 times per day, titrate to 60 mg 3 times per day	Hypersensitivity to pyridostigmine or bromides, mechanical intestinal or urinary obstruction
Droxidopa	Norepinephrine precursor	100 mg 3 times a day, with suggested dose increases of 100 mg 3 times a day every 24–48 h, up to a maximum recommended dose of 600 mg 3 times a day[87]	Supine hypertension May aggravate ischemic heart disease

been described after neck surgery and/or radiation therapy. The treatment of OH is conservative, but it is limited by the malfunction of baroreflexes.[89] The pharmacologic management of OH should be considered when nonpharmacologic attempts fail.[90]

DIFFERENTIATION SYNDROME (ALL-*TRANS*-RETINOIC ACID SYNDROME, RETINOIC ACID SYNDROME)

Cardiovascular Implications

Overview

Differentiation syndrome (DS) is a life-threatening complication in patients treated for acute promyelocytic leukemia (APL) that involves cardiac and respiratory distress and is associated with severe morbidity and mortality. DS was previously classified as retinoic acid syndrome, because all-*trans*-retinoic acid (ATRA) was the first agent to be involved in this complication. Nonetheless, there are other drugs, such as arsenic trioxide (ATO), that can cause this abnormality.[91] The combination of ATRA and ATO has been safe and effective in the frontline settings.[92]

The syndrome develops within a few days of initiated treatment for APL (mean of 7–12 days).[91] Induction treatment with ATRA and ATO, either as a single agent or in combination with cytotoxic drugs, leads to DS[91] in 2% to 31% of APL patients,[91] whereas the association with chemotherapy compared with ATRA as single-agent therapy is associated with lower risk of DS (9% vs 18%–25%).[93] Mortality due to DS has declined from 30% to 2% to 10% because of the early recognition and clinical intervention.[91] Notably, DS is rarely seen during consolidation and maintenance phases.

Pathophysiology

The pathophysiology of DS is not completely understood.[94] Both ATRA and ATO exert their action by degradation of the PML-RARα fusion product (Fig. 15.12). This causes a proinflammatory state, increasing the synthesis of cytokines, expression of adhesion molecules, and endothelial damage that leads to the extravasation of components from the blood, including leukocyte infiltration.[95]

In vitro, ATRA also leads to aggregation of APL cells, which appears to be mediated by induction by ATRA of the expression of high-affinity β2 integrins and their counterstructure on the cell surface (in particular, intercellular adhesion molecule-2). Methyl prednisolone rapidly inhibits

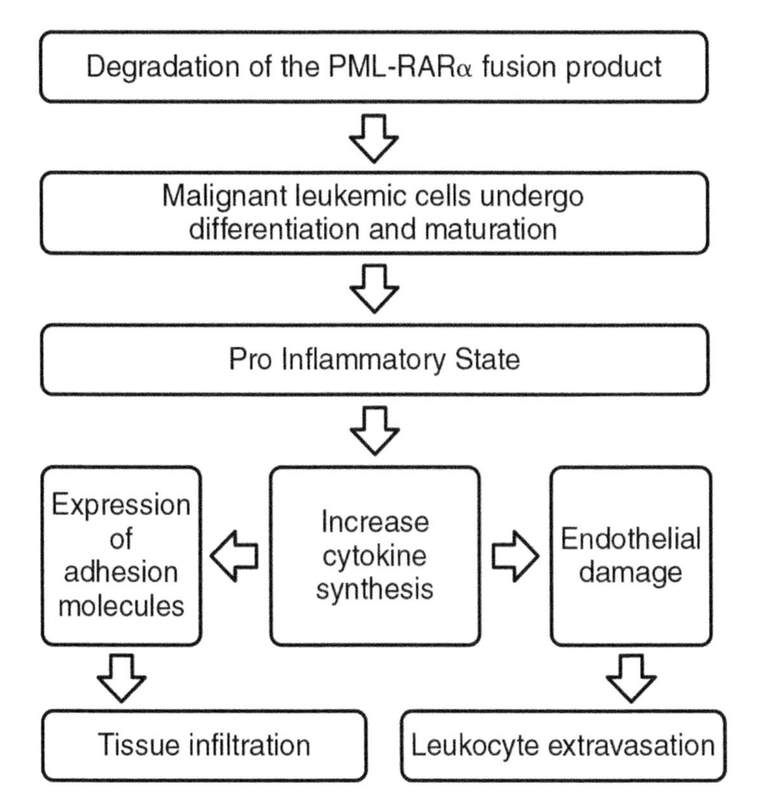

Fig. 15.12 Proposed pathophysiology for DS.

APL cell aggregation in a dose-dependent manner, consistent with its prompt clinical effectiveness in vivo.[96]

Risk factors

Risk factors for DS have not been completely defined.[97] Higher incidence of DS has been reported among patients who receive sequential, as compared with concurrent, chemotherapy.[93] Patients with a starting white blood cell (WBC) count greater than 5×10^9/L should be monitored closely for any signs and symptoms of DS during induction therapy, because it appears that an elevated baseline WBC may be a risk factor for the development of DS.[97]

Clinical manifestations

The onset of DS typically occurs 10 to 12 days (range 2–46 days) after treatment initiation.[91]

Main symptoms tend to be very diverse. Box 15.2 shows the most common clinical manifestations.

Leakage of fluid into the interstitial space may cause the pulmonary implications that may result in the development of respiratory distress syndrome as well as impact the renal and cardiovascular system, causing renal insufficiency and pericardial effusion, respectively. Fluid retention also occurs, and it is manifested as weight increase (around 80% of the cases).[91]

The incidence of complications by affected systems in DS is shown in Fig. 15.13.

BOX 15.2
Clinical manifestations of differentiation syndrome

Hematologic:
Rapidly rising white blood cell count
Respiratory:
Dyspnea
Respiratory distress
Pulmonary edema
Pulmonary infiltrates
Pleural effusion
Cardiovascular:
Pericardial effusion
Myopericarditis
Myocardial infarction
Bradycardia
QTc prolongation

Diagnosis and treatment

Initially, there are no clinical signs or laboratory tests to diagnose DS, nor is there a radiological finding that is pathognomonic for DS.

If the disease progresses, acute respiratory distress syndrome may develop. Diffuse alveolar damage and massive intra-alveolar hemorrhage were found in a necropsy patient study by Frankel and colleagues.[98]

Chest radiograph is the first imaging step. Radiologic features may be explained by the proposed hypotheses of pathophysiology of the DS. Some of the most common findings reported are cardiomegaly, widening of the vascular pedicle width, increased pulmonary blood volume, peribronchial cuffing, ground-glass opacity, septal lines, and pleural effusion. These findings are similar to those of congestive heart failure with pulmonary edema, but they could also probably be produced by leukemic lung infiltration and endothelial leakage in patients with diagnosed with progressive multifocal leukoencephalopathy.[99]

Finally, the diagnosis is made on clinical grounds with at least 3 of the following criteria being present (in the absence of other causes): weight gain, respiratory abnormalities, unexplained fever, interstitial pulmonary infiltrates, pleural or pericardial effusions.

After the diagnosis is made, the proper treatment is initiated typically with dexamethasone at a dosage of 10 mg twice daily intravenously as soon as DS is suspected. Steroid treatment should continue until DS resolves, and then the dosage can be gradually tapered in the following weeks.[100]

Also, discontinuation of ATRA and ATO is mandatory in moderate to severe cases.[100]

Differentiation Syndrome and Cardiovascular Implications

The use of ATRA could exacerbate the procoagulant state of APL and increase the incidence of thrombosis, which is estimated to be approximately 5%.[101] Ortega and colleagues[102] reported a few cases of acute cardiotoxicity when ATRA was combined with anthracycline therapy. However, as cases were related to retinoic acid syndrome, no patients developed late chronic cardiomyopathy. Mahadeo and colleagues[103] suggest the use of serial BNP levels for early diagnosis of cardiac complications and also to highlight the fact that ATRA might represent an independent risk factor for cardiotoxicity.

APL, per se, is often associated with a severe hemostatic disorder caused by the release of procoagulant and fibrinolytic substances from

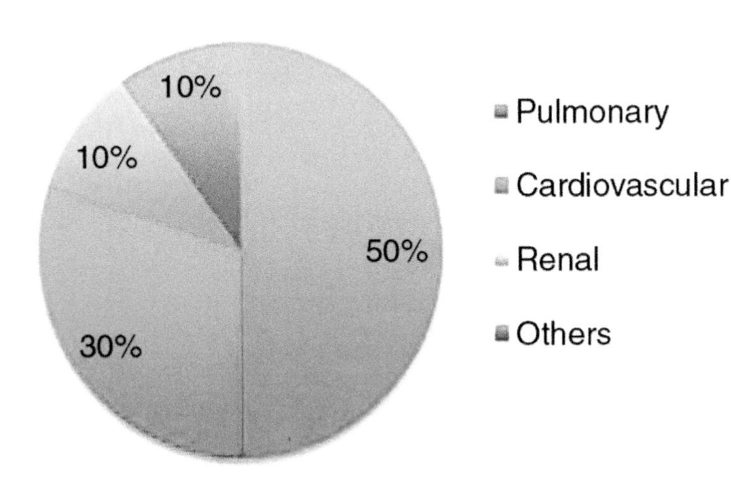

Fig. 15.13 Percentage of affected system in DS. (*Data from* Larson RS, Tallman MS. Retinoic acid syndrome: manifestations, pathogenesis, and treatment. Best Pract Res Clin Haematol 2003;16:453–61.)

leukemic blasts.[104] This state can also be induced by the treatment with ATRA as well as hyperleukocytosis.[105] Cahill and colleagues[106] reported a case of intracardiac thrombus formation complicating acute myocardial infarction as a rare presenting feature of APL.

Primary fibrinolysis due to leukocyte proteases plays a central role in the pathogenesis of the coagulopathy, favoring the use of antifibrinolytic agents.[107] The prothrombotic effect of ATRA has been attributed to the increase in thrombomodulin (an integral membrane protein expressed on the surface on endothelial cells which serves as a cofactor for thrombin).

Brown and colleagues[108] studied the consequences of using ATRA combined with tranexamic acid and found that 13% of patients died of a thrombotic event resulting in organ failure due to occlusion of the vasculature.

Catastrophic acute myocardial infarction has been reported in patients with APL treated with ATRA, with increased incidence in patients suspected of having DS.[109] Major thrombotic events in APL can happen before, during, or after induction therapy, with more than 80% of those occurring equally frequent either before or during induction therapy.

Several studies have shown that the most common cardiovascular finding in patients receiving treatment with ATRA is pericardial effusion (incidence of 30%),[110] that can be complicated by fatal pericardial tamponade, if pericardial effusion is not recognized on simple chest radiography and proper surveillance with computerized tomography or echocardiography is lacking.

In some patients, the DS can be accompanied by ECG and laboratory signs of myopericarditis, with or without radiological pericardial effusion, leading to transient cardiac ventricle dysfunction.[111]

Although not as frequent, other cardiac implications related to the use of ATRA, such as myocarditis, internodal conduction abnormalities, and persistent bradycardia, have been reported.[112]

The pathogenesis of myocarditis in patients under ATRA treatment depends on complex interactions between extravasation of acute promyelocytic leukemia cells, leukocyte infiltration, endothelial injury, and cytokine release, leading to myocardial cell lysis and release of cardiac biochemical markers into the blood.

Isik and colleagues[113] reported an ATRA treatment-related pancarditis and severe pulmonary edema in a child with acute promyelocytic leukemia, which started initially as an endomyocarditis during induction phase of the treatment and constituted the reason for initial discontinuation of ATRA. Subsequently, ATRA was resumed with the development of pancarditis, which resolved when the chemotherapeutic agent was removed.

Cardiac stunning after the initiation of ATRA treatment has also been reported in the literature as a manifestation of DS.[101]

ATO may also have cardiovascular implications. Studies have shown that it induces QT interval prolongation and arrhythmias in more than 50% of treated patients,[107] that makes the individual prone to the development of ventricular arrhythmias (nonsustained monomorphic ventricular tachycardia or isolated ventricular premature complexes). QT prolongation can lead to tTdP-type ventricular arrhythmias, which can be fatal. Patients who reach an absolute QT interval value >500 milliseconds should be reassessed and corrected for concomitant risk factors as

Soignet and colleagues[114] recommended. During ATO therapy, potassium concentration should be kept higher than 4 mEq/dL, and magnesium concentrations higher than 1.8 mg/dL. If ventricular tachycardia develops, patients should be monitored continuously, and serum electrolytes should be assessed. ATO therapy should temporarily be discontinued until the QT interval regresses to less than 460 milliseconds, electrolyte abnormalities are corrected, and irregular heartbeats cease. Decline in LVEF has also been reported.[115]

Cardiovascular care

Patients with cancer undergoing pharmacologic treatment with ATRA should receive proper cardiovascular evaluations with complete clinical examination, including an ECG and Doppler echocardiography.

Electrocardiogram. Abnormalities are often nonspecific in this clinical setting.[116] As mentioned earlier, findings, such as bradycardia, QTc interval prolongation, and ischemic changes, have been reported.

Doppler-echocardiography. A large amount of data demonstrates the importance of Doppler echocardiography for baseline cardiologic screening and follow-up of the oncologic patients during and after the completion of cancer therapy. In relation to its low cost, feasibility and reliability to diagnose LV systolic and diastolic dysfunction, regional wall motion abnormalities, valve disease, pericardial abnormalities, and carotid lesions, the ultrasound examination appears very useful to identify and monitor cancer therapy-related cardiac conditions over time.[116]

SUMMARY

DS is an unpredictable but frequent complication of ATRA and ATO therapy. Clinicians treating patients with APL should be aware of this disorder.[91] Complete recovery is possible with timely diagnosis and administration of high-dose steroid treatment.[117] Likewise, temporary discontinuation of ATRA and/or ATO may be warranted in severe cases of DS.[93] Patients should be closely monitored for cardiovascular complications because they may occur in up to 33% of the cases. Major cardiac thrombotic events may happen during or after induction therapy[118]; this argues for a low-threshold catheterization when myocardial ischemia is suspected.

REFERENCES

1. Hurst RT, Prasad A, Askew JW 3rd, et al. Takotsubo cardiomyopathy: a unique cardiomyopathy with variable ventricular morphology. JACC Cardiovasc Imaging 2010;3(6):641–9.
2. Scantlebury DC, Prasad A. Diagnosis of Takotsubo cardiomyopathy. Circ J 2014;78(9):2129–39.
3. Sherratt J, McDonald CE, York G, et al. A rare case report of mid cavitary Takotsubo: the role of magnetic resonance imaging. Case Rep Cardiol 2011; 2011:481394.
4. Ghadri JR, Ruschitzka F, Luscher TF, et al. Takotsubo cardiomyopathy: still much more to learn. Heart 2014;100(22):1804–12.
5. Lyon AR, Bossone E, Schneider B, et al. Current state of knowledge on Takotsubo syndrome: a Position Statement from the Taskforce on Takotsubo Syndrome of the Heart Failure Association of the European Society of Cardiology. Eur J Heart Fail 2016;18(1):8–27.
6. Wittstein IS, Thiemann DR, Lima JA, et al. Neurohumoral features of myocardial stunning due to sudden emotional stress. N Engl J Med 2005; 352(6):539–48.
7. Zielen P, Klisiewicz A, Januszewicz A, et al. Pheochromocytoma-related 'classic' Takotsubo cardiomyopathy. J Hum Hypertens 2010;24(5):363–6.
8. Lyon AR, Rees PS, Prasad S, et al. Stress (Takotsubo) cardiomyopathy–a novel pathophysiological hypothesis to explain catecholamine-induced acute myocardial stunning. Nat Clin Pract Cardiovasc Med 2008;5(1):22–9.
9. Paur H, Wright PT, Sikkel MB, et al. High levels of circulating epinephrine trigger apical cardiodepression in a beta2-adrenergic receptor/Gi-dependent manner: a new model of Takotsubo cardiomyopathy. Circulation 2012;126(6):697–706.
10. Spinelli L, Trimarco V, Di Marino S, et al. L41Q polymorphism of the G protein coupled receptor kinase 5 is associated with left ventricular apical ballooning syndrome. Eur J Heart Fail 2010;12(1):13–6.
11. Heubach JF, Blaschke M, Harding SE, et al. Cardiostimulant and cardiodepressant effects through overexpressed human beta2-adrenoceptors in murine heart: regional differences and functional role of beta1-adrenoceptors. Naunyn Schmiedebergs Arch Pharmacol 2003;367(4):380–90.
12. Liao P, Wang SQ, Wang S, et al. p38 Mitogen-activated protein kinase mediates a negative inotropic effect in cardiac myocytes. Circ Res 2002;90(2):190–6.
13. Kawano H, Okada R, Yano K. Histological study on the distribution of autonomic nerves in the human heart. Heart Vessels 2003;18(1):32–9.
14. Chesley A, Lundberg MS, Asai T, et al. The beta(2)-adrenergic receptor delivers an antiapoptotic

signal to cardiac myocytes through G(i)-dependent coupling to phosphatidylinositol 3'-kinase. Circ Res 2000;87(12):1172–9.
15. Liu R, Ramani B, Soto D, et al. Agonist dose-dependent phosphorylation by protein kinase A and G protein-coupled receptor kinase regulates beta2 adrenoceptor coupling to G(i) proteins in cardiomyocytes. J Biol Chem 2009;284(47):32279–87.
16. Prasad A, Lerman A, Rihal CS. Apical ballooning syndrome (Tako-Tsubo or stress cardiomyopathy): a mimic of acute myocardial infarction. Am Heart J 2008;155(3):408–17.
17. Vejpongsa P, Durand JB, Reyes M, et al. Takotsubo cardiomyopathy in cancer patients. Triggers, recovery, and resumption of therapy. J Am Coll Cardiol 2015.
18. Ting MH, Leslie S, Watson A. Postoperative Takotsubo's cardiomyopathy. Colorectal Dis 2012;14(12):e817–8.
19. Pai VB, Nahata MC. Cardiotoxicity of chemotherapeutic agents: incidence, treatment and prevention. Drug Saf 2000;22(4):263–302.
20. Grunwald MR, Howie L, Diaz LA Jr. Takotsubo cardiomyopathy and fluorouracil: case report and review of the literature. J Clin Oncol 2012;30(2):e11–4.
21. Sharkey SW, Windenburg DC, Lesser JR, et al. Natural history and expansive clinical profile of stress (Tako-Tsubo) cardiomyopathy. J Am Coll Cardiol 2010;55(4):333–41.
22. Song BG, Yang HS, Hwang HK, et al. The impact of stressor patterns on clinical features in patients with Tako-Tsubo cardiomyopathy: experiences of two tertiary cardiovascular centers. Clin Cardiol 2012;35(11):E6–13.
23. Singh SB, Harle IA. Takotsubo cardiomyopathy secondary in part to cancer-related pain crisis: a case report. J Pain Symptom Manage 2014;48(1):137–42.
24. Pelliccia F, Greco C, Vitale C, et al. Takotsubo syndrome (stress cardiomyopathy): an intriguing clinical condition in search of its identity. Am J Med 2014;127(8):699–704.
25. Kono T, Morita H, Kuroiwa T, et al. Left ventricular wall motion abnormalities in patients with subarachnoid hemorrhage: neurogenic stunned myocardium. J Am Coll Cardiol 1994;24(3):636–40.
26. Bybee KA, Kara T, Prasad A, et al. Systematic review: transient left ventricular apical ballooning: a syndrome that mimics ST-segment elevation myocardial infarction. Ann Intern Med 2004;141(11):858–65.
27. Bybee KA, Prasad A, Barsness GW, et al. Clinical characteristics and thrombolysis in myocardial infarction frame counts in women with transient left ventricular apical ballooning syndrome. Am J Cardiol 2004;94(3):343–6.
28. Bybee KA, Motiei A, Syed IS, et al. Electrocardiography cannot reliably differentiate transient left ventricular apical ballooning syndrome from anterior ST-segment elevation myocardial infarction. J Electrocardiol 2007;40(1):38.e31-6.
29. Kurisu S, Inoue I, Kawagoe T, et al. Time course of electrocardiographic changes in patients with Tako-Tsubo syndrome: comparison with acute myocardial infarction with minimal enzymatic release. Circ J 2004;68(1):77–81.
30. Nguyen TH, Neil CJ, Sverdlov AL, et al. N-terminal pro-brain natriuretic protein levels in Takotsubo cardiomyopathy. Am J Cardiol 2011;108(9):1316–21.
31. Citro R, Piscione F, Parodi G, et al. Role of echocardiography in Takotsubo cardiomyopathy. Heart Fail Clin 2013;9(2):157–66, viii.
32. Marwick TH, Leano RL, Brown J, et al. Myocardial strain measurement with 2-dimensional speckle-tracking echocardiography: definition of normal range. JACC Cardiovasc Imaging 2009;2(1):80–4.
33. Carasso S, Biaggi P, Rakowski H, et al. Velocity Vector Imaging: standard tissue-tracking results acquired in normals–the VVI-STRAIN study. J Am Soc Echocardiogr 2012;25(5):543–52.
34. Sosa S, Banchs J. Early recognition of apical ballooning syndrome by global longitudinal strain using speckle tracking imaging–the evil eye pattern, a case series. Echocardiography 2015;32(7):1184–92.
35. Bossone E, Lyon A, Citro R, et al. Takotsubo cardiomyopathy: an integrated multi-imaging approach. Eur Heart J Cardiovasc Imaging 2014;15(4):366–77.
36. Parodi G, Del Pace S, Carrabba N, et al. Incidence, clinical findings, and outcome of women with left ventricular apical ballooning syndrome. Am J Cardiol 2007;99(2):182–5.
37. Goldstein JA, Chinnaiyan KM, Abidov A, et al. The CT-STAT (Coronary Computed Tomographic Angiography for Systematic Triage of Acute Chest Pain Patients to Treatment) trial. J Am Coll Cardiol 2011;58(14):1414–22.
38. Halpern EJ. Triple-rule-out CT angiography for evaluation of acute chest pain and possible acute coronary syndrome. Radiology 2009;252(2):332–45.
39. Fernandez-Perez GC, Aguilar-Arjona JA, de la Fuente GT, et al. Takotsubo cardiomyopathy: assessment with cardiac MRI. AJR Am J Roentgenol 2010;195(2):W139–45.
40. Satoh H, Sano M, Suwa K, et al. Distribution of late gadolinium enhancement in various types of cardiomyopathies: significance in differential

diagnosis, clinical features and prognosis. World J Cardiol 2014;6(7):585–601.
41. Naruse Y, Sato A, Kasahara K, et al. The clinical impact of late gadolinium enhancement in Takotsubo cardiomyopathy: serial analysis of cardiovascular magnetic resonance images. J Cardiovasc Magn Reson 2011;13:67.
42. Redmond M, Knapp C, Salim M, et al. Use of vasopressors in Takotsubo cardiomyopathy: a cautionary tale. Br J Anaesth 2013;110(3):487–8.
43. Nishikawa S, Ito K, Adachi Y, et al. Ampulla ('Takotsubo') cardiomyopathy of both ventricles: evaluation of microcirculation disturbance using 99mTc-tetrofosmin myocardial single photon emission computed tomography and doppler guide wire. Circ J 2004;68(11):1076–80.
44. Villareal RP, Achari A, Wilansky S, et al. Anteroapical stunning and left ventricular outflow tract obstruction. Mayo Clin Proc 2001;76(1):79–83.
45. Citro R, Rigo F, D'Andrea A, et al. Echocardiographic correlates of acute heart failure, cardiogenic shock, and in-hospital mortality in Tako-Tsubo cardiomyopathy. JACC Cardiovasc Imaging 2014;7(2):119–29.
46. Chockalingam A, Dorairajan S, Bhalla M, et al. Unexplained hypotension: the spectrum of dynamic left ventricular outflow tract obstruction in critical care settings. Crit Care Med 2009;37(2):729–34.
47. Tse RW, Masindet S, Stavola T, et al. Acute myocardial infarction with dynamic outflow obstruction precipitated by intra-aortic balloon counterpulsation. Cathet Cardiovasc Diagn 1996; 39(1):62–6.
48. Schneider B, Athanasiadis A, Schwab J, et al. Complications in the clinical course of Tako-Tsubo cardiomyopathy. Int J Cardiol 2014;176(1): 199–205.
49. Madias C, Fitzgibbons TP, Alsheikh-Ali AA, et al. Acquired long QT syndrome from stress cardiomyopathy is associated with ventricular arrhythmias and torsades de pointes. Heart Rhythm 2011;8(4): 555–61.
50. Syed FF, Asirvatham SJ, Francis J. Arrhythmia occurrence with Takotsubo cardiomyopathy: a literature review. Europace 2011;13(6):780–8.
51. Kurisu S, Inoue I, Kawagoe T, et al. Torsade de pointes associated with bradycardia and Takotsubo cardiomyopathy. Can J Cardiol 2008;24(8): 640–2.
52. Kim J, Laird-Fick HS, Alsara O, et al. Pericarditis in Takotsubo cardiomyopathy: a case report and review of the literature. Case Rep Cardiol 2013; 2013:917851.
53. Yeh RW, Yu PB, Drachman DE. Takotsubo cardiomyopathy complicated by cardiac tamponade: classic hemodynamic findings with a new disease. Circulation 2010;122(12):1239–41.
54. Singh K, Carson K, Shah R, et al. Meta-analysis of clinical correlates of acute mortality in Takotsubo cardiomyopathy. Am J Cardiol 2014; 113(8):1420–8.
55. Singh K, Carson K, Usmani Z, et al. Systematic review and meta-analysis of incidence and correlates of recurrence of Takotsubo cardiomyopathy. Int J Cardiol 2014;174(3):696–701.
56. Peters MN, George P, Irimpen AM. The broken heart syndrome: Takotsubo cardiomyopathy. Trends Cardiovasc Med 2015;25(4):351–7.
57. Freeman R, Wieling W, Axelrod FB, et al. Consensus statement on the definition of orthostatic hypotension, neurally mediated syncope and the postural tachycardia syndrome. Auton Neurosci 2011;161(1–2):46–8.
58. Ricci F, De Caterina R, Fedorowski A. Orthostatic hypotension: epidemiology, prognosis, and treatment. J Am Coll Cardiol 2015;66(7):848–60.
59. Shibao C, Grijalva CG, Raj SR, et al. Orthostatic hypotension-related hospitalizations in the United States. Am J Med 2007;120(11):975–80.
60. Ricci F, Fedorowski A, Radico F, et al. Cardiovascular morbidity and mortality related to orthostatic hypotension: a meta-analysis of prospective observational studies. Eur Heart J 2015;36(25): 1609–17.
61. Chopra S, Baby C, Jacob JJ. Neuro-endocrine regulation of blood pressure. Indian J Endocrinol Metab 2011;15(Suppl 4):S281–8.
62. Diedrich A, Biaggioni I. Segmental orthostatic fluid shifts. Clin Auton Res 2004;14(3):146–7.
63. Morimoto S, Sasaki S, Itoh H, et al. Sympathetic activation and contribution of genetic factors in hypertension with neurovascular compression of the rostral ventrolateral medulla. J Hypertens 1999;17(11):1577–82.
64. Terlou A, Ruble K, Stapert AF, et al. Orthostatic intolerance in survivors of childhood cancer. Eur J Cancer 2007;43(18):2685–90.
65. Timmers HJ, Karemaker JM, Lenders JW, et al. Baroreflex failure following radiation therapy for nasopharyngeal carcinoma. Clin Auton Res 1999; 9(6):317–24.
66. Goodman BP, Schrader SL. Radiation-induced cranial neuropathies manifesting as baroreflex failure and progressive bulbar impairment. Neurologist 2009;15(2):102–4.
67. Huang CC, Huang TL, Hsu HC, et al. Long-term effects of neck irradiation on cardiovascular autonomic function: a study in nasopharyngeal carcinoma patients after radiotherapy. Muscle Nerve 2013;47(3):344–50.
68. Farach A, Fernando R, Bhattacharjee M, et al. Baroreflex failure following radiotherapy for head and neck cancer: a case study. Pract Radiat Oncol 2012;2(3):226–32.

69. Elerding SC, Fernandez RN, Grotta JC, et al. Carotid artery disease following external cervical irradiation. Ann Surg 1981;194(5):609–15.
70. Gianaros PJ, Jennings JR, Olafsson GB, et al. Greater intima-media thickness in the carotid bulb is associated with reduced baroreflex sensitivity. Am J Hypertens 2002;15(6):486–91.
71. Angell-James JE. Arterial baroreceptor activity in rabbits with experimental atherosclerosis. Circ Res 1974;34(1):27–39.
72. Angell-James JE, Lumley JS. The effects of carotid endarterectomy on the mechanical properties of the carotid sinus and carotid sinus nerve activity in atherosclerotic patients. Br J Surg 1974;61(10):805–10.
73. Zidar N, Ferluga D, Hvala A, et al. Contribution to the pathogenesis of radiation-induced injury to large arteries. J Laryngol Otol 1997;111(10):988–90.
74. Kong L, Lu JJ, Liss AL, et al. Radiation-induced cranial nerve palsy: a cross-sectional study of nasopharyngeal cancer patients after definitive radiotherapy. Int J Radiat Oncol Biol Phys 2011;79(5):1421–7.
75. King AD, Leung SF, Teo P, et al. Hypoglossal nerve palsy in nasopharyngeal carcinoma. Head Neck 1999;21(7):614–9.
76. Dermitzakis EV, Kimiskidis VK, Eleftheraki A, et al. The impact of oxaliplatin-based chemotherapy for colorectal cancer on the autonomous nervous system. Eur J Neurol 2014;21(12):1471–7.
77. Dineen J, Freeman R. Autonomic neuropathy. Semin Neurol 2015;35(4):458–68.
78. Moya A, Sutton R, Ammirati F, et al. Guidelines for the diagnosis and management of syncope (version 2009). Eur Heart J 2009;30(21):2631–71.
79. Fedorowski A, Melander O. Syndromes of orthostatic intolerance: a hidden danger. J Intern Med 2013;273(4):322–35.
80. Verheyden B, Gisolf J, Beckers F, et al. Impact of age on the vasovagal response provoked by sublingual nitroglycerine in routine tilt testing. Clin Sci 2007;113(7):329–37.
81. Robertson D. The epidemic of orthostatic tachycardia and orthostatic intolerance. Am J Med Sci 1999;317(2):75–7.
82. Naschitz JE, Rosner I. Orthostatic hypotension: framework of the syndrome. Postgrad Med J 2007;83(983):568–74.
83. Arnold AC, Shibao C. Current concepts in orthostatic hypotension management. Curr Hypertens Rep 2013;15(4):304–12.
84. Biaggioni I, Robertson RM. Hypertension in orthostatic hypotension and autonomic dysfunction. Cardiol Clin 2002;20(2):291–301, vii.
85. Figueroa JJ, Basford JR, Low PA. Preventing and treating orthostatic hypotension: as easy as A, B, C. Cleve Clin J Med 2010;77(5):298–306.
86. Gupta V, Lipsitz LA. Orthostatic hypotension in the elderly: diagnosis and treatment. Am J Med 2007;120(10):841–7.
87. Maule S, Papotti G, Naso D, et al. Orthostatic hypotension: evaluation and treatment. Cardiovasc Hematol Disord Drug Targets 2007;7(1):63–70.
88. Keating GM. Droxidopa: a review of its use in symptomatic neurogenic orthostatic hypotension. Drugs 2015;75(2):197–206.
89. Low PA, Tomalia VA. Orthostatic hypotension: mechanisms, causes, management. J Clin Neurol 2015;11(3):220–6.
90. Lee Y. Orthostatic hypotension in older people. J Am Assoc Nurse Pract 2013;25(9):451–8.
91. Patatanian E, Thompson DF. Retinoic acid syndrome: a review. J Clin Pharm Ther 2008;33(4):331–8.
92. Daver N, Kantarjian H, Marcucci G, et al. Clinical characteristics and outcomes in patients with acute promyelocytic leukaemia and hyperleucocytosis. Br J Haematol 2015;168(5):646–53.
93. De Botton S, Dombret H, Sanz M, et al. Incidence, clinical features, and outcome of all trans-retinoic acid syndrome in 413 cases of newly diagnosed acute promyelocytic leukemia. The European APL Group. Blood 1998;92(8):2712–8.
94. Gupta V, Yi QL, Brandwein J, et al. Role of all-trans-retinoic acid (ATRA) in the consolidation therapy of acute promyelocytic leukaemia (APL). Leuk Res 2005;29(1):113–4.
95. Luesink M, Pennings JL, Wissink WM, et al. Chemokine induction by all-trans retinoic acid and arsenic trioxide in acute promyelocytic leukemia: triggering the differentiation syndrome. Blood 2009;114(27):5512–21.
96. Larson RS, Brown DC, Sklar LA. Retinoic acid induces aggregation of the acute promyelocytic leukemia cell line NB-4 by utilization of LFA-1 and ICAM-2. Blood 1997;90(7):2747–56.
97. Rogers JE, Yang D. Differentiation syndrome in patients with acute promyelocytic leukemia. J Oncol Pharm Pract 2012;18(1):109–14.
98. Frankel SR, Eardley A, Lauwers G, et al. The "retinoic acid syndrome" in acute promyelocytic leukemia. Ann Intern Med 1992;117(4):292–6.
99. Chanarin N, Smith GB, Green A, et al. Retinoic acid syndrome. Lancet 1993;341(8855):1289–90.
100. Sanz MA, Grimwade D, Tallman MS, et al. Management of acute promyelocytic leukemia: recommendations from an expert panel on behalf of the European LeukemiaNet. Blood 2009;113(9):1875–91.
101. De Santis GC, Madeira MI, de Oliveira LC, et al. Cardiac stunning as a manifestation of ATRA differentiation syndrome in acute promyelocytic leukemia. Med Oncol 2012;29(1):248–50.
102. Ortega JJ, Madero L, Martin G, et al. Treatment with all-trans retinoic acid and anthracycline

monochemotherapy for children with acute promyelocytic leukemia: a multicenter study by the PETHEMA Group. J Clin Oncol 2005;23(30):7632–40.
103. Mahadeo KM, Dhall G, Ettinger LJ, et al. Exacerbation of anthracycline-induced early chronic cardiomyopathy with ATRA: role of B-type natriuretic peptide as an indicator of cardiac dysfunction. J Pediatr Hematol Oncol 2010;32(2):134–6.
104. Kocak U, Gursel T, Ozturk G, et al. Thrombosis during all-trans-retinoic acid therapy in a child with acute promyelocytic leukemia and factor VQ 506 mutation. Pediatr Hematol Oncol 2000; 17(2):177–80.
105. Warrell RP Jr, de The H, Wang ZY, et al. Acute promyelocytic leukemia. N Engl J Med 1993;329(3): 177–89.
106. Cahill TJ, Chowdhury O, Myerson SG, et al. Myocardial infarction with intracardiac thrombosis as the presentation of acute promyelocytic leukemia: diagnosis and follow-up by cardiac magnetic resonance imaging. Circulation 2011;123(10): e370–372.
107. Schwartz BS, Williams EC, Conlan MG, et al. Epsilon-aminocaproic acid in the treatment of patients with acute promyelocytic leukemia and acquired alpha-2-plasmin inhibitor deficiency. Ann Intern Med 1986;105(6):873–7.
108. Brown JE, Olujohungbe A, Chang J, et al. All-trans retinoic acid (ATRA) and tranexamic acid: a potentially fatal combination in acute promyelocytic leukaemia. Br J Haematol 2000;110(4):1010–2.
109. Escudier SM, Kantarjian HM, Estey EH. Thrombosis in patients with acute promyelocytic leukemia treated with and without all-trans retinoic acid. Leuk Lymphoma 1996;20(5–6):435–9.
110. Larson RS, Tallman MS. Retinoic acid syndrome: manifestations, pathogenesis, and treatment. Best practice & research. Clin Haematol 2003; 16(3):453–61.
111. Jung JI, Choi JE, Hahn ST, et al. Radiologic features of all-trans-retinoic acid syndrome. AJR Am J Roentgenol 2002;178(2):475–80.
112. Maruhashi K, Wada H, Taniguchi M, et al. Sinus bradyarrhythmia during administration of all-trans retinoic acid in a patient with acute promyelocytic leukemia. Rinsho ketsueki 1996;37(5):443–7.
113. Isik P, Cetin I, Tavil B, et al. All-transretinoic acid (ATRA) treatment-related pancarditis and severe pulmonary edema in a child with acute promyelocytic leukemia. J Pediatr Hematol Oncol 2010; 32(8):e346–348.
114. Soignet SL, Frankel SR, Douer D, et al. United States multicenter study of arsenic trioxide in relapsed acute promyelocytic leukemia. J Clin Oncol 2001;19(18):3852–60.
115. Tallman MS, Andersen JW, Schiffer CA, et al. Clinical description of 44 patients with acute promyelocytic leukemia who developed the retinoic acid syndrome. Blood 2000;95(1):90–5.
116. Galderisi M, Marra F, Esposito R, et al. Cancer therapy and cardiotoxicity: the need of serial Doppler echocardiography. Cardiovasc Ultrasound 2007;5:4.
117. Su YC, Dunn P, Shih LY, et al. Retinoic acid syndrome in patients following the treatment of acute promyelocytic leukemia with all-trans retinoic acid. Chang Gung Med J 2009;32(5):535–42.
118. Rashidi A, Silverberg ML, Conkling PR, et al. Thrombosis in acute promyelocytic leukemia. Thromb Res 2013;131(4):281–9.

CHAPTER 16

Diagnostic Tests in Cardio-oncology

Gina Biasillo, MD[a,*], Daniela Cardinale, MD, PhD, FESC[a], Lara F. Nhola, MD[b], Hector R. Villarraga, MD[b], Jennifer H. Jordan, PhD, MS[c], W. Gregory Hundley, MD[c]

BIOMARKERS

Cardiotoxicity

Modern anticancer therapies are highly effective in the treatment of malignancy and have significantly improved life expectancy. However, these kinds of drugs can lead to significant side effects, and among them, some involve the heart.[1]

At present, there is not a single and proper definition of chemotherapy-induced cardiac toxicity. In fact, the development of different cardiac events, such as acute coronary syndromes, loss of cardiac function, electrocardiogram changes and arrhythmias, even hypertension and thromboembolic events, may all be considered as an expressions of "cardiac toxicity."

However, the most frequent and typical manifestation of cardiotoxicity is the development of an asymptomatic or symptomatic left ventricular (LV) dysfunction, which may progress to overt heart failure. The current definition of cardiac toxicity is based on left ventricular ejection fraction (LVEF) evaluation. Cardiac toxicity is defined as a reduction of LVEF greater than 10% from baseline with a final value less than 50%, or as a reduction greater than 15% from baseline with a final LVEF value greater than 50%.[2] Modulated by different risk factors,[3] recent studies suggested that drug-induced cardiotoxicity is a continuum that starts with myocardial cell injury, followed by progressive LV dysfunction, which, if disregarded and not treated, leads to overt heart failure.[4]

The phenomenon of cardiac toxicity is expected to increase, because of the increasing number of patients undergoing anticancer treatment and because of increased survival of patients with cancer. This increasing incidence requires a more accurate diagnostic and therapeutic approach, in order to avoid limitations in indication, administration, and dose of anticancer drugs. Indeed, early identification of patients at risk of developing cardiac toxicity is mandatory.

At present, detection of cardiac toxicity is based on regular and periodic assessment of LVEF by echocardiography.[5,6] However, this approach has several limitations. It has relatively low sensitivity, because no considerable change in LVEF occurs until significant myocardial damage is present. Moreover, image quality depends on the acoustic windows, and there is a high interobserver variability. Other imaging modalities are available; however, radionuclide angiography detects only significant changes in cardiac function and entails exposure to radioactivity. Cardiac MRI represents the gold standard for the evaluation of volumes and function of LV, but it is limited by low availability, high costs, and long processing time. Furthermore, cardiac MRI is not a possibility for patients with cancer who received silicone or metal implants.

The limitations of LVEF assessment have led to the search for novel approaches. Among these, in particular, the use of biomarkers has emerged as a cost-effective diagnostic tool for early, real-time identification and monitoring of drug-induced cardiotoxicity. In comparison to the techniques described above, this approach seems to be more sensitive and specific, without intraobserver and interobserver variability, demands and risks for the patient, and with low costs and widespread availability.

Most of the existing data regarding use of cardiac biomarkers refer to troponins, directly reflective of cardiomyocyte integrity, and natriuretic peptides, released by the heart in response to volume expansion and increased wall stress.

[a] Cardioncology Unit, European Institute of Oncology, via Ripamonti 435, 20141 Milan, Italy; [b] Department of Cardiovascular Diseases, Mayo Clinic, Rochester, MN, USA; [c] Department of Internal Medicine, Section on Cardiovascular Medicine, Wake Forest School of Medicine, Winston-Salem, North Carolina, USA
* Corresponding author.
E-mail address: gina.biasillo@ieo.it

Troponins

The troponin complex, involved in the actin-myosin interaction in the cardiomyocytes, thus cardiac contraction and relaxation, is composed of 3 subunits, troponin C, troponin T, and troponin I (Fig. 16.1). It is mostly found in the sarcomeres of myocardial cells and in small quantities in the cytoplasm. With cardiomyocyte necrosis, there is a rapid depletion of the cytoplasmic pool, followed by a larger release of troponins into circulation after breakdown of the contractile apparatus. Accordingly, detection of cardiac troponins (cTns) in peripheral blood is indicative of cardiomyocyte necrosis. CTns have high tissue specificity and an evolving sensitivity for the detection of (even small amounts of) myocardial necrosis with the new highly sensitive (HS) assays. Historically, only one assay has been patented for cardiac troponin T (cTnT), but multiple assays are available for cardiac troponin I (cTnI). These assays will be collectively referred to as cTns unless otherwise specified.

Initially, cTns emerged as very useful markers in the diagnosis and risk stratification of patients with suspected and proven acute coronary syndromes.[7] However, their use has been extended to detect cardiac damage in other clinical settings, such as cardiac hypertrophy, heart failure, acute pulmonary embolism, blunt trauma, sepsis, stroke, and renal insufficiency.[8] Moreover, in the 2 last decades, cTns have also been evaluated in oncologic settings, in particular to detect cardiac toxicity associated with anticancer drugs (Table 16.1).[21]

The role of cTns as indicators of anthracycline-induced cardiotoxicity was first studied in animal models. CTnT elevation correlated with administered drug dose and with the degree of cardiac damage, as demonstrated by histology.[22] A large number of studies suggest the translation of these findings to patients receiving potentially cardiotoxic therapies. In one of the first larger-scale studies, Lipshultz and colleagues[9] observed an increase in the plasma concentrations of cTns in about 30% of children treated with doxorubicin, thus confirming that cTns are sensitive and specific markers of drug-induced myocardial injury, even months before its clinical recognition by symptoms or decline in ejection fraction.[9] Data from the European Institute of Oncology (EIO) group confirmed these data in the adult population (Fig. 16.2) and the role of cTns in predicting cardiac dysfunction in adult patients undergoing a high dose of anticancer drugs for different malignancies (Fig. 16.3). Importantly, this was not confined to high-dose chemotherapy regimens with anthracyclines (Fig. 16.4).

In these studies, cTnI increase predicted the development of LV dysfunction in the month following the completion of chemotherapy as

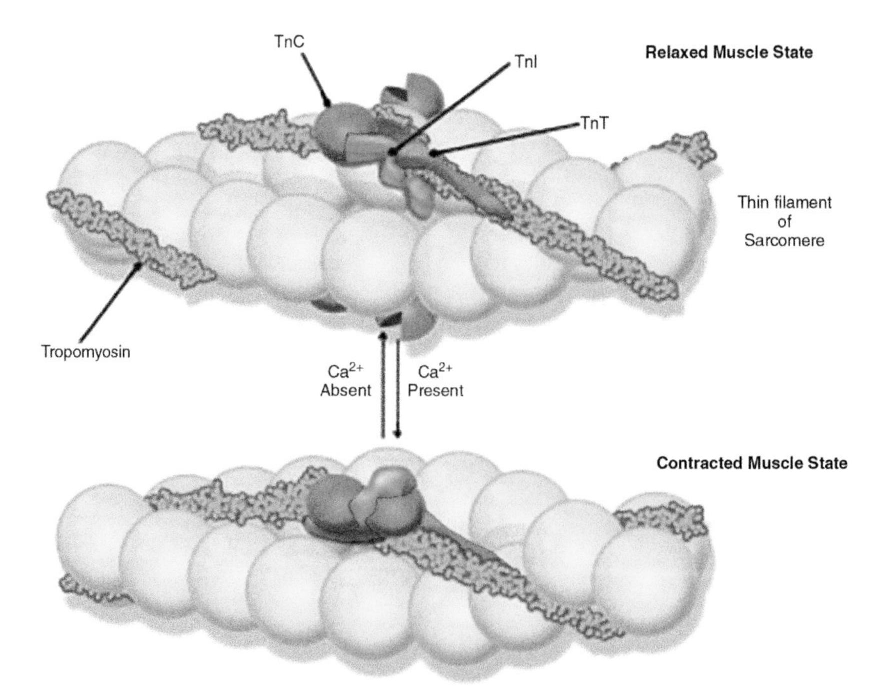

Fig. 16.1 Cardiac muscle showing location of cardiac troponin I (TnI), cardiac troponin T (TnT), and troponin C (TnC) in relation to actin and tropomyosin. (*Adapted from* Shave R, Baggish A, George K, et al. Exercise-induced cardiac troponin elevation: evidence, mechanisms, and implications. J Am Coll Cardiol 2010;56:170; with permission.)

TABLE 16.1
Studies demonstrating troponin as predictor of anticancer drug-induced cardiotoxicity

Study, Year	Patients (no.)	Cancer Type	Drugs	Troponin Type	Cutoff	Timing of Assessment
Lipshultz et al,[9] 1997	15[a]	ALL	AC	T	0.03 ng/mL	Before CT; 1–3 d after each dose
Cardinale et al,[10] 2000	201	Various	HD CT	I	0.04 ng/mL	0–12–24–36–72 h after CT
Cardinale et al,[11] 2002	232	Breast cancer	HD CT	I	0.04 ng/mL	0–12–24–36–72 h after CT
Auner et al,[12] 2002	30	Hematological	HD Cycl	T	0.03 ng/mL	Before CT; 1–14 d after CT
Sandri et al,[13] 2003	179	Various	HD CT	I	0.04 ng/mL	0–12–24–36–72 h after CT
Cardinale et al,[14] 2004	703	Various	HD CT	I	0.04 ng/mL	0–12–24–36–72 h after CT
Specchia et al,[15] 2005	79	Hematological	AC	I	0.15 ng/mL	Before CT; weekly × 4
Cardinale et al,[16] 2010	251	Breast cancer	TRZ	I	0.04 ng/mL	Before and after each cycle
Morris et al,[17] 2011	95	Breast cancer	AC + taxanes + TRZ/LAP	I	0.30 ng/mL	Every 2 wk during CT
Sawaya et al,[18] 2011	43	Breast cancer	AC + taxanes + TRZ	HS-I	0.015 ng/mL	Before CT; after 3 and 6 mo during CT
Sawaya et al,[19] 2012	81	Breast cancer	AC + taxane + TRZ	HS-I	30 pg/mL	Before CT; after 3 and 6 mo during CT
Ky et al,[20] 2014	78	Breast cancer	AC + taxanes + TRZ	HS-I	NA	Before CT; after 3 and 6 mo during CT

Abbreviations: AC, anthracycline-containing chemotherapy; ALL, acute lymphoblastic leukemia; CT, chemotherapy; Cycl, cyclophosphamide; HD, high dose; HS, ultrasensitive; I, troponin I; LAP, lapatinib; NA, not available; T, troponin T; TRZ, trastuzumab.
[a] Pediatric population.

well as its severity (Fig. 16.5).[10,11,14] The magnitude of cTnI elevation was on the order of 0.5 to 2.0 ng/mL (ie, 1–4 times the upper limit of reference), which is on the order of what is seen, for instance, with nonsevere myocarditis and small myocardial infarctions.

Troponin measurements are useful not only for the determination of cardiac toxicity induced by high-dose chemotherapy but also in prediction and monitoring of cardiac damage induced by standard dose chemotherapy.[12,15] In addition, increases in cTns are also observed in patients receiving newer anticancer drugs such as trastuzumab (Fig. 16.6). However, it has been debated whether this is due to trastuzumab itself or the interaction and unmasking of prior chemotherapy-induced myocardial injury as these drugs are often given in sequence in clinical practice. In agreement, most of the elevations are noted at baseline or with the first cycle. Still, even in these patients treated with different newer targeted cancer therapies, cTn

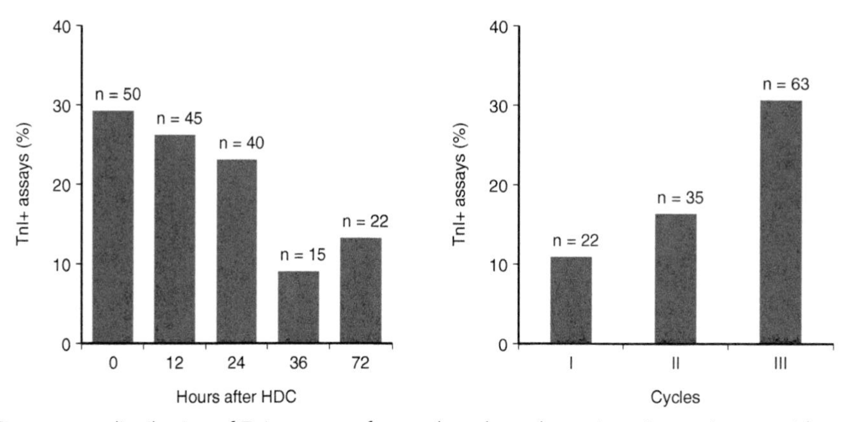

Fig. 16.2 Percentage distribution of TnI+ assays after each cycle at the various time points considered (*left*), and percentage distribution of TnI+ patients with breast cancer after each cycle of high-dose chemotherapy (HDC) (*right*). (*From* Cardinale D, Sandri MT, Martinoni A, et al. Myocardial injury revealed by plasma troponina I in breast cancer treated with high-dose chemotherapy. Ann Oncol 2002;13:710–5; with permission.)

elevation is predictive of development of late cardiac dysfunction and occurrence of cardiac events.[17] Data from the EIO group, in particular, suggest that cTnI identifies patients at risk of developing LV dysfunction (see Fig. 16.6). Moreover, cTnI helps to identify those patients who will less likely recover from toxicity despite heart failure treatments (see Fig. 16.6).[16] Interestingly, cTns provide important information also in the absence of detectable levels, helping to identify patients at low risk; in fact, the negative predictive value of cTns is in excess of 90% (Fig. 16.7). Finally, repeat assessment of cTn levels 1 month after chemotherapy allows for risk restratification of patients with cTn elevation during cancer therapy: those with persistent elevation represent the highest risk group, whereas those with normalization cTn levels by 1 month are at intermediate risk (Fig. 16.8).

Based on these data, cTns were given a central role in the European Society for Medical Oncology (ESMO) 2012 guidelines on the surveillance of patients undergoing chemotherapy with cardiotoxic agents (Fig. 16.9). Determination of cTnI at baseline and periodically during anticancer therapy gives the opportunity to schedule a strength surveillance of cardiac function in selected high-risk patients. On the other hand, the aforementioned high negative predictive value allows to safely identify patients at low risk, who could be excluded from the programs of long-term cardiac monitoring, with a respective lowering of costs.[23]

Currently, measurement of troponin levels only immediately before and immediately after each cycle seems to be effective and is transferable

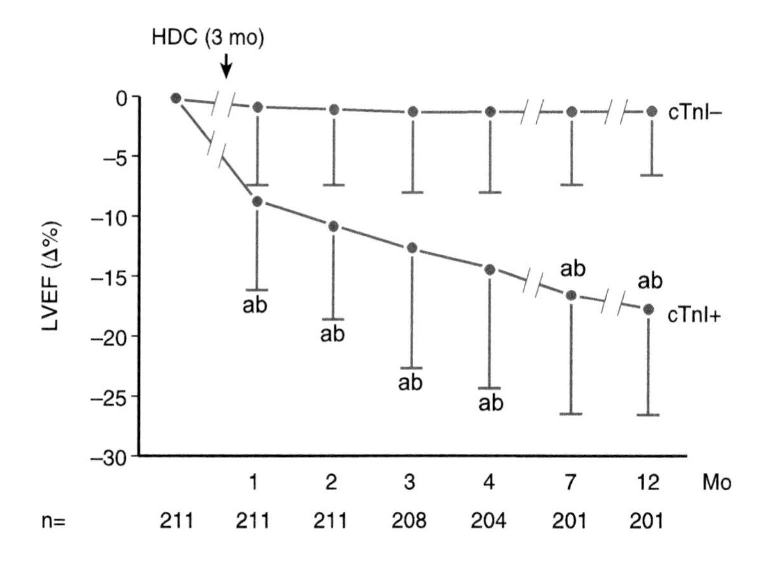

Fig. 16.3 LVEF percentage changes during the follow-up in TnI+ (*squares*) and TnI– (*circles*) patients. [a] $P<.001$ versus before HDC; [b] $P<.01$ versus TnI– group. (*From* Cardinale D, Sandri MT, Martinoni A, et al. Myocardial injury revealed by plasma troponina I in breast cancer treated with high-dose chemotherapy. Ann Oncol 2002;13:710–5; with permission.)

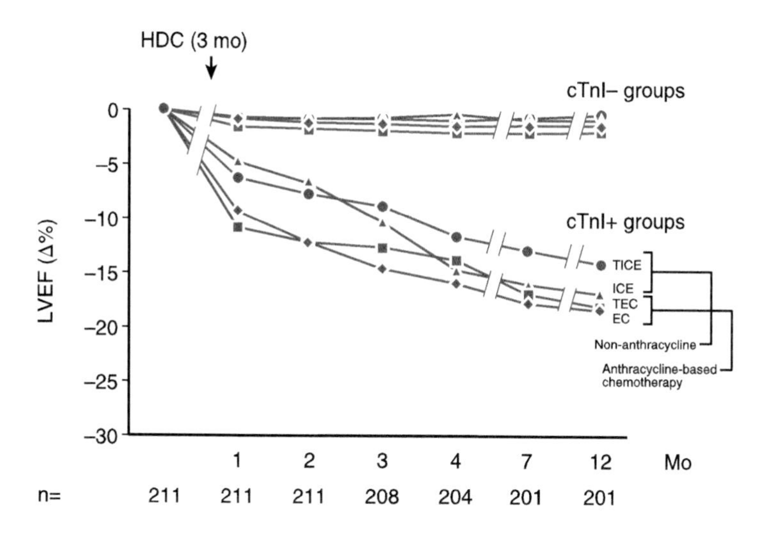

Fig. 16.4 LVEF pattern in TnI+ (*filled symbols*) and TnI– patients (*open symbols*), according to the 4 different chemotherapeutic regimens. EC, epirubicin–cyclophosphamide; ICE, ifosfamide–carboplatin–etoposide; TEC, taxotere–epirubicin–cyclophosphamide; TICE, taxotere–ifosfamide–carboplatin–etoposide. Standard deviations were omitted for clarity. (*From* Cardinale D, Sandri MT, Martinoni A, et al. Myocardial injury revealed by plasma troponina I in breast cancer treated with high-dose chemotherapy. Ann Oncol 2002;13:710–5; with permission.)

from research to clinical practice. Indeed, repeated troponin measurements and early treatment with cardioprotective agents, in patients showing increased levels, are very effective in preventing cardiac dysfunction and associated adverse events Indeed, in a randomized trial including 114 patients, showing persistent elevation of cTnI after chemotherapy, a treatment with enalapril, an angiotensin-converting enzyme inhibitor, prevented the development of cardiac dysfunction in all patients and significantly reduced the incidence of major adverse cardiac events[24] (Fig. 16.10).

However, there are still some limitations for the general use of cTns in clinical practice. Some studies failed to detect changes in troponins during or after anticancer treatments.[25,26] This could be related to different factors: various anticancer protocols used, varying times of sampling associated with different drugs administration schedule, lack of standardization of different assays, cardiac end-points definition and follow-up length taken into consideration, and imprecision in the estimation of LVEF.[27] Furthermore, one has to consider the possibility of cTn elevations not related to the myocardial injury caused by chemotherapy but other factors. Accordingly, patients with cancer may still have cTn elevation because of myocardial ischemia or pulmonary embolism or may have so-called false elevations because of liver function impairment. The development of HS assays, able to detect very low amounts of cTns in the systemic circulation, may be more problematic in this regard as most patients with cancer have, in fact, cTn levels just slightly above the cutoff values of upper limit of normal with the current levels. In the first study to use these new assays, neither an advantage

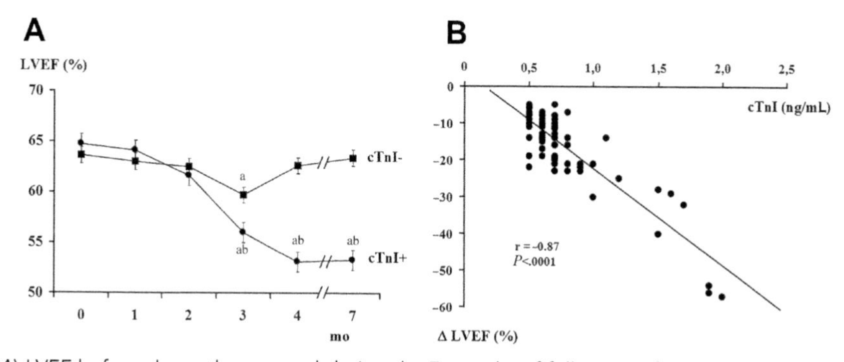

Fig. 16.5 (*A*) LVEF before chemotherapy and during the 7 months of follow-up of troponin I positive (cTnI+) and negative (cTnI–) patients. (*B*) Scatterplot of LVEF changes against troponin I value in cTnI+ patients. [a] $P<.001$ versus baseline (month 0); [b] $P<.001$ versus cTnI– group. (*Adapted from* Cardinale D, Sandri MT, Martinoni A, et al. Left ventricular dysfunction predicted by early troponin I release after high-dose chemotherapy. J Am Coll Cardiol 2000;36:517–22; with permission.)

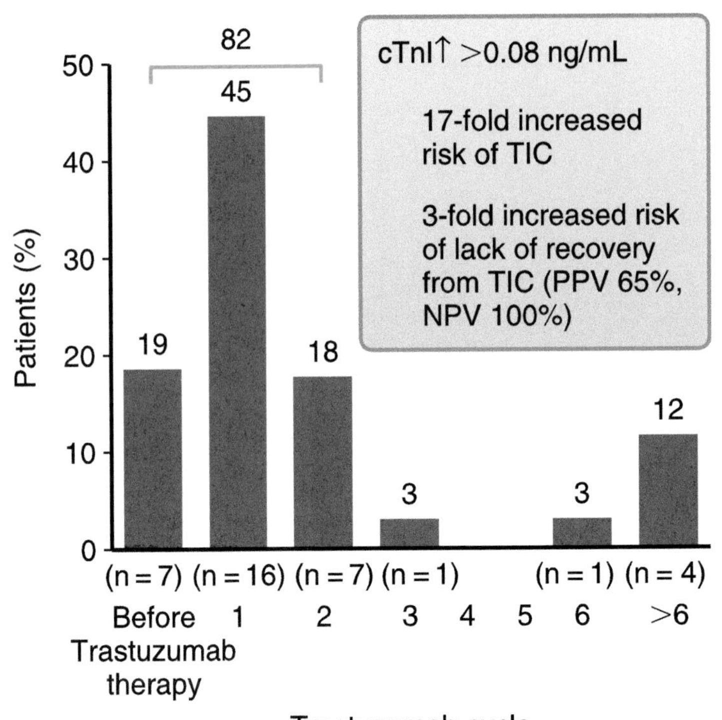

Fig. 16.6 Incidence of cTnI elevation in patients undergoing trastuzumab therapy and predictive value for trastuzumab-induced cardiomyopathy (TIC) and lack of recovery. NNV, negative predictive value; PPV, positive predictive value. (*From* Cardinale D, Colombo A, Torrisi R, et al. Trastuzumab-induced cardiotoxicity: clinical and prognostic implications of troponin I evaluation. J Clin Oncol 2010;28:3910–6; with permission.)

nor a disadvantage was noted. Decrease in peak longitudinal strain and increase in HS-troponin I levels were predictive of development of LV dysfunction.[19] Whether both parameters need to be obtained in routine clinical practice remains debatable. Furthermore, standardization of cTn assessment is needed; both are important areas for research in the future.

Natriuretic Peptides

Natriuretic peptides (ANP, BNP, and their NT fragments) are hormones produced by cardiomyocytes and released into the circulation in response to wall strain. They are involved in the maintenance of cardiovascular homeostasis, which includes regulation of electrolytes and water balance, inhibition of the renin-angiotensin

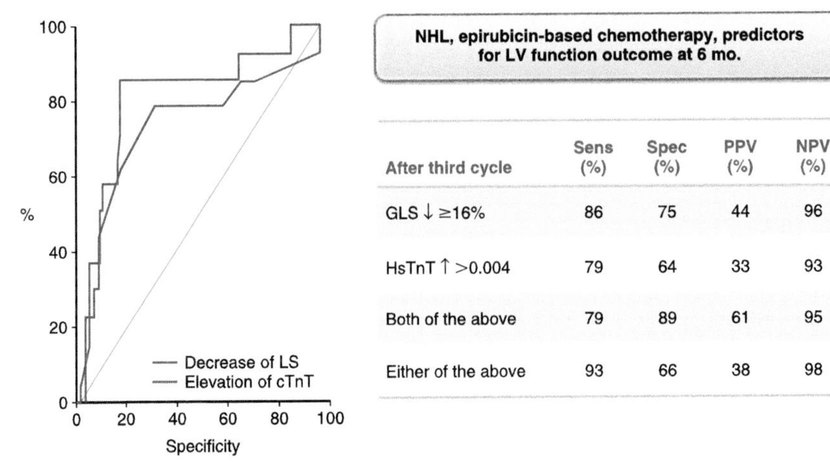

After third cycle	Sens (%)	Spec (%)	PPV (%)	NPV (%)
GLS ↓ ≥16%	86	75	44	96
HsTnT ↑ >0.004	79	64	33	93
Both of the above	79	89	61	95
Either of the above	93	66	38	98

Fig. 16.7 Diagnosis of CTRCD. LS, longitudinal strain; NHL, non-Hodgkin lymphoma; sens, sensitivity; spec, specificity. (*From* Kang Y, Xu X, Cheng L, et al. Two-dimensional speckle tracking echocardiography combined with high-sensitive cardiac troponin T in early detection and prediction of cardiotoxicity during epirubicine-based chemotherapy. Eur J Heart Fail 2014;16(3):300–8; with permission.)

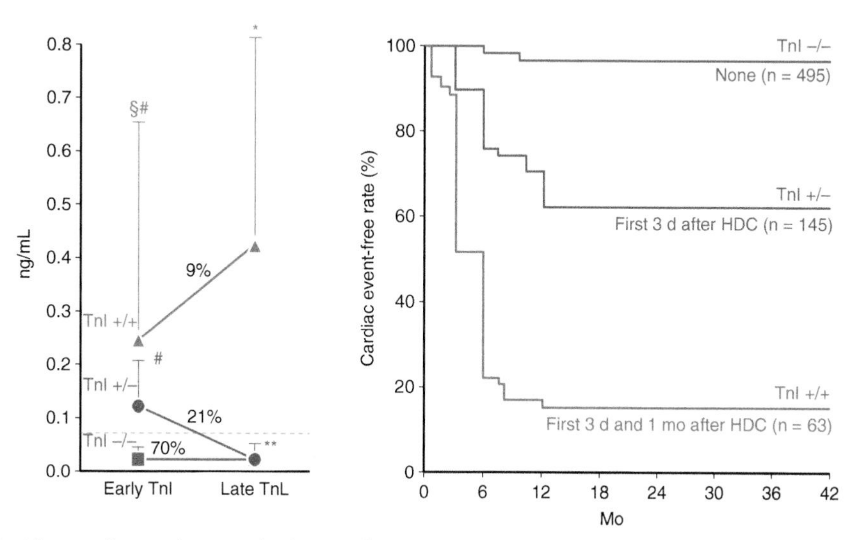

Fig. 16.8 Incidence of cTnI elevation by hours after start and cycles of HDC. HDC, high dose chemo-therapy. (*From* Cardinale D, Sandri MT, Colombo A, et al. Prognostic value of troponin I in cardiac risk stratification of cancer patients undergoing high-dose chemotherapy. Circulation 2004;109:2749–54; with permission.)

system, regulation of vascular permeability, and inhibition of the sympathetic nervous system. Because of their role in cardiovascular homeostasis, natriuretic peptides seem to play a pivotal role as markers of systolic dysfunction and myocardial damage.[28,29]

Indeed, BNP is a very important biomarker for diagnosis, prognosis, and evaluation of treatment efficacy in patients with heart failure. Intuitively, there has also been a high level of interest in investigating the role of natriuretic peptides in cardio-oncologic settings. In the 1990s, Suzuki and colleagues[30] first observed an association between persistent elevations of BNP and reduced cardiac tolerance to anticancer cardiotoxic drugs. In subsequent decades, many investigators observed that in patients with different malignancies, ages, and anticancer treatments, increased levels of natriuretic peptides were associated with cardiac dysfunction[26,31–33] (Table 16.2). Other groups demonstrated that early and persistent increases in BNP and NT-proBNP levels after anticancer treatment are predictive of late diastolic

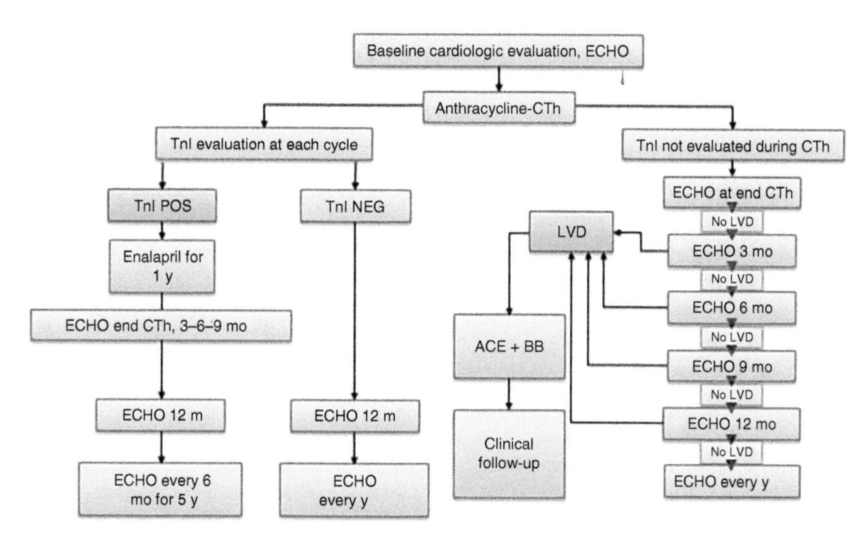

Fig. 16.9 Incidence of cTnI elevation by hours after start and cycles of HDC. BB, beta-blockers, CTh, chemo-therapy; ECHO, echocardiographic evaluation; LVD, left ventricular dysfunction; POS, positivity; y, year. (*From* Curigliano G, Cardinale D, Suter T, et al, ESMO Guidelines Working Group. Cardiovascular toxicity induced by chemotherapy, targeted agents and radiotherapy: ESMO Clinical Practice Guidelines. Ann Oncol 2012;23(Suppl 7):vii155–66; with permission.)

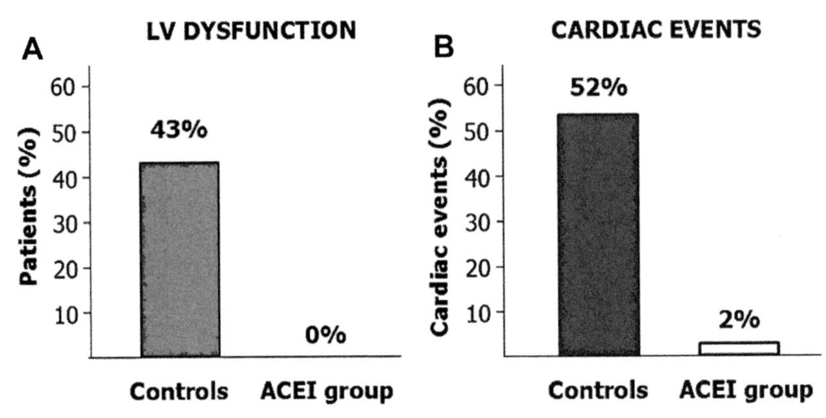

Fig. 16.10 (*A*) Percentage of patients developing cardiac dysfunction in Enalapril-treated group (angiotensin-converting enzyme inhibitor [ACEI] group) and in controls. (*B*) Incidence of cardiac events in patients treated with ACEI group and in controls. (*Adapted from* Cardinale D, Colombo A, Sandri MT, et al. Prevention of high-dose chemotherapy-induced cardiotoxicity in high-risk patients by angiotensin-converting enzyme inhibition. Circulation 2006;114:2474–81; with permission.)

and systolic LV dysfunction.[34] Increases in natriuretic peptides levels are predictive of left ventricular dysfunction also in patients treated with newer targeted therapies.[35,36] On the other hand, other investigators failed to reveal the clinical utility of natriuretic peptides in the same setting.[18] Therefore, despite available data, it is not yet possible to draw definite conclusions or indications for the clinical practice because of important limitations: small studies

TABLE 16.2
Studies demonstrating natriuretic peptides as predictor of anticancer drug-induced cardiotoxicity

Study, Year	Patients (no.)	Cancer Type	Drugs	Natriuretic Peptide Type	Timing of Assessment
Suzuki et al,[30] 1998	27	Hematological	AC	BNP	Before and after CT
Soker et al,[26] 2005	31[a]	Hematological	Doxorubicin	NT-proBNP	At least 1 mo after CT
Nousiainen et al,[31] 2002	28	Non-Hodgkin lymphoma	Doxorubicin	BNP	Baseline, before every treatment course and 4 wk after the last dose
Aggarwal et al,[32] 2007	37[a]	Various	AC	BNP	At least 1 y after CT
Mavinkurve-Groothuis et al,[33] 2009	122[a]	Various	AC	NT-proBNP	5 y after CT
Romano et al,[34] 2011	71	Breast cancer	AC	NT-proBNP	Before and 24 h after each cycle
Peric et al,[35] 2006	17	Breast cancer	TRZ	NT-proBNP	Before treatment, and after 4 and 6 cycles
Knobloch et al,[36] 2008	48	Breast cancer	TRZ	NT-proBNP	Before and after cycle

[a] Indicates pediatric population.

performed, different anticancer protocols used, use of different kinds of natriuretic peptides (BNP, NT-proBNP, ANP, NT-proANP), use of different immunoassays with no comparable values, different time sampling, and lack of standardized cardiac end points.

New prospective and multicenter studies, including large populations, using well-standardized methods for dosage and with well-defined timing of sampling and cardiac end points, are needed to define the appropriate use of natriuretic peptides in cardio-oncologic settings.

Other Proposed Biomarkers

Other biomarkers that have been proposed in the cardio-oncology setting include myeloperoxidase (MPO), an enzyme secreted by polymorphonuclear leukocytes and marker of oxidative stress. Some studies observed that MPO increases in patients treated with anticancer drugs, in particular with anthracyclines and trastuzumab. Placental growth factor (PlGF) and growth differentiation factor (GDF-15) have also gained interest. They belong to the same growth factor family and are released by different types of cells in response to ischemic, oxidative, and mechanical stress. PlGF seems to have prognostic value in pre-eclampsia and acute coronary syndrome, whereas GDF is associated with increased risk of heart failure,[20,37] but their role in cardio-oncology is not defined.

Because of the large number of mitochondria in myocardiocytes and the tight relationship linking oxidative metabolism with myocardial viability, mitochondrial dysfunction is considered as an expression of cardiotoxicity. Therefore, biomarkers related to mitochondrial dysfunction could be studied for monitoring the occurrence and extent of cardiac damage. Indeed, they could be investigated in the prevention of mitochondrial cardiotoxic effects of anticancer drugs. Among them, cytochrome C, mitochondrial DNA, and oxidized albumin seem to be early and reliable markers of mitochondrial dysfunction.[38]

Multiple-Marker Approach in Management of Cardiac Toxicity

In the complex field of drug-induced cardiac toxicity, an increasing number of biomarkers has been assessed, covering both the biochemical and imaging domain. Recently, different investigators have proposed evaluation strategies based on multiple-marker approaches.[19,20,37,39] The goal is to improve the positive predictive value as well as to provide novel insight into the mechanisms of drug-induced cardiac toxicity. Multimarker approach will aid in both stratification of risk and identification of more efficient strategies for cardioprotection.

ECHOCARDIOGRAPHY IN THE EVALUATION OF CARDIAC STRUCTURE AND FUNCTION IN PATIENTS WITH CANCER UNDERGOING TREATMENT

Echocardiography is a key diagnostic tool to assess cardiac structure and function in the care of patients with cancer before, during, and after chemotherapy or radiotherapy (RT).[40] This modality is preferred because it is noninvasive, radiation free, easily available, and cost-effective. It provides information of LV systolic and diastolic function and assesses cardiac valves and the pericardium.[40] Recently, 3-dimensional (3D) echocardiography (3DE) and 2-dimensional (2D) speckle-tracking echocardiography (2D-STE) have emerged to further enhance the role of this technique in the serial evaluation of LV function[41] and for the early detection of subclinical LV dysfunction.[42]

LVEF is an important parameter in monitoring algorithms for cancer therapeutics–related cardiac dysfunction (CTRCD)[43] and to guide the decision process in patients under cancer therapy.[44] Therefore, it is important that the assessment of LVEF is accurate with minimal temporal variability.

The 2D assessment of ejection fraction (EF) has high intermeasurement variability (10%, range 9.1–11.8),[41] and this magnitude of variability is similar to the 10% drop in LVEF, which defines CTRCD. According to the Joint Consensus from the American Society of Echocardiography (ASE) and the European Association of Cardiovascular Imaging (EACVI), CTRCD is defined as a decrease in the LVEF of greater than 10%, to a value less than 53%.[43,45] To be able to detect a 10% change in EF with confidence, the measurement technique should have intermeasurement variability less than 10%, making 2D echocardiography (2DE) a less reliable method for the detection of CTRCD.

Using cardiac magnetic resonance (CMR) imaging as the gold standard, several studies have shown that 3D echocardiographic measurements of LV volumes and EF have better accuracy,[46–49] better reproducibility,[41,50] and lower temporal variability,[41] compared with 2DE. This advantage rises from the fact that 3DE measurements do not rely on geometric assumptions, are not affected by foreshortened views,[51] and are quantified by an automated border-tracking algorithm.[52] In the breast cancer setting for serial monitoring of LVEF, the correlation of 3DE with CMR (end-diastolic volume [EDV] $r = 0.87$ at baseline; $r = 0.82$ at 6 months; and $r = 0.95$ at 12 months; end-systolic volume [ESV] $r = 0.89$ at baseline; $r = 0.87$ at 6 months; and $r = 0.93$ at 12 months; EF $r = 0.91$ at baseline; $r = 0.97$ at 6 months; and $r = 0.90$ at 12 months) was significantly higher than 2DE approach (EDV $r = 0.64$ at baseline; $r = 0.50$ at 6 months; and $r = 0.69$ at 12 months; ESV $r = 0.55$ at baseline; $r = 0.40$ at 6 months; and $r = 0.59$ at 12 months; EF $r = 0.31$ at baseline; $r = 0.53$ at 6 months; and $r = 0.42$ at 12 months) for all measurements. Comparison between RT3D TTE and cardiac MRI are show in Fig. 16.11.[49] In contrast, a cross-sectional study comparing CMR imaging and 3DE found that patients with reduced LVEF are underestimated with 3DE (Fig. 16.12).[53] The current group consensus[43] has suggested that 3DE should be the preferred imaging modality for monitoring LV systolic function in patients with cancer.

When 3DE is not available, or when the image quality is suboptimal, 2DE-modified biplane Simpson's method with the use of ultrasound contrast agents has been shown to improve the accuracy and reproducibility of LV volumes and EF measurements.[54,55] However, these agents have not been shown to have incremental value when combined with 3DE; thus, it has not been recommended in conjunction with 3DE for serial follow-up of patients with cancer.[43]

2D-STE is an accurate imaging technique that measures myocardial deformation (strain and strain rate [SR]) in all 3 domains of contractility (longitudinal, circumferential, and radial) independent of the translational motion of the heart (Fig. 16.13).[56,57] Moreover, it has incremental prognostic value over EF for the prediction of all-cause mortality in the general population[58] as well as in the prediction of CTRCD in patients undergoing cancer therapy.[59] Importantly, 2D-STE is easy to perform and reproducible when performed by expert operators on images with good quality. The interobserver and intraobserver variability for the relative mean error for global longitudinal strain (GLS) values ranged from 4.9% to 8.6%.[60] This mean error is lower than for LVEF.

The ability of 2D-STE–derived strain and SR to detect subclinical LV dysfunction and predict subsequent CTRCD and to detect late

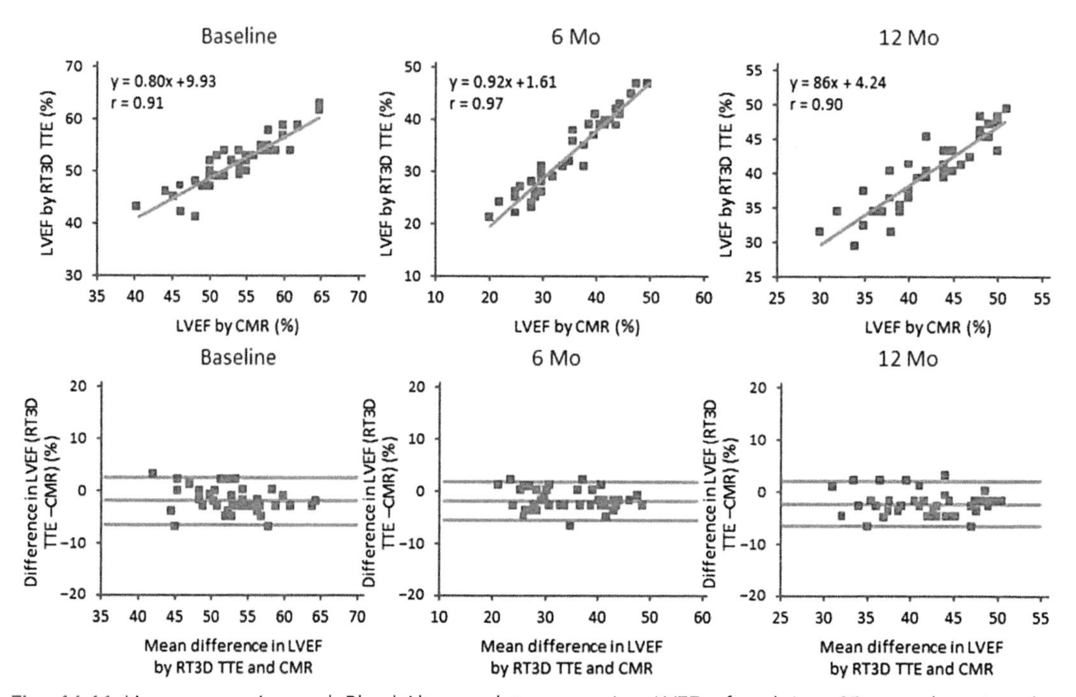

Fig. 16.11 Linear regression and Bland-Altman plots comparing LVEF of real-time 3D transthoracic echocardiography (RT3D TTE) versus CMR imaging at baseline, 6 months and 12 months. (*From* Walker J, Bhullar N, Fallah-Rad N, et al. Role of three-dimensional echocardiography in breast cancer: comparison with two-dimensional echocardiography, multiple-gated acquisition scans, and cardiac magnetic resonance imaging. J Clin Oncol 2010;28(21):3429–36; with permission.)

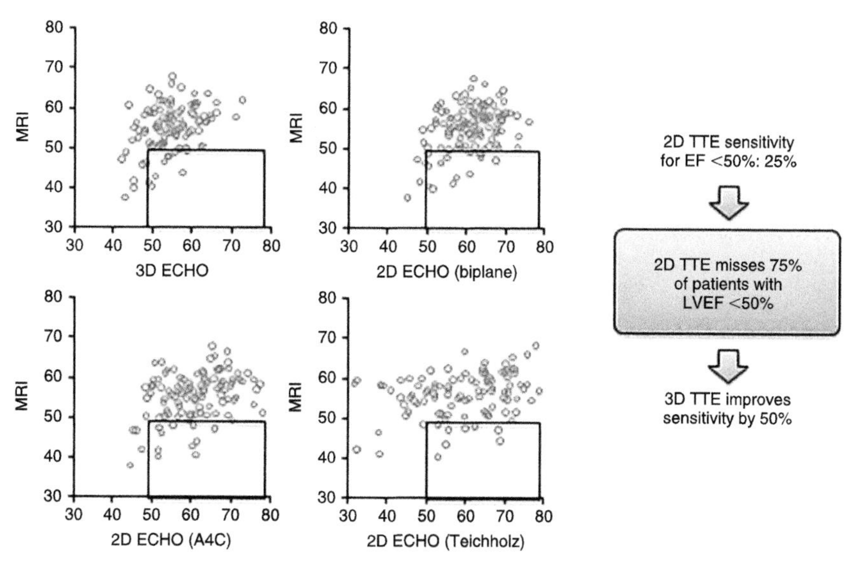

Fig. 16.12 Assessment of LVEF by different transthoracic echocardiogram (TTE) techniques versus cardiac MRI. A4C, apical 4-chamber; ECHO, echocardiography; 2D, two-dimensional; 3D, three-dimensional. (*From* Armstrong GT, Plana JC, Zhang N, et al. Screening adult survivors of childhood cancer for cardiomyopathy: comparison of echocardiography and cardiac magnetic resonance imaging. J Clin Oncol 2012;30(23):2876–84; with permission.)

consequences of cancer therapy has been extensively investigated, especially in breast cancer and hematological malignancies treated with anthracycline therapy, with or without trastuzumab. The decrease in strain during or early after anthracycline therapy[61–63] has been shown to occur before a drop in LVEF, with peak systolic GLS being the most sensitive

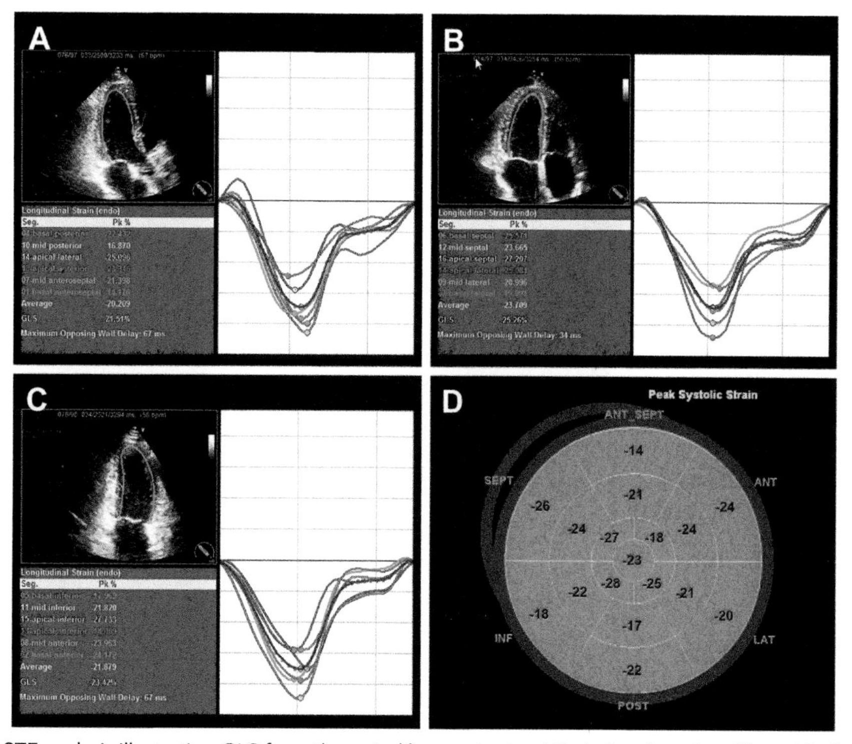

Fig. 16.13 STE analysis illustrating GLS from the apical long-axis view (*A*), 4-chamber view (*B*), and 2-chamber view (*C*) using TomTec 2D cardiac performance analysis, and bull's-eye plot (*D*) in a patient with Hodgkin lymphoma before receiving anthracycline based–chemotherapy. Each segment has a numeric and color-coded strain value.

parameter of the deformation markers. This signal has also been seen in patients undergoing treatment with vascular endothelial growth factor inhibitors for renal cell and colorectal metastatic cancer.[64] Kang and colleagues[39] reported in patients with non-Hodgkin lymphoma that GLS ($-18.48 \pm 1.72\%$ vs $-15.96 \pm 1.6\%$) was significantly reduced and HS cTnT was elevated from 0.0010 ± 0.0020 to 0.0073 ± 0.0038 ng/mL ($P<.01$ for all), whereas LVEF remained within normal limits at the completion of epirubicin-based chemotherapy compared with baseline (Fig. 16.14).

The prognostic value of early measurements of strain in the prediction of CTRCD has major importance for clinical practice. Early reduction in GLS in patients treated with anthracycline mostly followed by trastuzumab is the most robust predictor of CTRCD, compared with radial or circumferential strain.[18,19,59,65–67] A relative percentage reduction greater than 15% of GLS from the baseline has been shown to be the best predictor of CTRCD,[59] and this is specified in the ASE/EACVI consensus document (Fig. 16.15).[43]

In long-term cancer survivors receiving anthracycline, cross-sectional studies detected a decrease in GLS compared with age-matched healthy control patients.[68–70] RT also affects myocardial deformation. Tsai and colleagues[71] reported that patients who had received anthracycline and chest RT had a significantly reduced GLS compared with those who had undergone RT alone.

The aforementioned expert consensus statement from the ASE and the EACVI[43] recommends 2D-STE as the imaging technique of choice for detection of subclinical LV dysfunction in patients receiving cancer therapy and emphasizes the need for strain imaging during baseline assessment and follow-up. A distinction is made between agents causing type I and those associated with type II CTRCD, and the algorithms recommended for cardiac surveillance are summarized in Figs. 16.16–16.18.

A realistic limitation to the use of strain imaging in clinical practice has been intervendor variability. However, Farsalinos and colleagues[60] recently published a study comparing GLS measurements among 9 different vendors. Their main findings were absolute values of the averaged GLS ranging from −18.0% (3.4) to −21.5% (4.0) with a maximum absolute difference between vendors for GLS of 3.7% strain units, a strong correlation among them (R^2 between 0.84 and 0.89), and the Bland-Altman test revealed no value-dependent bias. The authors think that an absolute change greater than 3.7% in GLS will yield a high likelihood of showing a change in systolic function. The same machine and software version should be used for serial studies to assure comparability because of moderate but statistically significant variation between vendors. Another questionable pitfall of strain imaging is the load dependency of this measurement. Some studies have shown that afterload can influence strain, and strain rate values to a less extent, but this has been controversial.[72,73] Studies from the authors' group

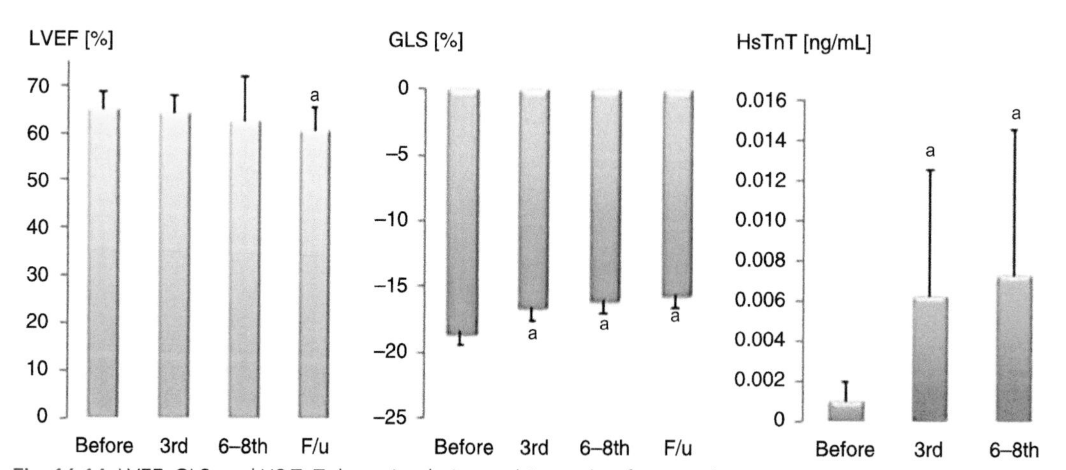

Fig. 16.14 LVEF, GLS, and HS TnT dynamics during and 6 months after epirubicin-based chemotherapy. [a] $P<.05$ vs baseline. F/U, follow-up. (*From* Kang Y, Xu X, Cheng L, et al. Two-dimensional speckle tracking echocardiography combined with high-sensitive cardiac troponin T in early detection and prediction of cardiotoxicity during epirubicine-based chemotherapy. Eur J Heart Fail 2014;16(3):300–8; with permission.)

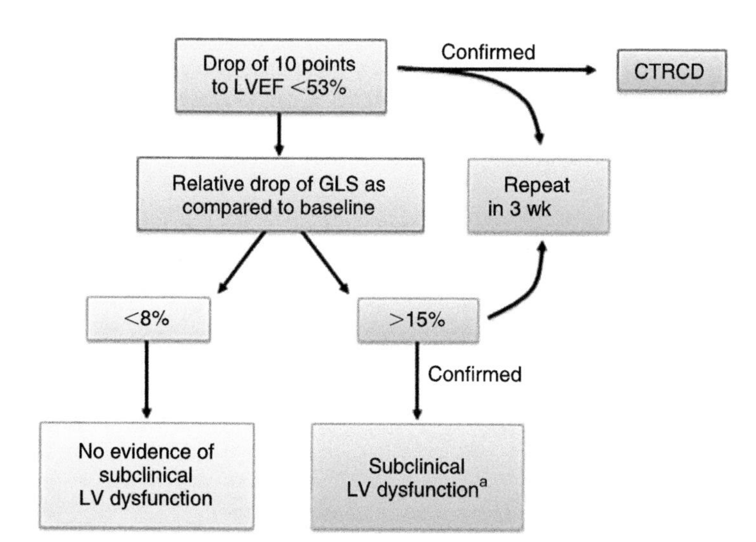

Fig. 16.15 Diagnosis of CTRCD. [a] The data supporting the initiation of cardioprotection for the treatment of subclinical LV dysfunction are limited. (*From* Plana JC, Galderisi M, Barac A, et al. Expert consensus for multimodality imaging evaluation of adult patients during and after cancer therapy: a report from the American Society of Echocardiography and the European Association of Cardiovascular Imaging. J Am Soc Echocardiogr 2014;27(9):911–96; with permission.)

(preliminary data) in patients with breast cancer have not shown that GLS is affected by preload and afterload parameters in a 2-year follow-up.

LV diastolic function conventionally assessed by Doppler and tissue Doppler techniques plays a limited role in the oncologic setting. Changes in E and e′ velocities may reflect alterations in loading conditions because of side effects associated with the chemotherapy instead of being a consequence of diastolic dysfunction.[74] Moreover, an early reduction in indexes of diastolic function in patients receiving anthracycline have not shown to be prognostic for CTRCD.[18,69]

In radiation-induced heart disease, 2DE is the method of choice for evaluating the wide range of effects, such as pericardial disease (constrictive pericarditis, pericardial effusion), valvular heart disease, and myocardial disease.[75] It is highly sensitive in detecting small amounts of pericardial effusion as well as in detecting any degree of valvular heart disease. The typical echocardiographic features of valve disease include calcification of the aortic root, aortic valve, intervalvular fibrosa, and mitral valve.[75,76] The prevalence of valve disease increases with time following irradiation and is significantly higher at 20 years after RT.[75–77] Coronary artery disease could manifest at an early age and generally 10 years after radiation exposure.[77] Stress echocardiography could be a useful tool for its diagnosis.

In summary, monitoring of LVEF by echocardiography, ideally 3DE, is a very useful strategy

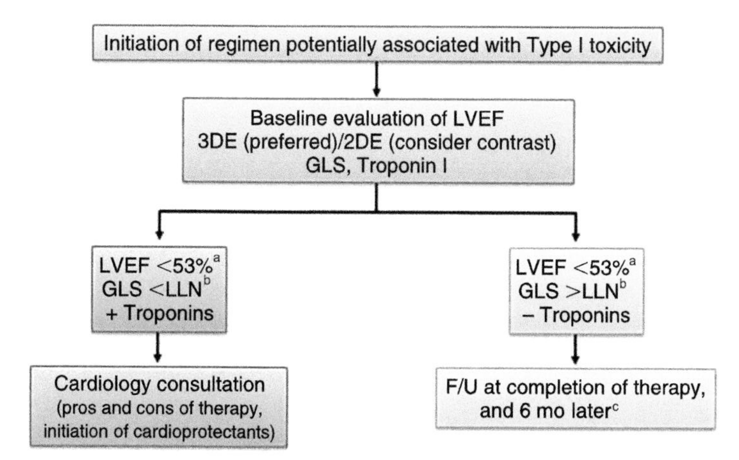

Fig. 16.16 Cardiac surveillance with chemotherapy with type I toxicity. [a] Consider confirmation with CMR. [b] LLN, lower limit of normal. [c] If the dose is higher than 240 mg/m^2 (or its equivalent), recommend measurement of LVEF, GLS, and troponin before each additional 50 mg/m^2. (*From* Plana JC, Galderisi M, Barac A, et al. Expert Consensus for multimodality imaging evaluation of adult patients during and after cancer therapy: a report from the American Society of Echocardiography and the European Association of Cardiovascular Imaging. J Am Soc Echocardiogr 2014;27(9):911–96; with permission.)

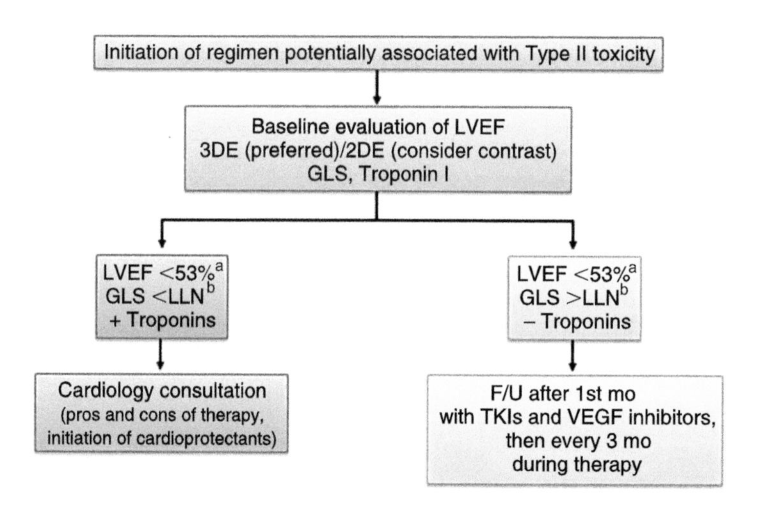

Fig. 16.17 Cardiac surveillance with chemotherapy with type II toxicity. [a] Consider confirmation with CMR. [b] LLN, Lower limit of normal. (*From* Plana JC, Galderisi M, Barac A, et al. Expert consensus for multimodality imaging evaluation of adult patients during and after cancer therapy: a report from the American Society of Echocardiography and the European Association of Cardiovascular Imaging. J Am Soc Echocardiogr 2014;27(9):911–96; with permission.)

to detect CTRCD during and after the administration of cancer therapy. GLS by 2D-STE is the best deformation parameter for the early detection of subclinical LV dysfunction and as a tool to initiate cardioprotective medication. Prospective studies with long-term follow-up are important to address whether the early deformation measurements will predict persistent decreases in LVEF or symptomatic heart failure. Echocardiography can also aid in the diagnosis of complications due to RT.

CARDIOVASCULAR MAGNETIC RESONANCE

Therapies for cancer may promote type I and II cardiotoxicity that involve LV systolic and diastolic dysfunction, decrements in LV mass, and increases in aortic stiffening. Type I cardiotoxicity, traditionally associated with anthracycline chemotherapy, is a dose-dependent injury that is associated with irreversible damage to the myocytes, whereas type II cardiotoxicity (traditionally associated with trastuzumab) is not dose-dependent and is often reversible.[43,78,79] CMR is an imaging methodology that allows one to assess the left ventricle (volumes, ejection fraction, mass, contractility), myocardial tissue characteristics, and aortic pulse wave velocity or distensibility (measures of aortic stiffness) during a single imaging session without exposure to ionizing radiation.[80] Contraindications to using this technology include ferromagnetic implants or fragments, cardiac pacemakers or devices, certain breast tissue expanders, or known claustrophobia[81]; also those receiving gadolinium (Gd)-enhanced contrast examinations should be screened for renal dysfunction (avoid,

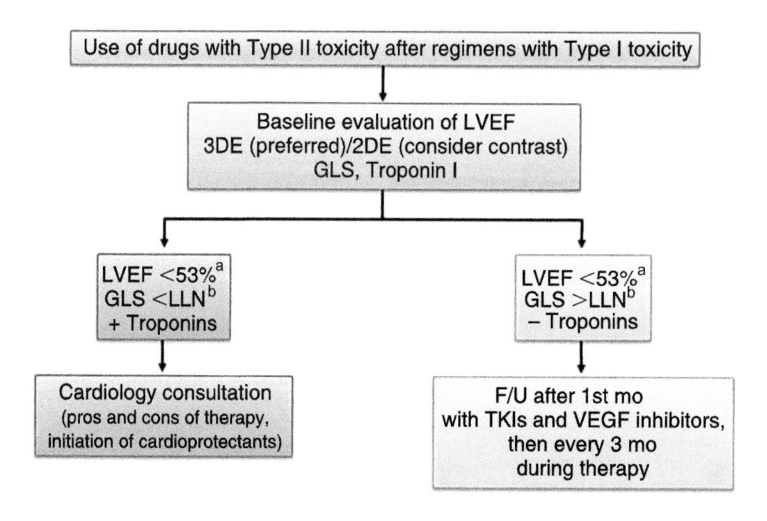

Fig. 16.18 Cardiac surveillance with chemotherapy with type II toxicity after treatment with type I toxicity agents. [a] Consider confirmation with CMR. [b] LLN, Lower limit of normal. TKI, tyrosine kinase inhibitor. (*From* Plana JC, Galderisi M, Barac A, et al. Expert consensus for multimodality imaging evaluation of adult patients during and after cancer therapy: a report from the American Society of Echocardiography and the European Association of Cardiovascular Imaging. J Am Soc Echocardiogr 2014;27(9):911–96; with permission.)

because of the risk of nephrogenic systemic fibrosis, in patients on dialysis, estimated glomerular filtration rate [eGFR] <30 mL/min/1.73 m^2 not on dialysis, and eGFR <40 mL/min/1.73 m^2 while in-patient).[82,83] This chapter reviews the use of CMR to identify cancer therapy associated type I and II cardiotoxicity, changes in myocardial mass and tissue characteristics, and increases in aortic stiffness.

Structural and Functional Assessments

Cardiac function—left ventricular ejection fraction

LVEF is the most widely used noninvasive imaging marker of systolic dysfunction associated with type I and type II cardiotoxicity.[84] Radionuclide ventriculography (RNV), 2D and 3D echocardiography, and CMR are regularly used to assess LVEF.[4,41,49,80,85] With CMR, cine imaging of the left ventricle with steady-state free-precession in multiple nonoverlapping short-axis planes covering the LV cavity from mitral plane to the cardiac apex are used for LVEF quantification (Fig. 16.19). After end-systolic and EDVs are identified using LV endocardial contours in each slice, the volumes are added by Simpson's rule to provide the cavity volumes for LVEF calculation.[80,85]

Serial monitoring of LVEF with CMR is particularly advantageous due to its high resolution, reproducibility, and accuracy compared with echocardiography.[86,87] The sensitivity of CMR to detect a 3% change in LVEF would require a sample size of 15 participants, representing an 85% reduction in sample size required to detect the same change by echocardiography (Table 16.3).[88]

Early subclinical declines in LVEF after receipt of treatment of cancer have been identified with CMR.[86,87,89] Importantly, declines in LVEF have been observed within 6 months of anthracycline receipt and were independent of cumulative dose.[86] More research is necessary to determine the relative importance and cause of these early changes in LVEF, and whether these early LVEF changes relate to long-term measures of LVEF in cancer survivors. Although LVEF monitoring algorithms with echocardiography and RNV have been proposed, these have yet to be proposed with CMR imaging.[43,90–97]

Cardiac structure—left ventricular volumes and mass

Measurements of LVEF are derived from calculation of the EDV and ESV. As shown in Fig. 16.20, declines in LVEF from 60% to 52% could be from potential reductions in EDV or increases in ESV. Identifying the changes in these volumes (and their indices normalized to body surface area) should support clinical decisions regarding the withholding of treatment due to LVEF drop. A reduction in the EDV may signal either hypovolemia from poor oral intake and nausea, which many patients undergoing cancer therapies experience, or early diastolic dysfunction. Cardiotoxic effects on the contractility of the myocytes and systolic function of the left ventricle may manifest as an increase in the ESV. In addition, other conditions such as sepsis could also impair LV systolic function and raise ESV and LVEF independent of cardiomyocyte injury from chemotherapy. Thus, when reporting LVEF declines in patients treated for cancer, it is important to evaluate the component measures of

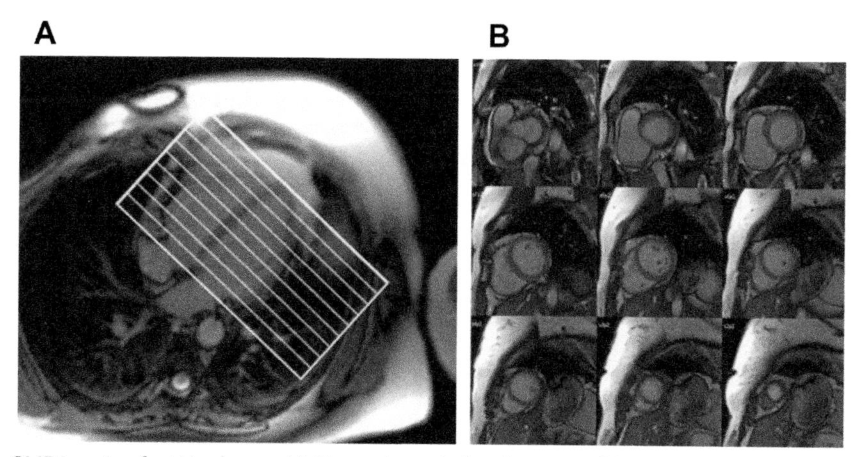

Fig. 16.19 CMR imaging for LV volumes. (*A*) Planned on a 4-chamber view of the left ventricle. (*B*) Contiguous short-axis slices covering the left ventricle are acquired for ventricular volume quantification and calculation of LVEF.

TABLE 16.3
Reduction in sample size by imaging modality for 90% power with $P<.05$

Measure	Clinical Change	Echo (no.)	CMR (no.)	Reduction in Sample Size (%)
EDV	10 mL	121	12	90
ESV	10 mL	53	10	81
EF	3%	102	15	85
Mass	10 g	273	9	97

From Bellenger NG, Davies LC, Francis JM, et al. Reduction in sample size for studies of remodeling in heart failure by the use of cardiovascular magnetic resonance. J Cardiovasc Magn Reson 2000;2(4):276; with permission.

LVEF (EDV and ESV) to gain insight into mechanisms associated with the decline. For example, individuals experiencing declines in LVEF due to reductions in EDV may need intravascular volume resuscitation as opposed to discontinuation of their chemotherapy due to cardiotoxicity.

LV mass measured with CMR may provide important insights into loss of myocytes and diminished myocyte size associated with many cancer therapies resulting in reduced LV mass (**Box 16.1**). In particular, myocellular death by doxorubicin chemotherapy is mediated by topoisomerase-IIβ, causing oxidative stress or apoptosis through the mitochondrial pathway from reactive oxygen species production,[98,99] DNA oxidant damage,[100] and downregulation of myocellular GATA4 expression.[101–103] In addition, diminished myocyte size in the setting of cancer and anthracycline therapies[104,105] and inhibition of myocyte turnover in the presence of diffuse cellular death and fibrosis[106,107] may be key contributors to LV atrophic remodeling and reduced LV mass. Although early transient increases in LV mass index have been observed in several studies,[108,109] LV mass reductions may occur late after cancer therapy when most cardio-oncology patients have completed standard CV monitoring.[53,110–112] Importantly, reductions in LV mass are associated with an increased risk of future cardiac events independent of cumulative anthracycline dose (**Fig. 16.21**).[110]

Ventricular function—strain imaging

Myocardial strain is a functional measurement of the deformation, or contractility, of myocardial tissue. CMR strain imaging is most often accomplished in CMR imaging with either displacement encoding with stimulated echoes CMR or spatial modulation of magnetization to measure the Eulerian circumferential strain (**Fig. 16.22**).[113–117]

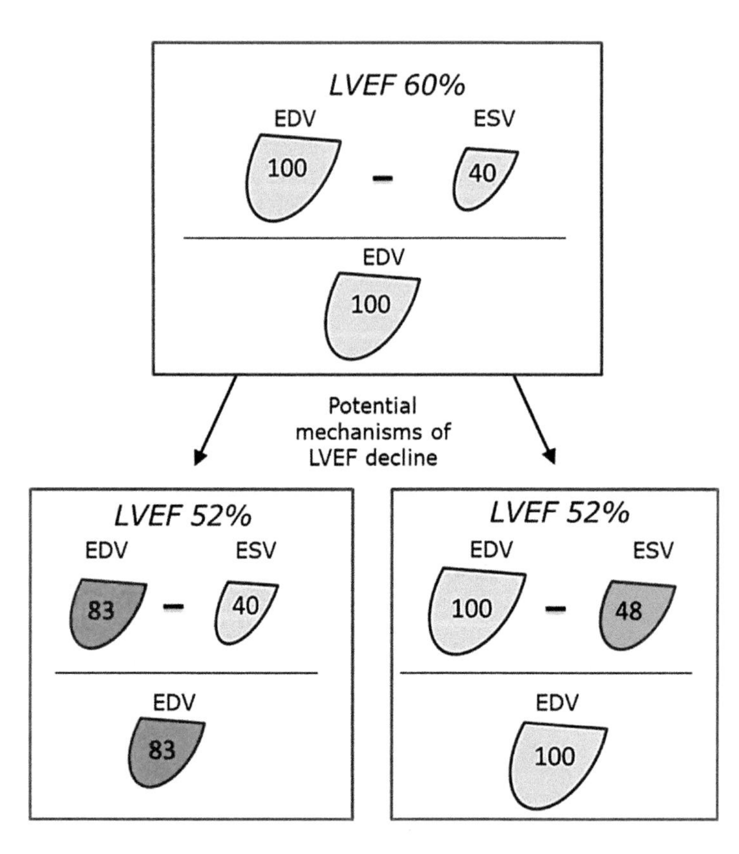

Fig. 16.20 LV volume changes leading to decrement in LVEF. LVEF is calculated by measuring the left ventricular EDV and subtracting the left ventricular ESV and then dividing by the EDV. As shown in the top cartoon with an EDV of 100 and an ESV of 40, a resultant LVEF of 60% is achieved. As shown, LVEF can decline to 52% through 1 of 2 primary mechanisms. As shown on the left, the EDV may decline from 100 mL to 83 mL while the ESV remains constant at 40 mL. This situation is reflective of intravascular hypovolemia and a decreased LV preload. In patients with cancer, this can be associated with poor oral intake, nausea, vomiting, or diarrhea. Alternatively on the right, the ESV may increase to 48 mL with the EDV remaining constant at 100 mL. Declines in LVEF due to increases in ESV are more likely associated with impairments of LV myocardial contractility, one of the hallmarks of cardiotoxicity after the administration of chemotherapy.

BOX 16.1
Mechanisms of left ventricular mass decline after cancer therapy

- Apoptosis from reactive oxygen species production, DNA damage, altered GATA4 expression
- Diminished myocyte size
- Inhibited myocyte turnover

Several studies have observed significant changes in myocardial strain 3 months after doxorubicin treatment.[86,118] Furthermore, in individuals treated with low-to-moderate doses of anthracyclines, a significant increase in circumferential strain (loss of contractility) occurred during a period of no or subclinical declines in LVEF.[86] In studies using transthoracic echocardiography, an early reduction of 10% to 15% in GLS is predictive of LVEF decline or heart failure used to diagnose cardiotoxicity.[42]

Vascular function—phase contrast imaging and angiography

Phase contrast–CMR (PC-CMR) may be used to measure aortic pulse wave velocity, compliance, or distensibility, all measures of aortic stiffness (Fig. 16.23).[119] With aging, the aorta stiffens, thereby reducing compliance and distensibility, and increasing the pulse wave velocity of blood ejected from the left ventricle.[120,121] Measures of increased aortic stiffening are associated with future CV events.[121–123] CMR measures of pulse wave velocity and distensibility have been shown to occur 1 to 6 months following initiation of potentially cardiotoxic chemotherapy.[86,124,125] At present, the implications of the findings of these relatively small studies are unknown. However, given the independent association of abnormal aortic stiffness with CV events in other disease processes, future research in larger multicenter studies is needed to determine if these single-center observations are reproducible, reversible, or associated with adverse CV events in individuals receiving treatment for cancer.

Myocardial tissue characterization

After receipt of anthracycline-based chemotherapy, early intracellular and extracellular myocardial edema occur in association with myocyte injury. This histopathologic feature is a hallmark of cardiotoxicity. Should the injury progress, myocellular death ensues followed by increased collagen deposition, reduced contractile performance, and LV remodeling—all resulting in a decline in LVEF.[126,127] Although echocardiography and RVN may appreciate changes in LVEF after potentially cardiotoxic chemotherapy, these modalities miss the opportunity to detect the early, reversible manifestations of myocardial injury associated with intracellular and extracellular edema and the subsequent development of myocardial fibrosis.[128,129] CMR technologies based on appreciating the behavior of hydrogen protons within a magnetic field possess the ability to characterize myocardial tissue that results from receipt of potentially cardiotoxic chemotherapy. Together with structural and functional measures, these tissue characterization techniques may further enhance one's ability to identify the cardiotoxic manifestations of cancer-treatment regimens.

Identifying myocardial tissue characteristics with CMR relies on measurement of intrinsic LV

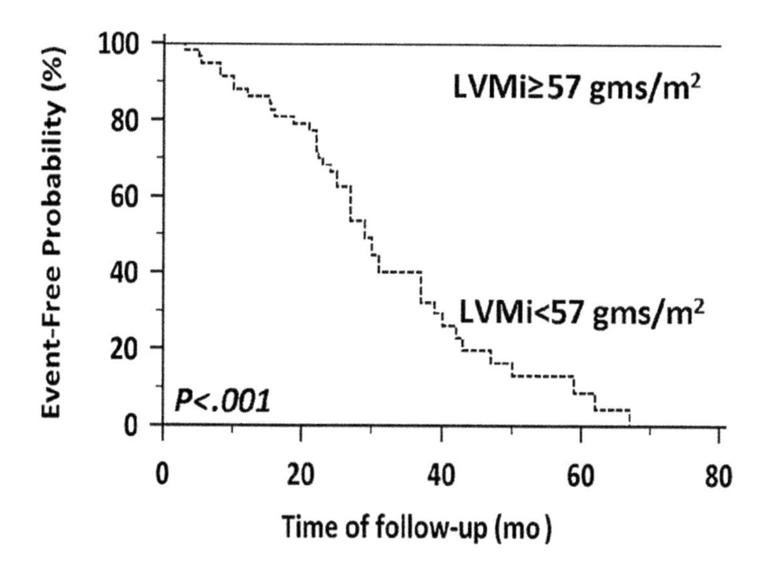

Fig. 16.21 Reduced LV mass is associated with cardiac events in cancer survivors. Anthracycline-treated cancer survivors with an indexed left ventricular mass (LVMi) <57 g/m^2 are at greater risk for future cardiac events. (*From* Neilan TG, Coelho-Filho OR, Pena-Herrera D, et al. Left ventricular mass in patients with a cardiomyopathy after treatment with anthracyclines. Am J Cardiol 2012;110(11):1684; with permission.)

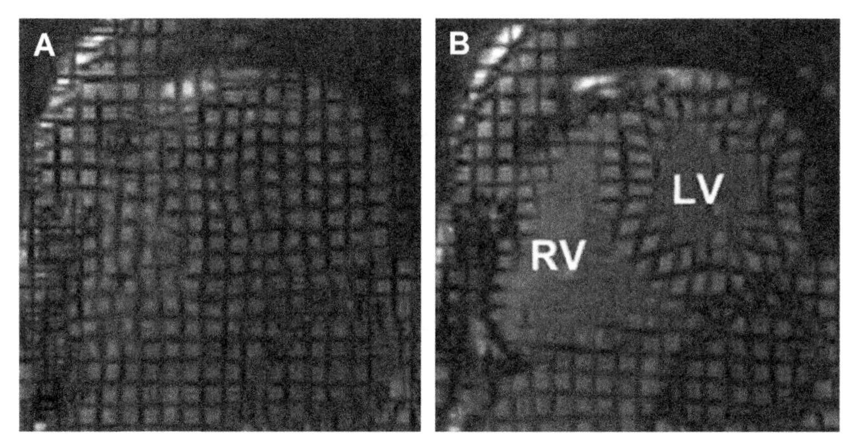

Fig. 16.22 Example of short-axis grid tagged images during cardiac cycle for myocardial strain quantification. Typically, tagging is applied just before contraction starts (end diastole, *A*). Because the taglines are a temporary property of the tissue, taglines move along with the tissue in which they are created. The lines will deform if the myocardium contracts (*B*), and become undeformed during relaxation. LV, left ventricle, RV, right ventricle. (*From* Götte MJW, Germans T, Rüssel IK, et al. Myocardial strain and torsion quantified by cardiovascular magnetic resonance tissue tagging: studies in normal and impaired left ventricular function. JACC 2006;48(10):2004; with permission.)

tissue properties, including T1 and T2 relaxation. The first time constant, T1 relaxation, is the longitudinal recovery of magnetization in the tissue to equilibrium after an applied radiofrequency pulse, whereas the second time constant, T2 relaxation, is transverse decay of magnetization in the tissue. Imaging sequences that "weight" the contributions of these time constants produce a variety of tissue contrasts in images.[130] Qualitative T_1-weighted and T_2-weighted CMR techniques have been successful in identifying inflammation and edema—the histopathologic changes that occur in early cardiotoxicity after receipt of anthracycline-based chemotherapy.[131–133] Increased myocardial T1 using a variety of CMR imaging or spectroscopy techniques has been associated with cancer treatment–related edema, inflammation, intracellular vacuolization, and extracellular matrix fibrosis in small-animal and single-center human studies.[87,134–137] In contrast-enhanced T_1-weighted images, myocardial relative signal

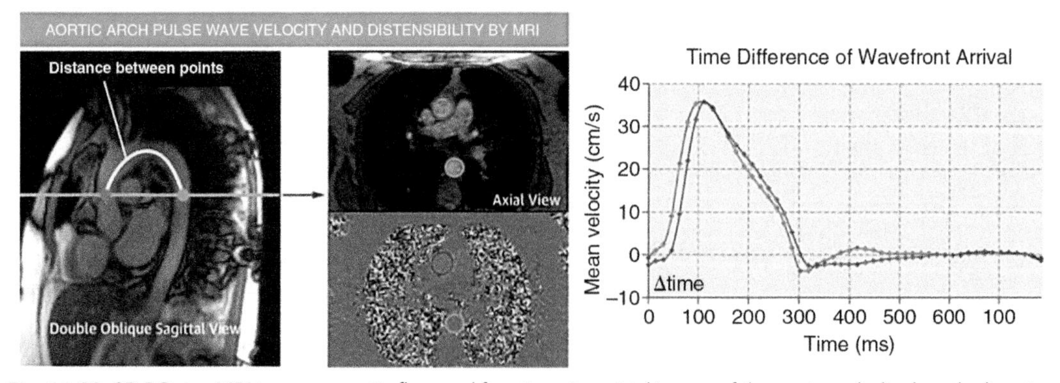

Fig. 16.23 2D PC cine MRI to assess aortic flow and function. A sagittal image of the aorta arch displays the location of the axial plane and is used to calculate the vessel centerline distance between the ascending and descending aorta. Through plane PC and magnitude, images in the axial plane are segmented for the ascending and descending aorta, and velocity versus time flow curves are generated (red is from the ascending aorta, blue is from the descending). The time difference between the arrival of 2 waveforms is determined. Pulse wave velocity is calculated by dividing the distance by the arrival time difference. Distensibility of the ascending and descending aorta can be calculated from the change in diastolic and systolic areas from the magnitude images and the central blood pressure. (*From* Whitlock MC, Hundley WG. Noninvasive imaging of flow and vascular function in disease of the aorta. JACC Cardiovasc Imaging 2015;8(9):1098; with permission.)

intensity increased following anthracycline chemotherapy and a greater than 5 times increase in relative signal intensity predicted a decrease LVEF of 16%.[87] In addition, increased signal intensity on contrast-enhanced T_1-weighted images is associated with measurements of LV systolic performance (LV ESV and LVEF) and histopathologic evidence of vacuolization and extracellular volume (ECV) in animals treated with doxorubicin anthracycline (Fig. 16.24)[134] occurred concurrently with LVEF declines (Fig. 16.25) in patients receiving anthracycline chemotherapy.[89]

Late gadolinium enhancement (LGE) is a term relating to the appearance of the effects of an extracellular contrast agent, Gd, several minutes after its administration on gradient-echo inversion recovery images. After administration, Gd diffuses throughout the body. In regions containing healthy tissue, Gd is removed from the extracellular space through renal excretion. Within the heart, Gd accumulates in regions of disrupted cell membranes when myocytes are injured or killed, and in areas of replacement fibrosis. In these 2 situations, this Gd accumulation reduces T1 relaxation. On gradient-echo inversion recovery images performed 5 minutes after Gd administration, regions of Gd accumulation appear "bright" or with high signal intensity relative to regions of healthy myocardium that appear dark.[138]

LGE has been reported in individuals receiving anthracycline-based chemotherapy, trastuzumab,

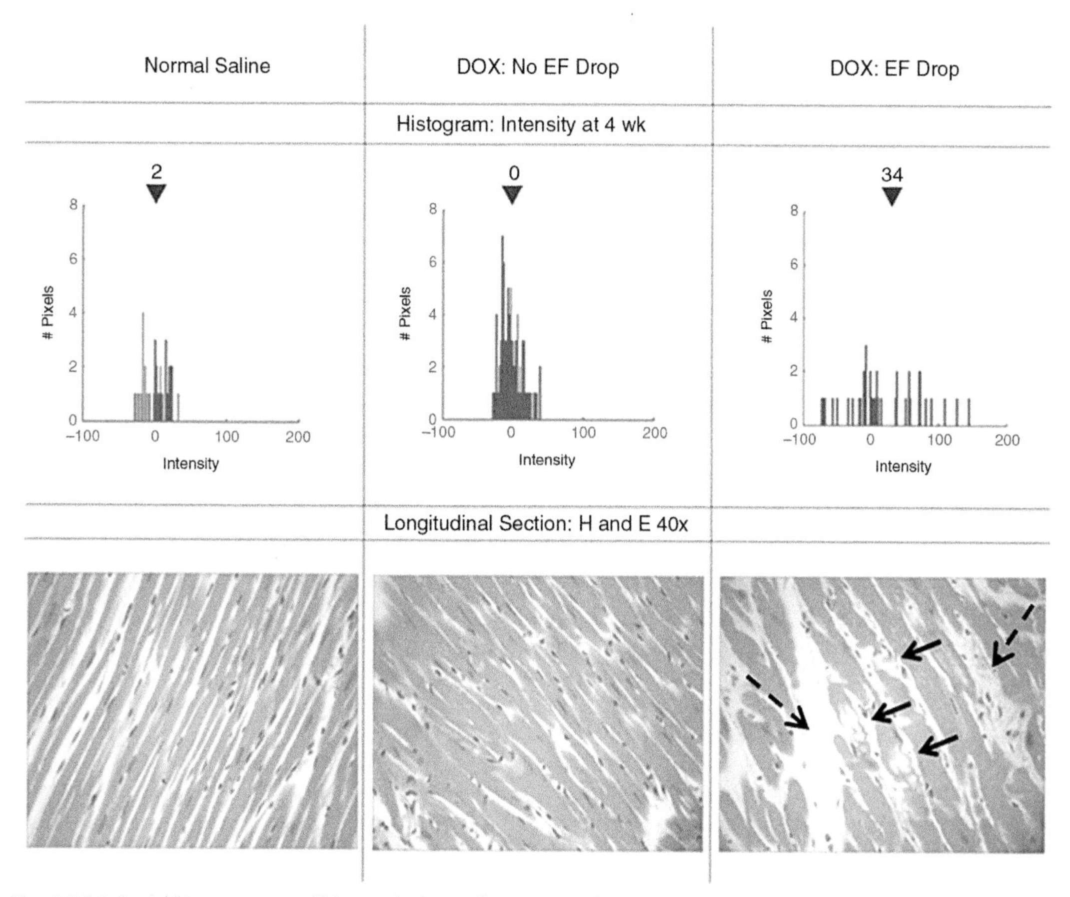

Fig. 16.24 Serial histograms and histopathology of contrast-enhanced T_1-weighted imaging following doxorubicin administration. On the top portion of the figure are 4-week histograms of the number of pixels (y-axes) and intensities (x-axes) in individual animals after receipt of normal saline (*top left*), doxorubicin (DOX) without an EF drop (*top middle*), and DOX with an EF drop (*top right*). Below the histograms are hematoxylin-eosin, original magnification ×40 histopathologic images from the same animals. Mean intensity in the animals that had a drop in EF corresponding to vacuolization (*arrows, bottom right*) and increased ECV (*dashed arrows, bottom right*). (*From* Lightfoot JC, D'Agostino RB Jr, Hamilton CA, et al. Novel approach to early detection of doxorubicin cardiotoxicity by gadolinium-enhanced cardiovascular magnetic resonance imaging in an experimental model. Circ Cardiovasc Imaging 2010;3(5):554; with permission.)

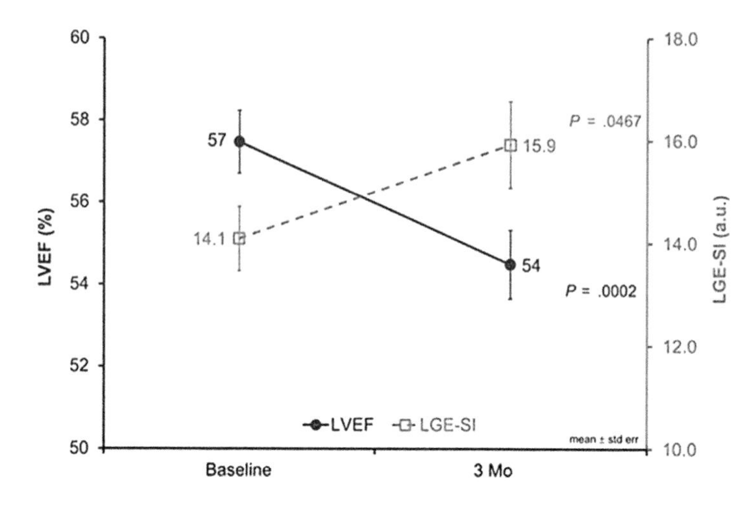

Fig. 16.25 Contrast-enhanced T_1-weighted signal intensity changes early after anthracycline administration with subclinical LVEF changes in cardio-oncology patients. LVEF dropped from 57 ± 1% to 54 ± 1% in the 3 months after chemotherapy exposure (*blue solid line*, *P*<.001). Concurrently, late Gd contrast-enhanced T_1-weighted signal intensity (LGE-SI) increased from 14.1 ± 0.6 to 15.9 ± 0.8 in the study population (*red dashed line*, *P*<.05). (*From* Jordan JH, D'Agostino RB, Hamilton CA, et al. Longitudinal assessment of concurrent changes in left ventricular ejection fraction and left ventricular myocardial tissue characteristics after administration of cardiotoxic chemotherapies using T_1-weighted and T_2-weighted cardiovascular magnetic resonance. Circ Cardiovasc Imaging 2014;7:876; with permission.)

and/or RT.[65,86,89,110,118,139–141] Although most studies report no qualitative findings of focal LGE,[86,89] several small case series and pilot studies have identified midmyocardial LGE (>2 standard deviations in signal intensity greater than remote healthy myocardium) predominantly in the lateral and inferolateral wall following adjuvant anthracycline or trastuzumab chemotherapy (Fig. 16.26).[65,110,118,139–142]

However, it is important to note that there are inconsistencies in the reported incidence (6%–30%) and spatial distribution of LGE across these single-center cohorts. Reasons for this are undetermined. Possible explanations for these findings include (a) the heterogeneity of patient populations studied, (b) the presence of confounding cardiovascular risk factors in the respective populations, (c) failure of these studies to exclude other causes of LGE pertaining to patients with cancer (eg, myocarditis), or (d) the LGE image acquisitions themselves possess inherent acquisition limitations related to factors that affect contrast clearance.[133] As such, further investigations are warranted to explore the mechanisms by which LGE occurs in patients treated for cancer.

Over the past 6 years, newer quantitative mapping CMR techniques have become available that depict voxel-by-voxel measures of magnetic relaxation values (T_1 and T_2). With this new technology, T_1/T_2 values can be directly compared on different scanners and followed longitudinally over time in an individual patient regardless of change in renal clearance of Gd.[133] Myocardial T_1 mapping can identify intracellular and extracellular tissue changes, including inflammation, edema, and focal and diffuse fibrosis without the need for healthy reference tissue, as is typically required in qualitative T_1-weighted sequences.[133,143–146]

In addition to T1 maps, T2 mapping may also be useful in trying to identify myocardial injury

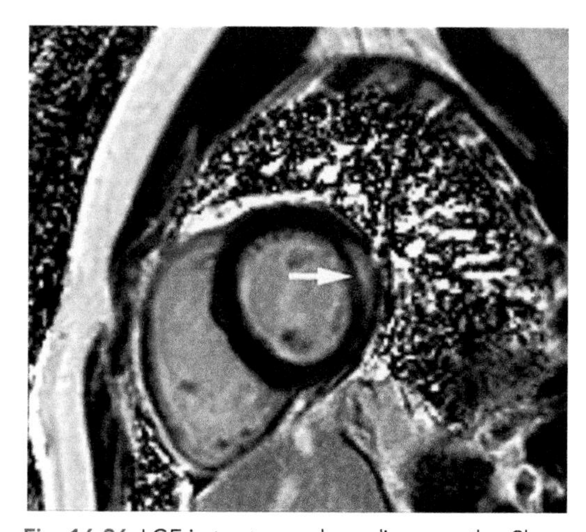

Fig. 16.26 LGE in trastuzumab cardiomyopathy. Short-axis phase-sensitive reconstructed inversion recovery-TrueFISP image through the midventricle demonstrates subepicardial linear LGE (*arrow*) in the lateral wall of a patient who had received trastuzumab. (*From* Fallah-Rad N, Walker JR, Wassef A, et al. The utility of cardiac biomarkers, tissue velocity and strain imaging, and cardiac magnetic resonance imaging in predicting early left ventricular dysfunction in patients with human epidermal growth factor receptor II–positive breast cancer treated with adjuvant trastuzumab therapy. J Am Coll Cardiol 2011;57(22):2268; with permission.)

after chemotherapy. T2 mapping measures increased water content in and around the myocytes after they die or their membranes become disrupted due to injury.[135,136] T_2 mapping of HER2+ patients with breast cancer receiving sequential anthracycline and trastuzumab identified a subset of patients with acute cardiotoxicity as defined by an impaired LVEF and myocardial edema (multiple segments with T_2 map values >59 ms) (Fig. 16.27).[142]

A consequence of myocyte injury includes the development of replacement fibrosis within the myocardial extracellular space. Through the evaluation of T1 maps before and after the administration of Gd, one can more precisely quantify the volume of the extracellular space, and within the heart, estimate the degree of extracellular replacement fibrosis. The term applied to this technique is (ECV) mapping (Box 16.2).[147–149] In ECV mapping, precontrast and postcontrast T_1 maps are acquired and adjusted for hematocrit values to remove contrast kinetic dependencies to calculate the myocardial ECV (Fig. 16.28).[147–151] Increased ECV quantified with ECV mapping can identify the burden or amount of diffuse fibrosis in myocardial diseases. In these subjects, ECV measures correlate strongly with biopsy evidence of histologic fibrosis (r^2 = 0.80).[149] Importantly, this technique can identify diffuse fibrosis that is undetected by LGE.[147]

ECV mapping is a novel tool to characterize the extracellular space of myocardial tissue from the development of myocardial fibrosis, which can occur late after cancer treatment.[148,150] Several small cross-sectional cardio-oncology studies have reported late ECV findings in cancer survivors previously treated with anthracyclines. In one study, adult cancer survivors (aged 55 ± 17 years) underwent a clinically indicated CMR examination on a 3-T Siemens scanner (Siemens Medical; Erlangen, Germany) 89 ± 40 months after treatment with anthracyclines.[152] Compared with healthy controls, the myocardial ECV of cancer survivors was elevated (36 ± 3% vs 28 ± 2%, $P<.0001$) and highest among survivors with a reduced LVEF, suggesting that incremental increases in ECV may be related to LVEF reductions.

Similarly, a group of asymptomatic pediatric survivors (n = 30, aged 15 ± 3 years) previously treated with anthracyclines an average of 7.6 ± 4.5 years before were evaluated for changes in ECV measured using a 1.5-T Siemens CMR scanner.[109] In this study, the ECV was measured

BOX 16.2
Tissue characterization with mapping techniques

- ↑ Native (precontrast) T1: Inflammation, edema, fibrosis, acute and chronic injury
- ↑ T2: Edema, acute injury
- ↑ Postcontrast T1: Extracellular injury, fibrosis
- ↑ ECV: Increased extracellular: intracellular space, fibrosis (chronic)

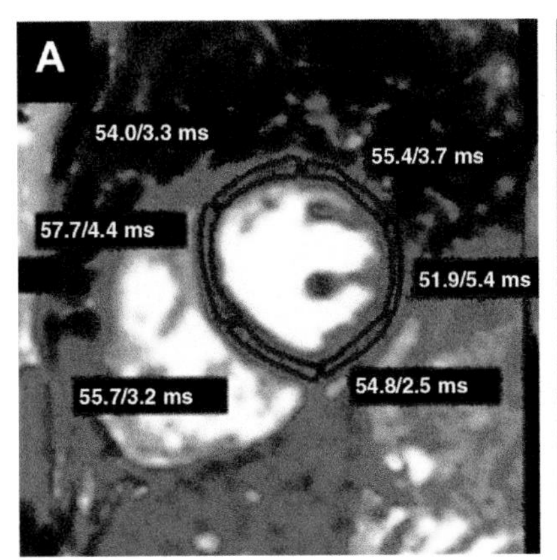

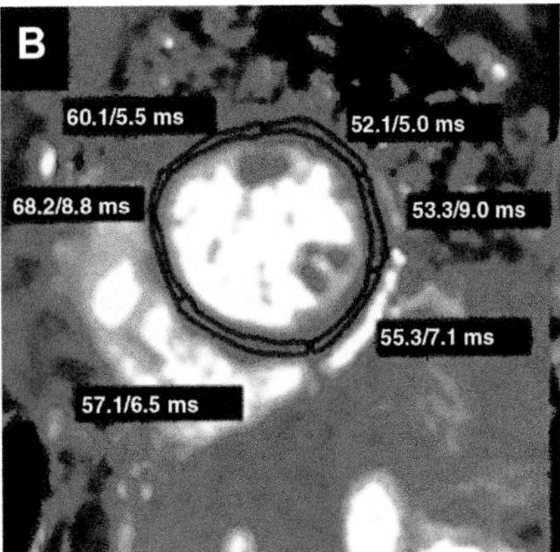

Fig. 16.27 T2 mapping for acute injury and edema following chemotherapy to evaluate acute cardiotoxicity. Mid short-axis T2 map demonstrating normal T2 values in patient with LVEF of 57% preinitiation of therapy (*A*). In a second patient, multiple segments demonstrated abnormal T2 values (>59 ms) and the LVEF dropped from 63% preinitiation to 46% following chemotherapy (*B*). The mean T2 for each segment and the standard deviation (mean/standard deviation ms) are shown. (*From* Thavendiranathan P, Amir E, Bedard P, et al. Regional myocardial edema detected by T2 mapping is a feature of cardiotoxicity in breast cancer patients receiving sequential therapy with anthracyclines and trastuzumab. J Cardiovasc Magn Reson 2014;16(Suppl 1):2; with permission.)

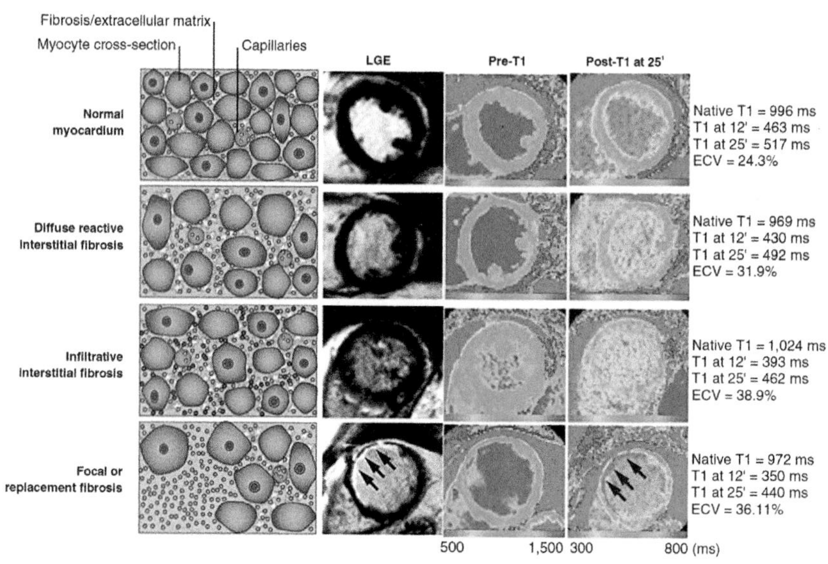

Fig. 16.28 The utility of using LGE, T1, and ECV CMR techniques to identify and discriminate fibrotic from normal myocardium in different pathologies. The increase in fibrosis leads to Gd-contrast retention that follows a different pattern depending on the nature of fibrosis (interstitial or focal myocardial fibrosis). Late-Gd enhancement and post-contrast T1 mapping performed 25 minutes after contrast administration offer a direct view of the amount and distribution of myocardial fibrosis. Blue circles indicate Gd contrast molecules; gray circles represent cellular infiltrates; arrows indicate an ischemic myocardial scar. (*From* Ambale-Venkatesh B, Lima JA. Cardiac MRI: a central prognostic tool in myocardial fibrosis. Nat Rev Cardiol 2015;12(1):21; with permission.)

to be within the normal range for young adults (20.7 ± 3.6%). Increased ECV, however, did correlate significantly with increased cumulative dose of anthracyclines, reduced exercise capacity (peak VO_2), and LV remodeling measures. Another study evaluated the ECV in n = 27 asymptomatic pediatric survivors aged 22 (12-42) years previously treated with anthracyclines an average of 9.6 (2.5–26.9) years before CMR examination.[153] ECV was found to be within the normal range for this age group (25 ± 10%); however, 5 asymptomatic subjects exhibited tissue characterization consistent with myocardial fibrosis (elevated mean ECV of 38 ± 7%). These studies, however, were limited by a major confounder in the survivors—the history of both cancer and cancer treatments—that could not be fully unraveled as each has been shown to cause systemic and myocardial tissue changes.

Most recently, a cross-sectional analysis of cancer survivors, newly diagnosed and untreated patients with cancer, and healthy controls observed native T1 and ECV were higher in cancer survivors treated 3 years before with anthracycline chemotherapy even after accounting for demographics, cardiovascular risk factors, demographics, and other markers of myocardial remodeling (*P*<.01 for all) (Fig. 16.29).[154] This finding suggests that elevated ECV is associated with anthracycline-based chemotherapy treatment and not necessarily the presence of cancer itself, and thus, treatment-associated fibrosis may be a factor in the higher rates of CV events in cancer survivors. Although more prospective longitudinal studies are required to determine the full utility of newer quantitative T1, T2, and ECV mapping techniques in cardio-oncology, preliminary work has shown that myocardial tissue characterization with CMR can identify changes related to the pathophysiology of cancer treatments in cardio-oncology patients.

Future Directions

Technological advances in CMR have produced the ability to obtain accurate, highly reproducible measures of cardiovascular structure and function, including LV volumes, mass, EF, strain as well as aortic stiffness measures (phase contrast and distensibility). Furthermore, emerging tissue characterization techniques (T1, T2, ECV mapping) are able to identify underlying substrate changes in the myocardium and can be acquired in a single, comprehensive CMR examination protocol (Table 16.4). Future scientific advances in noncontrasted measures of tissue characterization, such as T1-rho and magnetization transfer mapping,[155,156] may aid in discriminating causes of injury for patients with renal dysfunction who are unable to receive Gd contrast. In addition to the manifestations of cardiotoxicity discussed

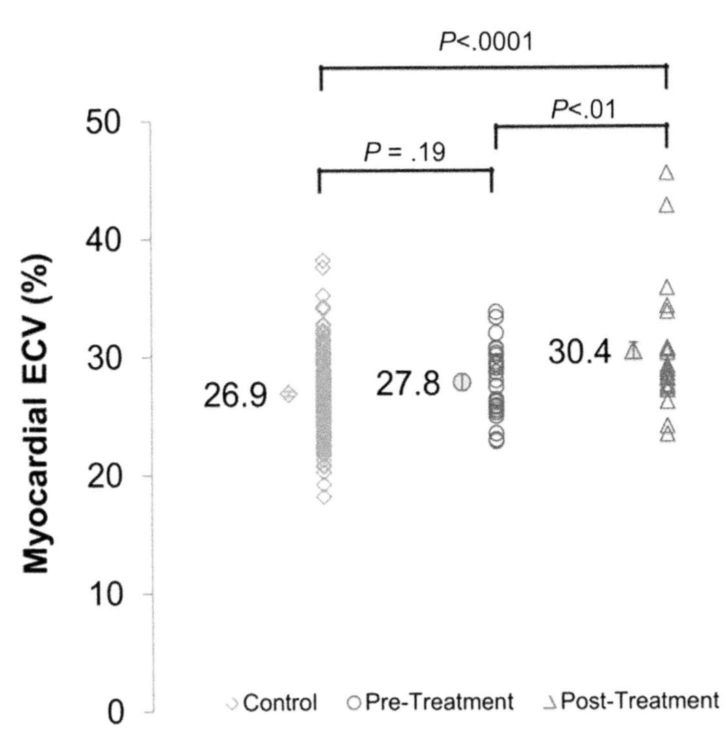

Fig. 16.29 Cardiovascular magnetic resonance (CMR) assessments of myocardial extracellular volume (ECV). Myocardial ECV measured by cardiovascular magnetic resonance in controls (26.9±0.2%) and cancer pretreatment participants (27.8±0.7%) compared with cancer survivors treated with anthracycline chemotherapy (30.4±0.7%). ECV incrementally increases across the groups ($P<0.0001$) with a significant increase in post-treatment ECV values compared with pretreatment ECV values ($P<0.01$). (*From* Jordan JH, Vasu S, Morgan TM, et al. Anthracycline-associated T1 mapping characteristics are elevated independent of the presence of cardiovascular comorbidities in cancer survivors. Circ Cardiovasc Imaging. 2016;9(8):e004325; with permission.)

within this chapter, cancer treatments may also damage the microcirculation in the heart or myocellular mitochondrial energetics.[157–159] Future CMR research could determine the utility of quantitative perfusion or phosphorous (adenosine triphosphate metabolites) to assess the microcirculation and mitochondrial bioenergetics in individuals treated for cancer.[160–162]

In addition to emerging technologic advances in CMR that facilitate new understanding of the mechanisms of cardiac injury after cancer treatment, other research focused on the clinical utility of CMR for monitoring patients receiving potentially cardiotoxic chemotherapy is underway. For example, current work is underway to reduce the standard cardio-oncology CMR protocol (see Table 16.4) by 75% to rapidly acquire the most clinically useful CMR biomarkers of cardiotoxicity (Fig. 16.30) for optimal management and surveillance of cardio-oncology patients. This advancement could lower costs associated with using CMR in clinical medicine. In addition, research is underway to determine the appropriate algorithm for selecting the imaging and serum biomarkers tests that most readily identify those at risk of CV events after receipt of potentially cardiotoxic chemotherapy.

TABLE 16.4
Cardio-oncology cardiac magnetic resonance protocol

Sequence	Assessment
Localizer scans	Extra-cardiac abnormalities
Cines: 2-, 3-, and 4-chamber	Wall motion abnormalities
Short axis (SAX) grid tagging	Contractility, circumferential strain
SAX dark blood STIR T_2-weighted	Myocardial edema
SAX Native T1 mapping	Edema, inflammation, fibrosis
SAX T2 mapping	Myocardial edema
Gd Contrast	Optional
SAX cine stack	Wall motion abnormalities, LV volumes and mass
PC-CMR, aortic arch	Aortic distensibility and pulse wave velocity
SAX postcontrast T1 mapping	Myocardial fibrosis, ECV
LGE	Myocardial fibrosis

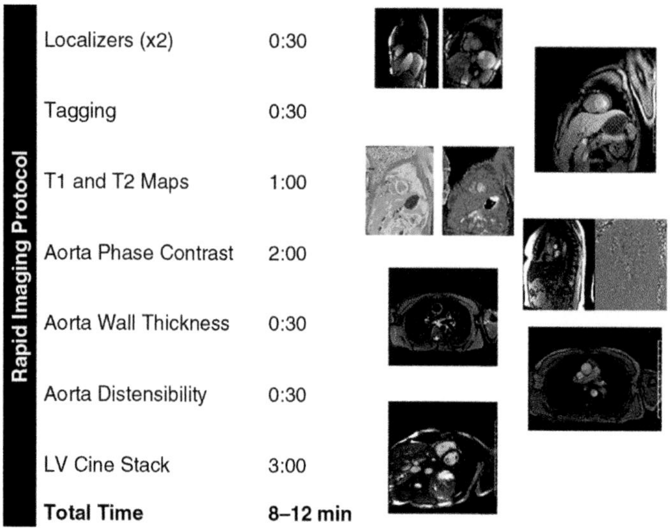

Rapid Imaging Protocol

Localizers (x2)	0:30
Tagging	0:30
T1 and T2 Maps	1:00
Aorta Phase Contrast	2:00
Aorta Wall Thickness	0:30
Aorta Distensibility	0:30
LV Cine Stack	3:00
Total Time	**8–12 min**

Fig. 16.30 Proposed rapid imaging CMR protocol for cardio-oncology evaluation. Technological advances in fast scanning methods and reduction of images collected can reduce the CMR protocol by 75%, thus improving clinical utility and facilitating the integration of surveillance with CMR into cardio-oncology management of cancer survivors.

SUMMARY

Structural, functional, and compositional assessments of the heart and vasculature may be performed in a single, comprehensive CMR examination. Recent study results demonstrate abnormalities of CMR measures of LVEF, mass, strain, aortic stiffening, and evidence of changes in myocardial tissue substrate in patients receiving treatment for cancer. These metrics forecast adverse cardiac events in other patient populations, but the long-term sequelae of their presence during treatment for cancer remain unknown. Future research is needed to determine the importance of these findings in patients treated for cancer and to determine the utility of new evolving CMR techniques that enable (<10 minute) assessments of the cardiotoxic effects of current and emerging therapies for cancer treatment.

REFERENCES

1. Truong J, Yan AT, Cramarossa G, et al. Chemotherapy-induced cardiotoxicity: detection, prevention, and management. Can J Cardiol 2014;30:869–78.
2. Bird BR, Swain SM. Cardiac toxicity in breast cancer survivors: review of potential cardiac problems. Clin Cancer Res 2008;14:14–24.
3. Cardinale D, Bacchiani G, Beggiato M, et al. Strategies to prevent and treat cardiovascular risk in cancer patients. Semin Oncol 2013;40:186–98.
4. Cardinale D, Colombo A, Bacchiani G, et al. Early detection of anthracycline cardiotoxicity and improvement with heart failure therapy. Circulation 2015;131(22):1981–8.
5. Hunt SA, Abraham WT, Chin MH, et al. Focused update incorporated into the ACC/AHA 2005 guidelines for the diagnosis and management of heart failure in adults: a report of the American College of Cardiology Foundation/American Heart Association task force on practice guidelines developed in collaboration with the International Society for Heart and Lung Transplantation. J Am Coll Cardiol 2009;14(53):e1–90.
6. Eschenhagen T, Force T, Ewer MS, et al. Cardiovascular side effects of cancer therapies: a position statement from the Heart Failure Association of the European Society of Cardiology. Eur J Heart Fail 2011;13:1–10.
7. Thygesen K, Alpert JS, Jaffe AS, et al. Joint ESC/ACCF/AHA/WHF task force for universal definition of myocardial infarction. Third universal definition of myocardial infarction. J Am Coll Cardiol 2012;60:1581–98.
8. Newby LK, Jesse RL, Babb JD, et al. ACCF 2012 expert consensus document on practical clinical considerations in the interpretation of troponin elevations: a report of the American College of Cardiology Foundation task force on Clinical Expert Consensus Documents. J Am Coll Cardiol 2012;60:2427–63.
9. Lipshultz SE, Rifai N, Sallan SE, et al. Predictive value of cardiac troponin T in pediatric patients at risk for myocardial injury. Circulation 1997;96:2641–8.
10. Cardinale D, Sandri MT, Martinoni A, et al. Left ventricular dysfunction predicted by early troponin I release after high-dose chemotherapy. J Am Coll Cardiol 2000;36:517–22.
11. Cardinale D, Sandri MT, Martinoni A, et al. Myocardial injury revealed by plasma troponin

I in breast cancer treated with high-dose chemotherapy. Ann Oncol 2002;13:710–5.
12. Auner HW, Tinchon C, Brezinschek RI, et al. Monitoring of cardiac function by serum cardiac troponin T levels, ventricular repolarisation indices, and echocardiography after conditioning with fractionated total body irradiation and high-dose cyclophosphamide. Eur J Haematol 2002; 69:1–6.
13. Sandri MT, Cardinale D, Zorzino L, et al. Minor increases in plasma troponin I predict decreased left ventricular ejection fraction after high dose chemo-therapy. Chin Chem 2003;49(2):248–52.
14. Cardinale D, Sandri MT, Colombo A, et al. Prognostic value of troponin I in cardiac risk stratification of cancer patients undergoing high-dose chemotherapy. Circulation 2004;109:2749–54.
15. Specchia G, Buquicchio C, Pansini N, et al. Monitoring of cardiac function on the basis of serum troponin I levels in patients with acute leukemia treated with anthracyclines. J Lab Clin Med 2005; 145:212–20.
16. Cardinale D, Colombo A, Torrisi R, et al. Trastuzumab-induced cardiotoxicity: clinical and prognostic implications of troponin I evaluation. J Clin Oncol 2010;28:3910–6.
17. Morris PG, Chen C, Steingart R, et al. Troponin I and C-reactive protein are commonly detected in patients with breast cancer treated with dose-dense chemotherapy incorporating trastuzumab and lapatinib. Clin Cancer Res 2011;17:3490–9.
18. Sawaya H, Sebag IA, Plana JC, et al. Early detection and prediction of cardiotoxicity in chemotherapy-treated patients. Am J Cardiol 2011;107:1375–80.
19. Sawaya H, Sebag IA, Plana JC, et al. Assessment of echocardiography and biomarkers for the extended prediction of cardiotoxicity in patients treated with anthracyclines, taxanes, and trastuzumab. Circ Cardiovasc Imaging 2012;5(5): 596–603.
20. Ky B, Putt M, Sawaya H, et al. Early increases in multiple biomarkers predict subsequent cardiotoxicity in patients with breast cancer treated with doxorubicin, taxanes, and trastuzumab. J Am Coll Cardiol 2014;63:809–16.
21. O'Brien PJ. Cardiac troponin is the most effective translational safety biomarker for myocardial injury in cardiotoxicity. Toxicology 2008;245:206–18.
22. Herman EH, Zhang J, Lipshultz SE, et al. Correlation between serum levels of cardiac troponin-T and the severity of the chronic cardiomyopathy induced by doxorubicin. J Clin Oncol 1999;17:2237–43.
23. Curigliano G, Cardinale D, Suter T, et al, ESMO Guidelines Working Group. Cardiovascular toxicity induced by chemotherapy, targeted agents and radiotherapy: ESMO Clinical Practice Guidelines. Ann Oncol 2012;23(Suppl 7): vii155–66.
24. Cardinale D, Colombo A, Sandri MT, et al. Prevention of high-dose chemotherapy-induced cardiotoxicity in high-risk patients by angiotensin-converting enzyme inhibition. Circulation 2006;114:2474–81.
25. Kismet E, Varan A, Ayabakan C, et al. Serum troponin T levels and echocardiographic evaluation in children treated with doxorubicin. Pediatr Blood Cancer 2004;42:220–4.
26. Soker M, Kervancioglu M. Plasma concentrations of NT-pro-BNP and cardiac troponin-I in relation to doxorubicin-induced cardiomyopathy and cardiac function in childhood malignancy. Saudi Med J 2005;26:1197–202.
27. Christenson ES, James T, Agrawal V, et al. Use of biomarkers for the assessment of chemotherapy-induced cardiac toxicity. Clin Biochem 2015;48: 223–35.
28. Kimura K, Yamaguchi Y, Horii M, et al. ANP is cleared much faster than BNP in patients with congestive heart failure. Eur J Clin Pharmacol 2007;63:699–702.
29. Chowdhury P, Kehl D, Choudhary R, et al. The use of biomarkers in the patient with heart failure. Curr Cardiol Rep 2013;15:372.
30. Suzuki T, Hayashi D, Yamazaki T, et al. Elevated B-type natriuretic peptide levels after anthracycline administration. Am Heart J 1998;136:362–3.
31. Nousiainen T, Vanninen E, Jantunen E, et al. Natriuretic peptides during the development of doxorubicin-induced left ventricular diastolic dysfunction. J Intern Med 2002;251:228–34.
32. Aggarwal S, Pettersen MD, Bhambhani K, et al. B-type natriuretic peptide as a marker for cardiac dysfunction in anthracycline-treated children. Pediatr Blood Cancer 2007;49:812–6.
33. Mavinkurve-Groothuis AM, Groot-Loonen J, Bellersen L, et al. Abnormal NT-pro-BNP levels in asymptomatic long-term survivors of childhood cancer treated with anthracyclines. Pediatr Blood Cancer 2009;52:631–6.
34. Romano S, Fratini S, Ricevuto E, et al. Serial measurements of NT-proBNP are predictive of not-high-dose anthracycline cardiotoxicity in breast cancer patients. Br J Cancer 2011;105: 1663–8.
35. Perik PJ, Lub-De Hooge MN, Gietema JA, et al. Indium-111-labeled trastuzumab scintigraphy in patients with human epidermal growth factor receptor 2-positive metastatic breast cancer. J Clin Oncol 2006;24:2276–82.
36. Knobloch K, Tepe J, Lichtinghagen R, et al. Simultaneous hemodynamic and serological cardiotoxicity monitoring during immunotherapy with trastuzumab. Int J Cardiol 2008;125:113–5.

37. Putt M, Hahn VS, Januzzi JL, et al. Longitudinal changes in multiple biomarkers are associated with cardiotoxicity in breast cancer patients treated with Doxorubicin, Taxanes, and Trastuzumab. Clin Chem 2015;61:1164–72.
38. Force T, Krause DS, Van Etten RA. Molecular mechanisms of cardiotoxicity of tyrosine kinase inhibition [review]. Nat Rev Cancer 2007;7:332–44.
39. Kang Y, Xu X, Cheng L, et al. Two-dimensional speckle tracking echocardiography combined with high-sensitive cardiac troponin T in early detection and prediction of cardiotoxicity during epirubicine-based chemotherapy. Eur J Heart Fail 2014;16(3):300–8.
40. American College of Cardiology Foundation Appropriate Use Criteria Task Force, American Society of Echocardiography, American Heart Association, et al. ACCF/ASE/AHA/ASNC/HFSA/HRS/SCAI/SCCM/SCCT/SCMR 2011 Appropriate Use Criteria for Echocardiography. A Report of the American College of Cardiology Foundation Appropriate Use Criteria Task Force, American Society of Echocardiography, American Heart Association, American Society of Nuclear Cardiology, Heart Failure Society of America, Heart Rhythm Society, Society for Cardiovascular Angiography and Interventions, Society of Critical Care Medicine, Society of Cardiovascular Computed Tomography, Society for Cardiovascular Magnetic Resonance American College of Chest Physicians. J Am Soc Echocardiogr 2011;24(3):229–67.
41. Thavendiranathan P, Grant AD, Negishi T, et al. Reproducibility of echocardiographic techniques for sequential assessment of left ventricular ejection fraction and volumes: application to patients undergoing cancer chemotherapy. J Am Coll Cardiol 2013;61(1):77–84.
42. Thavendiranathan P, Poulin F, Lim K-D, et al. Use of myocardial strain imaging by echocardiography for the early detection of cardiotoxicity in patients during and after cancer chemotherapy: a systematic review. J Am Coll Cardiol 2014;63(25 Pt A):2751–68.
43. Plana JC, Galderisi M, Barac A, et al. Expert consensus for multimodality imaging evaluation of adult patients during and after cancer therapy: a report from the American Society of Echocardiography and the European Association of Cardiovascular Imaging. J Am Soc Echocardiogr 2014;27(9):911–39.
44. Herrmann J, Lerman A, Sandhu NP, et al. Evaluation and management of patients with heart disease and cancer: cardio-oncology. Mayo Clin Proc 2014;89(9):1287–3065.
45. Lang RM, Badano LP, Mor-Avi V, et al. Recommendations for cardiac chamber quantification by echocardiography in adults: an update from the American Society of Echocardiography and the European Association of Cardiovascular Imaging. J Am Soc Echocardiogr 2015;28(1):1–39.e14.
46. Dorosz JL, Lezotte DC, Weitzenkamp DA, et al. Performance of 3-dimensional echocardiography in measuring left ventricular volumes and ejection fraction: a systematic review and meta-analysis. J Am Coll Cardiol 2012;59(20):1799–808.
47. Jenkins C, Chan J, Hanekom L, et al. Accuracy and feasibility of online 3-dimensional echocardiography for measurement of left ventricular parameters. J Am Soc Echocardiogr 2006;19(9):1119–28.
48. Sugeng L, Mor-Avi V, Weinert L, et al. Quantitative assessment of left ventricular size and function: side-by-side comparison of real-time three-dimensional echocardiography and computed tomography with magnetic resonance reference. Circulation 2006;114(7):654–61.
49. Walker J, Bhullar N, Fallah-Rad N, et al. Role of three-dimensional echocardiography in breast cancer: comparison with two-dimensional echocardiography, multiple-gated acquisition scans, and cardiac magnetic resonance imaging. J Clin Oncol 2010;28(21):3429–36.
50. Jacobs LD, Salgo IS, Goonewardena S, et al. Rapid online quantification of left ventricular volume from real-time three-dimensional echocardiographic data. Eur Heart J 2006;27(4):460–8.
51. Jenkins C, Moir S, Chan J, et al. Left ventricular volume measurement with echocardiography: a comparison of left ventricular opacification, three-dimensional echocardiography, or both with magnetic resonance imaging. Eur Heart J 2009;30(1):98–106.
52. Muraru D, Badano LP, Piccoli G, et al. Validation of a novel automated border-detection algorithm for rapid and accurate quantitation of left ventricular volumes based on three-dimensional echocardiography. Eur J Echocardiogr 2010;11(4):359–68.
53. Armstrong GT, Plana JC, Zhang N, et al. Screening adult survivors of childhood cancer for cardiomyopathy: comparison of echocardiography and cardiac magnetic resonance imaging. J Clin Oncol 2012;30(23):2876–84.
54. Hoffmann R, von Bardeleben S, ten Cate F, et al. Assessment of systolic left ventricular function: a multi-centre comparison of cineventriculography, cardiac magnetic resonance imaging, unenhanced and contrast-enhanced echocardiography. Eur Heart J 2005;26(6):607–16.
55. Malm S, Frigstad S, Sagberg E, et al. Accurate and reproducible measurement of left ventricular volume and ejection fraction by contrast echocardiography: a comparison with magnetic

resonance imaging. J Am Coll Cardiol 2004;44(5):1030–5.
56. Mor-Avi V, Lang RM, Badano LP, et al. Current and evolving echocardiographic techniques for the quantitative evaluation of cardiac mechanics: ASE/EAE consensus statement on methodology and indications: endorsed by the Japanese Society of Echocardiography. J Am Soc Echocardiogr 2011;24(3):277–313.
57. Villarraga HR, Herrmann J, Nkomo VT. Cardio-oncology: role of echocardiography. Prog Cardiovasc Dis 2014;57(1):10–8.
58. Stanton T, Leano R, Marwick TH. Prediction of all-cause mortality from global longitudinal speckle strain: comparison with ejection fraction and wall motion scoring. Circ Cardiovasc Imaging 2009;2(5):356–64.
59. Negishi K, Negishi T, Hare JL, et al. Independent and incremental value of deformation indices for prediction of trastuzumab-induced cardiotoxicity. J Am Soc Echocardiogr 2013;26(5):493–8.
60. Farsalinos KE, Daraban AM, Ünlü S, et al. Head-to-head comparison of global longitudinal strain measurements among nine different vendors: the EACVI/ASE inter-vendor comparison study. J Am Soc Echocardiogr 2015;28(10):1171–81. e2.
61. Poterucha JT, Kutty S, Lindquist RK, et al. Changes in left ventricular longitudinal strain with anthracycline chemotherapy in adolescents precede subsequent decreased left ventricular ejection fraction. J Am Soc Echocardiogr 2012;25(7):733–40.
62. Stoodley PW, Richards DAB, Boyd A, et al. Left ventricular systolic function in HER2/neu negative breast cancer patients treated with anthracycline chemotherapy: a comparative analysis of left ventricular ejection fraction and myocardial strain imaging over 12 months. Eur J Cancer 2013;49(16):3396–403.
63. Stoodley PW, Richards DAB, Hui R, et al. Two-dimensional myocardial strain imaging detects changes in left ventricular systolic function immediately after anthracycline chemotherapy. Eur J Echocardiogr 2011;12(12):945–52.
64. Nhola LF, Mulvagh SL, Abdelmoneim SS, et al. Is there a change in myocardial mechanical function in patients on vascular endothelial grow factor axis inhibitor therapy for genitourinary and gastrointestinal cancer? J Am Soc Echocardiogr 2015;28:B41–2.
65. Fallah-Rad N, Walker JR, Wassef A, et al. The utility of cardiac biomarkers, tissue velocity and strain imaging, and cardiac magnetic resonance imaging in predicting early left ventricular dysfunction in patients with human epidermal growth factor receptor II–positive breast cancer treated with adjuvant trastuzumab therapy. J Am Coll Cardiol 2011;57(22):2263–70.
66. Sandhu N, Spoon J, Herrmann J, et al. Two dimensional speckle tracking echocardiography predicts preclinical cardiotoxicity in breast cancer patients. J Am Coll Cardiol 2014;63:A199.
67. Xu Y, Herrmann J, Pellikka PA, et al. Early changes in 2D-speckle-tracking echocardiography may predict a decrease in left ventricular ejection fraction in lymphoma patients undergoing anthracycline chemotherapy: a pilot study. J Clin Exp Oncol 2015;4:1.
68. Cheung Y-F, Hong W-J, Chan GCF, et al. Left ventricular myocardial deformation and mechanical dyssynchrony in children with normal ventricular shortening fraction after anthracycline therapy. Heart 2010;96(14):1137–41.
69. Ho E, Brown A, Barrett P, et al. Subclinical anthracycline- and trastuzumab-induced cardiotoxicity in the long-term follow-up of asymptomatic breast cancer survivors: a speckle tracking echocardiographic study. Heart 2010;96(9):701–7.
70. Mavinkurve-Groothuis AMC, Groot-Loonen J, Marcus KA, et al. Myocardial strain and strain rate in monitoring subclinical heart failure in asymptomatic long-term survivors of childhood cancer. Ultrasound Med Biol 2010;36(11):1783–91.
71. Tsai H-R, Gjesdal O, Wethal T, et al. Left ventricular function assessed by two-dimensional speckle tracking echocardiography in long-term survivors of Hodgkin's lymphoma treated by mediastinal radiotherapy with or without anthracycline therapy. Am J Cardiol 2011;107(3):472–7.
72. Burns AT, La Gerche A, D'hooge J, et al. Left ventricular strain and strain rate: characterization of the effect of load in human subjects. Eur J Echocardiogr 2010;11(3):283–9.
73. Marwick TH. Measurement of strain and strain rate by echocardiography: ready for prime time? J Am Coll Cardiol 2006;47(7):1313–27.
74. Nagueh SF, Appleton CP, Gillebert TC, et al. Recommendations for the evaluation of left ventricular diastolic function by echocardiography. J Am Soc Echocardiogr 2009;22(2):107–33.
75. Lancellotti P, Nkomo VT, Badano LP, et al. Expert consensus for multi-modality imaging evaluation of cardiovascular complications of radiotherapy in adults: a report from the European Association of Cardiovascular Imaging and the American Society of Echocardiography. J Am Soc Echocardiogr 2013;26(9):1013–32.
76. Heidenreich PA, Hancock SL, Lee BK, et al. Asymptomatic cardiac disease following mediastinal irradiation. J Am Coll Cardiol 2003;42(4):743–9.
77. Hull MC, Morris CG, Pepine CJ, et al. Valvular dysfunction and carotid, subclavian, and coronary

artery disease in survivors of Hodgkin lymphoma treated with radiation therapy. JAMA 2003; 290(21):2831–7.
78. Singal PK, Iliskovic N. Doxorubicin-induced cardiomyopathy. N Engl J Med 1998;339(13):900–5.
79. Ewer MS, Yeh ET. Cancer and the heart. Shelton, Connecticut: People's Medical Publishing House; 2013.
80. Hundley WG, Bluemke DA, Finn JP, et al. ACCF/ACR/AHA/NASCI/SCMR 2010 expert consensus document on cardiovascular magnetic resonance: a report of the American College of Cardiology Foundation Task Force on Expert Consensus Documents. Circulation 2010;121(22):2462–508.
81. Shellock FG, Crues JV. MR procedures: biologic effects, safety, and patient care. Radiology 2004; 232(3):635–52.
82. Nacif MS, Arai AE, Lima J, et al. Gadolinium-enhanced cardiovascular magnetic resonance: administered dose in relationship to United States Food and Drug Administration (FDA) guidelines. J Cardiovasc Magn Reson 2012;14:18.
83. Wang Y, Alkasab TK, Narin O, et al. Incidence of nephrogenic systemic fibrosis after adoption of restrictive gadolinium-based contrast agent guidelines. Radiology 2011;260(1):105–11.
84. U.S. Department of Health and Human Services. Common terminology criteria for adverse events (CTCAE) version 4.0, vol. 4. National Institutes of Health; National Cancer Institute; 2009.
85. Bellenger N, Burgess M, Ray S, et al. Comparison of left ventricular ejection fraction and volumes in heart failure by echocardiography, radionuclide ventriculography and cardiovascular magnetic resonance. Are they interchangeable? Eur Heart J 2000;21(16):1387–96.
86. Drafts BC, Twomley KM, D'Agostino R Jr, et al. Low to moderate dose anthracycline-based chemotherapy is associated with early noninvasive imaging evidence of subclinical cardiovascular disease. JACC Cardiovasc Imaging 2013;6(8): 877–85.
87. Wassmuth R, Lentzsch S, Erdbruegger U, et al. Subclinical cardiotoxic effects of anthracyclines as assessed by magnetic resonance imaging- A pilot study. Am Heart J 2001;141(6):1007–13.
88. Bellenger NG, Davies LC, Francis JM, et al. Reduction in sample size for studies of remodeling in heart failure by the use of cardiovascular magnetic resonance. J Cardiovasc Magn Reson 2000;2(4): 271–8.
89. Jordan JH, D'Agostino RB, Hamilton CA, et al. Longitudinal assessment of concurrent changes in left ventricular ejection fraction and left ventricular myocardial tissue characteristics after administration of cardiotoxic chemotherapies using T1-weighted and T2-weighted cardiovascular magnetic resonance. Circ Cardiovasc Imaging 2014;7:872–9.
90. Panjrath GS, Jain D. Trastuzumab-induced cardiac dysfunction. Nucl Med Commun 2007; 28(2):69–73.
91. Hall PS, Harshman LC, Srinivas S, et al. The frequency and severity of cardiovascular toxicity from targeted therapy in advanced renal cell carcinoma patients. JACC Heart Fail 2013;1(1):72–8.
92. Steinherz LJ, Graham T, Hurwitz R, et al. Guidelines for cardiac monitoring of children during and after anthracycline therapy: report of the Cardiology Committee of the Childrens Cancer Study Group. Pediatrics 1992;89(5 Pt 1):942–9.
93. Alexander J, Dainiak N, Berger HJ, et al. Serial assessment of doxorubicin cardiotoxicity with quantitative radionuclide angiocardiography. N Engl J Med 1979;300(6):278–83.
94. Kostler WJ, Schwab B, Singer CF, et al. Monitoring of serum Her-2/neu predicts response and progression-free survival to trastuzumab-based treatment in patients with metastatic breast cancer. Clin Cancer Res 2004;10(5):1618–24.
95. Lipshultz SE, Sanders SP, Goorin AM, et al. Monitoring for anthracycline cardiotoxicity. Pediatrics 1994;93(3):433–7.
96. Altena R, Perik PJ, van Veldhuisen DJ, et al. Cardiovascular toxicity caused by cancer treatment: strategies for early detection. Lancet Oncol 2009; 10(4):391–9.
97. Schwartz RG, Jain D, Storozynsky E. Traditional and novel methods to assess and prevent chemotherapy-related cardiac dysfunction noninvasively. J Nucl Cardiol 2013;20(3):443–64.
98. Childs AC, Phaneuf SL, Dirks AJ, et al. Doxorubicin treatment in vivo causes cytochrome C release and cardiomyocyte apoptosis, as well as increased mitochondrial efficiency, superoxide dismutase activity, and Bcl-2:Bax ratio. Cancer Res 2002; 62(16):4592–8.
99. An J, Li P, Li J, et al. ARC is a critical cardiomyocyte survival switch in doxorubicin cardiotoxicity. J Mol Med (Berl) 2009;87(4):401–10.
100. Sorensen BS, Sinding J, Andersen AH, et al. Mode of action of topoisomerase II-targeting agents at a specific DNA sequence: uncoupling the DNA binding, cleavage and religation events. J Mol Biol 1992;228(3):778–86.
101. Zhu S-G, Kukreja RC, Das A, et al. Dietary nitrate supplementation protects against doxorubicin-induced cardiomyopathy by improving mitochondrial function. J Am Coll Cardiol 2011;57(21): 2181–9.
102. Kim Y, Ma AG, Kitta K, et al. Anthracycline-induced suppression of GATA-4 transcription factor: implication in the regulation of cardiac myocyte apoptosis. Mol Pharmacol 2003;63(2):368–77.

103. Menna P, Salvatorelli E, Minotti G. Anthracycline degradation in cardiomyocytes: a journey to oxidative survival. Chem Res Toxicol 2010; 23(1):6–10.
104. Cosper PF, Leinwand LA. Cancer causes cardiac atrophy and autophagy in a sexually dimorphic manner. Cancer Res 2011;71(5):1710–20.
105. Zhao Y, McLaughlin D, Robinson E, et al. Nox2 NADPH oxidase promotes pathologic cardiac remodeling associated with Doxorubicin chemotherapy. Cancer Res 2010;70(22):9287–97.
106. Huang C, Zhang X, Ramil JM, et al. Juvenile exposure to anthracyclines impairs cardiac progenitor cell function and vascularization resulting in greater susceptibility to stress-induced myocardial injury in adult mice. Circulation 2010;121(5): 675–83.
107. Zhang S, Liu X, Bawa-Khalfe T, et al. Identification of the molecular basis of doxorubicin-induced cardiotoxicity. Nat Med 2012;18(11):1639–42.
108. Ganame J, Claus P, Eyskens B, et al. Acute cardiac functional and morphological changes after anthracycline infusions in children. Am J Cardiol 2007;99(7):974–7.
109. Tham EB, Haykowsky MJ, Chow K, et al. Diffuse myocardial fibrosis by T1-mapping in children with subclinical anthracycline cardiotoxicity: relationship to exercise capacity, cumulative dose and remodeling. J Cardiovasc Magn Reson 2013; 15:48.
110. Neilan TG, Coelho-Filho OR, Pena-Herrera D, et al. Left ventricular mass in patients with a cardiomyopathy after treatment with anthracyclines. Am J Cardiol 2012;110(11):1679–86.
111. De Wolf D, Suys B, Maurus R, et al. Dobutamine stress echocardiography in the evaluation of late anthracycline cardiotoxicity in childhood cancer survivors. Pediatr Res 1996;39(3):504–12.
112. Iarussi D, Galderisi M, Ratti G, et al. Left ventricular systolic and diastolic function after anthracycline chemotherapy in childhood. Clin Cardiol 2001; 24(10):663–9.
113. Aletras AH, Ding SJ, Balaban RS, et al. DENSE: displacement encoding with stimulated echoes in cardiac functional MRI. J Magn Reson 1999; 137(1):247–52.
114. Kim D, Gilson WD, Kramer CM, et al. Myocardial tissue tracking with two-dimensional cine displacement-encoded MR imaging: development and initial evaluation. Radiology 2004; 230(3):862–71.
115. Osman NF, Kerwin WS, McVeigh ER, et al. Cardiac motion tracking using CINE harmonic phase (HARP) magnetic resonance imaging. Magn Reson Med 1999;42(6):1048–60.
116. Young AA, Imai H, Chang CN, et al. 2-Dimensional left-ventricular deformation during systole using magnetic-resonance-imaging with spatial modulation of magnetization. Circulation 1994; 89(2):740–52.
117. Götte MJ, van Rossum AC, Twisk JW, et al. Quantification of regional contractile function after infarction: strain analysis superior to wall thickening analysis in discriminating infarct from remote myocardium. J Am Coll Cardiol 2001; 37(3):808–17.
118. Lunning MA, Kutty S, Rome ET, et al. Cardiac magnetic resonance imaging for the assessment of the myocardium after doxorubicin-based chemotherapy. Am J Clin Oncol 2013;21(12):1283–9.
119. Whitlock MC, Hundley WG. Noninvasive imaging of flow and vascular function in disease of the aorta. JACC Cardiovasc Imaging 2015;8(9):1094–106.
120. Rogers WJ, Hu YL, Coast D, et al. Age-associated changes in regional aortic pulse wave velocity. J Am Coll Cardiol 2001;38(4):1123–9.
121. Benetos A, Waeber B, Izzo J, et al. Influence of age, risk factors, and cardiovascular and renal disease on arterial stiffness: clinical applications. Am J Hypertens 2002;15(12):1101–8.
122. Laurent S, Boutouyrie P, Asmar R, et al. Aortic stiffness is an independent predictor of all-cause and cardiovascular mortality in hypertensive patients. Hypertension 2001;37(5):1236–41.
123. Sutton-Tyrrell K, Najjar SS, Boudreau RM, et al. Elevated aortic pulse wave velocity, a marker of arterial stiffness, predicts cardiovascular events in well-functioning older adults. Circulation 2005; 111(25):3384–90.
124. Chaosuwannakit N, D'Agostino R Jr, Hamilton CA, et al. Aortic stiffness increases upon receipt of anthracycline chemotherapy. J Clin Oncol 2010; 28(1):166–72.
125. Grover S, Lou PW, Bradbrook C, et al. Early and late changes in markers of aortic stiffness with breast cancer therapy. Intern Med J 2015;45(2): 140–7.
126. Ferrans VJ. Overview of cardiac pathology in relation to anthracycline cardiotoxicity. Cancer Treat Rep 1978;62(6):955–61.
127. Olson HM, Young DM, Prieur DJ, et al. Electrolyte and morphologic alterations of myocardium in adriamycin-treated rabbits. Am J Pathol 1974; 77(3):439–54.
128. Gottdiener JS, Mathisen DJ, Borer JS, et al. Doxorubicin cardiotoxicity—assessment of late left-ventricular dysfunction by radionuclide cineangiography. Ann Intern Med 1981;94(4):430–5.
129. DeVita VT, Hellman S, Rosenberg SA. Cancer, principles & practice of oncology. 7th edition. Philadelphia: Lippincott Williams & Wilkins; 2005.
130. Bernstein MA, King KF, Zhou ZJ. Handbook of MRI pulse sequences. Amsterdam (the Netherlands): Academic Press; 2004.

131. Higgins DM, Ridgway JP, Radjenovic A, et al. T1 measurement using a short acquisition period for quantitative cardiac applications. Med Phys 2005; 32(6):1738–46.
132. Kehr E, Sono M, Chugh SS, et al. Gadolinium-enhanced magnetic resonance imaging for detection and quantification of fibrosis in human myocardium in vitro. Int J Cardiovasc Imaging 2008;24(1):61–8.
133. Messroghli DR, Niendorf T, Schulz-Menger J, et al. T1 mapping in patients with acute myocardial infarction. J Cardiovasc Magn Reson 2003;5(2): 353–9.
134. Lightfoot JC, D'Agostino RB Jr, Hamilton CA, et al. Novel approach to early detection of doxorubicin cardiotoxicity by gadolinium-enhanced cardiovascular magnetic resonance imaging in an experimental model. Circ Cardiovasc Imaging 2010; 3(5):550–8.
135. Thompson RC, Canby RC, Lojeski EW, et al. Adriamycin cardiotoxicity and proton nuclear-magnetic-resonance relaxation properties. Am Heart J 1987; 113(6):1444–9.
136. Cottin Y, Ribuot C, Maupoil V, et al. Early incidence of adriamycin treatment on cardiac parameters in the rat. Can J Physiol Pharmacol 1994; 72(2):140–5.
137. Anderson B, Sawyer DB. Predicting and preventing the cardiotoxicity of cancer therapy. Expert Rev Cardiovasc Ther 2008;6(7):1023–33.
138. Kim RJ, Fieno DS, Parrish TB, et al. Relationship of MRI delayed contrast enhancement to irreversible injury, infarct age, and contractile function. Circulation 1999;100(19):1992–2002.
139. Wadhwa D, Fallah-Rad N, Grenier D, et al. Trastuzumab mediated cardiotoxicity in the setting of adjuvant chemotherapy for breast cancer: a retrospective study. Breast Cancer Res Treat 2009; 117(2):357–64.
140. Fallah-Rad N, Lytwyn M, Fang T, et al. Delayed contrast enhancement cardiac magnetic resonance imaging in trastuzumab induced cardiomyopathy. J Cardiovasc Magn Reson 2008; 10(1):1–4.
141. Lawley C, Wainwright C, Segelov E, et al. Pilot study evaluating the role of cardiac magnetic resonance imaging in monitoring adjuvant trastuzumab therapy for breast cancer. Asia Pac J Clin Oncol 2012;8(1):95–100.
142. Thavendiranathan P, Amir E, Bedard P, et al. Regional myocardial edema detected by T2 mapping is a feature of cardiotoxicity in breast cancer patients receiving sequential therapy with anthracyclines and trastuzumab. J Cardiovasc Magn Reson 2014;16(Suppl 1):P273.
143. Messroghli DR, Radjenovic A, Kozerke S, et al. Modified Look-Locker Inversion recovery (MOLLI) for high-resolution T1 mapping of the heart. Magn Reson Med 2004;52(1):141–6.
144. Messroghli DR, Plein S, Higgins DM, et al. Human myocardium: single-breath-hold MR T1 mapping with high spatial resolution: a reproducibility study. Radiology 2006;238(3):1004–12.
145. Messroghli DR, Greiser A, Frohlich M, et al. Optimization and validation of a fully-integrated pulse sequence for modified look-locker inversion-recovery (MOLLI) T1 mapping of the heart. J Magn Reson Imaging 2007;26(4):1081–6.
146. Messroghli DR, Walters K, Plein S, et al. Myocardial T1 mapping: application to patients with acute and chronic myocardial infarction. Magn Reson Med 2007;58(1):34–40.
147. Broberg CS, Chugh SS, Conklin C, et al. Quantification of diffuse myocardial fibrosis and its association with myocardial dysfunction in congenital heart disease. Circ Cardiovasc Imaging 2010;3(6): 727–34.
148. Ugander M, Oki AJ, Kellman P, et al. Myocardial extracellular volume imaging allows quantitative assessment of atypical late gadolinium enhancement. J Cardiovasc Magn Reson 2010; 12(1):100.
149. Flett AS, Hayward MP, Ashworth MT, et al. Equilibrium contrast cardiovascular magnetic resonance for the measurement of diffuse myocardial fibrosis: preliminary validation in humans. Circulation 2010; 122(2):138–44.
150. Ugander M, Oki AJ, Hsu LY, et al. Myocardial extracellular volume imaging by CMR quantitatively characterizes myocardial infarction and subclinical myocardial fibrosis. J Cardiovasc Magn Reson 2011;13(1):148.
151. Ambale-Venkatesh B, Lima JA. Cardiac MRI: a central prognostic tool in myocardial fibrosis. Nat Rev Cardiol 2015;12(1):18–29.
152. Neilan TG, Coelho-Filho OR, Shah RV, et al. Myocardial extracellular volume by cardiac magnetic resonance imaging in patients treated with anthracycline-based chemotherapy. Am J Cardiol 2013;111(5):717–22.
153. Toro-Salazar OH, Gillan E, O'Loughlin MT, et al. Occult cardiotoxicity in childhood cancer survivors exposed to anthracycline therapy. Circ Cardiovasc Imaging 2013;6(6):873–80.
154. Jordan JH, Vasu S, Morgan TM, et al. Anthracycline-associated T1 mapping characteristics are elevated independent of the presence of cardiovascular comorbidities in cancer survivors. Circ Cardiovasc Imaging 2016;9(8): e004325.
155. Wang C, Zheng J, Sun J, et al. Endogenous contrast T1rho cardiac magnetic resonance for myocardial fibrosis in hypertrophic cardiomyopathy patients. J Cardiol 2015;66(6):520–6.

156. Stromp TA, Leung SW, Andres KN, et al. Gadolinium free cardiovascular magnetic resonance with 2-point Cine balanced steady state free precession. J Cardiovasc Magn Reson 2015;17:90.
157. Eckman DM, Stacey RB, Rowe R, et al. Weekly doxorubicin increases coronary arteriolar wall and adventitial thickness. PLoS One 2013;8(2):e57554.
158. Berthiaume JM, Wallace KB. Adriamycin-induced oxidative mitochondrial cardiotoxicity. Cell Biol Toxicol 2007;23(1):15–25.
159. Wallace KB. Adriamycin-induced interference with cardiac mitochondrial calcium homeostasis. Cardiovasc Toxicol 2007;7(2):101–7.
160. Neubauer S. The failing heart—an engine out of fuel. N Engl J Med 2007;356(11):1140–51.
161. Hamon M, Fau G, Nee G, et al. Meta-analysis of the diagnostic performance of stress perfusion cardiovascular magnetic resonance for detection of coronary artery disease. J Cardiovasc Magn Reson 2010;12:29.
162. Klem I, Heitner JF, Shah DJ, et al. Improved detection of coronary artery disease by stress perfusion cardiovascular magnetic resonance with the use of delayed enhancement infarction imaging. J Am Coll Cardiol 2006;47(8):1630–8.

CHAPTER 17

Pretherapy Cardiology Evaluation

Richard M. Steingart, MD*, Howard Weinstein, MD, John Sasso, MS, Lee W. Jones, PhD, Michelle Johnson, MD, MPH, Carol Chen, MD, Jennifer Liu, MD, Nancy Roistacher, MD, Shawn C. Pun, MD, Jonathan W. Weinsaft, MD, Eileen McAleer, MD, Dipti Gupta, MD, MPH, Anthony Yu, MD, Michael Baum, MD, Wendy Schaffer, MD, PhD

 **Video content accompanies this chapter.**

INTRODUCTION

Cancer therapies have succeeded tremendously in improving outcomes for diseases uniformly perceived as fatal. With an expanding armamentarium available to improve cancer survival, however, came the recognition that it might pose problems on its own. These problems included significant cardiovascular side effects such as heart failure (HF) that were not only therapy limiting but also even antagonizing the overall outcome by imposing significant morbidity and mortality.

Furthermore, cancer is increasingly a disease of the elderly,[1] and the potential for drug interactions in this population is high, not even considering chemotherapeutic drugs.[2] Two-thirds of patients with cancer older than 50 years of age have a high Framingham risk and more than 25% have heart disease (HD).[3,4] Importantly, coexisting HD is associated with a survival disadvantage in patients with cancer equivalent to an advance in age of 10 years. Typically, patients with HD and cancer were treated less aggressively for their cancers than those without HD.[3] Indeed, the presence of these 2 disease processes together may temper the enthusiasm for the aggressive treatment of either. However, it is possible to adequately manage these patients although with greater complexity and demands and largely unsupported by trial data.

The evidence base available to prevent or treat cardiovascular disease (CVD) in patients with cancer is limited in part due to the youth of the field, and in part due to the traditional practice of excluding patients with cancer from the best science of clinical trials. Professional consensus guidelines for the management of CVD in patients with cancer are sparse. Thus, herein, the authors extrapolate from clinical trials done in patients without cancer, use the limited evidence-based data on CVD in patients with cancer available, but admittedly rely largely on their collective experience caring for tens of thousands of patients with cancer over the years at the Memorial Sloan-Kettering Cancer Center. The authors reason that simple and safe measures to treat CVD should be applied whenever possible on the assumption that control of cardiac disease and its risk factors will make cancer therapy safer and more effective and stimulate the patient and the doctor to have a more favorable view of the attempted cancer palliation or cure.

PRECANCER THERAPY CARDIOVASCULAR EVALUATION

In principle, patients with cancer undergo 3 main treatment modalities: surgery, radiation therapy, or chemotherapy, or a combination of these, as, for instance, with stem cell or bone marrow transplantation (Fig. 17.1). The goal of the cardio-oncologic pretreatment evaluation is to define and mitigate the cardiovascular risk these patients might be experiencing. This risk is determined by the cardiovascular reserve at baseline, which can be reduced by cardiovascular risk factors and pre-existing cardiovascular reserve (Fig. 17.2). Any planned cancer therapy may challenge this reserve, unveiling underlying HD as well as by itself

1275 York Avenue, New York, NY 10065, USA
* Corresponding author.
E-mail address: steingar@mskcc.org

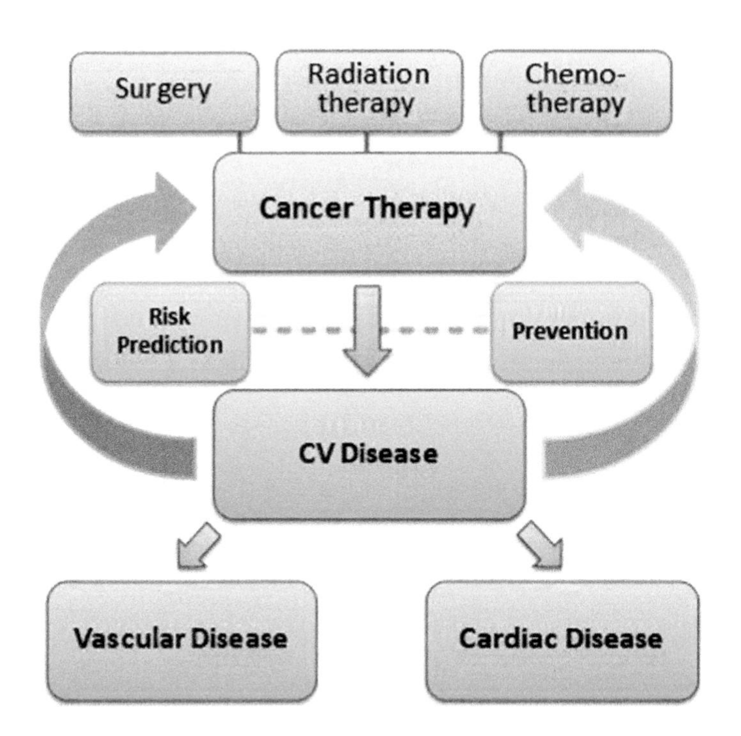

Fig. 17.1 Key elements of cancer therapy, which can induce and worsen CVD, which in itself can impact cancer therapy. The goal of cardio-oncology is to allow for cancer therapy to proceed without detrimental cardiovascular consequences.

being a cause for HD. Genetics and environmental factors play into this equation. For instance, patients with greater exercise tolerance and lower Karnofsky or Eastern Cooperative Oncology Group scores do better with cancer therapies in general. As patients with cancer are seen by their primary oncologist or hematologist, some parameters may be set as to when these patients are referred for a cardio-oncology evaluation (Fig. 17.3). This evaluation is to address the question of the referring provider and should keep a broader scope with regards to the cardiovascular consequences of cancer therapy (Fig. 17.4). Importantly, the cardio-oncology team approach remains multidisciplinary with communication among all providers involved in the care of the patient with the goal to complete the best possible cancer therapy at the lowest possible risk of CVD manifestations or complications (Fig. 17.5).

CARDIO-ONCOLOGY EVALUATION BEFORE CANCER SURGERY, ENDOSCOPIC AND INTERVENTIONAL RADIOLOGY PROCEDURES

The preanesthesia medical evaluation serves as a prime illustrating example for the cardio-oncologic precancer therapy evaluation. The goals are to a degree generic but more complex and nuanced, because not uncommonly 2 life-threatening diseases are being managed

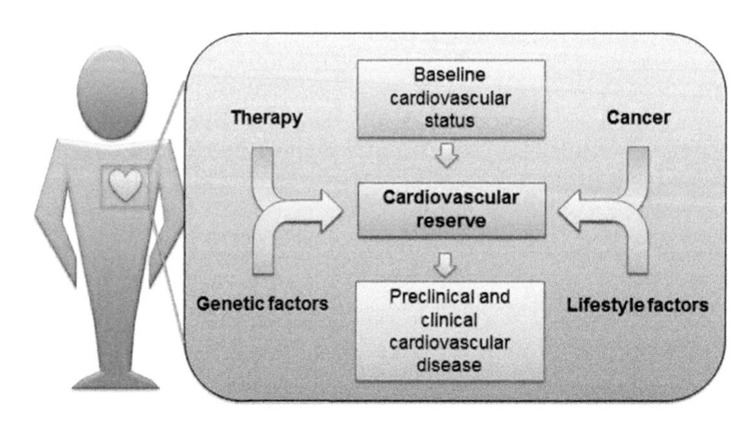

Fig. 17.2 Cardiovascular reserve in any given patient, which, if exhausted, leads to CVD manifestations. This risk is determined by the underlying (baseline) cardiovascular status and impacting factors as outlined.

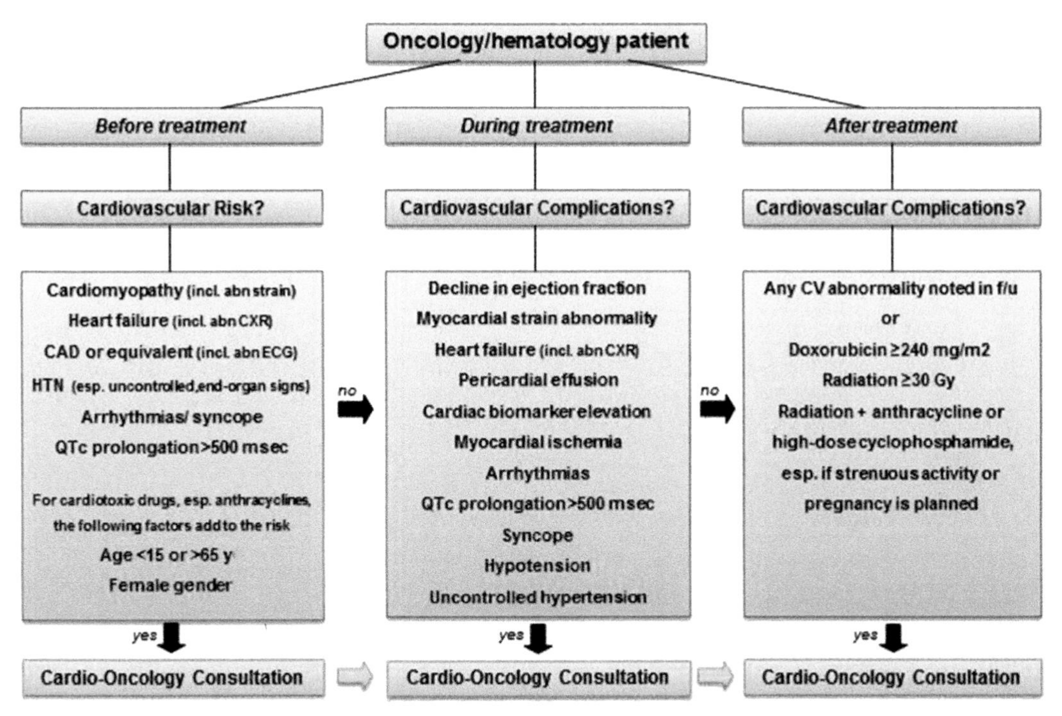

Fig. 17.3 Cardio-oncology practice referral models over the course of cancer treatment. Abn., abnormal; CAD, coronary artery disease; CXR, chest x-ray; HTN, hypertension.

concurrently, and not uncommonly at cross-purposes. Hence, preoperative evaluations in cardio-oncology should be comprehensive and transcend the commonplace advice of "cleared for surgery."[5] Indeed, most preoperative cardiology and medical consultations may fail to meet their intended purpose,[5,6] which should not be the case here.

Perioperative myocardial ischemia is most common in the early postoperative period and can result in myocardial infarction (MI) and other cardiac complications.[7,8] In contrast, intraoperative ischemia is less common and is infrequently associated with postoperative events. Perioperative MI typically is preceded by ST depression and can evolve into a non-ST elevation acute coronary syndrome (ACS) within 24 to 48 hours of surgery, incurring an in-hospital mortality of 10% to 15%. Acute ischemia results from either supply/demand mismatch (type 2 MI, more prevalent with severe underlying coronary stenoses and peaking relatively early after surgery) or from plaque rupture (type 1 MI, affecting midgrade coronary lesions and developing throughout the perioperative period).[7]

The American College of Cardiology/American Heart Association (ACC/AHA) preoperative guidelines[9] can be adapted when considering patients referred for cancer surgery (Fig. 17.6). Procedure risk in cardio-oncology can be defined as high (emergent major operations, particularly in the elderly, and prolonged procedures with large fluid shifts and blood loss), intermediate (head and neck, intraperitoneal and intrathoracic, orthopedic and prostate surgery), and low (endoscopic, superficial, and breast). The comprehensive suite of interventional radiology and endoscopic procedures in cardio-oncology is undefined in risk by guidelines, calling for local experience in understanding their morbidity. The central question of what constitutes prohibitive risk has no fixed definition; risk is considered in relation to alternative treatments. Many patients prefer an intervention with high initial risk with a chance for cure to the alternative of an inexorable downhill cancer course without surgery.

Clinical risk factors from the Revised Cardiac Risk Index, including ischemic HD, compensated or prior HF, cerebrovascular disease, diabetes mellitus, and renal insufficiency, have been used historically. The new AHA/ACC guideline favors the MICA (myocardial infarction and cardiac arrest) risk calculator, which integrates type of surgery and functional level. Exercise tolerance is crucial; patients able to climb the equivalent of 2 flights of stairs or more can generally tolerate most necessary cancer surgery.[9] If further risk stratification is indicated, stress electrocardiography, stress echo, or myocardial perfusion imaging[10] may be performed (Videos 1 and 2). The

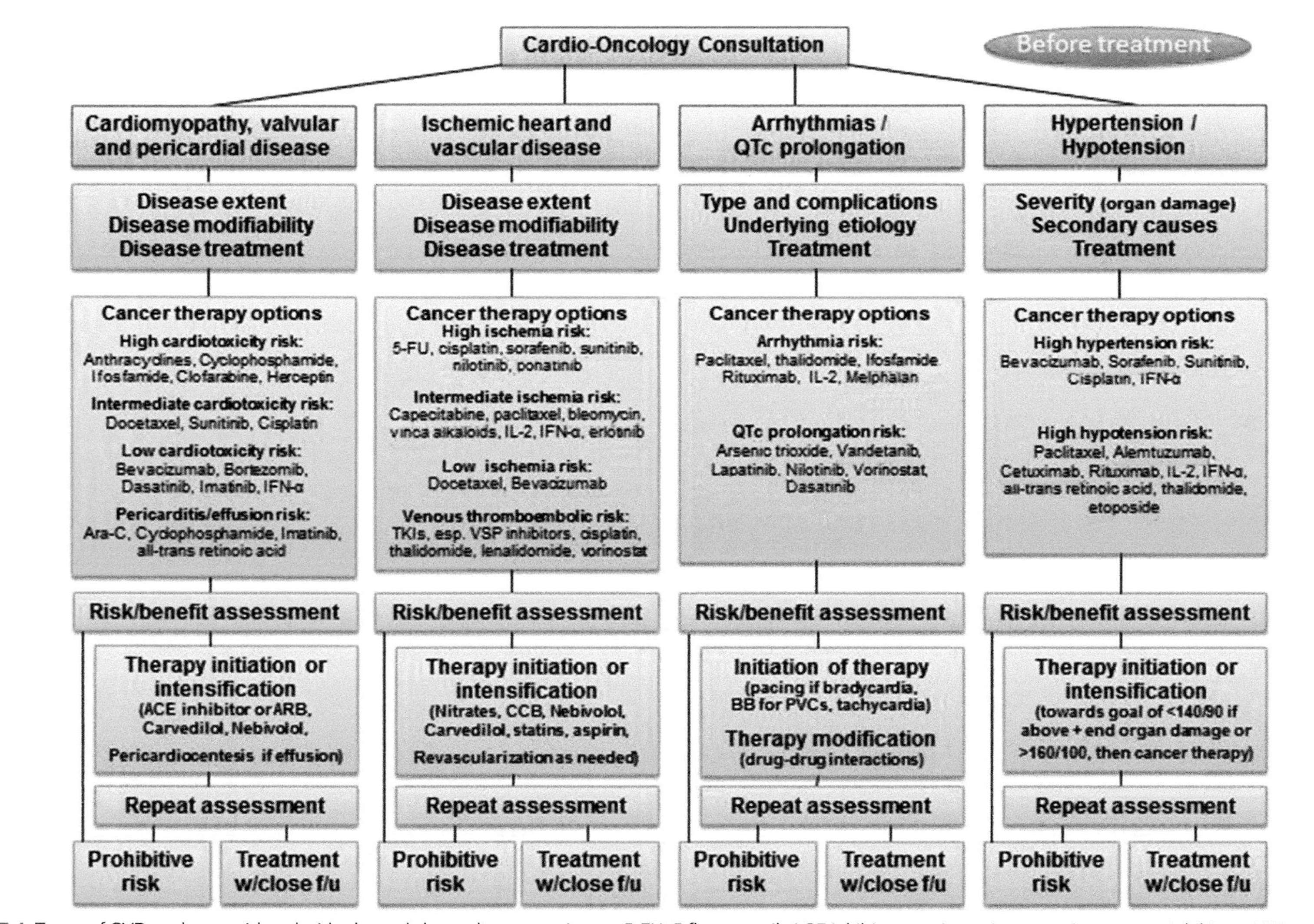

Fig. 17.4 Types of CVDs to be considered with planned chemotherapy regimens. 5-FU, 5 fluorouracil; ACE inhibitor, angiotensin converting enzyme inhibitor; ARB, angiotensin receptor blocker; Ara-C, beta-cytosine arabinoside; BB, beta blocker; CCB, calcium channel blocker; IFN-α, interferon-α; IL-2, interleukin-2; PVCs, premature ventricular complexes; TKI, tyrosine kinase inhibitor.

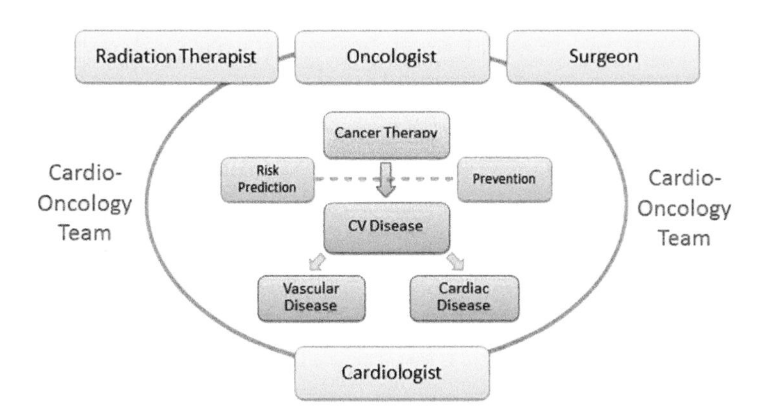

Fig. 17.5 The cardio-oncology care team model.

authors find they are using these adjuncts to assess perioperative risk in patients with cancer less often in recent years, with acceptably low operative morbidity and mortality.

Management strategies for functionally severe coronary artery disease (CAD) are limited by the uncertain utility of preoperative coronary revascularization in reducing perioperative risk. The authors therefore support the dictum that revascularization should be performed before cancer surgery only if appropriate for the long-term benefit of the patient, which for patients with cancer is a decision that is often best made after the cancer surgical results are known. If catheter-based coronary interventions are considered in patients with cancer, one must first consider the patient's tolerance for dual antiplatelet therapy. Although there are cases where active/recent bleeding or thrombocytopenia precludes revascularization or shortens the course of antiplatelet therapy, there are also instances whereby an early window of opportunity for revascularization presents itself before cancer treatment begins.

Surgeons and patients often inquire about the anesthetic risk as synonymous with the procedural risk; therein lies a misconception, because anesthetic mortality is roughly 1 in 13,000 and is stable over time.[11] Poor functional status is a critical factor that defines a high perioperative risk.[12] In patients with thoracic cancer, length of stay is strongly influenced by objective preoperative

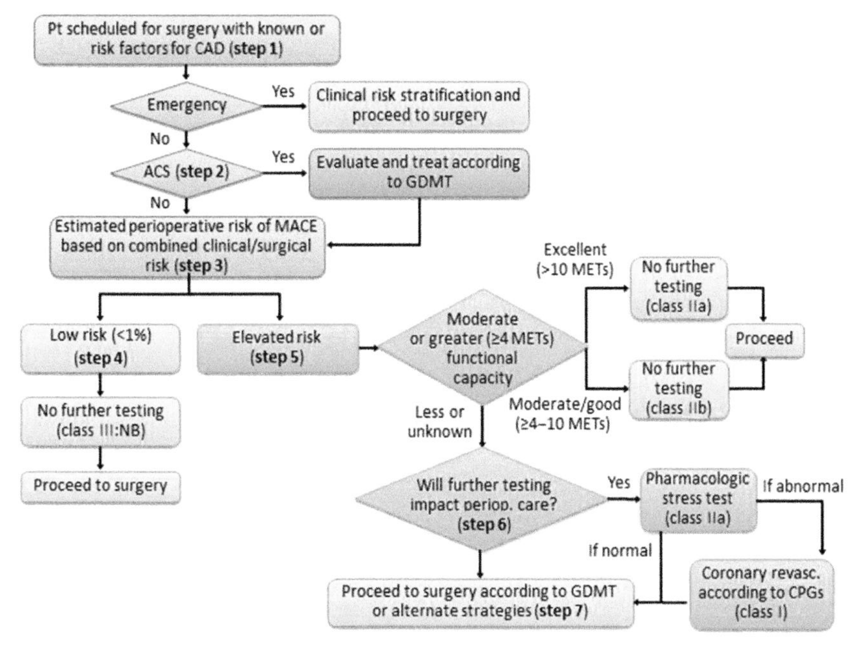

Fig. 17.6 Preoperative evaluation algorithm by the AHA/ACC. (*From* Fleisher LA, Fleischmann KE, Auerbach AD, et al. 2014 ACC/AHA Guideline on perioperative cardiovascular evaluation and management of patients undergoing noncardiac surgery. Journal of the American College of Cardiology 2014;9;64(22):e77–137; with permission.)

exercise tolerance.[13] The assessment of perioperative risk should incorporate both cardiac and total morbidity. The risk/benefit of a procedure is often weighed differently by operators, cardiologists, and patients, and risk tolerance will evolve with the perception of diminishing alternatives and the need for palliation. In the authors' practice, in medically optimized patients, cancer therapeutic procedures of low or moderate risk (estimated morbidity $\leq$10%) typically proceed, whereas those with high-risk estimates (>10%) are subject to negotiation among all parties involved (Fig. 17.7).

The thrombogenicity of tumors, the duration and complexity of tumor resection and of needed restorative surgical components (eg, head/neck and breast surgery), and the potential for interventions to release cardiotoxic agents (eg, hepatic embolization) are unique to cancer surgery. Performance status is often compromised by cancer, as weight loss, anemia, and hypoproteinemia impair metabolic status, and chemotherapy and radiation promote deconditioning and effort intolerance. Host factors can add risk in specific cancers: alcohol abuse and smoking (head/neck, hepatocellular, bladder); smoking and lung disease (lung); and advanced age and cardiac risk factors (prostate).[4]

Compelling surgical indications not uncommonly drive the decision making. When palliation is needed such as when there is impending loss of function (eg, spinal compression, obstructive uropathy, gastrointestinal tract obstruction) or intractable pain, the imperative is to determine the least invasive option to achieve treatment goals. At times palliative (colostomy) rather than curative (low anterior resection) surgery is the treatment of choice.

The time imperative for surgery must also be considered in the options available for investigations and interventions. Prostate, renal, and benign tumors generally have low time imperative, accommodating standard cardiac treatment and stabilization. Lung, colon, and head/neck cancers typically permit a delay of several weeks, permitting revascularization with bare-metal stents or open heart surgery for valvular or coronary disease when indicated (Fig. 17.8). Aggressive tumors or, as noted, impending loss of function, may restrict options for cardiac investigation and treatment severely.

The indications for prophylactic perioperative β-blockers have diminished, with current guidelines mandating only that these be maintained perioperatively if previously started.[9] Initiation of β-blocker therapy perioperatively is a class IIb recommendation for those with intermediate- or high-risk myocardial ischemia noted in preoperative risk stratification or 3 or greater Revised Cardiac Risk Index factors. This class of drugs also remains desirable, however, for the perioperative treatment of CAD, HF, and arrhythmias. β-Blocker therapy should not be started on the day of surgery in β-blocker-naïve patients but rather 2 to 7 days before surgery with optimal dosing and titration perioperatively to avoid hemodynamic instability. Angiotensin-converting enzyme (ACE) inhibitors and angiotensin receptor blockers (ARBs) as well as statins can and should be continued if patients had been on these medications.

HF and severe valvular HD merit special consideration. Clinical HF and pulmonary hypertension are associated with a high perioperative risk. In patients with cancer, HF can be precipitated by cancer treatments and its diagnosis confounded because dyspnea, fatigue, and edema are so common in cancer. These confounders can result in underdiagnosis of HF. The importance of HF is underscored by the

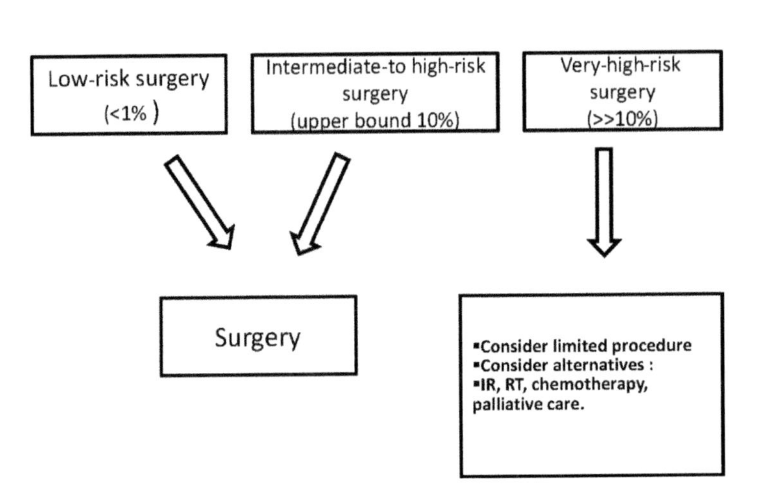

Fig. 17.7 Cancer surgical risk categories. IR, interventional radiology; RT, radiation therapy.

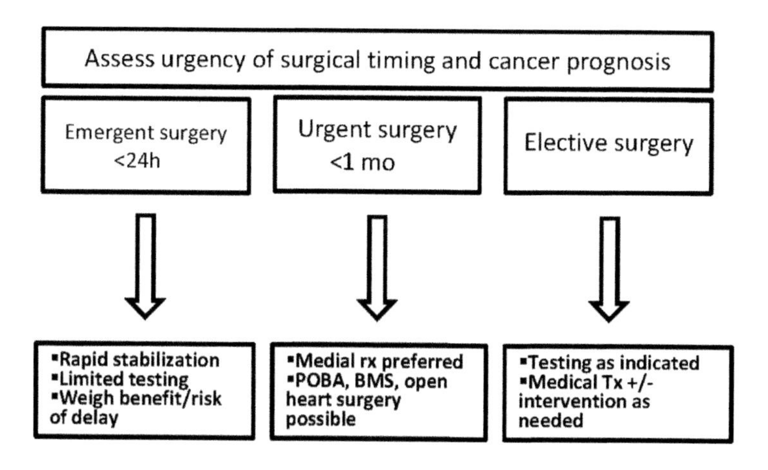

Fig. 17.8 The impact of the timing of cancer surgery on cardiac management choices. BMS, bare-metal stent; POBA, plain old balloon angioplasty; rx, therapy; Tx, treatment.

striking 30-day perioperative mortality of greater than 9% for HF versus 2.9% for CAD.[14] This risk appears to be mitigated somewhat in stable HF patients when treated within a structured preoperative treatment program.[15] Left ventricular dysfunction (LVD) is a strong perioperative risk marker independent of HF.[16] HF with preserved left ventricular ejection fraction (LVEF) incurs an intermediate risk, meriting close attention as well.[17] Limited data in vascular patients support natriuretic peptide measurement to diagnose and follow HF perioperatively.[18]

The once prohibitive perioperative risk of severe aortic stenosis (AS) has declined of late (2.1% mortality for moderate and severe AS, vs 1% for matched controls[19]), with a somewhat elevated risk of MI. The advent of transcatheter aortic valve replacement (TAVR) now offers an alternative to intensive conservative care and balloon valvuloplasty in patients with cancer with severe AS, albeit with limited data supporting its perioperative use. Analogous strategies may be considered in patients with severe symptomatic mitral stenosis. Severe regurgitant lesions incur an elevated perioperative risk but are better tolerated than stenotic lesions,[20,21] particularly severe mitral regurgitation, and are typically managed conservatively in patients with cancer around the time of their cancer treatments.

Preoperative arrhythmias appear to incur minimal incremental perioperative risk[21] but may warrant investigation for underlying HD. Atrial fibrillation (AF) is relatively common in the elderly patient with cancer[22] and is managed with continued ventricular rate control medications and, if needed, interruption of anticoagulation. Bridging anticoagulation is rarely required. Premature ventricular complexes and nonsustained ventricular tachycardia incur a higher risk of perioperative arrhythmias but not of MI or cardiac death[23] and, hence, do not require specific therapy. Underlying structural or ischemic HD should be treated.

In the current era of sensitive biomarkers, patients are increasingly diagnosed with myocardial injury with a troponin elevation. Some data support routine troponin monitoring in the postoperative period. For now, the authors reserve this for selective patients undergoing cancer surgery with uninterpretable electrocardiograms (ECGs, [eg, left bundle branch block]) and high cardiac risk. When postoperative troponin elevation is seen, a clinical judgment is made about the presence of a true ACS with markers of high risk (eg, ongoing ischemia, HF, malignant arrhythmias, and inducible ischemia on stress testing) and the appropriateness of coronary intervention. This judgment should consider the patient's cancer prognosis and need for further intensive therapy or surgery, their tolerance for further interventions, and the poor prognosis of myocardial injury after noncardiac surgery.[24]

Embolization procedures are generally short in duration and do not involve significant blood loss and therefore lack the traditional risk factors associated with high periprocedural risk. Clearance typically involves ensuring that there is no evidence for uncontrolled arrhythmias, ACSs, or decompensated HF. Substantial hemodynamic perturbations can be produced when larger volumes of tissue are embolized, particularly in proximity to the diaphragm with the release of physiologically active substances or stimulation of nearby sympathetic and/or parasympathetic nerve fibers. For example, hepatic embolization can be associated with significant bradycardia and hypotension with an appearance similar to the -Jarisch reflex. Embolization of significant amounts of hemostatic material(s) to the lung is a rare but catastrophic complication.

Finally, high-quality perioperative care requires close postoperative follow-up. At Memorial Sloan Kettering, in addition to routine postoperative cardiac consultations for suggestive signs and symptoms, a dedicated postoperative cardiology service follows all surgical inpatients and selected outpatients who have undergone preoperative cardiology evaluation to ensure continuity of care, adherence to preoperative recommendations, and appropriate discharge planning.

CARDIO-ONCOLOGY EVALUATION BEFORE CANCER CHEMOTHERAPY

The cardio-oncology evaluation of patients before the initiation of chemotherapy is based on the details of the planned therapy and the associated risks of CVD. Given the complexity that often can be encountered, a very practical approach might be a review of and focus on the specific cardiovascular disease domains linked to the specific chemotherapeutic agents and/or the patient's baseline presentation.

Cardiomyopathy and Heart Failure

Historically, the greatest concerns have been with regards to impairment of cardiac function and HF with anthracyclines in particular. These and related compounds remain key components of treatment regimens for many childhood and adult cancers, such as breast cancer, sarcoma, lymphoma, and leukemia. Cumulative dose is the strongest predictor for cardiotoxicity (traditionally >240 mg/m^2 doxorubicin, >500 mg/m^2 epirubicin); type of administration (pegylated and continuous vs bolus infusions) furthermore influences the risk. Other proposed risk factors include combination chemotherapy (eg, trastuzumab), chest radiation, age (<15 or >65 years), and female gender. Any patient undergoing anthracycline therapy is at least intermediate risk for cardiomyopathy, in combination with chest radiation at high risk (Fig. 17.9). Additional risk factors for anthracycline cardiotoxicity that should be screened for especially in the adult population constitute any pre-existing CVD and risk factors, particularly hypertension; African Americans may also be at higher risk. An integrative approach to patients who are considered for anthracycline-based therapy is in outlined in Fig. 17.10.

Before initiation of anthracycline chemotherapy, a baseline assessment of cardiac function should be performed. Two-dimensional (2D) echocardiography is the preferred imaging technique because of its widespread availability and safety profile and is endorsed by the 2011 American College of Cardiology Foundation (ACCF) Appropriate Use Criteria for Echocardiography.[25] Alternative options such as radionuclide ventriculography or cardiac MRI can be considered to overcome the technical limitations of echocardiography. The rationale for performing a baseline cardiac assessment is to screen for asymptomatic left ventricular dysfunction (ALVD). However, there are no guidelines to inform the decision on whether anthracyclines can be safely administered to patients with ALVD. Furthermore, although not widely reported, in the authors' experience, patients with significant mitral or aortic regurgitation or AS, even in the absence of obvious HF, are at risk for anthracycline

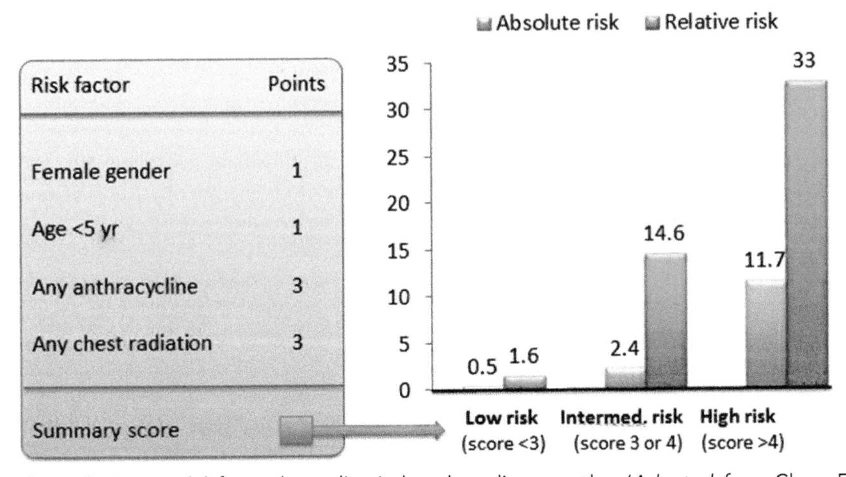

Fig. 17.9 Risk prediction model for anthracycline-induced cardiomyopathy. (*Adapted from* Chow EJ, Chen Y, Kremer LC, et al. Individual prediction of heart failure among childhood cancer survivors. J Clin Oncol 2015;33(5):394–402; with permission.)

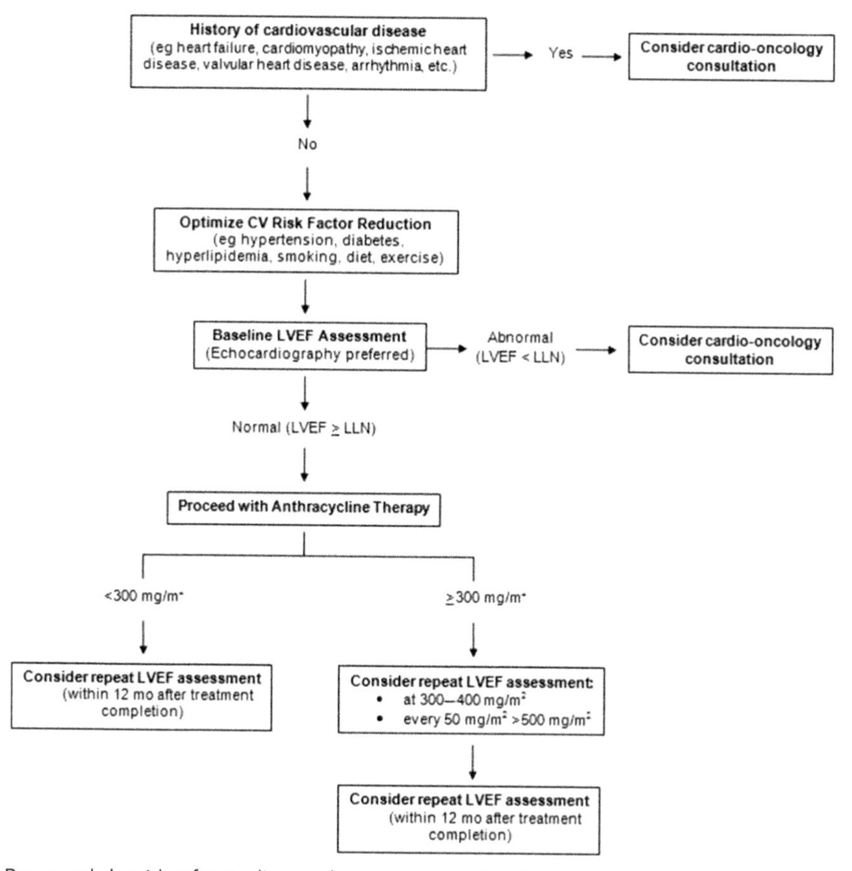

Fig. 17.10 Proposed algorithm for cardiovascular assessment of patients treated with anthracycline chemotherapy. LLN, lower limit of normal.

cardiotoxicity. The decision about whether to use anthracyclines under these circumstances should be made by an oncologist in consultation with a cardiologist versed in cancer care taking into consideration the stage of disease, magnitude of potential benefit from anthracycline treatment, efficacy of alternative nonanthracycline regimens, the options available for treatment of the cardiovascular abnormalities, other comorbidities, and, of course, patient preferences.

Multiple strategies are available to reduce the risk of anthracycline cardiotoxicity. Given that damage caused by anthracyclines occurs in a cumulative dose-dependent fashion,[26] it is generally recommended that the maximum cumulative doxorubicin equivalent dose for adults be limited to 450 to 500 mg/m^2. Prolonged infusion protocols have also been shown to lower the incidence of cardiotoxicity when compared with conventional bolus therapy.[27] In a *Cochrane Database Review* of 6 randomized controlled trials in which different anthracycline dosage schedules were used, the rate of HF was significantly lower with a long infusion (≥6 hours) as compared with a shorter infusion (relative risk [RR] = 0.27; 95% confidence interval 0.09–0.81).[28] This strategy has not been shown to adversely affect the cancer response rate or overall survival (OS).

Use of liposome-encapsulated preparations of anthracyclines is another strategy to reduce the risk of cardiotoxicity and has been effective for the treatment of breast cancer, ovarian cancer, and multiple myeloma.[29–34] Liposomal encapsulation of anthracyclines modifies the tissue distribution and pharmacokinetics of these agents, resulting in decreased penetration to cardiac structures without compromising anticancer effects.[33] Decreased cardiac damage at the tissue level was demonstrated by endomyocardial biopsy among patients receiving pegylated liposomal doxorubicin compared with patients receiving nonliposomal doxorubicin.[35] Liposomal doxorubicin is currently approved by the US Food and Drug Administration (FDA) for the treatment of ovarian cancer and multiple myeloma, but its use is limited by significantly higher cost and fewer supporting studies of efficacy and toxicity compared with conventional doxorubicin. Use of liposomal doxorubicin for the treatment of metastatic breast cancer is currently an off-label use in the United States, but is approved for this indication in Canada.

Dexrazoxane is the only FDA-approved agent for cardioprotection against anthracycline cardiotoxicity. Dexrazoxane is an EDTA-like chelator that binds to iron, reduces the formation of superhydroxide radicals, and prevents anthracycline binding to topoisomerase 2 beta.[36,37] Treatment with dexrazoxane has been shown to reduce the incidence of HF in multiple cancer types among adults.[38] In contrast, studies in children have mainly shown the reduction of surrogate markers for HF.[39,40] The potential risk that dexrazoxane may compromise tumor response to chemotherapy or increase risk of secondary malignant disease has raised uncertainty about the use of this medication[41]; however, a meta-analysis showed no significant difference in tumor response rate, progression-free survival, OS, adverse effects, or secondary malignant disease with dexrazoxane treatment.[38] Dexrazoxane is only FDA approved for use in patients with metastatic breast cancer who have received more than 300 mg/m^2 of doxorubicin and who need additional doxorubicin.[42] Guidelines for the use of dexrazoxane published by the American Society of Clinical Oncology also suggest that dexrazoxane be considered in patients with nonbreast malignancies who have received 300 mg/m^2 or more of doxorubicin-based therapy.[43]

The second agent most commonly associated with cardiotoxicity is trastuzumab, a monoclonal antibody that targets the human epidermal growth factor 2 (HER2, or ErbB2) receptor. HER2 is overexpressed in up to 25% of breast cancers, and trastuzumab in combination with adjuvant chemotherapy improves disease-free survival and OS in women with HER2-positive breast cancer.[44,45] Several other anti-HER2-targeted therapies have been developed with slightly variable binding properties (eg, lapatinib, pertuzumab, TDM-1) and are used alone or in combination with trastuzumab. In early trials of trastuzumab for metastatic breast cancer, cardiotoxicity was unexpectedly observed in 27% of patients treated concurrently with anthracyclines and trastuzumab.[46] In subsequent adjuvant trials of trastuzumab, HF (New York Heart Association class III or IV) and asymptomatic LVEF decline was observed in 0.4% to 4.1% and 7.1% to 18.6%, respectively.[47–51] Blockade of downstream HER2 signaling that leads to inhibition of normal cellular repair mechanisms in cardiomyocytes is one proposed mechanism of trastuzumab-induced cardiac injury.[52] Concurrent or sequential anthracycline chemotherapy has been identified as an important risk factor for trastuzumab cardiotoxicity. Other proposed risk factors include older age (>65 years), hypertension, diabetes mellitus, CAD, arrhythmia, and low normal baseline LVEF. Patients with a frankly depressed baseline LVEF have been excluded from clinical trials, and these patients are not captured in validated trastuzumab cardiotoxicity prediction models (Fig. 17.11).

An approach similar to anthracyclines can be taken for patients considered for trastuzumab therapy (Fig. 17.12). A baseline assessment of cardiac function is recommended to evaluate for pre-existing structural HD. 2D echocardiography remains the most common modality for this purpose, although other options include 3-dimensional echocardiography (with or without echo contrast), radionuclide ventriculography, or

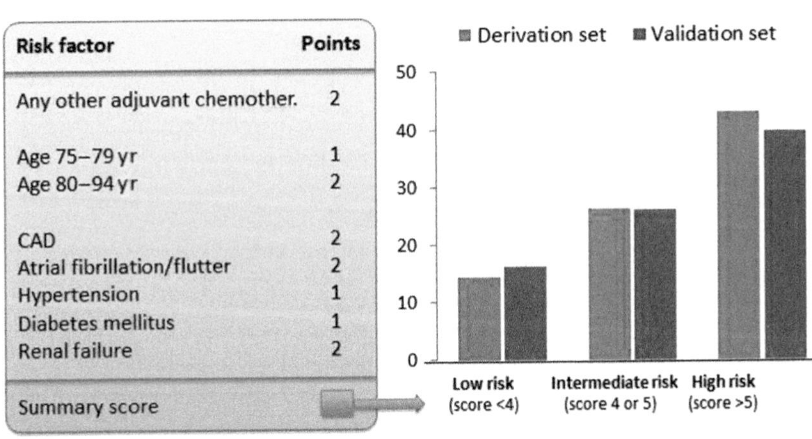

Fig. 17.11 Risk prediction model for trastuzumab cardiotoxicity. (*Adapted from* Ezaz G, Long JB, Gross CP, et al. Risk prediction model for heart failure and cardiomyopathy after adjuvant trastuzumab therapy for breast cancer. J Am Heart Assoc 2014;3(1):e000472.)

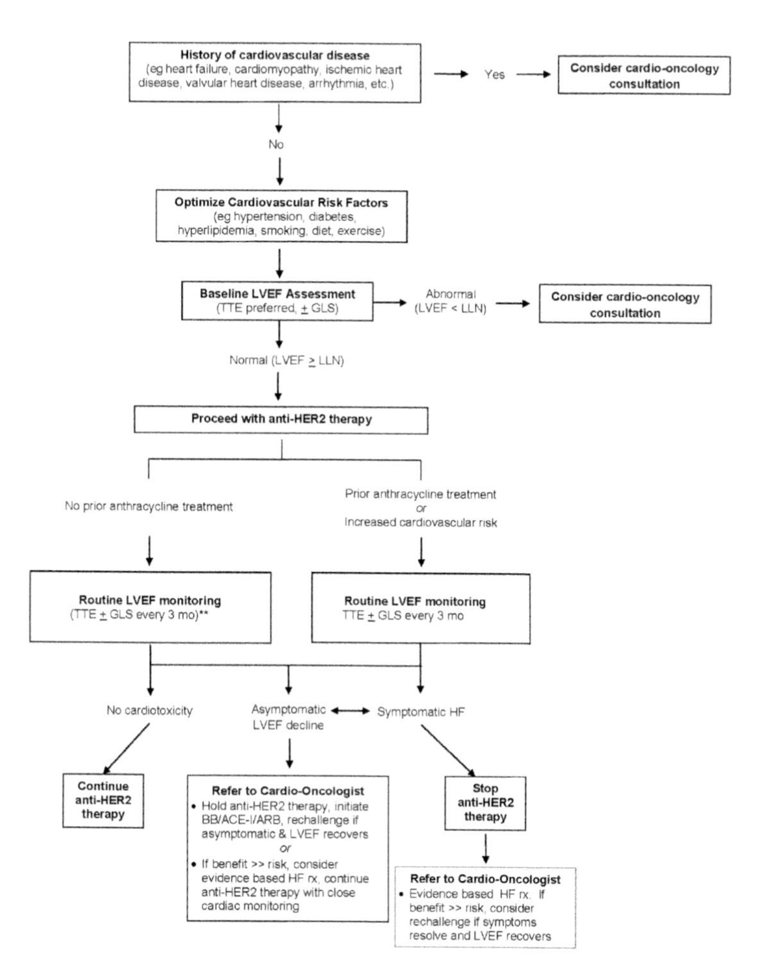

Fig. 17.12 Proposed algorithm for cardiovascular assessment of patients treated with anti-HER2 targeted therapy. LLN, lower limit of normal; TTE, transthoracic echocardiogram. [a] Alternative LVEF monitoring schedules could be considered given low risk of cardiac toxicity from anti-HER2 therapy without prior anthracycline exposure.

cardiac MRI.[53–55] The cardiac safety of trastuzumab therapy for patients with pre-existing left ventricular (LV) systolic dysfunction or HF with preserved ejection fraction (EF) requires further investigation. The authors recommend against initiation of trastuzumab for patients with symptomatic HF and/or moderate to severe LV systolic dysfunction (LVEF <40%). For asymptomatic patients with mild LV systolic dysfunction (LVEF ≥40%), the risks and benefits of trastuzumab therapy should be considered with consultation between the oncologist and cardiologist. Some have suggested that women with multiple risk factors for trastuzumab cardiotoxicity but relatively lower-risk HER2-positive breast cancer be spared anthracycline-containing regimens.[56] However, in most patients, the authors remain unable to accurately predict who will develop cardiotoxicity. As such, there is increasing effort to identify alternative biomarkers that can identify vulnerable patients in preclinical stages of cardiotoxicity. Global longitudinal strain (GLS) using speckle tracking echocardiography has been identified as the most robust parameter for subclinical detection of trastuzumab cardiotoxicity. In a prospective study by Sawaya and colleagues[54] of women with HER2-positive breast cancer, a GLS less than 19% after completion of anthracycline treatment was predictive of HF during trastuzumab therapy. Similarly, a study by Negishi and colleagues[55] of women receiving adjuvant trastuzumab demonstrated that an 11% reduction in GLS was the strongest predictor of subsequent cardiotoxicity.

Trastuzumab cardiotoxicity may lead to cardiovascular morbidity and mortality as well as to the potential deleterious effects of premature trastuzumab interruption on cancer outcomes.[57] Thus, there are increasing efforts to prevent cardiotoxicity and minimize the unnecessary interruption of trastuzumab therapy. Several randomized clinical trials are ongoing to evaluate whether prophylactic β-blockers and/or ACE inhibitors can prevent trastuzumab-induced cardiotoxicity in patients with HER2-positive breast cancer (NCT01009918, NCT01434134).

Not only HER-2-directed therapies but also tyrosine kinase inhibitors (TKIs) in general and especially multitargeted TKIs and vascular endothelial growth factor (VEGF) signaling pathway (VSP) inhibitors are also associated with a higher risk of cardiotoxicity. This is due to so-called on-target effects wherein the target of the drug in the cancer cell is also present in the heart and associated with cardiovascular toxicity as well as off-target effects on noncancer pathways that are involved in cardiovascular function.[58–68]

Although there are convincing data that VSP inhibitors are associated with LVD and clinical HF, in practice there is a paucity of data indicating frequency and severity and in how these considerations should impact management decisions.[69] CAD and hypertension have been noted as risk factors for cardiotoxicity with VSP inhibitor therapy (RR 16–18 and 2.5–3, respectively) (Table 17.1), as has been a history of HF but not with as precise estimates of RR. Some studies suggest that drug-induced hypertension may be related to cardiotoxicity; others do not. Clearly, hypertension should be controlled, but there is no clear evidence to support prophylactic therapy to prevent LVD. Age and prior chemotherapy may also be contributing factors.[66]

Approach to the Patient with Heart Failure and/or Reduced Ejection Fraction at Baseline

Under these circumstances, the risks and benefits of therapy have to be carefully weighed in consultation with the patient, oncologist, and cardiologist. It is easiest to separate anthracyclines and trastuzumab for the purposes of this discussion. Generally, patients who have experienced HF or a significant decrease of the EF into the abnormal range as a consequence of prior exposure to anthracyclines should not be rechallenged with anthracyclines. It has been suggested that a patient with a subnormal EF at baseline from causes other than anthracycline exposure who is without HF can be treated with anthracyclines with frequent EF monitoring.[70] It is the authors' experience that, although this is possible, it is rarely done. Rather, alternative chemotherapies are sought. Patients in HF should not receive anthracyclines.

The approach to the use of trastuzumab in patients with HF or reduced EF is more nuanced. Patients who are in HF should not receive trastuzumab until the HF is effectively treated. On the contrary, the authors do not think that withholding trastuzumab for an isolated decrease in the ejection within the normal range is justified if there is a strong clinical indication for its use. The patient should be well informed of the reasons for this decision and the possible risks, with careful monitoring for any signs or symptoms of HF, including more frequent cardiac EF monitoring and biomarker determination as needed. For patients with a resting EF between the lower limit of normal and greater than or equal to 40% who are not in HF, the authors recommend treating with trastuzumab as indicated for breast cancer, ideally with β-blockers and ACE inhibitors/ARBs in the context of a clinical trial. On rare occasions, in the metastatic setting, the authors have used trastuzumab for cancer control in the presence of an EF less than 40% with aggressive β-blocker, ACE inhibitors/ARB therapy, and careful clinical and EF monitoring.

Pericardial and Valvular Heart Disease

Cytarabine is the chemotherapeutic classically associated with pericarditis and pericardial effusion, a reputation gained by case reports. Cytarabine is used for the treatment of acute nonlymphocytic leukemia in adults and children. It is also used in the treatment of acute lymphocytic leukemia and the acute blast phase of chronic myelocytic leukemia. High-dose therapy is the only defined risk factor. The underlying mechanism is unknown, but a hypersensitivity reaction is suspected.

Serosal inflammation has also been attributed to cases of pericarditis with bleomycin, immununotherapies such as anti-PD-1 and anti-CTLA-4 antibodies, and dasatinib, which are difficult to predict.[71–73] The best studied is dasatinib because it has become a well-recognized and anticipated side effect similar to pleural effusion and pulmonary hypertension. Thus, echocardiography might be a useful screening technique in these patients. Risk factors for the development of pericardial effusion may include pre-existing comorbidities, such as cardiac or pulmonary disorders, viral reactivation, or infection, and an increase in activated lymphocytes.

One of the most concerning chemotherapeutics remains cyclophosphamide, which can cause a hemorrhagic myopericarditis, related HF, even with fatal outcomes.[74] It is broadly used in combination chemotherapy for non–Hodgkin lymphoma, leukemia, Hodgkin disease, Burkitt lymphoma, multiple myeloma, endometrial cancer, lung cancer, and breast cancer. At high dosages, alone or in combination with bone marrow transplant, it is used in the treatment of solid tumors and lymphomas. The incidence of symptomatic and fatal cardiotoxicity is 20% to 25% and 11%, respectively. The most robust predictor of toxicity is dose, typically 180 to 200 mg/kg over 2 to 4 days, but cardiotoxicity is seen even with

TABLE 17.1
Vascular endothelial growth factor signaling pathway inhibitors: cardiotoxicity

Agent	Mechanism	Total Hypertension (%)	Grade 3–4 Hypertension (%)	Symptomatic CHF and LV Dysfunction (%)	ATE (%)	VTE (%)	QT Prolongation (%)	Tumor Target
Bevacizumab	mAb to VEGFA	24	8	1.6–2.9	3	12	—	CR, Cer, GBM, NSCLC, Ov, RCC
Aflibercept	VEGF trap	42	17	2.4 grade 3/4 "dyspnea"	3	9	—	CR
Ramucirumab	VEGFR2 inhibitor	20	9	0.4 (1 trial)	2	4	—	CR, NSCLC, AdSGE
Sunitinib	TKI	22	7	3.60	1	*	2	RCC, Pan
Sorafenib	TKI	23	6	3.4 Myocardial ischemia 2.9	2	*	—	RCC, T
Axitinib	TKI	40	13	2.70	1	*	0.30	RCC
Regorafenib	TKI	44	13	0–18 "dyspnea"	NA	NA	—	CR, GIST
Pazopanib	TKI	36	7	6.10	1	*	0.40	RCC, STSarc
Vandetanib	TKI	24	6	0.40	0	*	12 at high dose	MT
Cabozantinib	TKI	33	8	NA	2	6	—	MT
Levantinib	TKI	69	43	7	5	5	—	T

Abbreviations: *, not reported; AdSGE, advanced gastric, gastroesophageal; ATE, arterial thromboembolism; Cer, cervical; CR, colorectal; GBM, glioblastoma multiforme; GIST, gastrointestinal stromal tumor; MT, medullary thyroid; NSCLC, non–small-cell lung cancer; Ov, ovarian; Pan, pancreatic; RCC, renal cell carcinoma; STSarc, soft tissue sarcoma; T, thyroid; VTE, venous thromboembolism.

doses as low as 120 mg/kg. A better parameter may be dose per body surface area, and the cardiotoxicity risk is 25% at 1.5 $g/m^2/d$ or more. Other risk factors include prior anthracycline or mitoxantrone therapy and chest irradiation. The precise mechanisms of cyclophosphamide cardiotoxicity are unknown. A leading theory, however, is that cyclophosphamide causes injury to the endothelial layer with transudation of toxic metabolite, resulting in myocyte damage, interstitial hemorrhage, and edema. Furthermore, intracapillary microthrombi can contribute to the ischemic toxicity spectrum. Damage to the endothelium and interstitial transudation may result in decreased electrical activity and decreased QRS complex, thus compromising LV systolic function. Myocardial ischemia due to coronary artery vasospasm is also proposed to lead to cyclophosphamide-induced cardiotoxicity.[75–79]

Induction of acute injury of the heart valves has not been reported with chemotherapy. Thus, the main focus is related to conditions that can contribute to valve disease such as endocarditis and the management of pre-existing valvular HD. These conditions are largely treated conservatively in the absence of refractory HF or the need for extensive noncardiac surgery. TAVR now offers definitive management of severe AS in selected patients with cancer as does the Mitral Clip for mitral insufficiency. Mechanical valvular prostheses present treatment dilemmas when anticoagulation must be interrupted, with priority given to morbidity from acute bleeding. When feasible, intravenous or subcutaneous heparin may be used as a partial bridge. Subacute bacterial endocarditis prophylaxis follows standard guidelines.

Ischemic Heart Disease and Vascular Disease

The drugs traditionally associated with myocardial ischemia are 5-fluorouracil (5-FU) and its oral derivate, capecitibine. These drugs are key elements in the treatment of gastrointestinal malignancies and are widely used for breast cancer and other malignancies. Coronary vasospasm during 5-FU infusion was first noted during angiography by Luwaert and colleagues.[80] 5-FU causes increased brachial artery contraction in humans as well as spasms of proximal coronary arteries and infarct in animal models.[81,82] 5-FU also causes cardiac hypertrophy, myocardial necrosis, apoptosis of myocardial and endothelial cells consistent with a toxic myocarditis, as well as vascular damage and thrombus formation.[82–85] In keeping with the complexity of the pathophysiology, 5-FU causes a spectrum of clinical syndromes, including chest pain/angina, ischemia, ST-elevation myocardial infarction (STEMI), and non-STEMI, silent ischemia noted on ECG or ambulatory monitoring, bradyarrhythmias, ventricular arrhythmias, QT prolongation, HF, stress cardiomyopathy, and "ventricular dysfunction" with negative cardiac enzymes.[86–90] The great variation in the clinical manifestations of 5-FU cardiotoxicity and definitions, cohorts, and time eras complicates the task of accurately assessing cardiac risk with 5-FU administration.[90,91]

Polk and colleagues,[92] however, systematically identified 30 studies and found the incidence of cardiac events up to 20%, with a mean of 5%. Symptoms of chest pain (often with ECG abnormalities) are noted in as many as 19% of patients, dyspnea, or hypotension in up to 6%. The incidence of life-threatening complications, including MI, HF, cardiogenic shock, and cardiac arrest, is less than 2%.[92] The overall mortality associated with 5-FU was well less than 1% (0%–0.5%).[92]

Early studies noted cardiac events, defined as anginal chest pain with ECG changes with or without elevated cardiac enzymes, in a little more than 1% of patients with no CAD, and 4.5% to 15% of patients with known CAD.[90,91] Another study reported asymptomatic ischemic ST-segment changes during 5-FU infusion in 56% of patients without known CAD and in 100% of patients with CAD.[93] A prospective study from the 1990s, with almost 500 patients treated inpatient with approximately 1000 mg/m^2 of 5-FU over 4 to 5 days, reported a 10% risk of cardiotoxicity in patients with CAD compared with 1% risk in patients without.[94] Two recent studies, one with 5-FU and the other with capecitabine, failed to demonstrate an increase in cardiotoxicity among patients with CAD, but the numbers of patients included and/or the event rates were too small to achieve significance.[95,96] Overall, one may still conclude though that cardiotoxicity with 5-FU is likely higher in patients with ischemic HD.[91]

When assessing the risk of an individual without known ischemic HD, the authors cite a cardiac event risk on the lower end of the spectrum at about 1% and for patients with ischemic HD on the higher end at about 5%.[91,92,94] Several reports document examples of dramatic left ventricular dysfunction with 5-FU.[97–102] It is important when counseling patients to emphasize that although the risk of mortality with 5-FU is very low, any syndrome suggesting ischemia (eg, shortness of breath, discomfort above the diaphragm) with 5-FU or capecitabine may represent a potentially life-threatening event and must be reported to health care providers immediately. If there is significant ischemia despite optimal management, the authors recommend inpatient administration of 5-FU with appropriate cardiac monitoring. 5-FU administration should probably be avoided in patients who have experienced recent MI or ACSs (spontaneously or associated with prior 5-FU administration), or in those with uncontrolled HF or arrhythmias. However, even in these patients, the risks and benefits of 5-FU administered under carefully monitored conditions must be individualized.

Continuous infusion 5-FU may carry a higher risk of cardiac events than bolus infusion.[103] Whether the incidence of events with capecitabine is lower than or similar to with 5-FU is not entirely clear because of differences in patient selection, dosing schedules, and definitions of outcomes.[89,92,104–107] Limited case studies suggest dose-reduction and/or prophylaxis with antianginal therapy (usually nitrates and/or calcium channel blockers) may be helpful[108–110] (Appendix 1). Given the complex pathophysiology of 5-FU cardiotoxicity, prophylaxis to address coronary vasospasm alone is probably not sufficient to prevent all recurrent events.

Another class of chemotherapy agents classically associated with myocardial ischemia is the taxanes, especially paclitaxel. The reported incidences vary from less than 1% to less than 5%. Other agents with vascular toxicity and reported events of ACS include cisplatin and VSP inhibitors. The incidence is on the order of nearly 2% with either and twice as high with combination therapies. Furthermore, TKIs seem to be associated with a higher incidence of ACS events, in fact, in as high as 10% in the initial reports. Finally, and most recently, similar rate of ACS events were reported for the BCR-Abl inhibitors nilotinib and ponatinib, a risk that seemingly persisted even after therapy was discontinued and involved other vascular territories as well. Aspirin may mitigate the ischemic event risk, at least for those on bevacizumab, 65 years or older, and with a history of an arterial thrombotic event, however, at a 1.3 times higher risk of grade 3 and 4 bleeding events.[111] How soon these therapies can be initiated after an ACS event is not well defined. Historically, patients were excluded from therapy if they had any ischemic event within the past year.

In general, it is not too uncommon to encounter ischemic HD in patients with cancer because there is some overlap in risk factor profile and pathogenesis.[112–115] The management of stable CAD in patients with cancer centers on symptom reduction and event prophylaxis, ideally per guidelines.[116–123] It is the authors' practice to manage coronary disease with medical therapy rather than an interventional or a surgical approach whenever possible in the patient with active cancer or those recently treated. Once the cancer has been treated and the prognosis is better defined, the role of interventional cardiology or cardiac surgery can be reassessed. This approach avoids the need for prolonged antiplatelet therapy, which could complicate future cancer surgery or chemotherapy. It also minimizes the morbidity and early disability of surgical approaches to coronary disease in patients whose lifespan may be limited by cancer. Medical therapy is more problematic in patients with unstable coronary syndromes or uncontrolled HF or arrhythmias. In such patients especially, the approach must be individualized after discussions with the patient, family, surgeon, oncologist, and cardiologist.

Regarding risk factors for ischemic HD, hyperlipidemia may complicate targeted cancer therapies, and worse control is to be anticipated with certain therapies. For instance, mammalian target of rapamycin inhibitors significantly increase serum triglycerides, low-density lipoprotein, and glucose. TKIs such as nilotinib alter glucose metabolism.[124] The net benefit of statins in overall and cancer-specific survival[125] supports their use in hyperlipidemia or vascular disease in patients with cancer without elevated transaminases. This issue is pertinent, for example, in those with liver metastases. Moreover, similar to antihypertensives, it is important to consider the drug-drug interaction potential of these medications. Furthermore, in patients with an estimated life expectancy of between 1 month and 1 year and a recent deterioration in functional status, discontinuing statins improved quality of life without affecting mortality.[9,126]

Thromboembolic Disease

Cancer is a prothrombotic state, and endothelial cells may develop procoagulant activity in the presence of some tumors.[127] VSP inhibitors and other vasotoxic agents may exacerbate this risk by damaging the endothelium. Arterial thrombotic events have been reported with several agents; the evidence for increased risk of venous thrombosis is less clear.[111,128] Patients with prior history of arterial thrombosis and age greater than 65 appear to be at higher risk. Risk may also vary with the type of tumor (higher for colon cancer than breast cancer) and with the agent, for example, bevacizumab. Before drug therapy, cardiac risk factors should be managed. Antiplatelet agents may be considered in patients with prior arterial thromboembolism. Drug therapy should be discontinued for new thromboembolic event grade 3/4 (National Cancer Institute Common Terminology Criteria for Adverse Events [CTCAE] v4.0), and the patient treated appropriately.[129] There is a concern for continuation of therapy with anticoagulation because these agents are associated with increased risk of bleeding. Of note, a retrospective review of bevacizumab use in metastatic colon cancer and non–small-cell lung cancer indicated full anticoagulation may be safe for the prevention of venous thrombosis.[130]

In regards to the prediction of thromboembolism with chemotherapy, several drugs have been associated with a higher risk. These drugs include cisplatin (8.5%), thalidomide (up to 58%), lenalidomide (up to 75%), vorinostat (5%–8%), and erlotinib (4%–11%). A risk score for venous thromboembolism in patients undergoing chemotherapy has been developed (Fig. 17.13), interestingly, not including any specific classes of chemotherapeutics, thus underscoring that the risk may largely be driven by the underlying milieu rather than the cancer therapy itself.

Systemic Hypertension

Hypertension has been reported with all VSP inhibitors and is usually in the early stages of treatment. It may appear abruptly (within 24 hours) and can be of severe degree. As long as VSP inhibitor therapy is continued without change, the blood pressure increase can be sustained. On the contrary, a rapid decrease in blood pressure may occur when the agent is stopped, requiring vigilant monitoring of antihypertensive therapy. Pre-existing hypertension, age 60 years or greater, and body mass index 25 kg/m^2 or higher are independent risk factors for VSP inhibitor-related hypertension. Consensus guidelines indicate that blood pressure treatment should be individualized, taking into account pretreatment blood pressure status and underlying cardiovascular risk factors and disease. Home blood pressure monitoring is recommended starting at the beginning of VSP inhibitor therapy for diagnosis and to fine-tune dosing.[131–140]

Systemic hypertension is one of the main comorbidities and one of the key risk factors for cardiovascular toxicity in patients with cancer, but its management can be challenging. Blood pressure variability can be accentuated by autonomic nervous system dysfunction, inflammation, endothelial dysfunction, and metabolic abnormalities,[141] states commonly seen in patients with cancer. A wide variation in blood pressure is typically observed during chemotherapy with marked changes in fluid status (hypovolemia, fluid loading, anemia), adjuvant steroids, physical and emotional stress, and sepsis. Rarely, hypertension may signal a paraneoplastic syndrome.[142–144]

Antihypertensives are often withheld in postural hypotension and renal insufficiency. All major classes of antihypertensives improve outcomes similarly in the general population[145] and are frequently used in cardio-oncology. Diuretics may be particularly helpful in treating coexisting edema but should be used cautiously when hypovolemia is suspected. ACE inhibitors and ARBs, Carvedilol, or Nebivolol may be preferred in those at an estimated high risk for cardiotoxicity with anthracyclines.

Arrhythmias/QTc Prolongation

Paclitaxel, namely its Cremophor EL formulation, was found to be associated with hypersensitivity reactions, and it was routine continuous cardiac monitoring for these that led to the documentation of cardiac arrhythmias. The most frequent is asymptomatic bradycardia in nearly 30% of patients, ventricular tachycardia and ventricular fibrillation in 0.26%, supraventricular tachycardia,

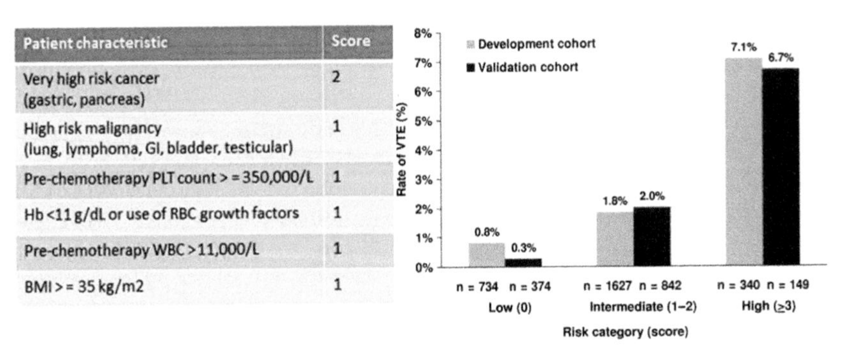

Patient characteristic	Score
Very high risk cancer (gastric, pancreas)	2
High risk malignancy (lung, lymphoma, GI, bladder, testicular)	1
Pre-chemotherapy PLT count > = 350,000/L	1
Hb <11 g/dL or use of RBC growth factors	1
Pre-chemotherapy WBC >11,000/L	1
BMI > = 35 kg/m2	1

Fig. 17.13 Risk prediction model of thromboembolism in patients with cancer on chemotherapy. BMI, body mass index; GI, gastrointestinal; Hb, hemoglobin; PLT, platelets; RBC, red blood cells; WBC, white blood cells. (*From* Khorana AA, Kuderer NM, Culakova E, et al. Development and validation of a predictive model for chemotherapy-associated thrombosis. Blood 2008;111(10):4904–5; with permission.)

AF, and atrial flutter in 0.24%, and heart block in 0.11%; ischemic events were also noted, grade 4 and 5 in 0.29%.[146,147] The most concerning arrhythmias, ventricular arrhythmias, become evident within the first 24 hours of infusion of paclitaxel, occasionally already during the first cycle but most often during the second or subsequent cycles.[74] Atrial arrhythmias occur within the first hours to days (2.5 hours to 6 days) and first cycles (range 1–7). These rhythm abnormalities are most commonly self-limiting or resolve over 48 to 72 hours and as early as 4 hours after discontinuation of therapy. Some patients may continue to exhibit rare and brief episodes of supraventricular tachycardia or rare premature ventricular contractions even 10 days after discontinuing paclitaxel. However, there are no clinically significant sequela, and there is no cumulative or long-term effect. This being said, MI and ischemia were seen during and up to 14 days following paclitaxel therapy but unrelated to arrhythmias.

The precise mechanisms are not clear, and it is not clear whether they are related to paclitaxel or its Cremophor EL formulation vehicle. This vehicle induces histamine release, and stimulation of H1 and H2 receptors can increase myocardial oxygen demand, induce coronary vasoconstriction (H1), and cause chronotropic effects (H2). In particular, selective activation of histamine receptors in the cardiac tissue may result in bradycardia, atrioventricular conduction prolongation, bundle branch block, ventricular irritability, and even cardiac ischemia. On the other hand, the H1 and H2 antagonists used to prevent the hypersensitivity reactions may also cause these events. Arrhythmias, especially bradyarrhythmias, have been reported with cimetidine, ranitidine, and famotidine, and hypotension, palpitations, tachycardia, and extrasystoles have been reported with diphenhydramine. However, many of the cardiac abnormalities associated with paclitaxel appeared later during the infusion. They were usually self-limited or resolved soon after the discontinuation of the paclitaxel infusion.

Which patients precisely are at risk is not well defined. Nevertheless, those with a history of MI, angina, or CHF, unable to tolerate bradycardias, with evidence of pre-existing cardiac conduction abnormalities (bundle branch block, first-degree atrioventricular block), requiring negatively dromotropic and chronotropic medications (β-blockers, digoxin, calcium antagonists) may be at a higher risk of arrhythmias during paclitaxel therapy. Such patients may require careful cardiac evaluation and continuous monitoring during therapy. Furthermore, patients on higher-risk chemotherapy combination may require monitoring. Paclitaxel can enhance doxorubicin-induced cardiotoxicity by increasing doxorubicinol, the major metabolite of doxorubicin, in cardiomyocytes. Thus, temporal separation of therapy by at least 1 day and/or restriction of the cumulative doxorubicin dose to 380 mg/m^2 is recommended. This interaction was not observed for epirubicin, so this drug should be selected preferentially when combined with taxanes. Still, Cremophor EL lowers the renal and hepatic clearance of anthracyclines, resulting in their increased plasma concentrations.

The combination of docetaxel with thalidomide is another higher-risk combination for bradycardias. Thalidomide by itself can cause bradycardia, in up to 50% of patients with multiple myeloma. The underlying mechanisms are unclear, including induction of overreactivity of the parasympathetic nervous system, resulting in bradycardia and conduction disturbances and thalidomide-induced hypothyroidism. The risk of bradycardia is increased in the elderly and in patients with comorbidities and in combination with β-blockers, calcium channel blockers, digoxin, antiarrhythmic drugs, doxorubicin, or cyclophosphamide, or following chest radiation therapy. Therefore, these patients should be monitored closely for signs and symptoms of bradycardia during the administration of thalidomide, and a thyroid-stimulating hormone level should be obtained to rule out hypothyroidism.

It has to be mentioned that the real incidence of chemotherapy-induced arrhythmias is uncertain and likely underestimated because routine cardiac monitoring may not be performed or include only 12-lead ECGs. Also, patients with cancer may have baseline ECG abnormalities and arrhythmias for various reasons, challenging any causal relationship conclusions. This being said, chemotherapeutics can induce cardiac arrhythmias due to direct electrophysiological effects or cardiac indirect effects.

In the cardio-oncology clinic, the goal and challenge are to identify patients most susceptible to cardiac arrhythmias, to define their clinical monitoring, and to optimize their treatment strategy in an effort to reduce morbidity and mortality.[148] As always, a careful cardiovascular evaluation should be performed in all patients undergoing chemotherapy, including physical examination, family and personal history of cardiac diseases, and cardiovascular risk factors or pre-existing CVDs (CAD, hypertension, HF, cardiomyopathies, thromboembolic events), endocrine and metabolic abnormalities (hypothyroidism/hyperthyroidism, especially with neck radiation), or electrolyte abnormalities, as well as previous treatments with chemotherapy and radiation therapy. The electrophysiological evaluation may include a baseline ECG, chest radiograph, exercise testing, and LV function assessment by echocardiography, and/or MRI, if necessary. A 12-lead ECG and Holter monitor are relatively available and inexpensive methods to detect bradyarrhythmias/tachyarrhythmias, conduction disturbances, and repolarization abnormalities (QTc interval prolongation) as well as signs of myocardial ischemia, LV hypertrophy, and cardiomyopathy before and during the treatment. As a key goal of cardiac monitoring, it should remain to identify signs of cardiac diseases early enough to prevent, reverse, or decrease them and their consequences.

Increased susceptibility to chemotherapy-induced arrhythmias should be assumed to be present in patients with cancer with basal ECG abnormalities, impaired exercise capacity, or pre-existing CVDs, and those undergoing treatment regimens with known cardiotoxicity potential and its risk factors. Comorbidities that could represent a possible arrhythmogenic substrate should be identified and treated aggressively before and during chemotherapy. ACE and aldosterone inhibitors, β-blockers, or statins are considered to improve the arrhythmogenic substrate in patients with CAD, arterial hypertension, LV dysfunction, or HF. Amelioration of cardiotoxicity by alternative formulation or administration should also be considered, especially with anthracyclines. Early identification and aggressive treatment to prevent and/or reverse cardiac remodeling are likely also the best strategy to modulate the arrhythmogenic substrate and improve outcomes in patients with chemotherapy-induced arrhythmias.

Atrial and ventricular ectopy is commonly observed in cancer therapy with underlying HD. Amiodarone is the most effective prophylactic agent against postoperative AF after lung cancer surgery[149]; accordingly, thoracic surgery patients at the authors' institution receive a 3-day perioperative course of amiodarone. Thoracic tumors, mediastinal irradiation, cardiotoxins, bone marrow transplant, sepsis, pneumonia, surgery, pericarditis and pericardial effusion, chronic inflammation, and other sympathetic stressors precipitate and aggravate arrhythmias. Persistence of arrhythmic substrates during active cancer treatment limits the utility of cardioversion for AF, and this should wait if possible until the precipitating/enabling factors have been controlled and there has been a satisfactory period of anticoagulation.[22] The onset of AF during cancer treatment incurs a high risk of thromboembolism and a 6-fold risk of HF, yet risk scores for initiating antithrombotic treatment do not account for cancer-induced hypercoagulability. Cancer per se though did not seem to affect the predictive utility of the CHADS2 score in a large cohort of patients with baseline (but not incident) AF.[150] Oral anticoagulation with warfarin is problematic in patients with cancer, typically requiring its suspension, because of wide fluctuations in international normalized ratio. Thus, low-molecular-weight heparin (LMWH) is frequently used by oncologists to treat or prevent thromboembolism in cancer.[151] The new oral anticoagulants (NOACs) have been increasingly prescribed in patients with cancer, where thromboembolism incurs a poor prognosis,[152,153] but their limited experience in cancer and multiple drug interactions preclude firm recommendations.[154] For patients with cancer with HD, NOACs are limited to thromboprophylaxis in nonvalvular AF.

A team approach to managing implantable cardiac devices is particularly useful in the periprocedural period, in collaboration with anesthesiology,[155] and for radiation therapy,[156] when the device may need relocation either at the outset or, with temporary support from a defibrillator jacket, after completion of therapy.[157]

More than before, with the introduction of TKIs came the recognition of QTc prolongation attributed to inhibition of hERG channels and prolongation of the ventricular action potential duration. Overall, the effect is relatively mild (on average 15-ms increase in QTc interval), except for sunitinib, lapatinib, nilotinib, and vandetanib (average 22.4-, 23.4-, 25.8-, and 36.4-ms increase, respectively).[163] QTc prolongation to 500 ms was noted in as many as 2.3% and torsades de pointes in 0.1% of patients on dasatinib, nilotinib, sunitinb, or pazopanib. The incidence of all-grade and high-grade QTc interval prolongation with vandetanib is 16.4% and 3.7%, respectively, among patients with nonthyroid cancer, and 18.0% and 12.0%, respectively, among patients with thyroid cancer. Patients with thyroid cancer who have longer treatment duration also have a higher incidence of high-grade events. Crizotinib, dasatinib, lapatinib, nilotinib, pazopanib, sorafenib, sunitinib, vandetanib and vemurafenib should be administered with caution in patients with pre-existing QT prolongation or QT-related risk factors.

Another class of chemotherapeutics associated with QTc prolongation and arrhythmias are histone deacetylase (HDAC) inhibitors.[148] For instance, QTc prolongation can be seen in 10%

of patients, SVT in 38%, VT in 14%, and atrial and ventricular ectopy in 65% and 38%, respectively, in patients on romidepsin. Both QTc prolongation and arrhythmias usually resolve before the next cycle. However, cases of sudden death have been reported, underscoring the need for vigilance. QTc prolongation has also been reported in 10% of patients on dacinostat, 6.3% to 28% on panobinostat, and 3.5% to 6% on vorinostat. The observations are consistent with a class effect, and HDAC inhibitors block hERG channels as a mechanistic explanation for the QT prolongation. The risk of QT prolongation increases as a function of peak dose, that is, it is highest with short bolus administrations. The risk for torsades de pointes is higher in women, the elderly, and those with bradyarrhythmias, electrolyte abnormalities, structural HDs, and baseline QTc prolongation.

Cardio-Oncology Evaluation Before Radiation Therapy

Radiation therapy has been and remains an integral component in the treatment of cancers, especially breast cancer and lymphomas, with regards to the chest and head, and neck cancer, with regards to the upper body. Although significant advances in terms of protection of noncancerous tissue have been made, it remains harmful to the cardiovascular system (Fig. 17.14). A pivotal culprit is the endothelial lining of viscera and vessels, and endothelial cell damage then activates an acute inflammatory response followed by release of profibrotic cytokines.[158,159] There is also activation of the coagulation cascade that contributes to fibrin deposition. Treatment- and patient-related risk factors that contribute to radiation-induced heart disease (RIHD) are outlined in Box 17.3.[160–172] An important concept is that radiation is essentially an additional potent cardiovascular risk factor. Thus, those with underlying CVD and risk factors are at greatest risk for clinical progression and events. This has been shown in patients with breast cancer undergoing chest radiation therapy with the highest risks for acute coronary events in those with baseline ischemic HD and especially a history of MI. For this very reason, there should be a thorough review and evaluation of the patient's baseline CVD status and a thoughtful discussion of the risks and benefits of radiation therapy. Those who proceed should have sound control of their cardiovascular risk factors. This is emphasized in the new algorithm by the Society of Cardiac Angiography and Intervention. The preventive merit of antiplatelet and statin therapy, possibly even ACE inhibitor therapy, in this patient population is not defined. Decisions on withholding therapy cannot be based on currently available risk calculators because they do not take into account radiation therapy as an additional risk factor. However, those who do meet treatment criteria for treatment of heart disease or its risk factors by traditional criteria should be initiated on appropriate therapy. Interventions beyond limiting radiation exposure to cardiovascular structures that would change the development of HF (restrictive cardiomyopathy) and valvular HD are unknown. All of these are later manifestations of RIHD. The main acute complication to evaluate for in the pretherapy setting is pericarditis.

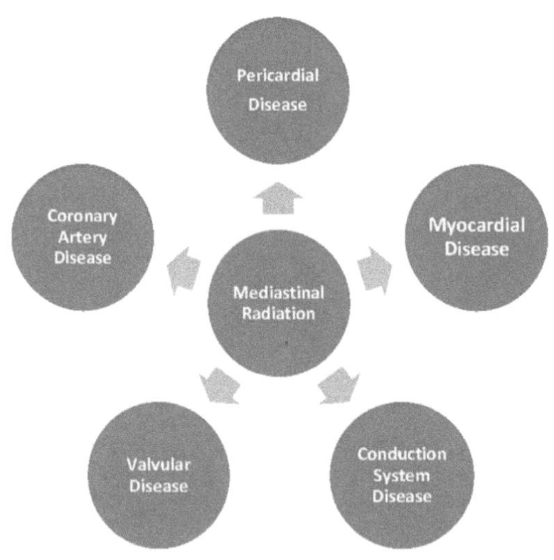

Fig. 17.14 The spectrum of RIHD.

Pericardial disease was one of the earliest recognized and most common cardiac complications of mediastinal radiation therapy. Autopsy studies of young patients showed that more than two-thirds have evidence of radiation-induced pericardial disease.[173,174] Acute pericarditis typically presents with chest pain, fever, and ECG changes within the first few of weeks of radiation. Cardiac monitoring is often recommended because of concerns regarding associated arrhythmias. Fortunately, with the advent of contemporary radiation techniques the incidence of pericarditis has drastically decreased.[175] Symptomatic pericarditis usually responds well to nonsteroidal anti-inflammatory agents and colchicine. Also commonly seen are pericardial effusions, generally asymptomatic identified on chest radiograph or computed tomographic scan as an enlarging cardiac silhouette. The authors monitor asymptomatic effusions with careful clinical and echocardiographic surveillance and avoid withholding needed cancer therapy and anticoagulant therapy in these cases.

CARDIO-ONCOLOGY EVALUATION BEFORE TRANSPLANTATION

Hematopoietic stem cell transplantation (HCT) presents an extended period of physiologic stress that patients with cardiac comorbidities may not tolerate, but recent advances have made HCT an option even for older adults who are more likely to have concurrent cardiac disease.[176,177] The management of CAD, abnormalities of LV function, valvular HD, and arrhythmias during HCT is problematic. Patients face significant thrombocytopenia, anemia, tachycardia, hypotension, fluid challenges, and electrolyte imbalance.[176] Transfusion requirements depend on the underlying cancer, prior treatments, and conditioning, but a study of patients with non-Hodgkin lymphoma or multiple myeloma gives a sense of the magnitude of the physiologic stress, with a median 21 days to platelets greater than 50,000, median platelet transfusions 5, range 1 to 74, median blood transfusions 3, range 0 to 30. As many as 10% to 20% of patients undergoing HCT will be admitted to the intensive care unit (ICU) with mortalities greater than 50%.[176,178,179] Polypharmacy is common, with potential drug interactions further complicated by renal dysfunction in 20% of patients and hepatic dysfunction in 30%.[180] Optimal cardiac care during HCT, including management of antiplatelet therapy, β-blockers, and fluids, is challenging.

Prehematopoietic Stem Cell Transplantation Screening

Age, performance status, resting LVEF, and pulmonary function tests are used to evaluate patients before HCT. The HCT-comorbidity index (HCT-CI) measures organ system dysfunction, with cardiac dysfunction, CAD requiring medical treatment or revascularization, congestive heart failure (CHF), MI or LVEF $\leq$50%, and arrhythmias each given a weight of 1, and significant valvular HD given a weight of 3.[181] Nonrelapse mortality at 2 years with an HCT-CI of 1 to 2 is 21%, and increases to 41% with a score of 3 or higher.[178] Routine stress testing does not add significant prognostic information.[182–184] A single study found patients with both reduced resting LV function and an inability to increase LVEF 5% or greater with exercise were at increased peritransplant mortality, but with more than 30% of the study population transplanted for breast or ovarian cancer, unexpectedly high transplant mortality and no deaths due to cardiac causes, the relevance of this study to current transplant patients is limited.[185]

Coronary Artery Disease

Few data can be found on patients with CAD during HCT: a retrospective study of about 70 patients with established CAD and a 1994 case report.[186,187] In the retrospective study, 25% of patients had coronary artery bypass graft (CABG), 50% had percutaneous coronary intervention (PCI), and about 50% had prior MI.[186] Slightly more than half of the transplants were autologous, almost all peripheral stem cell grafts, with more than 85% receiving myeloablative conditioning predominantly for lymphoma, leukemia, and multiple myeloma. ICU admission, transplant related mortality, and OS at 1 year were similar to a matched group without CAD.[186] This study provides evidence that patients with stable CAD can receive HCT without prohibitively increased risk.

If a patient has unstable or high-risk CAD, stress testing and/or cardiac catheterization before HCT may be warranted. The decision to perform cardiac catheterization should be made by a cardio-oncologist in collaboration with the transplant oncologist and the interventional cardiologist, weighing the risk of delaying transplant with the benefit of revascularization. The method of revascularization, PCI (and then bare-metal vs drug-eluting stent) versus CABG, should be discussed. At least 4 weeks of dual antiplatelet therapy is recommended for bare-metal stents, with continuation of aspirin thereafter.[188] The recommended duration of dual antiplatelet therapy with drug-eluting stents depends on the generation of the stent, but is up to 1 year from stent placement.[188] It is common to discontinue aspirin when platelets drop to less than 50,000, but platelets less than 20,000 may be a more appropriate cutoff.[189] Further informing the discussion of aspirin use with severe thrombocytopenia, there is one study of aspirin use for ACS in patients with cancer with thrombocytopenia (median platelet count 32,000, range 4000–100,000) that suggests benefit.[190] Aspirin should be restarted when the patient has engrafted with platelets above the chosen cutoff. Statins are often discontinued for HCT because of multiple drug interactions and restarted after transplant admission.

Reduced Left Ventricular Function

For many years, patients with LVEF less than 50% were ineligible for HCT.[191] Reduced LVEF is a concern with HCT given the fluid challenge and risk for infection. Carefully selected patients with impaired LV systolic function can undergo HCT without prohibitively increased risk, including those with anthracycline-related cardiomyopathy.[192–195] Although there were more CTCAE v3.2 cardiac complications grade 2 or more in patients with LVEF ≤45% who also had at least one cardiac risk factor (prior smoking, hypertension, hyperlipidemia, CAD, arrhythmia, or prior CHF) that underwent allogeneic HCT, 100-day nonrelapsed mortality was similar to a control group with LVEF ≥50%.[193] About 20% of patients had an EF ≤35%, about 40% had EF 36% to 40%, and about 40% had EF 41% to 45%. In a study of 49 patients who underwent allogeneic HCT with mildly depressed LVEF (LVEF range 28%–49%, median LVEF 45%), TRM was not significantly different than in patients with normal LV function.[195] TRM was increased in patients with CAD and reduced LV function, and OS at 2 years was decreased in patients with LVEF less than 43%, but the number of patients in these subgroups was small.[194] The most common cardiac complications were CHF and AF.[193,194] The vast majority of patients received reduced intensity conditioning, which begs the question whether these patients with reduced LV function are being undertreated with respect to their oncologic disease, out of deference to their compromised cardiac status. The answer is unclear, but warrants consideration by the cardio-oncologist and the transplant oncologist when assessing patients for HCT who have reduced LVEF.

During the transplant admission, patients with moderate or severe LV dysfunction warrant inpatient consultation with the cardio-oncology team, with aggressive efforts to normalize fluid status. A brain natriuretic peptide test (BNP) on admission can be helpful as a baseline.

Arrhythmias

Atrial arrhythmias during HCT are a poor prognostic indicator.[196–198] Patients with a history of arrhythmias are at increased risk.[198] Arrhythmias during HCT are associated with increased length of transplant admission, increased TRM, and decreased OS at 1 year. Arrhythmias complicate allogeneic more frequently than autologous transplants, 8% versus 3% to 5%. Myeloablative conditioning is not more arrhythmogenic than nonmyeloablative conditioning. Adequate control of arrhythmias before transplant, continuation of antiarrhythmic agents with consideration of renal/hepatic dysfunction and drug interactions, and aggressive management of arrhythmias during HCT is recommended. There are no data on rhythm versus rate control for AF. Underlying stressors, such as infection, should be addressed, with efforts to avoid severe anemia, fluid overload, and severe electrolyte imbalance.[197,199]

Medication interactions should also be considered in patients with QT prolongation (QTc ≥500 milliseconds). An informed risk assessment is necessary, as many of the QT prolonging medications used during HCT cannot be discontinued. Telemetry monitoring, repletion of electrolytes, and avoiding bradycardia are recommended as are daily ECGs when QTc is prolonging or if new medications are added.

Valvular Heart Disease

There are no data on the management of severe valvular HD during HCT. Extrapolating from the extensive data on valvular HD in the setting of noncardiac surgery, regurgitant lesions can often be managed with careful fluid management.[200] Severe stenotic lesions are problematic, and a formal evaluation by a cardio-oncologist is recommended, to weigh the risks and benefits of intervention on the valve before HCT.

Pre-exercise/Cardiovascular Screening Guidelines

In light of the recently released national guidelines as well as increasing interest from patients and cardio-oncology professionals,[201] a clinically important question is how to appropriately screen/clear patients for exercise participation.[202] The risk of an adverse cardiovascular event during light-to-moderate-intensity exercise in healthy individuals is low; thus, the benefits of regular exercise far outweigh the potential risks, even in patients with cancer (**Fig. 17.15**).[203,204] Nevertheless, the incidence of serious adverse events (SAEs) (eg, MI, sudden cardiac death) during structured exercise training in cardiac patients is 10 times that of healthy individuals.[205] Hence, the risk of an exercise-related event depends on the extent of underlying concomitant comorbid disease. Such considerations may be important in the oncology setting because patients with cancer are often older and either have overt CVD or are at risk of developing of CVD at the time of cancer diagnosis in 30% to 80%.[206] In addition, normal age-related abnormalities are also compounded by the direct adverse effects of the various anticancer therapies on cardiac function and other components of the cardiovascular system as well as effects secondary to therapy such as deconditioning.[207] Consequently, patients

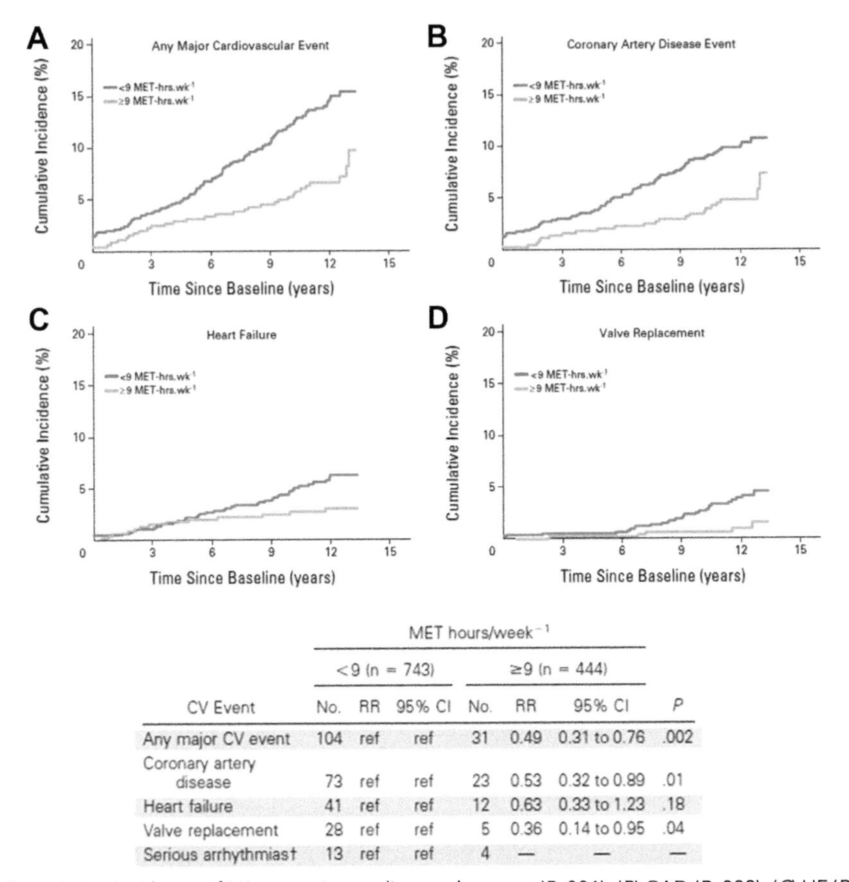

	MET hours/week⁻¹						
	<9 (n = 743)			≥9 (n = 444)			
CV Event	No.	RR	95% CI	No.	RR	95% CI	P
Any major CV event	104	ref	ref	31	0.49	0.31 to 0.76	.002
Coronary artery disease	73	ref	ref	23	0.53	0.32 to 0.89	.01
Heart failure	41	ref	ref	12	0.63	0.33 to 1.23	.18
Valve replacement	28	ref	ref	5	0.36	0.14 to 0.95	.04
Serious arrhythmias†	13	ref	ref	4	—	—	—

Fig. 17.15 Cumulative incidence of (*A*) any major cardiovascular event (*P* .001), (*B*) CAD (*P* .002), (*C*) HF (*P* .028), and (*D*) valve replacement (*P* .006) according to meeting national guidelines for vigorous intensity exercise (ie, 9 vs 9 metabolic equivalent [MET] h/wk). ref, referent; RR, rate ratio. Adjusted for attained age, age at diagnosis, sex, race, smoking status, education, and CV disease risk factor profile as time-dependent variables, anthracycline exposure, chest radiation exposure, and baseline (grade 3 or 4) chronic (non-CV) conditions. [a] Result from multivariable analysis was not available as a result of the small number of events. (*From* Jones LW, Liu Q, Armstrong GT, et al. Exercise and risk of major cardiovascular events in adult survivors of childhood Hodgkin lymphoma: a report from the childhood cancer survivor study. J Clin Oncol 2014;32(32):3647; with permission.)

with cancer may be at heightened risk of an exercise-related event, creating the rationale for appropriate preexercise screening guidelines.

Pre-exercise/cardiovascular screening guidelines are established for noncancer clinical populations.[208] Most guidelines stratify individuals into low-, moderate-, and high-risk categories based on demographic and medical variables. The appropriateness of existing guidelines and/or the development of oncology-specific pre-exercise clearance guidelines have received scant attention in the oncology setting. In the only study to date, Kenjale and colleagues[209] investigated the utility of established exercise clearance guidelines to predict exercise-related events in adult patients with cancer. Patients (n = 413) with histologically confirmed solid or hematologic malignancy were categorized into pre-exercise risk stratification (ie, low, moderate, or high risk) based on American College Sports Medicine (ACSM) clearance guidelines. Risk of an exercise-related event was evaluated during a symptom-limited cardiopulmonary exercise test (CPET) with 12-lead ECG. A first important finding was that the vast majority of patients with cancer (>80%) were categorized as moderate or high risk, and exercise capacity (VO_{2peak}) was, on average, ~20% less than that of age-matched sedentary, but otherwise healthy individuals; 15% had a VO_{2peak} <14 mL kg^{-1} min^{-1}, the threshold criteria for referral for heart transplantation in patients with HF. In terms of safety, no major SAEs or fatal events were observed during CPET procedures. However, a total of 31 positive ECG tests were observed, for an overall event rate of 8%. Importantly, ACSM risk stratification did not predict the risk of a positive test, suggesting that widely used screening recommendations developed in noncancer clinical populations may have suboptimal utility in adults with cancer. Given this, Kenjale and colleagues[209] also explored medical and demographic predictors of exercise-related events to inform evidence-based, oncology-specific screening guidelines. These analyses indicated that age, statin use, antiplatelet therapy use, CVD, prior treatment with adriamycin or radiation therapy, and being sedentary were predictors of a positive test.

There is currently a lack of consensus regarding the level of pre-exercise screening required in any clinical population, particularly incorporation of formalized exercise testing.[211–213] There is currently no evidence to support any absolute or relative contraindications to exercise participation in adults with cancer.[210] Nevertheless, based on the data of Kenjale and colleagues,[209] the authors recommend that formalized pre-exercise screening be required for all sedentary oncology patients planning to engage in an exercise program/prescription. Such screening can be readily achieved using validated tools such as the Physical Activity Readiness Questionnaire (PAR-Q) or PAR-med-X. The PAR-Q is a self-screening tool that asks participants about prior medical history, whereas the PARmed-X is an exercise-specific checklist used by a physician in patients with positive responses to the PAR-Q. Initial use of the PAR-Q should be undertaken when a patient opts to do any of the following: (1) undergo a fitness assessment, (2) join a health club or sports team, (3) work with a personal trainer, or (4) decide to become much more physically active than current levels (that is, above their habitual [daily] physical activity level or adopting a structured physical activity/exercise program).[210] Initial screening can be performed by a qualified exercise professional or any allied health professional. In terms of the need for formalized exercise stress testing, some organizations advocate for exercise testing in patients at high risk of CVD before engaging in moderate-intensity exercise,[212] whereas others recommend that exercise testing is not required.[211] The results of Kenjale and colleagues indicate that formal exercise testing is likely not required for the vast majority of patients with cancer. However, patients presenting with overt CVD or CVD risk factors as well as those undergoing or previously treated with known cardiotoxic agents (eg, anthracyclines, trastuzumab) require PARmed-X referral to a physician or other allied health professional for consideration of blood and ECG tests and possibly exercise testing and cardiac imaging, as appropriate.

Exercise Prescription/Program Guidelines

All cancer-specific exercise guidelines for adult patients with cancer recommend participation in at least 150 minutes per week of moderate-intensity (eg, brisk walking, light swimming) or 75 minutes per week of vigorous-intensity (eg, jogging, running, hard swimming) exercise both during and following the completion of cancer therapy.[214–217] However, the authors contend that this recommendation should be viewed as a long-term goal, and one that is likely not achievable for most sedentary patients. A key aspect of providing safe and effective exercise prescriptions is "individualization" of the program to the patient, particularly in light of the stark differences in pathophysiology, therapeutic management, and prognosis between malignancies and individual patients.[218–220] It is possible to effectively achieve this goal through the use of the fundamental principles of exercise prescription: *F*requency (sessions per week), *I*ntensity (how hard per session), *T*ime (session duration), and *T*ype (exercise modality), more commonly referred to as the *F.I.T.T* principle.[202]

A general approach to exercise prescriptions incorporating the *F.I.T.T.* principle is provided in Fig. 17.16. The first question should focus on how much (leisure-time) exercise the patient is currently performing. Patients meeting the national guidelines should be encouraged to maintain this level of behavior, although it is important to remember that exercise beyond 150 minutes per week of moderate or 75 minutes per week of vigorous exercise is associated with greater health benefits; this can be effectively achieved by varying the intensity, frequency, duration, and type of exercise every 2 to 3 weeks.

For patients not meeting the guidelines, Fig. 17.16 provides a simple framework to guide the recommendation of exercise during routine clinical visits. Walking will likely be the preferred choice of exercise behavior for most patients, although stationary cycling may be more appropriate for older/frail patients. The addition of resistance training is a critical component of a comprehensive exercise prescription to augment muscle mass and/or prevent atrophy, particularly in those patients at high risk of cachexia. There are several methods to explain exercise intensity. The most accurate methods involve use of ratings

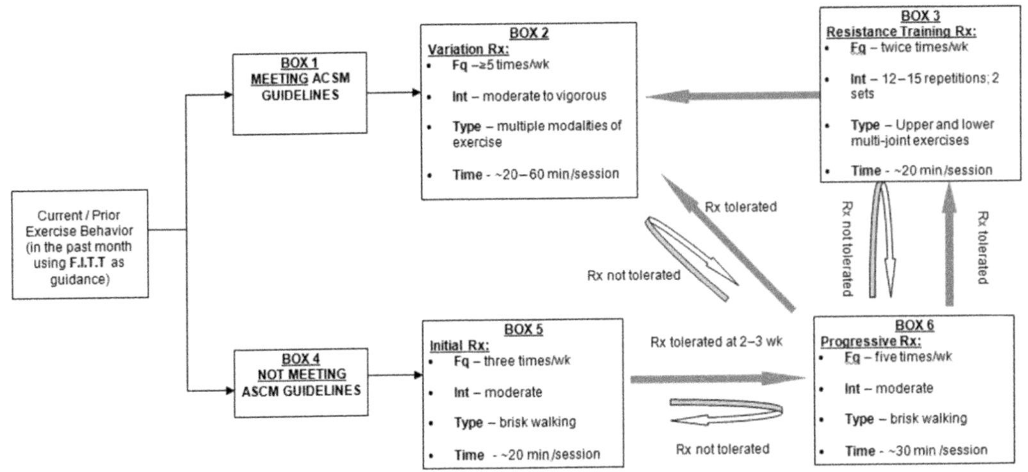

Fig. 17.16 Patients meeting the ACSM guidelines (ie, ≥150 minutes per week of moderate or ≥75 minutes per week vigorous exercise; Box 17.1) should be encouraged to either maintain (eg, if undergoing therapy) or preferably increase exercise levels; this can be achieved by varying the intensity, frequency, duration, and type of exercise every 2 to 3 weeks (Box 17.2). Resistance training should also be recommended to these patients once aerobic training has become part of habitual activity (Box 17.3). Those not meeting the ACSM guidelines (Box 17.4) should be initially recommended an introductory prescription as described (Box 17.5). If adequately tolerated, the patient can progressively increase the frequency and/or duration of exercise every week until 150 minutes per week or more of moderate exercise is achieved. In those patients maintaining exercise behavior consistent with the guidelines for 12 or more weeks, resistance training should be added to the prescription (see Box 17.3) as well as exercise variation (see Box 17.2). F.I.T.T., frequency, intensity, type, and time; Rx, prescription. (*Adapted from* Jones LW, Liu Q, Armstrong GT, et al. Exercise and risk of major cardiovascular events in adult survivors of childhood Hodgkin lymphoma: a report from the childhood cancer survivor study. J Clin Oncol 2014;32(32):3643–50; with permission.)

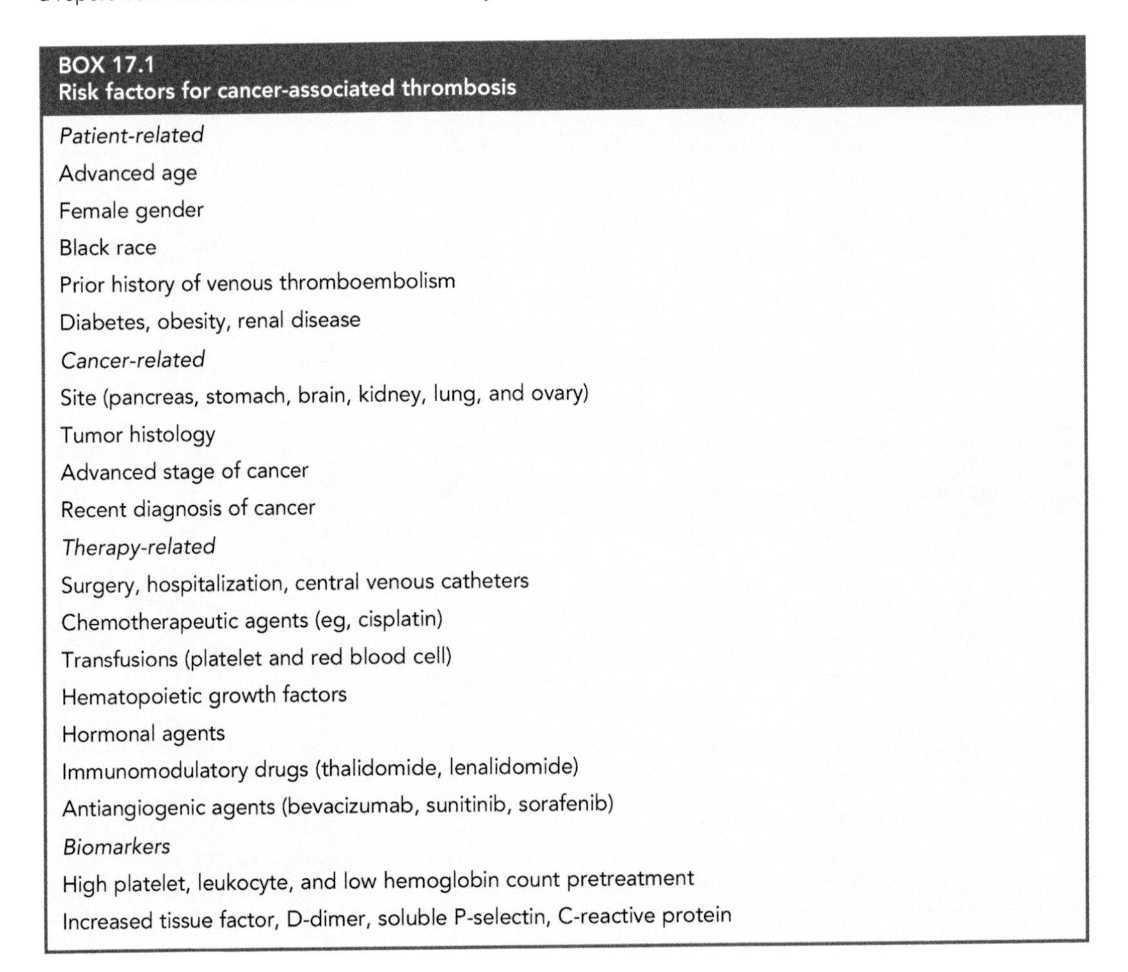

BOX 17.1
Risk factors for cancer-associated thrombosis

Patient-related

Advanced age

Female gender

Black race

Prior history of venous thromboembolism

Diabetes, obesity, renal disease

Cancer-related

Site (pancreas, stomach, brain, kidney, lung, and ovary)

Tumor histology

Advanced stage of cancer

Recent diagnosis of cancer

Therapy-related

Surgery, hospitalization, central venous catheters

Chemotherapeutic agents (eg, cisplatin)

Transfusions (platelet and red blood cell)

Hematopoietic growth factors

Hormonal agents

Immunomodulatory drugs (thalidomide, lenalidomide)

Antiangiogenic agents (bevacizumab, sunitinib, sorafenib)

Biomarkers

High platelet, leukocyte, and low hemoglobin count pretreatment

Increased tissue factor, D-dimer, soluble P-selectin, C-reactive protein

BOX 17.2
Venous thromboembolism prophylaxis for patients with cancer

Hospitalized surgical patients

Consider UFH, LMWH, or fondaparinux in all patients undergoing major cancer surgery. Consider extended (4 week) prophylaxis with LMWH after major surgery, obesity, and a history of VTE.

Hospitalized nonsurgical patients

Consider UFH, LMWH, or fondaparinux (strongly consider if decreased mobility and active cancer)

Ambulatory patients receiving chemotherapy

Routine prophylaxis not recommended

VTE prophylaxis should be considered in the following subgroups:

- Patients receiving highly thrombogenic thalidomide or lenalidomide-based combination chemotherapy regimens.
- Higher-risk ambulatory patients receiving chemotherapy (eg, those with a Khorana score ≥3).
- Prior history of unprovoked VTE

Abbreviations: UFH, unfractionated heparin; VTE, venous thromboembolism.

of perceived exertion or heart rate training zones. Such training zones can be calculated using either age-sex-predicted equations or, preferably, heart rate responses obtained from the exercise stress test.

BOX 17.3
Risk factors for radiation-induced heart disease

Total radiation exposure greater than 30 to 35 Gy

Daily fractions greater than 2 Gy

Older radiation protocols (eg, cobalt)

Left-sided and anterior chest exposure

No cardiac shielding

Pre-existing coronary artery disease or cardiac risk factors

Adjuvant cardiotoxic chemotherapy (eg, anthracycline)

Younger age

BOX 17.4
Second cancer therapy evaluation in patients with prior mediastinal radiation exposure

Complete physical examination and risk factor screening: lipid profile, fasting blood glucose, ECG

Resting echocardiogram (MUGA or CMRI)

Evaluation for premature atherosclerosis (consider >5 years after radiation therapy)

Carotid Dopplers

Stress echocardiography or coronary computed tomographic angiography

Abbreviations: CMRI, cardiac magnetic resonance imaging; MUGA, multigated acquisition.

In summary, evidence indicates that insufficient exercise levels are associated with deconditioning, poor symptom control, and possibly inferior clinical outcome following a cancer diagnosis.[221–223] Exercise tolerance and several patient-reported outcomes can be improved with structured exercise training across a broad range of oncology settings; with appropriate screening and prescription, exercise is safe, well-tolerated, and efficacious for patients with cancer. A positive recommendation for exercise participation from cardiology-oncology professionals can lead to considerable increases in exercise levels; thus, the authors stress the importance of providing exercise guidance to patients whenever appropriate.

BOX 17.5
Management considerations in patients with prior mediastinal radiation exposure before second cancer therapy

Smoking cessation, blood pressure control, maintaining normal weight, heart-healthy diet, aerobic exercise

Consider aspirin and statin therapy in select patients

Appropriate surveillance and management of asymptomatic valvular, carotid, and coronary disease

Percutaneous or surgical interventions for symptomatic and/or high-risk lesions depending on anatomic considerations, comorbidities, and individual candidacy

SUPPLEMENTARY DATA

Supplementary data related to this article can be found online at http://dx.doi.org/10.1016/j.chtm.2016.07.016.

REFERENCES

1. Balducci L, Extermann M. Cancer and aging. An evolving panorama. Hematol Oncol Clin North Am 2000;14(1):1–16.
2. Popa MA, Wallace KJ, Brunello A, et al. Potential drug interactions and chemotoxicity in older patients with cancer receiving chemotherapy. J Geriatr Oncol 2014;5(3):307–14.
3. Janssen-Heijnen ML, Szerencsi K, van de Schans SA, et al. Cancer patients with cardiovascular disease have survival rates comparable to cancer patients within the age-cohort of 10 years older without cardiovascular morbidity. Crit Rev Oncol Hematol 2010;76(3):196–207.
4. Davis MK, Rajala JL, Tyldesley S, et al. The prevalence of cardiac risk factors in men with localized prostate cancer undergoing androgen deprivation therapy in British Columbia, Canada. J Oncol 2015;2015:820403.
5. Katz RI, Barnhart JM, Ho G, et al. A survey on the intended purposes and perceived utility of preoperative cardiology consultations. Anesth Analg 1998;87(4):830–6.
6. Katz RI, Cimino L, Vitkun SA. Preoperative medical consultations: impact on perioperative management and surgical outcome. Can J Anaesth 2005; 52(7):697–702.
7. Landesberg G, Beattie WS, Mosseri M, et al. Perioperative myocardial infarction. Circulation 2009; 119(22):2936–44.
8. Landesberg G. The pathophysiology of perioperative myocardial infarction: facts and perspectives. J Cardiothorac Vasc Anesth 2003;17(1):90–100.
9. Fleisher LA, Fleischmann KE, Auerbach AD, et al. 2014 ACC/AHA guideline on perioperative cardiovascular evaluation and management of patients undergoing noncardiac surgery: a report of the American College of Cardiology/American Heart Association Task Force on practice guidelines. J Am Coll Cardiol 2014;64(22):e77–137.
10. Weinstein H, Steingart R. Myocardial perfusion imaging for preoperative risk stratification. J Nucl Med 2011;52(5):750–60.
11. Lagasse RS. Anesthesia safety: model or myth? A review of the published literature and analysis of current original data. Anesthesiology 2002;97(6):1609–17.
12. Reilly DF, McNeely MJ, Doerner D, et al. Self-reported exercise tolerance and the risk of serious perioperative complications. Arch Intern Med 1999;159(18):2185–92.
13. Weinstein H, Bates AT, Spaltro BE, et al. Influence of preoperative exercise capacity on length of stay after thoracic cancer surgery. Ann Thorac Surg 2007;84(1):197–202.
14. van Diepen S, Bakal JA, McAlister FA, et al. Mortality and readmission of patients with heart failure, atrial fibrillation, or coronary artery disease undergoing noncardiac surgery: an analysis of 38 047 patients. Circulation 2011;124(3):289–96.
15. Xu-Cai YO, Brotman DJ, Phillips CO, et al. Outcomes of patients with stable heart failure undergoing elective noncardiac surgery. Mayo Clin Proc 2008;83(3):280–8.
16. Healy KO, Waksmonski CA, Altman RK, et al. Perioperative outcome and long-term mortality for heart failure patients undergoing intermediate- and high-risk noncardiac surgery: impact of left ventricular ejection fraction. Congest Heart Fail 2010;16(2):45–9.
17. Meta-analysis Global Group in Chronic Heart Failure (MAGGIC). The survival of patients with heart failure with preserved or reduced left ventricular ejection fraction: an individual patient data meta-analysis. Eur Heart J 2012;33(14):1750–7.
18. Rodseth RN, Lurati Buse GA, Bolliger D, et al. The predictive ability of pre-operative B-type natriuretic peptide in vascular patients for major adverse cardiac events: an individual patient data meta-analysis. J Am Coll Cardiol 2011;58(5): 522–9.
19. Agarwal S, Rajamanickam A, Bajaj NS, et al. Impact of aortic stenosis on postoperative outcomes after noncardiac surgeries. Circ Cardiovasc Qual Outcomes 2013;6(2):193–200.
20. Lai HC, Lai HC, Lee WL, et al. Impact of chronic advanced aortic regurgitation on the perioperative outcome of noncardiac surgery. Acta Anaesthesiol Scand 2010;54(5):580–8.
21. Hollenberg M, Mangano DT, Browner WS, et al. Predictors of postoperative myocardial ischemia in patients undergoing noncardiac surgery. The Study of Perioperative Ischemia Research Group. Jama 1992;268(2):205–9.
22. Farmakis D, Parissis J, Filippatos G. Insights into onco-cardiology: atrial fibrillation in cancer. J Am Coll Cardiol 2014;63(10):945–53.
23. O'Kelly B, Browner WS, Massie B, et al. Ventricular arrhythmias in patients undergoing noncardiac surgery. The Study of Perioperative Ischemia Research Group. JAMA 1992;268(2):217–21.
24. Botto F, Alonso-Coello P, Chan MT, et al. Myocardial injury after noncardiac surgery: a large, international, prospective cohort study establishing diagnostic criteria, characteristics, predictors, and 30-day outcomes. Anesthesiology 2014;120(3): 564–78.

25. American College of Cardiology Foundation Appropriate Use Criteria Task Force, American Society of Echocardiography, American Heart Association, et al. ACCF/ASE/AHA/ASNC/HFSA/HRS/SCAI/SCCM/SCCT/SCMR 2011 Appropriate Use Criteria for Echocardiography. A Report of the American College of Cardiology Foundation Appropriate Use Criteria Task Force, American Society of Echocardiography, American Heart Association, American Society of Nuclear Cardiology, Heart Failure Society of America, Heart Rhythm Society, Society for Cardiovascular Angiography and Interventions, Society of Critical Care Medicine, Society of Cardiovascular Computed Tomography, and Society for Cardiovascular Magnetic Resonance Endorsed by the American College of Chest Physicians. J Am Coll Cardiol 2011;57:1126–66.
26. Bristow MR, Mason JW, Billingham ME, et al. Dose-effect and structure-function relationships in doxorubicin cardiomyopathy. Am Heart J 1981;102:709–18.
27. Legha SS, Benjamin RS, Mackay B, et al. Reduction of doxorubicin cardiotoxicity by prolonged continuous intravenous infusion. Ann Intern Med 1982; 96:133–9.
28. van Dalen EC, van der Pal HJ, Caron HN, et al. Different dosage schedules for reducing cardiotoxicity in cancer patients receiving anthracycline chemotherapy. Cochrane Database Syst Rev 2006;(4):CD005008.
29. Young AM, Dhillon T, Bower M. Cardiotoxicity after liposomal anthracyclines. Lancet Oncol 2004; 5:654.
30. Jones RL, Berry GJ, Rubens RD, et al. Clinical and pathological absence of cardiotoxicity after liposomal doxorubicin. Lancet Oncol 2004;5:575–7.
31. Harris KA, Harney E, Small EJ. Liposomal doxorubicin for the treatment of hormone-refractory prostate cancer. Clin Prostate Cancer 2002;1: 37–41.
32. Harris L, Batist G, Belt R, et al. Liposome-encapsulated doxorubicin compared with conventional doxorubicin in a randomized multicenter trial as first-line therapy of metastatic breast carcinoma. Cancer 2002;94:25–36.
33. O'Brien ME, Wigler N, Inbar M, et al. Reduced cardiotoxicity and comparable efficacy in a phase III trial of pegylated liposomal doxorubicin HCl (CAELYX/Doxil) versus conventional doxorubicin for first-line treatment of metastatic breast cancer. Ann Oncol 2004;15:440–9.
34. Batist G, Ramakrishnan G, Rao CS, et al. Reduced cardiotoxicity and preserved antitumor efficacy of liposome-encapsulated doxorubicin and cyclophosphamide compared with conventional doxorubicin and cyclophosphamide in a randomized, multicenter trial of metastatic breast cancer. J Clin Oncol 2001;19:1444–54.
35. Berry G, Billingham M, Alderman E, et al. The use of cardiac biopsy to demonstrate reduced cardiotoxicity in AIDS Kaposi's sarcoma patients treated with pegylated liposomal doxorubicin. Ann Oncol 1998;9:711–6.
36. Jones RL. Utility of dexrazoxane for the reduction of anthracycline-induced cardiotoxicity. Expert Rev Cardiovasc Ther 2008;6:1311–7.
37. Lyu YL, Kerrigan JE, Lin CP, et al. Topoisomerase IIbeta mediated DNA double-strand breaks: implications in doxorubicin cardiotoxicity and prevention by dexrazoxane. Cancer Res 2007;67:8839–46.
38. van Dalen EC, Caron HN, Dickinson HO, et al. Cardioprotective interventions for cancer patients receiving anthracyclines. Cochrane Database Syst Rev 2011;(6):CD003917.
39. Lipshultz SE, Rifai N, Dalton VM, et al. The effect of dexrazoxane on myocardial injury in doxorubicin-treated children with acute lymphoblastic leukemia. N Engl J Med 2004;351:145–53.
40. Kremer LC, van Dalen EC. Dexrazoxane in children with cancer: from evidence to practice. J Clin Oncol 2015;33:2594–6.
41. Swain SM, Whaley FS, Gerber MC, et al. Cardioprotection with dexrazoxane for doxorubicin-containing therapy in advanced breast cancer. J Clin Oncol 1997;15:1318–32.
42. U.S. Food and Drug Administration. Drug safety and availability. FDA statement on dexrazoxane. Jul 20 AahwfgDDuh.
43. Hensley ML, Hagerty KL, Kewalramani T, et al. American Society of Clinical Oncology 2008 clinical practice guideline update: use of chemotherapy and radiation therapy protectants. J Clin Oncol 2009;27:127–45.
44. Romond EH, Perez EA, Bryant J, et al. Trastuzumab plus adjuvant chemotherapy for operable HER2-positive breast cancer. N Engl J Med 2005; 353:1673–84.
45. Slamon D, Eiermann W, Robert N, et al. Adjuvant trastuzumab in HER2-positive breast cancer. N Engl J Med 2011;365:1273–83.
46. Seidman A, Hudis C, Pierri MK, et al. Cardiac dysfunction in the trastuzumab clinical trials experience. J Clin Oncol 2002;20:1215–21.
47. Piccart-Gebhart MJ, Procter M, Leyland-Jones B, et al. Trastuzumab after adjuvant chemotherapy in HER2-positive breast cancer. N Engl J Med 2005;353:1659–72.
48. Cote GM, Sawyer DB, Chabner BA. ERBB2 inhibition and heart failure. N Engl J Med 2012;367: 2150–3.
49. Herceptin prescribing information. South San Francisco, CA: Genetech Inc; 2016.

50. National Comprehensive Cancer Network. NCCN clinical practice guidelines in oncology. Breast Cancer. Version 1. 2012. Available at: www.nccn.org. Accessed June 30, 2015.
51. Swain SM, Baselga J, Kim SB, et al. Pertuzumab, trastuzumab, and docetaxel in HER2-positive metastatic breast cancer. N Engl J Med 2015; 372:724–34.
52. Ewer MS, Vooletich MT, Durand JB, et al. Reversibility of trastuzumab-related cardiotoxicity: new insights based on clinical course and response to medical treatment. J Clin Oncol 2005;23:7820–6.
53. Plana JC, Galderisi M, Barac A, et al. Expert consensus for multimodality imaging evaluation of adult patients during and after cancer therapy: a report from the American Society of Echocardiography and the European Association of Cardiovascular Imaging. J Am Soc Echocardiogr 2014;27: 911–39.
54. Sawaya H, Sebag IA, Plana JC, et al. Assessment of echocardiography and biomarkers for the extended prediction of cardiotoxicity in patients treated with anthracyclines, taxanes, and trastuzumab. Circ Cardiovasc Imaging 2012;5:596–603.
55. Negishi K, Negishi T, Hare JL, et al. Independent and incremental value of deformation indices for prediction of trastuzumab-induced cardiotoxicity. J Am Soc Echocardiogr 2013;26:493–8.
56. Burstein HJ, Piccart-Gebhart MJ, Perez EA, et al. Choosing the best trastuzumab-based adjuvant chemotherapy regimen: should we abandon anthracyclines? J Clin Oncol 2012;30:2179–82.
57. Gong IY, Verma S, Yan AT, et al. Long-term cardiovascular outcomes and overall survival of early-stage breast cancer patients with early discontinuation of trastuzumab: a population-based study. Breast cancer research and treatment 2016;157(3):535–44.
58. Folkman J. Tumor angiogenesis: therapeutic implications. N Engl J Med 1971;285(21):1182–6.
59. Dy GK, Adjei AA. Understanding, recognizing, and managing toxicities of targeted anticancer therapies. CA Cancer J Clin 2013;63(4):249–79.
60. de Jesus-Gonzalez N, Robinson E, Moslehi J, et al. Management of antiangiogenic therapy-induced hypertension. Hypertension 2012;60(3):607–15.
61. Steeghs N, Gelderblom H, Roodt JO, et al. Hypertension and rarefaction during treatment with telatinib, a small molecule angiogenesis inhibitor. Clin Cancer Res 2008;14(11):3470–6.
62. Facemire CS, Nixon AB, Griffiths R, et al. Vascular endothelial growth factor receptor 2 controls blood pressure by regulating nitric oxide synthase expression. Hypertension 2009;54(3):652–8.
63. Eremina V, Jefferson JA, Kowalewska J, et al. VEGF inhibition and renal thrombotic microangiopathy. N Engl J Med 2008;358(11):1129–36.
64. Granger JP. Vascular endothelial growth factor inhibitors and hypertension: a central role for the kidney and endothelial factors? Hypertension 2009;54(3):465–7.
65. Vigneau C, Lorcy N, Dolley-Hitze T, et al. All anti-vascular endothelial growth factor drugs can induce 'pre-eclampsia-like syndrome': a RARe study. Nephrol Dial Transplant 2014; 29(2):325–32.
66. Maitland ML, Kasza KE, Karrison T, et al. Ambulatory monitoring detects sorafenib-induced blood pressure elevations on the first day of treatment. Clin Cancer Res 2009;15(19):6250–7.
67. Chu TF, Rupnick MA, Kerkela R, et al. Cardiotoxicity associated with tyrosine kinase inhibitor sunitinib. Lancet 2007;370(9604):2011–9.
68. Groarke JD, Choueiri TK, Slosky D, et al. Recognizing and managing left ventricular dysfunction associated with therapeutic inhibition of the vascular endothelial growth factor signaling pathway. Curr Treat Options Cardiovasc Med 2014;16(9):335.
69. Steingart RM, Bakris GL, Chen HX, et al. Management of cardiac toxicity in patients receiving vascular endothelial growth factor signaling pathway inhibitors. Am Heart J 2012;163(2):156–63.
70. Schwartz RG, McKenzie WB, Alexander J, et al. Congestive heart failure and left ventricular dysfunction complicating doxorubicin therapy. Seven-year experience using serial radionuclide angiocardiography. Am J Med 1987; 82(6):1109–18.
71. White DA, Schwartzberg LS, Kris MG, et al. Acute chest pain syndrome during bleomycin infusions. Cancer 1987;59(9):1582–5.
72. Breccia M, Alimena G. Pleural/pericardic effusions during dasatinib treatment: incidence, management and risk factors associated to their development. Expert Opin Drug Saf 2010;9(5): 713–21.
73. Krauth MT, Herndlhofer S, Schmook MT, et al. Extensive pleural and pericardial effusion in chronic myeloid leukemia during treatment with dasatinib at 100 mg or 50 mg daily. Haematologica 2011;96(1):163–6.
74. Pai VB, Nahata MC. Cardiotoxicity of chemotherapeutic agents: incidence, treatment and prevention [review]. Drug Saf 2000;22(4):263–302.
75. Madeddu C, Deidda M, Piras A, et al. Pathophysiology of cardiotoxicity induced by nonanthracycline chemotherapy. J Cardiovasc Med 2016; 17(Suppl 1):S12–8.
76. Ishida S, Doki N, Shingai N, et al. The clinical features of fatal cyclophosphamide-induced cardiotoxicity in a conditioning regimen for allogeneic hematopoietic stem cell transplantation (allo-HSCT). Ann Hematol 2016;95(7):1145–50.

77. Wadia S. Acute cyclophosphamide hemorrhagic myopericarditis: dilemma case report, literature review and proposed diagnostic criteria. J Clin Diagn Res 2015;9(11):OE01–3.
78. de Azambuja E, Ameye L, Diaz M, et al. Cardiac assessment of early breast cancer patients 18 years after treatment with cyclophosphamide-, methotrexate-, fluorouracil- or epirubicin-based chemotherapy. Eur J Cancer 2015;51(17):2517–24.
79. Fields PA, Townsend W, Webb A, et al. De novo treatment of diffuse large B-cell lymphoma with rituximab, cyclophosphamide, vincristine, gemcitabine, and prednisolone in patients with cardiac comorbidity: a United Kingdom National Cancer Research Institute trial. J Clin Oncol 2014;32(4): 282–7.
80. Luwaert RJ, Descamps O, Majois F, et al. Coronary artery spasm induced by 5-fluorouracil. Eur Heart J 1991;12(3):468–70.
81. Sudhoff T, Enderle MD, Pahlke M, et al. 5-Fluorouracil induces arterial vasocontractions. Ann Oncol 2004;15(4):661–4.
82. Tsibiribi P, Bui-Xuan C, Bui-Xuan B, et al. Cardiac lesions induced by 5-fluorouracil in the rabbit. Hum Exp Toxicol 2006;25(6):305–9.
83. Cwikiel M, Zhang B, Eskilsson J, et al. The influence of 5-fluorouracil on the endothelium in small arteries. An electron microscopic study in rabbits. Scanning Microsc 1995;9(2):561–76.
84. Cwikiel M, Eskilsson J, Wieslander JB, et al. The appearance of endothelium in small arteries after treatment with 5-fluorouracil. An electron microscopic study of late effects in rabbits. Scanning Microsc 1996;10(3):805–18 [discussion: 819].
85. Cwikiel M, Eskilsson J, Albertsson M, et al. The influence of 5-fluorouracil and methotrexate on vascular endothelium. An experimental study using endothelial cells in the culture. Ann Oncol 1996;7(7):731–7.
86. Stewart T, Pavlakis N, Ward M. Cardiotoxicity with 5-fluorouracil and capecitabine: more than just vasospastic angina. Intern Med J 2010;40(4): 303–7.
87. Heidelberger C, Chaudhuri NK, Danneberg P, et al. Fluorinated pyrimidines, a new class of tumour-inhibitory compounds. Nature 1957; 179(4561):663–6.
88. Talapatra K, Rajesh I, Rajesh B, et al. Transient asymptomatic bradycardia in patients on infusional 5-fluorouracil. J Cancer Res Ther 2007;3(3): 169–71.
89. Wacker A, Lersch C, Scherpinski U, et al. High incidence of angina pectoris in patients treated with 5-fluorouracil. A planned surveillance study with 102 patients. Oncology 2003;65(2):108–12.
90. Schober C, Papageorgiou E, Harstrick A, et al. Cardiotoxicity of 5-fluorouracil in combination with folinic acid in patients with gastrointestinal cancer. Cancer 1993;72(7):2242–7.
91. Labianca R, Beretta G, Clerici M, et al. Cardiac toxicity of 5-fluorouracil: a study on 1083 patients. Tumori 1982;68(6):505–10.
92. Polk A, Vaage-Nilsen M, Vistisen K, et al. Cardiotoxicity in cancer patients treated with 5-fluorouracil or capecitabine: a systematic review of incidence, manifestations and predisposing factors. Cancer Treat Rev 2013;39(8):974–84.
93. Rezkalla S, Kloner RA, Ensley J, et al. Continuous ambulatory ECG monitoring during fluorouracil therapy: a prospective study. J Clin Oncol 1989; 7(4):509–14.
94. Meyer CC, Calis KA, Burke LB, et al. Symptomatic cardiotoxicity associated with 5-fluorouracil. Pharmacotherapy 1997;17(4):729–36.
95. Grunwald MR, Howie L, Diaz LA Jr. Takotsubo cardiomyopathy and Fluorouracil: case report and review of the literature. J Clin Oncol 2012; 30(2):e11–14.
96. Meydan N, Kundak I, Yavuzsen T, et al. Cardiotoxicity of de Gramont's regimen: incidence, clinical characteristics and long-term follow-up. Jpn J Clin Oncol 2005;35(5):265–70.
97. Ng M, Cunningham D, Norman AR. The frequency and pattern of cardiotoxicity observed with capecitabine used in conjunction with oxaliplatin in patients treated for advanced colorectal cancer (CRC). Eur J Cancer 2005;41(11):1542–6.
98. Akhtar SS, Wani BA, Bano ZA, et al. 5-Fluorouracil-induced severe but reversible cardiogenic shock: a case report. Tumori 1996;82(5):505–7.
99. Kim L, Karas M, Wong SC. Chemotherapy-induced takotsubo cardiomyopathy. J Invasive Cardiol 2008;20(12):E338–40.
100. Ozturk MA, Ozveren O, Cinar V, et al. Takotsubo syndrome: an underdiagnosed complication of 5-fluorouracil mimicking acute myocardial infarction. Blood Coagul Fibrinolysis 2013;24(1):90–4.
101. Y-Hassan S, Tornvall P, Tornerud M, et al. Capecitabine caused cardiogenic shock through induction of global Takotsubo syndrome. Cardiovasc Revasc Med 2013;14(1):57–61.
102. Lim SH, Wilson SM, Hunter A, et al. Takotsubo cardiomyopathy and 5-fluorouracil: getting to the heart of the matter. Case Rep Oncol Med 2013; 2013:206765.
103. Akhtar SS, Salim KP, Bano ZA. Symptomatic cardiotoxicity with high-dose 5-fluorouracil infusion: a prospective study. Oncology 1993;50(6):441–4.
104. Kelly C, Bhuva N, Harrison M, et al. Use of raltitrexed as an alternative to 5-fluorouracil and capecitabine in cancer patients with cardiac history. Eur J Cancer 2013;49(10):2303–10.
105. Kosmas C, Kallistratos MS, Kopterides P, et al. Cardiotoxicity of fluoropyrimidines in different

schedules of administration: a prospective study. J Cancer Res Clin Oncol 2008;134(1):75–82.
106. Tsavaris N, Kosmas C, Vadiaka M, et al. 5-Fluorouracil cardiotoxicity is a rare, dose and schedule-dependent adverse event: a prospective study. J BUON 2005;10(2):205–11.
107. Van Cutsem E, Hoff PM, Blum JL, et al. Incidence of cardiotoxicity with the oral fluoropyrimidine capecitabine is typical of that reported with 5-fluorouracil. Ann Oncol 2002;13(3):484–5.
108. Jensen SA, Sorensen JB. Risk factors and prevention of cardiotoxicity induced by 5-fluorouracil or capecitabine. Cancer Chemother Pharmacol 2006;58(4):487–93.
109. Cianci G, Morelli MF, Cannita K, et al. Prophylactic options in patients with 5-fluorouracil-associated cardiotoxicity. Br J Cancer 2003;88(10):1507–9.
110. Aleman BM, van den Belt-Dusebout AW, Klokman WJ, et al. Long-term cause-specific mortality of patients treated for Hodgkin's disease. J Clin Oncol 2003;21(18):3431–9.
111. Scappaticci FA, Skillings JR, Holden SN, et al. Arterial thromboembolic events in patients with metastatic carcinoma treated with chemotherapy and bevacizumab. J Natl Cancer Inst 2007;99(16):1232–9.
112. Ross R. Atherosclerosis–an inflammatory disease. N Engl J Med 1999;340(2):115–26.
113. Libby P, Ridker PM, Hansson GK, Leducq Transatlantic Network on Atherothrombosis. Inflammation in atherosclerosis: from pathophysiology to practice. J Am Coll Cardiol 2009;54(23):2129–38.
114. Thompson PA, Khatami M, Baglole CJ, et al. Environmental immune disruptors, inflammation and cancer risk. Carcinogenesis 2015;36(Suppl 1):S232–53.
115. Kundu JK, Surh YJ. Inflammation: gearing the journey to cancer. Mutat Res 2008;659(1–2):15–30.
116. Fihn SD, Gardin JM, Abrams J, et al. 2012 ACCF/AHA/ACP/AATS/PCNA/SCAI/STS guideline for the diagnosis and management of patients with stable ischemic heart disease: a report of the American College of Cardiology Foundation/American Heart Association task force on practice guidelines, and the American College of Physicians, American Association for Thoracic Surgery, Preventive Cardiovascular Nurses Association, Society for Cardiovascular Angiography and Interventions, and Society of Thoracic Surgeons. Circulation 2012;126(25):e354–471.
117. Boden WE, O'Rourke RA, Teo KK, et al. Optimal medical therapy with or without PCI for stable coronary disease. N Engl J Med 2007;356(15):1503–16.
118. Group BDS, Frye RL, August P, et al. A randomized trial of therapies for type 2 diabetes and coronary artery disease. N Engl J Med 2009;360(24):2503–15.
119. O'Rourke RA. Optimal medical therapy is a proven option for chronic stable angina. J Am Coll Cardiol 2008;52(11):905–7.
120. McFalls EO, Ward HB, Moritz TE, et al. Coronary-artery revascularization before elective major vascular surgery. N Engl J Med 2004;351(27):2795–804.
121. Chandra S, Lenihan DJ, Wei W, et al. Myocardial perfusion imaging and cardiovascular outcomes in a cancer population. Tex Heart Inst J 2009;36(3):205–13.
122. Thygesen K, Alpert JS, Jaffe AS, et al. Third universal definition of myocardial infarction. Circulation 2012;126(16):2020–35.
123. Amsterdam EA, Wenger NK, Brindis RG, et al. 2014 AHA/ACC guideline for the management of patients with non-ST-elevation acute coronary syndromes: a report of the American College of Cardiology/American Heart Association Task Force on Practice Guidelines. Circulation 2014;130(25):e344–426.
124. Verges B, Walter T, Cariou B. Endocrine side effects of anti-cancer drugs: effects of anti-cancer targeted therapies on lipid and glucose metabolism. Eur J Endocrinol 2014;170(2):R43–55.
125. Zhong S, Zhang X, Chen L, et al. Statin use and mortality in cancer patients: systematic review and meta-analysis of observational studies. Cancer Treat Rev 2015;41(6):554–67.
126. Kutner JS, Blatchford PJ, Taylor DH Jr, et al. Safety and benefit of discontinuing statin therapy in the setting of advanced, life-limiting illness: a randomized clinical trial. JAMA Intern Med 2015;175(5):691–700.
127. Falanga A, Schieppati F, Russo D. Cancer tissue procoagulant mechanisms and the hypercoagulable state of patients with cancer. Semin Thromb Hemost 2015;41(7):756–64.
128. Sonpavde G, Je Y, Schutz F, et al. Venous thromboembolic events with vascular endothelial growth factor receptor tyrosine kinase inhibitors: a systematic review and meta-analysis of randomized clinical trials. Crit Rev Oncol Hematol 2013;87(1):80–9.
129. Li W, Croce K, Steensma DP, et al. Vascular and metabolic implications of novel targeted cancer therapies: focus on kinase inhibitors. J Am Coll Cardiol 2015;66(10):1160–78.
130. Leighl NB, Bennouna J, Yi J, et al. Bleeding events in bevacizumab-treated cancer patients who received full-dose anticoagulation and remained on study. Br J Cancer 2011;104(3):413–8.
131. Maitland ML, Bakris GL, Black HR, et al. Initial assessment, surveillance, and management of blood pressure in patients receiving vascular

endothelial growth factor signaling pathway inhibitors. J Natl Cancer Inst 2010;102(9):596–604.
132. Rini BI, Quinn DI, Baum M, et al. Hypertension among patients with renal cell carcinoma receiving axitinib or sorafenib: analysis from the randomized phase III AXIS trial. Target Oncol 2015;10(1):45–53.
133. McKay RR, Rodriguez GE, Lin X, et al. Angiotensin system inhibitors and survival outcomes in patients with metastatic renal cell carcinoma. Clin Cancer Res 2015;21(11):2471–9.
134. Khakoo AY, Sidman RL, Pasqualini R, et al. Does the renin-angiotensin system participate in regulation of human vasculogenesis and angiogenesis? Cancer Res 2008;68(22):9112–5.
135. Rini BI, Cohen DP, Lu DR, et al. Hypertension as a biomarker of efficacy in patients with metastatic renal cell carcinoma treated with sunitinib. J Natl Cancer Inst 2011;103(9):763–73.
136. Estfan B, Byrne M, Kim R. Sorafenib in advanced hepatocellular carcinoma: hypertension as a potential surrogate marker for efficacy. Am J Clin Oncol 2013;36(4):319–24.
137. Jubb AM, Harris AL. Biomarkers to predict the clinical efficacy of bevacizumab in cancer. Lancet Oncol 2010;11(12):1172–83.
138. Langenberg MH, van Herpen CM, De Bono J, et al. Effective strategies for management of hypertension after vascular endothelial growth factor signaling inhibition therapy: results from a phase II randomized, factorial, double-blind study of Cediranib in patients with advanced solid tumors. J Clin Oncol 2009;27(36):6152–9.
139. Porta C, Gore ME, Rini BI, et al. Long-term safety of sunitinib in metastatic renal cell carcinoma. Eur Urol 2016;69:345–51.
140. Chintalgattu V, Rees ML, Culver JC, et al. Coronary microvascular pericytes are the cellular target of sunitinib malate-induced cardiotoxicity. Sci Transl Med 2013;5(187):187ra169.
141. Krzych LJ, Bochenek A. Blood pressure variability: epidemiological and clinical issues. Cardiol J 2013;20(2):112–20.
142. Arai H, Saitoh S, Matsumoto T, et al. Hypertension as a paraneoplastic syndrome in hepatocellular carcinoma. J Gastroenterol 1999;34(4):530–4.
143. Rickman T, Garmany R, Doherty T, et al. Hypokalemia, metabolic alkalosis, and hypertension: Cushing's syndrome in a patient with metastatic prostate adenocarcinoma. Am J Kidney Dis 2001;37(4):838–46.
144. von Stempel C, Perks C, Corcoran J, et al. Cardiorespiratory failure secondary to ectopic Cushing's syndrome as the index presentation of small-cell lung cancer. BMJ Case Rep 2013;2013.
145. Law MR, Morris JK, Wald NJ. Use of blood pressure lowering drugs in the prevention of cardiovascular disease: meta-analysis of 147 randomised trials in the context of expectations from prospective epidemiological studies. BMJ 2009;338:b1665.
146. Rowinsky EK, McGuire WP, Guarnieri T, et al. Cardiac disturbances during the administration of taxol. J Clin Oncol 1991;9:1704–12.
147. Arbuck SG, Strauss H, Rowinsky E, et al. A reassessment of cardiac toxicity associated with taxol. J Natl Cancer Inst Monogr 1993;15:117–30.
148. Tamargo J, Caballero R, Delpón E. Cancer chemotherapy and cardiac arrhythmias: a review. Drug Saf 2015;38(2):129–52.
149. Riber LP, Larsen TB, Christensen TD. Postoperative atrial fibrillation prophylaxis after lung surgery: systematic review and meta-analysis. Ann Thorac Surg 2014;98(6):1989–97.
150. Hu YF, Liu CJ, Chang PM, et al. Incident thromboembolism and heart failure associated with new-onset atrial fibrillation in cancer patients. Int J Cardiol 2013;165(2):355–7.
151. Lyman GH, Bohlke K, Khorana AA, et al. Venous thromboembolism prophylaxis and treatment in patients with cancer: American Society of Clinical Oncology clinical practice guideline update 2014. J Clin Oncol 2015;33(6):654–6.
152. Short NJ, Connors JM. New oral anticoagulants and the cancer patient. Oncologist 2014;19(1):82–93.
153. den Exter PL, van der Hulle T, Klok FA, et al. The newer anticoagulants in thrombosis control in cancer patients. Semin Oncol 2014;41(3):339–45.
154. Sanford D, Naidu A, Alizadeh N, et al. The effect of low molecular weight heparin on survival in cancer patients: an updated systematic review and meta-analysis of randomized trials. J Thromb Haemost 2014;12(7):1076–85.
155. Crossley GH, Poole JE, Rozner MA, et al. The Heart Rhythm Society (HRS)/American Society of Anesthesiologists (ASA) Expert Consensus Statement on the perioperative management of patients with implantable defibrillators, pacemakers and arrhythmia monitors: facilities and patient management this document was developed as a joint project with the American Society of Anesthesiologists (ASA), and in collaboration with the American Heart Association (AHA), and the Society of Thoracic Surgeons (STS). Heart Rhythm 2011;8(7):1114–54.
156. Munshi A, Agarwal JP, Pandey KC. Cancer patients with cardiac pacemakers needing radiation treatment: a systematic review. J Cancer Res Ther 2013;9(2):193–8.
157. Bowers RW, Scott PA, Roberts PR. Use of external defibrillator jacket to facilitate safe delivery of radiotherapy for lung cancer—a report of two cases. Indian Heart J 2014;66(1):111–4.

158. Taunk NK, Haffty BG, Kostis JB, et al. Radiation-induced heart disease: pathologic abnormalities and putative mechanisms. Front Oncol 2015;5:39.
159. Hatoum OA, Otterson MF, Kopelman D, et al. Radiation induces endothelial dysfunction in murine intestinal arterioles via enhanced production of reactive oxygen species. Arterioscler Thromb Vasc Biol 2006;26(2):287–94.
160. Carver JR, Shapiro CL, Ng A, et al, ASCO Cancer Survivorship Expert Panel. American Society of Clinical Oncology clinical evidence review on the ongoing care of adult cancer survivors: cardiac and pulmonary late effects. J Clin Oncol 2007; 25(25):3991–4008.
161. Darby SC, Ewertz M, McGale P, et al. Risk of ischemic heart disease in women after radiotherapy for breast cancer. N Engl J Med 2013; 368(11):987–98.
162. Armstrong GT, Oeffinger KC, Chen Y, et al. Modifiable risk factors and major cardiac events among adult survivors of childhood cancer. J Clin Oncol 2013;31(29):3673–80.
163. Gupta D, Pun SC, Verma S, et al. Radiation-induced coronary artery disease: a second survivorship challenge? Future Oncol 2015;11(14): 2017–20.
164. Children's Oncology Group. Long-term follow-up guidelines for survivors of childhood, adolescent and young adult cancers, version 4.0. Monrovia (CA): Children's Oncology Group. 2013
165. Heidenreich PA, Hancock SL, Lee BK, et al. Asymptomatic cardiac disease following mediastinal irradiation. J Am Coll Cardiol 2003;42(4): 743–9.
166. Heidenreich PA, Hancock SL, Vagelos RH, et al. Diastolic dysfunction after mediastinal irradiation. Am Heart J 2005;150(5):977–82.
167. Chang AS, Smedira NG, Chang CL, et al. Cardiac surgery after mediastinal radiation: extent of exposure influences outcome. J Thorac Cardiovasc Surg 2007;133(2):404–13.
168. Liang JJ, Sio TT, Slusser JP, et al. Outcomes after percutaneous coronary intervention with stents in patients treated with thoracic external beam radiation for cancer. JACC Cardiovasc Interv 2014; 7(12):1412–20.
169. Schomig K, Ndrepepa G, Mehilli J, et al. Thoracic radiotherapy in patients with lymphoma and restenosis after coronary stent placement. Catheter Cardiovasc Interv 2007;70(3):359–65.
170. Sharabi Y, Dendi R, Holmes C, et al. Baroreflex failure as a late sequela of neck irradiation. Hypertension 2003;42(1):110–6.
171. Groarke JD, Tanguturi VK, Hainer J, et al. Abnormal exercise response in long-term survivors of Hodgkin lymphoma treated with thoracic irradiation: evidence of cardiac autonomic dysfunction and impact on outcomes. J Am Coll Cardiol 2015;65(6):573–83.
172. Plummer C, Henderson RD, O'Sullivan JD, et al. Ischemic stroke and transient ischemic attack after head and neck radiotherapy: a review. Stroke 2011;42(9):2410–8.
173. Brosius FC 3rd, Waller BF, Roberts WC. Radiation heart disease. Analysis of 16 young (aged 15 to 33 years) necropsy patients who received over 3,500 rads to the heart. Am J Med 1981;70(3):519–30.
174. Veinot JP, Edwards WD. Pathology of radiation-induced heart disease: a surgical and autopsy study of 27 cases. Hum Pathol 1996;27(8):766–73.
175. Carmel RJ, Kaplan HS. Mantle irradiation in Hodgkin's disease. An analysis of technique, tumor eradication, and complications. Cancer 1976; 37(6):2813–25.
176. Mileshkin LR, Seymour JF, Wolf MM, et al. Cardiovascular toxicity is increased, but manageable, during high-dose chemotherapy and autologous peripheral blood stem cell transplantation for patients aged 60 years and older. Leuk Lymphoma 2005;46(11):1575–9.
177. Sirohi B, Powles R, Treleaven J, et al. The role of autologous transplantation in patients with multiple myeloma aged 65 years and over. Bone Marrow Transplant 2000;25(5):533–9.
178. Afessa B, Azoulay E. Critical care of the hematopoietic stem cell transplant recipient. Crit Care Clin 2010;26(1):133–50.
179. Bayraktar UD, Shpall EJ, Liu P, et al. Hematopoietic cell transplantation-specific comorbidity index predicts inpatient mortality and survival in patients who received allogeneic transplantation admitted to the intensive care unit. J Clin Oncol 2013;31(33): 4207–14.
180. Gooley TA, Chien JW, Pergam SA, et al. Reduced mortality after allogeneic hematopoietic-cell transplantation. N Engl J Med 2010;363(22): 2091–101.
181. Sorror ML, Maris MB, Storb R, et al. Hematopoietic cell transplantation (HCT)-specific comorbidity index: a new tool for risk assessment before allogeneic HCT. Blood 2005;106(8):2912–9.
182. Bolwell BJ. Are predictive factors clinically useful in bone marrow transplantation? Bone Marrow Transplant 2003;32(9):853–61.
183. Hertenstein B, Stefanic M, Schmeiser T, et al. Cardiac toxicity of bone marrow transplantation: predictive value of cardiologic evaluation before transplant. J Clin Oncol 1994;12(5):998–1004.
184. Jain B, Floreani AA, Anderson JR, et al. Cardiopulmonary function and autologous bone marrow transplantation: results and predictive value for respiratory failure and mortality. The University of

Nebraska Medical Center Bone Marrow Transplantation Pulmonary Study Group. Bone Marrow Transplant 1996;17(4):561–8.
185. Zangari M, Henzlova MJ, Ahmad S, et al. Predictive value of left ventricular ejection fraction in stem cell transplantation. Bone Marrow Transplant 1999;23(9):917–20.
186. Stillwell EE, Wessler JD, Rebolledo BJ, et al. Retrospective outcome data for hematopoietic stem cell transplantation in patients with concurrent coronary artery disease. Biol Blood Marrow Transplant 2011;17:1182–6.
187. Schechter D, Drakos P, Nagler A. Underlying coronary artery disease and successful bone marrow transplantation: a case report. Bone Marrow Transplant 1994;13(5):665–6.
188. Levine GN, Bates ER, Bittl JA, et al. 2016 ACC/AHA guideline focused update on duration of dual antiplatelet therapy in patients with coronary artery disease. J Am Coll Cardiol 2016;6;68(10):1082–115.
189. Deloughery TG. Between Scylla and Charybdis: antithrombotic therapy in hematopoietic progenitor cell transplant patients. Bone Marrow Transplant 2012;47(10):1269–73.
190. Sarkiss MG, Yusuf SW, Warneke CL, et al. Impact of aspirin therapy in cancer patients with thrombocytopenia and acute coronary syndromes. Cancer 2007;109(3):621–7.
191. Bearman SI, Petersen FB, Schor RA, et al. Radionuclide ejection fractions in the evaluation of patients being considered for bone marrow transplantation: risk for cardiac toxicity. Bone Marrow Transplant 1990;5(3):173–7.
192. Itoh M, Iwai K, Kotone-Miyahara Y, et al. Successful allogeneic bone marrow transplantation for acute myelogenous leukemia after drug-induced cardiomyopathy. Tohoku J Exp Med 2004;204(1):85–91.
193. Qazilbash MH, Amjad AI, Qureshi S, et al. Outcome of allogeneic hematopoietic stem cell transplantation in patients with low left ventricular ejection fraction. Biol Blood Marrow Transplant 2009;15(10):1265–70.
194. Hurley P, Konety S, Cao Q, et al. Hematopoietic stem cell transplantation in patients with systolic dysfunction: can it be done? Biol Blood Marrow Transplant 2015;21(2):300–4.
195. Tang WH, Thomas S, Kalaycio M, et al. Clinical outcomes of patients with impaired left ventricular ejection fraction undergoing autologous bone marrow transplantation: can we safely transplant patients with impaired ejection fraction? Bone Marrow Transplant 2004;34(7):603–7.
196. Tonorezos ES, Stillwell EE, Calloway JJ, et al. Arrhythmias in the setting of hematopoietic cell transplants. Bone Marrow Transplant 2015;50(9):1212–6.
197. Hidalgo JD, Krone R, Rich MW, et al. Supraventricular tachyarrhythmias after hematopoietic stem cell transplantation: incidence, risk factors and outcomes. Bone Marrow Transplant 2004;34(7):615–9.
198. Feliz V, Saiyad S, Ramarao SM, et al. Melphalan-induced supraventricular tachycardia: incidence and risk factors. Clin Cardiol 2011;34(6):356–9.
199. Fatema K, Gertz MA, Barnes ME, et al. Acute weight gain and diastolic dysfunction as a potent risk complex for post stem cell transplant atrial fibrillation. Am J Hematol 2009;84(8):499–503.
200. Nishimura RA, Otto CM, Bonow RO, et al. 2014 AHA/ACC guideline for the management of patients with valvular heart disease: executive summary: a report of the American College of Cardiology/American Heart Association Task Force on Practice Guidelines. J Am Coll Cardiol 2014;63(22):2438–88.
201. Demark-Wahnefried W, Peterson B, McBride C, et al. Current health behaviors and readiness to pursue life-style changes among men and women diagnosed with early stage prostate and breast carcinomas. Cancer 2000;88(3):674–84.
202. Jones LW, Eves ND, Peppercorn J. Pre-exercise screening and prescription guidelines for cancer patients. Lancet Oncol 2010;11(10):914–6.
203. Thompson PD, Buchner D, Pina IL, et al. Exercise and physical activity in the prevention and treatment of atherosclerotic cardiovascular disease: a statement from the Council on Clinical Cardiology (Subcommittee on Exercise, Rehabilitation, and Prevention) and the Council on Nutrition, Physical Activity, and Metabolism (Subcommittee on Physical Activity). Circulation 2003;107(24):3109–16.
204. Thompson PD, Franklin BA, Balady GJ, et al. Exercise and acute cardiovascular events placing the risks into perspective: a scientific statement from the American Heart Association Council on Nutrition, Physical Activity, and Metabolism and the Council on Clinical Cardiology. Circulation 2007;115(17):2358–68.
205. Fletcher GF, Balady G, Froelicher VF, et al. Exercise standards. A statement for healthcare professionals from the American Heart Association. Writing Group. Circulation 1995;91(2):580–615.
206. Yancik R, Wesley MN, Ries LA, et al. Effect of age and comorbidity in postmenopausal breast cancer patients aged 55 years and older. JAMA 2001;285(7):885–92.
207. Jones LW, Eves ND, Haykowsky M, et al. Exercise intolerance in cancer and the role of exercise therapy to reverse dysfunction. Lancet Oncol 2009;10(6):598–605.
208. Balady GJ, Chaitman B, Driscoll D, et al. Recommendations for cardiovascular screening, staffing,

and emergency policies at health/fitness facilities. Circulation 1998;97(22):2283–93.

209. Kenjale AA, Hornsby WE, Crowgey T, et al. Pre-exercise participation cardiovascular screening in a heterogeneous cohort of adult cancer patients. Oncologist 2014;19(9):999–1005.
210. Jones LW. Evidence-based risk assessment and recommendations for physical activity clearance: cancer. Appl Physiol Nutr Metab 2011;36(Suppl 1):S101–12 [This paper is one of a selection of papers published in this Special Issue, entitled Evidence-based risk assessment and recommendations for physical activity clearance, and has undergone the Journal's usual peer review process].
211. U.S. Preventive Services Task Force. Screening for coronary heart disease: recommendation statement. Ann Intern Med 2004;140(7):569–72.
212. Gibbons RJ, Balady GJ, Bricker JT, et al. ACC/AHA 2002 guideline update for exercise testing: summary article: a report of the American College of Cardiology/American Heart Association Task Force on Practice Guidelines (Committee to Update the 1997 Exercise Testing Guidelines). Circulation 2002;106(14):1883–92.
213. Pescatello LS, American College of Sports Medicine. ACSM's guidelines for exercise testing and precription. 9th edition. Philadelphia: Wolters Kluwer/Lippincott Williams & Wilkins Health; 2014.
214. Schmitz KH, Courneya KS, Matthews C, et al. American College of Sports Medicine roundtable on exercise guidelines for cancer survivors. Med Sci Sports Exerc 2010;42(7):1409–26.
215. Rock CL, Doyle C, Demark-Wahnefried W, et al. Nutrition and physical activity guidelines for cancer survivors. CA Cancer J Clin 2012;62(4): 242–74.
216. Hayes SC, Spence RR, Galvao DA, et al. Australian Association for Exercise and Sport Science position stand: optimising cancer outcomes through exercise. J Sci Med Sport 2009;12(4):428–34.
217. van den Berg JP, Velthuis MJ, Gijsen BC, et al. Guideline cancer rehabilitation. Ned Tijdschr Geneeskd 2011;155(51):A4104.
218. Sasso JP, Eves ND, Christensen JF, et al. A framework for prescription in exercise-oncology research. J Cachexia Sarcopenia Muscle 2015;6(2):115–24.
219. Bach PB, Schrag D, Brawley OW, et al. Survival of blacks and whites after a cancer diagnosis. JAMA 2002;287:2106–13.
220. The unequal burden of cancer. 1999.
221. Knols R, Aaronson NK, Uebelhart D, et al. Physical exercise in cancer patients during and after medical treatment: a systematic review of randomized and controlled clinical trials. J Clin Oncol 2005; 23(16):3830–42.
222. McNeely ML, Campbell KL, Rowe BH, et al. Effects of exercise on breast cancer patients and survivors: a systematic review and meta-analysis. CMAJ 2006;175(1):34–41.
223. Speck RM, Courneya KS, Masse LC, et al. An update of controlled physical activity trials in cancer survivors: a systematic review and meta-analysis. J Cancer Surviv 2010;4(2):87–100.

CHAPTER 18

Intratherapy Cardiology Evaluation

Wendy Schaffer, MD, PhD, Dipti Gupta, MD, MPH, Anthony Yu, MD, Jennifer Liu, MD, Michael Baum, MD, Howard Weinstein, MD, Michelle Johnson, MD, MPH, Carol Chen, MD, Nancy Roistacher, MD, Shawn C. Pun, MD, Jonathan W. Weinsaft, MD, Eileen McAleer, MD, John Sasso, MS, Lee W. Jones, PhD, Richard M. Steingart, MD*

INTRODUCTION

Patients with cancer can develop signs and symptoms of cardiovascular diseases during their active treatment, which require prompt recognition, evaluation, and management.[1–14] Although a general cardiology consultation could be requested, there is benefit in a cardio-oncology referral given the nuances and ramifications of the interplay of cancer therapy and cardiovascular diseases. Key questions to answer are whether the cardiovascular disease process was caused by the cancer therapy, aggravated by the cancer therapy, or "naturally" occurring, unrelated to cancer therapy. The answers to these questions are crucial for determining if cancer therapy can proceed as planned. However, even if not caused or aggravated by cancer therapy, heart failure (HF) and myocardial infarction, for instance, can have a tremendous impact on the future course of cancer treatment. Herein, the spectrum of cardiovascular diseases as they may arise during cancer treatment (**Fig. 18.1**) is reviewed.

CARDIOMYOPATHY AND HEART FAILURE

In the cardio-oncology patient population, the diagnosis of HF is complicated by the overlap of symptoms between HF, cancer, and its therapy. Dyspnea/effort intolerance is typically multifactorial in patients with cancer, and the diagnosis of HF is often delayed. Natriuretic peptides tend to be nonspecifically elevated at baseline, and radiologic evidence of HF is often inconclusive by computed tomography (CT). In addition, the geriatric nature of cardio-oncology further complicates the diagnosis of HF.[15] Most elderly patients with cancer report fatigue,[16] confounding the diagnosis of HF. A sound level of clinical suspicion and evaluation is thus required. Following the diagnosis, further studies will have to conclude on the cause of the cardiomyopathy/HF (drug, ischemia, arrhythmia, and so forth). One nuance is Takotsubo (stress) cardiomyopathy,[17] which is increasingly appreciated in a wide range of cancers,[18–25] as its emotional and physical triggers are prevalent in oncology. Treatment of HF, by current American College of Cardiology/American Heart Association (AHA/ACC) guidelines, during cancer therapy often is limited by hypotension and renal insufficiency. In active HF, cancer therapy or surgery is typically deferred for cardiac investigation and management. Once HF is compensated and its cause understood, cancer treatment may proceed, with careful cardiology guidance.

A particular aspect and focus in cardio-oncology are related to the fact that several cancer therapeutics can induce HF, and in fact, it is this very topic that generated the momentum for the field. Two drugs in particular are mentioned in this context because they have been so influential. Anthracyclines were the first class for which it is was recognized that HF can be a dose-limiting side effect. It was subsequently noted that a drop in left ventricular ejection fraction (LVEF) preceded the onset of HF, and that interruption of therapy could halt this decline in cardiac function. These observations then led to

Cardiology Service, Department of Medicine Memorial Sloan Kettering Cancer Center, 1275 York Avenue, New York, NY 10065, USA
* Corresponding author.
E-mail address: steingar@mskcc.org

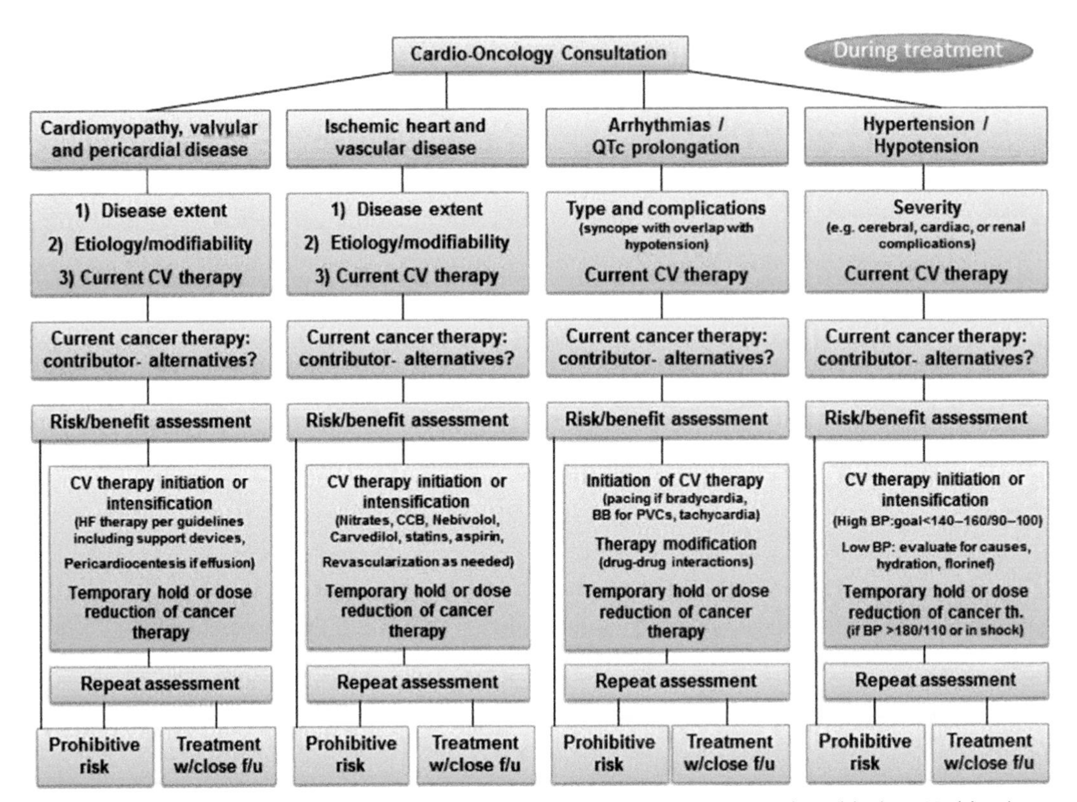

Fig. 18.1 Overview of the cardio-oncology consultation during cancer therapy. BB, beta blocker; BP, blood pressure; CCB, calcium channel blocker; CV, cardiovascular; PVC, premature ventricular complex.

the development of validated LVEF surveillance protocols (Fig. 18.2). Accordingly, all patients should have a baseline LVEF assessment, and if 30% or less, no chemotherapy is recommended. According to this algorithm, patients with an LVEF 30% or greater but less than 50% can receive anthracyclines, but with repeat LVEF assessment before each dose. However under these circumstances it is our practice to encourage the use of nonanthracycline therapies if possible, and certainly to avoid anthracyclines if there is any suspicion of clinical heart failure. With a baseline LVEF 50% or more, evaluations should be repeated after a cumulative dose of 250 to 300 mg/m^2 and thereafter at 450 mg/m^2 if no risk factors. If patients have known cardiovascular

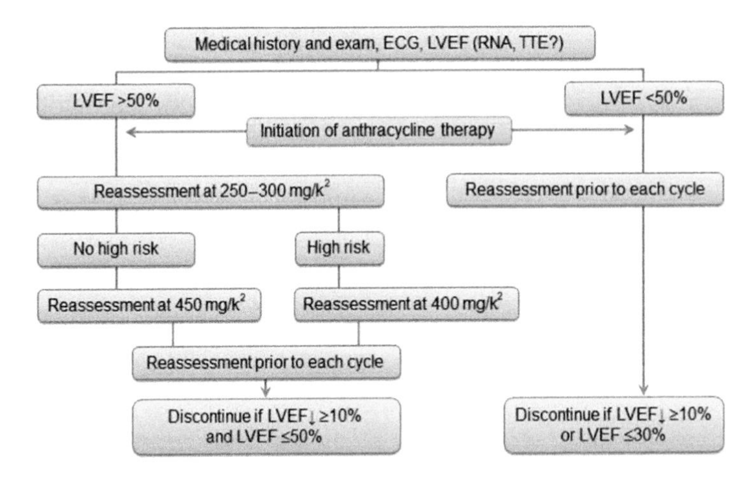

Fig. 18.2 First validated cardiac function surveillance algorithm for anthracycline therapy. ECG, electrocardiogram; LVEF, left ventricular ejection fraction; RNA, radionuclide angiocardiogram; TTE, transthoracic echocardiography. (*From* Herrmann J, Lerman A, Sandhu NP, et al. Evaluation and management of patients with heart disease and cancer: cardio-oncology. Mayo Clin Proc 2014; 89(9): 1287–1306; *Adapted from* Schwartz RG, McKenzie WB, Alexander J, et al. Congestive heart failure and left ventricular dysfunction complicating doxorubicin therapy. Seven-year experience using serial radionuclide angiocardiography. Am J Med 1987;82(6):1109–18; with permission.)

disease, prior chest radiation, abnormal electrocardiogram (ECG) changes, or concomitant cardiotoxic chemotherapy, LVEF assessment should be repeated at 400 mg/m^2 instead of 450 mg/m^2 and with each dose thereafter. Anthracycline therapy should be stopped in case of a 10% or greater absolute drop in the ejection fraction to 50% or less in patients with baseline LVEF 50% or greater, and to 30% or less in patients with baseline LVEF less than 50% but greater than 30%. The American Society of Echocardiography (ASE) recommendations state that if the cumulative doxorubicin dose is higher than 240 mg/m^2 (or its equivalent), LVEF, global longitudinal strain (GLS), and troponin should be measured before each additional 50 mg/m^2 (Fig. 18.3).[26] The American Society of Clinical Oncology guidelines recommend frequent cardiac monitoring after cumulative doxorubicin doses of 400 mg/m^2, suggesting a repeat study after 500 mg/m^2 and subsequently after every 50 mg/m^2 of doxorubicin.[27,28] Finally, the European Society for Medical Oncology recommends either a cardiac troponin (cTn)-based or an echocardiography-based approach and suggests angiotensin-converting enzyme (ACE) inhibitor therapy for those with cTn elevation and ACE inhibitor/β-blocker for those with left ventricular (LV) dysfunction (Fig. 18.4). Thus, the details on how to monitor cardiac function during anthracycline therapy, if at all, and when to discontinue anthracyclines remain uncertain.

These questions are very pertinent though because the clinical spectrum of acute/subacute anthracycline cardiotoxicity is quite broad and includes ECG abnormalities, arrhythmias, pericarditis/myocarditis, asymptomatic LVEF decline, and HF. Nonspecific ST- and T-wave changes, decreased QRS voltage, and prolongation of QT interval may be seen in 20% to 30% of the patients. Arrhythmias, including ventricular, supraventricular, and junctional tachycardia, are noted in 0.5% to 3% of the patients, with sinus tachycardia being the most common. More advanced arrhythmias, even atrial flutter or atrial fibrillation (AF), are rare. Would any of these events suffice to stop therapy? None may be captured by LVEF beforehand or even at the time and yet could be a reflection of the acute myocardial damage. In fact, there is no correlation with the extent of histologic injury on biopsy, and LVEF may remain normal even with substantial anthracycline-induced cardiac injury, at least early on. Cardiac troponin may be a useful asset in these cases. Also, echocardiographic parameters of LVEF and fractional shortening are influenced by the cardiac loading conditions, which can fluctuate significantly in patients with cancer due to fever, anemia, sepsis, volume infusions, renal failure, malnutrition, and central nervous system disease. The ASE recommends the measurement of GLS to detect subclinical declines in LV function during cardiotoxic therapy (Fig. 18.5).[26] Detection of abnormal GLS may provide an early opportunity to intervene with cardioprotective medications (eg, β-blockers, ACE inhibitors, or angiotensin receptor blockers [ARBs]) with the goal of preventing subsequent LVEF decline or HF; however, further investigation is needed in this area. However, even GLS is not without caveats, and the decision to discontinue anthracycline therapy based on LVEF or GLS alone should be balanced with the risk of reducing remission and increasing relapse rates. There is,

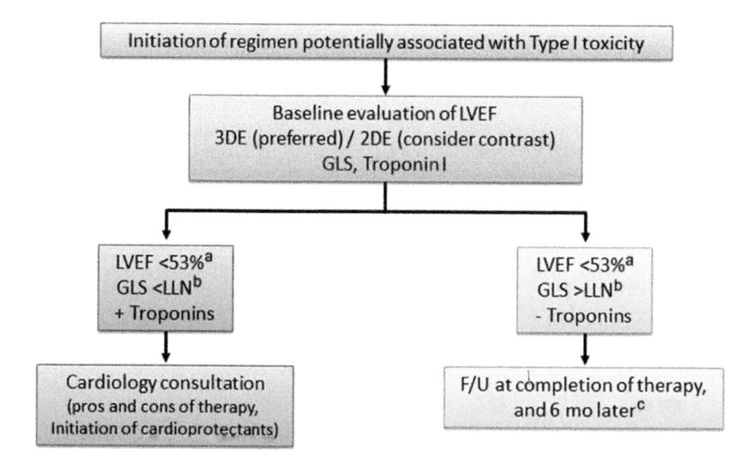

Fig. 18.3 ASE cardiac surveillance algorithm, with chemotherapy with type I toxicity (typically associated with anthracycline chemotherapy). [a] Consider confirmation with CMR (cardiac magnetic resonance). [b] LLN = lower limit of normal. [c] If the dose is higher than 240 mg/m^2 (or its equivalent), recommend measurement of LVEF, GLS and troponin prior to each additional 50 mg/m^2. 2DE, two dimensional echocardiography; 3DE, three dimensional echocardiography; GLS, global longitudinal strain; LVEF, left ventricular ejection fraction. (*From* Plana JC, Galderisi M, Barac A, et al. Expert consensus for multimodality imaging evaluation of adult patients during and after cancer therapy: a report from the American Society of Echocardiography and the European Association of Cardiovascular imaging. J Am Soc Echocardiogr 2014;27:931; with permission.)

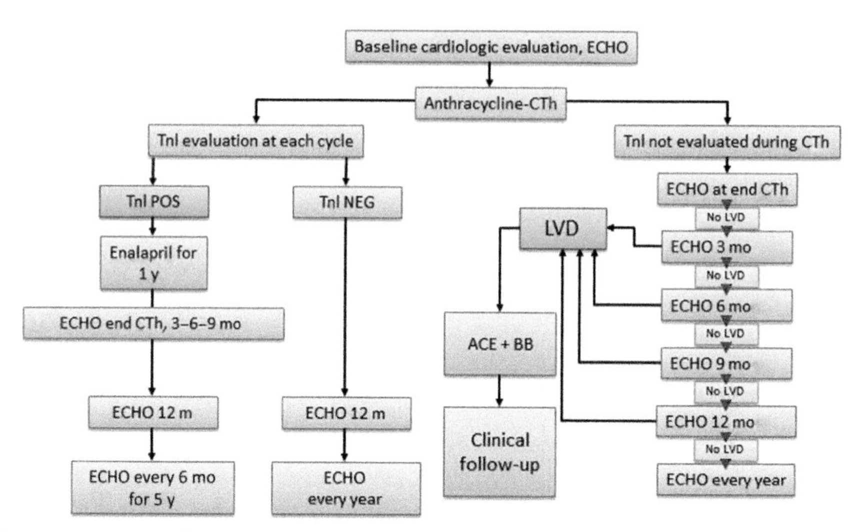

Fig. 18.4 European Society of Medical Oncology surveillance and management algorithm for cardiotoxicity with anthracycline therapy. ACE, angiotensin converting inhibitor; CTh, chemotherapy; ECHO, echocardiography; LVD, left ventricular dysfunction; NEG, negative; TnI, troponin I. (*From* Curigliano G, Cardinale D, Suter T, et al. Cardiovascular toxicity induced by chemotherapy, targeted agents and radiotherapy: ESMO Clinical Practice Guidelines. Ann Oncol 2012;23(Suppl 7):vii159; with permission.)

however, no controversy that anthracyclines should be discontinued for signs or symptoms of HF.

After completion of anthracycline chemotherapy, the National Comprehensive Cancer Network (NCCN) survivorship guidelines recommend that a follow-up echocardiogram be considered within 1 year after completion of anthracycline therapy (Appendix 1).[29] Other groups have recommended different screening intervals, and this remains an evolving topic, as reviewed (see Chapter 19).

Similar to anthracyclines, it was the unanticipated and thus "shocking" occurrence of cases of HF, even with fatal outcomes, with the use of trastuzumab that generated the call for routine echocardiograms every 3 months during therapy, as endorsed in the US Food and Drug Administration–approved package insert and the NCCN Breast Cancer Guidelines, and different algorithms (Figs. 18.6–18.8).[30–37] There are no published data on the efficacy of this strategy for cardiotoxicity prevention. Moreover, these recommendations apply regardless of whether trastuzumab is given with or without anthracyclines, even though cardiac toxicity is rarely reported when trastuzumab is given without anthracycline therapy.[38] Thus, although there is an evidence base to support LVEF monitoring when trastuzumab is given after anthracyclines, it is not clear

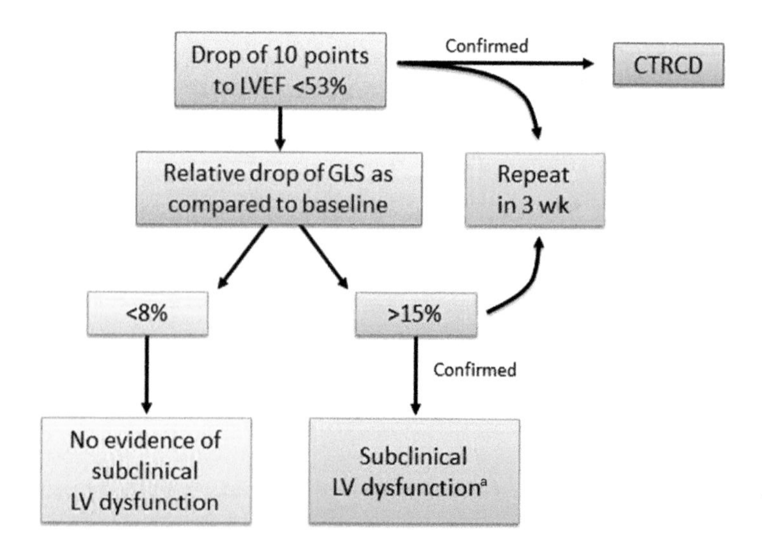

Fig. 18.5 ASE criteria for the diagnosis of cancer therapy-related cardiac dysfunction (CTRCD). [a] The data supporting the initiation of cardioprotection for the treatment of subclinical LV dysfunction is limited. GLS, global longitudinal strain; LVEF, left ventricular ejection fraction; LV, left ventricular. (*From* Plana JC, Galderisi M, Barac A, et al. Expert consensus for multimodality imaging evaluation of adult patients during and after cancer therapy: a report from the American Society of Echocardiography and the European Association of Cardiovascular Imaging. J Am Soc Echocardiogr 2014;27:931; with permission.)

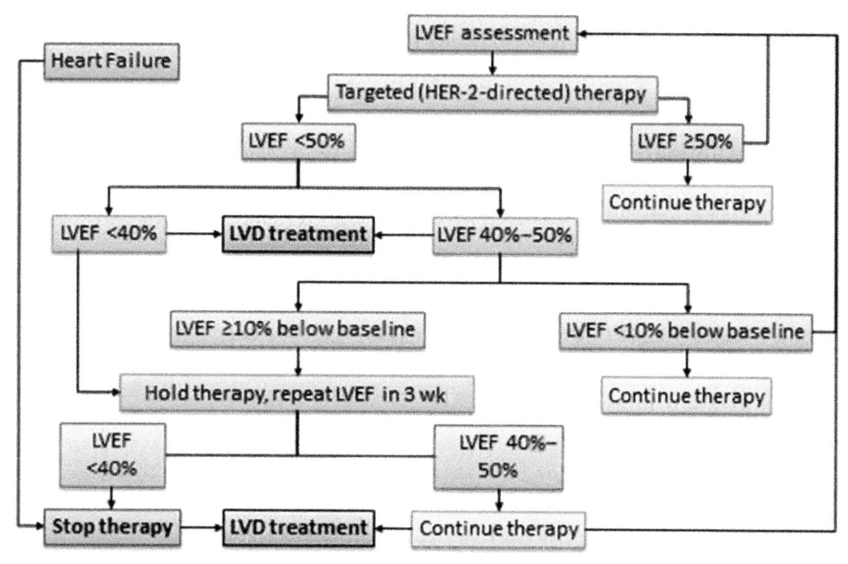

Fig. 18.6 European Society of Medical Oncology surveillance and management algorithm for cardiotoxicity with HER-2-directed (trastuzumab) therapy. LVEF, left ventricular ejection fraction, LVD, left ventricular dysfunction. (*Adapted from* Curigliano G, Cardinale D, Suter T, et al. Cardiovascular toxicity induced by chemotherapy, targeted agents and radiotherapy: ESMO Clinical Practice Guidelines. Ann Oncol 2012;23(Suppl 7):vii159; with permission.)

that LVEF monitoring is beneficial or even necessary for all patients treated with trastuzumab who never have received or never will receive an anthracycline.

Trastuzumab is temporarily interrupted for patients that develop an asymptomatic decline in LVEF, with or without prior exposure to anthracyclines (see Fig. 18.6). Although there is no consensus definition of an asymptomatic LVEF decline, one commonly used criterion is an absolute decrease of LVEF ≥16%, or ≥10% below the lower limit of normal, further specified by ASE (see Fig. 18.5). The significant oncologic benefit of trastuzumab therapy has raised the question of whether trastuzumab interruption is necessary in patients with an asymptomatic LVEF decline. The cardiac safety of uninterrupted trastuzumab therapy for patients with asymptomatic LVEF decline is currently under investigation in the Safe-Heart study (NCT01904903). When

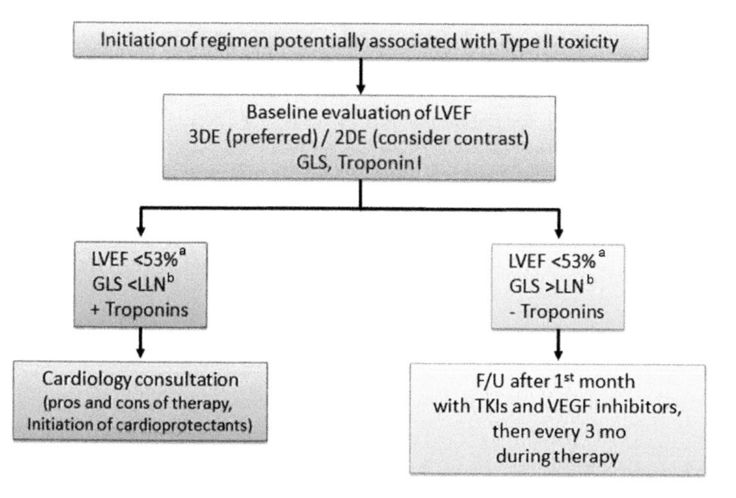

Fig. 18.7 ASE cardiac surveillance with chemotherapy with type II toxicity (typically associated with trastuzumab therapy). CMR, cardiac magnetic resonance. [a] Consider confirmation with CMR. [b] LLN = lower limit of normal. LVEF, left ventricular ejection fraction; GLS, global longitudinal strain; TKIs, tyrosine kinase inhibitors, VEGF, vascular endothelial growth factor; 3DE, three dimensional echocardiography; 2DE, two dimensional echocardiography. (*Adapted from* Plana JC, Galderisi M, Barac A, et al: Expert consensus for multimodality imaging evaluation of adult patients during and after cancer therapy: a report from the American Society of Echocardiography and the European Association of Cardiovascular Imaging. J Am Soc Echocardiogr 2014;27:930; with permission.)

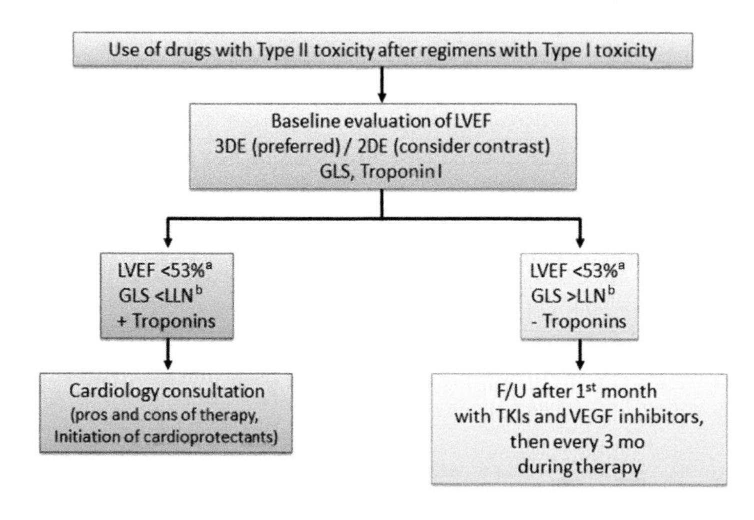

Fig. 18.8 ASE cardiac surveillance with chemotherapy with type II toxicity after treatment with type I toxicity agents. [a] Consider confirmation with CMR. [b] LLN = lower limit of normal. LVEF, left ventricular ejection fraction; GLS, global longitudinal strain; TKIs, tyrosine kinase inhibitors, VEGF, vascular endothelial growth factor; 3DE, three dimensional echocardiography; 2DE, two dimensional echocardiography. (*From* Plana JC, Galderisi M, Barac A, et al Expert consensus for multimodality imaging evaluation of adult patients during and after cancer therapy: a report from the American Society of Echocardiography and the European Association of Cardiovascular Imaging. J Am Soc Echocardiogr 2014;27:911–39; with permission.)

trastuzumab is interrupted, functional recovery of LV function is generally observed after which trastuzumab can be safely reintroduced in most patients under close cardiac surveillance.[39,40] Although there are limited data on the efficacy of HF medications for the treatment of mild asymptomatic LVEF decline during trastuzumab therapy, the authors adhere to ACC/AHA guidelines for the management of HF.[28] For patients that develop symptomatic HF, pharmacologic HF therapy (eg, β-blockers, ACE inhibitors, ARBs, aldosterone antagonists, diuretics) should be initiated. The development of symptomatic HF during adjuvant trastuzumab was a criterion for permanent discontinuation of therapy in the clinical trial setting. However, in clinical practice, the authors think that it is reasonable to consider reinitiation of trastuzumab along with close cardiac monitoring if HF symptoms resolve and LVEF recovers. This decision should take into consideration several factors, including baseline and nadir LVEF, time course of LVEF recovery, concomitant cardiovascular comorbidities, and estimated oncologic benefit from additional trastuzumab. The same considerations on LVEF as expressed above apply, and cardiac troponins may be particularly helpful in predicting which patients may face a worse prognosis. In a study by Cardinale and colleagues[41] of 251 women with HER2-positive breast cancer treated with trastuzumab, patients with an increase in troponin-I (>0.08 ng/mL) had a higher incidence of cardiac events and 3-fold lower chance of recovery from trastuzumab-induced cardiotoxicity. Similarly, a study by Sawaya and colleagues demonstrated that ultrasensitive troponin-I predicted the subsequent development of cardiotoxicity in women with HER2-positive breast cancer treated with adjuvant chemotherapy and trastuzumab.[42] Overall, these studies suggest that troponins may have a role in the clinical assessment of trastuzumab cardiotoxicity, but additional studies are needed before they can be recommended for general practice. Other biomarkers currently under investigation include brain natriuretic peptide, myeloperoxidase, galectin 3, and ST2.

There are no consensus guidelines for evaluating and managing vascular endothelial growth factor (VEGF) signaling pathway (VSP) inhibitor associated HF.[43–51] Consideration should be given to performing pretreatment multigated acquisition radionuclide angiograms or echocardiograms in patients thought to be at risk. Timing of follow-up studies to detect the development of asymptomatic LV dysfunction has been specified in the ASE consensus document. Because HF may appear early in the course of treatment (3 months with sunitinib), frequent clinical monitoring early on is indicated with particular attention to the nonspecific complaints of fatigue, dyspnea, and edema as potential indicators of HF. Accordingly, the recommendation is cardiac surveillance after the first month with tyrosine kinase inhibitors (TKIs) and VSP inhibitors and then every 3 months during therapy. The role of cardiac biomarkers has not been evaluated. There is no clear evidence to support prophylactic therapy to prevent LV dysfunction. Treatment of established HF should follow ACC/AHA recommendations because there is no specific evidence-based guideline for HF during treatment with the VSP inhibitors.[52–55]

PERICARDIAL AND VALVULAR HEART DISEASE

Any new onset or aggravation of chest pain in patients with cancer needs a thorough evaluation of various differential diagnostic considerations. These considerations include pulmonary embolism, acute coronary syndrome, acute aortic syndrome, pleuritis, and pericarditis. The signs and symptoms of pericarditis are distinct (somatic pain character, worse with deep inspiration or lying down, improved by shallow breathing and in the upright position). Analgesics and anti-inflammatory agents (preferably colchicine) are the drugs of choice. Prednisone is frequently given and might not be complicated by the same rate of recurrence and chronicity as is the case in noncancer patients.

Pericarditis with cyclophosphamide presents with chest pain, pericardial friction rub, and arrhythmias. The onset is acute within 1 to 10 days after the first dose and may last from 1 to 6 days. ECG changes may include typical widespread "tentlike" ST-segment elevation and PR depression or may show nonspecific changes, which may occur even in the absence of clinical cardiotoxicity. A decrease in QRS voltage may signal pericardial effusion but often constitutes a more ominous sign of myocarditis and cardiomyopathy. In fact, loss of QRS voltage is seen in 50% to 90% of the cases with significant congestive HF. The echocardiogram shows a dose-dependent decrease in LVEF with no decrease but rather an increase in LV mass index. Fulminant HF can develop, but there have been no reports of development of late cardiotoxicity (>3 weeks) in patients who survived the initial event, and restoration of cardiac function can be documented in more than half of the patients. However, cyclophosphamide-related cardiotoxicity can be fatal.[56–58]

In view of the gravity of these events, higher-risk groups such as those with previous anthracycline therapy, mitoxantrone exposure, and/or chest radiation (mantle radiation) and those receiving high doses of cyclophosphamide or ifosfamide should be monitored with serial 12-lead ECGs and echocardiogram. The time interval, however, is not defined, and these tests may remain negative even in patients with signs and symptoms of clinical cardiotoxicity. Baseline LVEF is not predictive of cardiotoxicity. Treatment should be initiated immediately to control the symptoms and improve outcomes. Patients in fulminant HF require intensive care, even mechanical assist device or extracorporeal membrane oxygenation, to support until the onset of the recovery phase. For pericarditis, corticosteroids and nonsteroidal anti-inflammatory drugs could be used but both with their own caveats, and colchicine would be the preferred initial approach. Large pericardial effusion may require pericardiocentesis, which is an emergent necessity in the case of cardiac tamponade. In patients with chest pain, myocardial infarction still needs to be ruled out because it might occur as well. Arrhythmias and ECG changes should be treated based on the seriousness of clinical signs and symptoms, following institutional or published guidelines.

Structurally related to cyclophosphamide, ifosfamide has been associated with HF (as high as 17% incidence in bone marrow transplant patients) and severe arrhythmias. The onset is typically between 6 to 23 days after the initiation of ifosfamide therapy, resolving within 4 to 7 days after starting supportive care and discontinuation of therapy without recurrences. The risk is dose-dependent and may be related to delayed renal elimination of cardiotoxic metabolites of the drug. Exposure to doxorubicin may also potentiate the cardiotoxicity risk.

Dasatinib[59–61] is an oral dual tyrosine kinase inhibitor active against ABL1 and Src-family kinases. It inhibits BCR-ABL1 with a 325-fold greater potency than imatinib. The incidence of grade 3/4 pleural/pericardial effusions in clinical trials and practice ranges from 14% to 34%. Factors associated with effusions include previous history of cardiac disease or autoimmune disorders, previous skin rash during imatinib treatment, hypertension, hypercholesterolemia, advanced phase leukemia, twice-a-day schedule, and a high dose of dasatinib. Postulated pathogenetic mechanisms include interference with the viability of pericytes and the regulation of angiogenesis via PDGFR-b inhibition, or through inhibition of src-kinases, which might regulate the stability of pleural and pericardial epithelium through regulation of cell adhesion or lymphocyte activation. Therapeutic measures include drug suspension, dose reduction, and the use of diuretics and steroids. In rare instances with large compromising effusions, drainage may be necessary.

ISCHEMIC HEART DISEASE AND VASCULAR DISEASE

5-Fluorouracil (5-FU) causes a spectrum of clinical syndromes, including chest pain/angina, ischemia, ST-elevation myocardial infarction (STEMI) and non-STEMI, silent ischemia noted on ECG or ambulatory monitoring, bradyarrhythmias, ventricular arrhythmias, QT prolongation, HF, and a stress cardiomyopathy.[62–68]

5-FU cardiotoxicity includes a reversible cardiomyopathy consistent with a stress cardiomyopathy.[69–78] Stress cardiomyopathy is likely the abnormality underlying reports of HF, hypotension, and cardiogenic shock with 5-FU infusion.[78] Patients with this syndrome present with hemodynamic instability, congestive HF, chest pain, sinus tachycardia, ST-segment alterations including elevation on ECGs, apical akinesis on echocardiogram with severely decreased ejection fraction, and normal or low-level increase in cardiac enzymes. Cardiac catheterization by definition demonstrates normal coronary arteries. LV function and wall motion normalize within a few days with intensive supportive care and discontinuation of 5-FU. This clinical syndrome has also been reported with capecitabine.

Cardiac events with 5-FU occur most frequently during the first cycle, with incidence 2 to 8 times the incidence during later cycles.[79–88] With the de Gramont regimen (fluorouracil and leucovorin), the incidence was 3.5% in the first cycle, 0.4% in later cycles.[81] Several studies report median onset within 72 hours of initiating 5-FU. Transformed to 5-FU, capecitabine results in a continuous low-dose infusion of 5-FU, although the incidence of cardiac events is also higher during the first cycle with capecitabine, 5.2% versus 1.3% in later cycles.

Patients at higher risk should receive 5-FU under controlled settings with telemetry and clinical monitoring. If cardiac events occur, 5-FU should be discontinued immediately. Treatment of 5-FU cardiotoxicity is usually based on the assumption that vasospasm may be playing an important role, although this is not always the case. Nitrates and/or calcium channel blockers are often administered but may not be effective. If underlying coronary artery disease (CAD) cannot be definitely ruled out, acute management should include aspirin and statin. Cardiac testing to be considered includes emergency cardiac catheterization to rule out acute coronary occlusion in the presence of significant ST-segment elevation, depression, or new left bundle branch block, or hemodynamic instability. For those with suggestive cardiac symptoms including discomfort or shortness of breath but without diagnostic ECG changes, immediate echocardiography for wall motion and ejection fraction, serial cardiac enzymes, and a focused cardiac care unit are indicated. In less urgent cases, CT angiogram or cardiac stress testing may also be helpful in evaluating whether ischemic heart disease (HD) is contributing. Patients in cardiogenic shock may require intensive care with vasopressor, inotropic, and ventilator support.

Whether to rechallenge a patient with a prior 5-FU cardiotoxicity is a complex decision made with the patient's oncologist that depends on the nature of the prior cardiotoxicity, potential benefit of 5-FU-based chemotherapy, and availability of alternative treatment modalities. For a patient who had chest pain without ECG changes or troponin elevation, and for whom 5-FU promises the best oncologic outcome, consider inpatient admission with cardiac monitoring for the subsequent dose. Prophylaxis includes nitrates or calcium-channel blockers if vasospasm is suspected but may not always succeed. Dose reduction and bolus rather than continuous infusion of 5-FU can be considered. If chest pain was exertional, exercise stress echo during the 5-FU infusion provides insight into the pathophysiology of the chest pain. For patients who have had more significant cardiotoxicity manifest as arrhythmia, HF, or objective evidence for ischemia, rechallenging is not advised, although there are individual cases where the potential for benefit is great, and comparable treatment options are not available. In these cases, inpatient admission with cardiac monitoring is required, with an appropriate consent process with the patient before proceeding.

TKIs such as nilotinib and ponatinib are also associated with an at least 7.5% incidence of acute coronary syndrome (ACS), occurring at any point in time during and even after treatment.[89] TKIs targeting the VSP also pose a significant risk that approaches 10%, whereas it might be as low as less than 2% for bevacizumab.[90–92] Elements of vasoconstriction as well as thrombosis have been documented in these patients and determine the management (dual antiplatelet therapy [DAPT], nitrates, and percutaneous coronary intervention as needed). The scenario is similar for patients with ACS events on cisplatin-based therapies. Whether these events can be prevented with antiplatelet therapy and vasodilator therapy is not known. Overall, these patients should be managed with current AHA/ACC guidelines.

ACS/myocardial infarction in patients with cancer may result from an ischemic imbalance (type 2), which includes vasoconstriction, as opposed to spontaneous plaque rupture/thrombosis (type 1), and its diagnosis can be difficult. Causes of troponin elevation from myocardial injury are protean[93]; many of these are prominent in cancer.

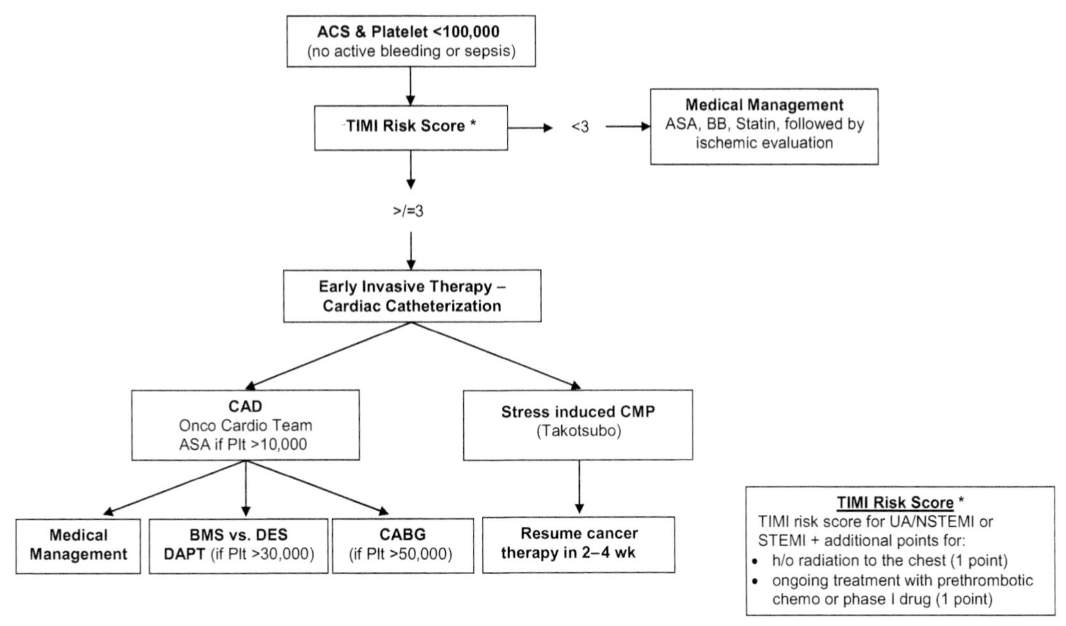

Fig. 18.9 Revascularization approach used at the MD Anderson Cancer Center. ACS, acute coronary syndrome; BB, beta blocker; BMS, bare metal stent; CABG, coronary artery bypass grafting; CMP, cardiomyopathy; DES, drug eluting stent; TIMI, thrombolysis in myocardial infarction; NSTEMI, non ST segment elevation myocardial infarction; PLT, platelets; STEMI, ST segment elevation myocardial infarction; DES, drug eluting stent. (*Adapted from* Iliescu CA, Grines CL, Herrmann J, et al. SCAI expert consensus statement: evaluation, management, and special considerations of cardio-oncology patients in the cardiac catheterization laboratory (endorsed by the Cardiological Society of India, and Sociedad Latino Americana de Cardiologıa Intervencionista). Catheter Cardiovasc Interv 2016;87(5):E202–23; with permission.)

Although treatment of ACS in patients with cancer is ideally risk based, referral for coronary intervention should also reflect the unique cancer aspects, the potential need for maintaining DAPT, and physician and patient preferences. A consensus document was recently released by the Society of Cardiac Angiography and Intervention (SCAI) that summarizes the approach to be taken (Fig. 18.9) and points out the decisions to be taken into consideration. For patients with cancer with an acceptable prognosis, general appropriate criteria apply. For those with an expected survival less than 1 year, percutaneous revascularization may be considered for patients with acute STEMI and high-risk NSTEMI; otherwise, every effort should be made to maximally optimize medical therapy before resorting to an invasive strategy as a palliative effort. The use of fractional flow reserve is encouraged to justify the need for revascularization. When an invasive approach is taken, balloon angioplasty should be considered for patients with cancer who are not candidates for DAPT (platelets <30,000/mL) or when a noncardiac procedure or surgery is necessary as soon as possible. A bare-metal stent (BMS) should be considered for patients with platelet counts greater than 30,000/mL who need a noncardiac procedure, surgery, or chemotherapy, which can be postponed for greater than 4 weeks. Newer-generation drug-eluting stents (DES) should be considered for patients with platelet counts greater than 30,000/mL who are not in immediate need for a noncardiac procedure, surgery, or chemotherapy. Bivalirudin and/or radial approach should be considered to minimize the risk of bleeding. Intravascular imaging, such as intravascular ultrasound (IVUS) or optical coherence tomography (OCT), is recommended after stent placement to ensure optimal expansion and an absence of complications given the potential for early DAPT interruption.

Aspirin is reasonable in those with established CAD and in those with ACS and platelet counts greater than 10,000. Thrombocytopenia may limit the use of antiplatelet agents during cancer treatment, but failure to treat with aspirin in thrombocytopenic (<100,000) patients with cancer with acute myocardial infarction (AMI) resulted in a markedly poor 7-day survival.[94] Although there is no minimum platelet count to perform a diagnostic coronary angiogram, for patients with platelet counts less than 30,000/mL, revascularization and DAPT should be decided after a preliminary multidisciplinary evaluation (interventional cardiology/oncology/hematology) and a risk/benefit analysis.

Prophylactic platelet transfusion in discussion with the oncology/hematology team can be considered for patients with a platelet count less than 20,000 and one of the following: (a) high fever, (b) leukocytosis, (c) rapid decrease in platelet count, (d) other coagulation abnormality, or (e) receiving therapy for bladder, gynecologic, or colorectal tumors, melanoma, or necrotic tumors. Therapeutic platelet transfusions are recommended in thrombocytopenic patients who develop bleeding during or after cardiac catheterization. Repeat platelet counts are recommended after platelet transfusions. DAPT with clopidogrel may be used when platelet counts are 30,000 to 50,000. Prasugrel, ticagrelor, and IIB-IIIA inhibitors should not be used in patients with platelet counts less than 50,000. If platelet counts are less than 50,000, the duration of DAPT may be restricted to 2 weeks following PTCA alone, 4 weeks after BMS, and 6 months after second- or third-generation DES if optimal stent expansion was confirmed by IVUS or OCT. Borrowing from the literature on elective surgery following an AMI, assuming the patient is clinically stable, the authors encourage waiting 4 to 6 weeks after an AMI before resuming cancer treatments. This timeframe poses the highest risk for recurrent adverse events, including death.[95–97] The cardiovascular event rate declines further up to 6 months following an acute coronary event, but waiting that long to resume cancer treatment is usually not practical.

Systemic Hypertension

Systemic hypertension has been reported with all VSP inhibitors. VSP hypertension is reproducible and may be sustained. It may appear abruptly (within 24 hours) and usually is seen in the early stages of treatment. It may be severe.[98] A rapid decrease in blood pressure may occur when the agent is stopped, requiring vigilant monitoring of antihypertensive therapy. Pre-existing hypertension, age greater than 60 years, and body mass index 25 kg/m^2 or greater are independent risk factors for VSP inhibitor-related hypertension. Consensus guidelines indicate that blood pressure treatment should be individualized, taking into account pretreatment blood pressure status and underlying cardiovascular risk factors and disease. Home blood pressure monitoring is recommended starting at the beginning of VSP inhibitor therapy for diagnosis and to fine-tune dosing.[99,100]

There is no specific preferred antihypertensive agent. Choice of agent should be in keeping with clinical status of the patient, that is, β-blocker in patients with ischemic HD, angiotensin system inhibitors (ASI) in patients with LV dysfunction, diabetes, and proteinuria. There is increasing evidence that angiotensin II plays a role in VEGF-dependent angiogenesis. A recent retrospective study of metastatic renal cell carcinoma (mRCC) demonstrated that patients treated with ASI had improved survival over patients whose drug-induced hypertension was treated with other agents. The authors hypothesize that ASI may have a synergistic effect on angiogenesis with the antiangiogenic agents. Prospective studies are necessary to validate.[101,102]

Hypertension is an on-target effect and therefore has been postulated as a marker of efficacy with patients without a hypertensive response having shorter survival. Retrospective studies have shown predictive value with sorafenib in hepatocellular carcinoma and in mRCC treated with sunitinib (Fig. 18.10). Studies with bevacizumab have shown conflicting results. Treatment of the hypertension does not appear to adversely affect the efficacy of VSP inhibitor therapy.[103–106]

There are limited data on long-term follow-up of hypertension with targeted agents. A pooled analysis of mRCC patients receiving sunitinib for 2 to 6 years indicated an incidence of 36% in the first year, falling to 29% in the second year, and then remaining stable. Grade 3 to 4 hypertension occurred in 8% of patients over the first year and declined thereafter.[107–109]

ARRHYTHMIAS/QTC PROLONGATION

Patients with cancer can have arrhythmias for various reasons and of various types, duration, and intensity. These arrhythmias may be associated with no symptoms, recognized only on routine ECG or precipitate symptoms ranging from palpitations, fatigue, and light-headedness to syncope and even sudden cardiac death (SCD). They might be a reflection of underlying HD or cardiotoxicity with cancer therapy (Table 18.1). One classical example is anthracyclines, as detailed above. These types of arrhythmias are more difficult to anticipate and are not routinely monitored for. All patients with concern for rhythm abnormalities need a thorough ECG evaluation, including Holter or event monitor, if not on a telemetry unit, and those with concerns for further cardiac injury also need echocardiography and cardiac troponin assessment. The differential diagnosis of cardiac arrhythmia should include primary cancers or metastatic

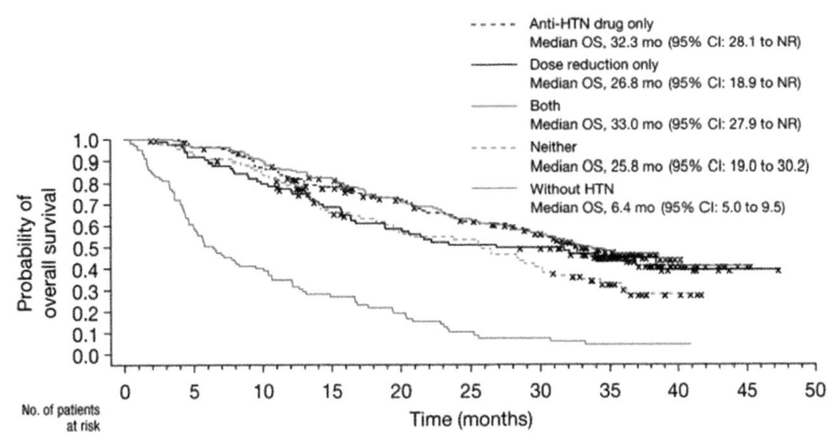

Fig. 18.10 Kaplan-Meier estimates of overall survival (OS) by hypertension (HTN) control and status. HTN was defined by a maximum systolic blood pressure of at least 140 mm Hg (after cycle 1, day 1). CI, confidence interval; NR, not reached. (*From* Rini BI, Cohen DP, Lu DR, et al. Hypertension as a biomarker of efficacy in patients with metastatic renal cell carcinoma treated with sunitinib. J Natl Cancer Inst 2011;103(9):763–73; with permission.)

TABLE 18.1
Main type of cardiac arrhythmias induced by chemotherapy drugs

Type of Arrhythmia	Causative Drug
Sinus bradycardia	Amsacrine, arsenic trioxide, bortezomib, capecitabine, cisplatin, combretastatin, crizotinib, cyclophosphamide, cytarabine, daunorubicin, fludarabine, 5-FU, mitoxantrone, paclitaxel, ponatinib, rituximab, taxanes, thalidomide, vinca alkaloids, vorinostat
AV block	Arsenic trioxide, bortezomib, capecitabine, cisplatin, cyclophosphamide, daunorubicin, doxorubicin, epirubicin, 5-FU, ifosfamide, IL-2, interferon-α, mitoxantrone, ponatinib, rituximab, taxanes, thalidomide
Intraventricular conduction block	Cisplatin, 5-FU, imatinib, paclitaxel, trastuzumab
Sinus tachycardia	Arsenic trioxide, bortezomib, bosutinib, capecitabine, carmustine, cyclophosphamide, epirubicin, 5-FU, paclitaxel, romidepsin, vorinostat
AF	Alemtuzumab, amsacrine, bortezomib, cetuximab, cisplatin, cyclophosphamide, doxorubicin, gemcitabine, ifosfamide, IL-2, interferon-α, melphalan, ponatinib, rituximab, sorafenib, sunitinib, taxanes, vinca alkaloids
Supraventricular tachycardias	Amsacrine, capecitabine, cisplatin, cyclophosphamide, daunorubicin, doxorubicin, ifosfamide, interferon-α, IL-2, melphalan, ponatini, taxanes
QT prolongation	Amsacrine, arsenic trioxide, bosutinib, cabozantinib, capecitabine, combretastatin, daunorubicin, doxorubicin, enzastaurin, eribulin mexilate, HDAC inhibitors (dacinostat, panobinostat, romidepsin, vorinostat), rituximab, small-molecule PKI (dasatinib, lapatinib, nilotinib, ponatinib, sorafenib, sunitinib, vandetanib)
PVCs	Capecitabine, doxorubicin, 5-FU, ifosfamide, interferon-α/γ, methotrexate, rituximab, taxanes, vincristine
VT/Vfib	Alkylating agents (cisplatin, cyclophosphamide, ifosfamide, melphalan), amsacrine, antimetabolites (capecitabine, 5-FU, gemcitabine, methotrexate), anthracyclines (daunorubicin, doxorubicin), arsenic trioxide, dasatinib, HDAC inhibitors (panobinostat, romidepsin), interferon-α/-c, IL-2, monoclonal antibodies (alemtuzumab, rituximab, trastuzumab), taxanes
Torsades de pointes	Arsenic trioxide, dacinostat, daunorubicin, HDAC inhibitors, vorinostat
SCD	Amsacrine, arsenic trioxide, cabozantinib, capecitabine, doxorubicin, 5-FU, interferon-α, nilotinib, romidepsin, rituximab

Abbreviations: AV, atrioventricular; HDAC, histone deacetylase; IL-2, interleukin-2; PKI, protein kinase inhibitor; PVC, packed cell volume; VT/Vfib, ventricular tachycardia/ventricular fibrillation.

disease[110,111] to the heart where after a preliminary echocardiographic examination cardiac magnetic resonance imaging is the diagnostic modality of choice. Furthermore, electrolyte levels and thyroid function should be checked in these patients as well as other concomitant processes such as infection. Finally, a detailed review of all medications should be performed. Paclitaxel is known to produce bradycardia. Patients on a combination regimen of doxorubicin and paclitaxel might experience enhanced doxorubicin cardiotoxicity, because paclitaxel may cause a decrease in doxorubicin clearance. In the absence of any concomitant anthracycline use, patients on paclitaxel who develop asymptomatic sinus bradycardia should continue with therapy and may not require further monitoring apart from vital sign assessment. Monitoring is recommended for patients with symptomatic bradycardia, and those with advanced or progressive conduction abnormalities may require temporary or permanent cardiac pacing, even prophylactically. In general, the indication for a temporary or permanent pacemaker is based on the severity of symptoms, hemodynamic consequences, and need of continued paclitaxel therapy. The use of any other negatively dromotropic and chronotropic cardiac medications needs to be reviewed, but continuation is advised if they meet indications with appropriate monitoring.

Sinus bradycardia can occur in multiple myeloma patients treated with thalidomide (up to 55%), of severe degree, although in the minority (<5%). The effect usually resolves by a decrease in dose or drug discontinuation, but approximately 4% to 5% of patients may require pacemaker implantation. In view of these numbers and the chronicity of treatment, patients should be monitored closely for signs and symptoms of bradycardia (fatigue, limitations in physically activity, syncope, light-headedness, or dizziness) while on therapy. This should be pursued especially in elderly patients and those on β-blockers, calcium channel blockers, digoxin, or any other antiarrhythmic drugs. Prior anthracycline, cyclophosphamide, or chest radiation therapy may also increase the risk.[112]

Atrial and ventricular ectopy is commonly observed in cancer therapy with underlying HD and receiving cardiotoxins and or perioperatively. Persistence of arrhythmic substrates during active cancer treatment limits the utility of cardioversion for AF, and this should wait if possible until the precipitating/enabling factors have been controlled and there has been a satisfactory period of anticoagulation.[113,114] The onset of AF during cancer treatment incurs a high risk of thromboembolism and a 6-fold risk of HF, yet risk scores for initiating antithrombotic treatment do not account for cancer-induced hypercoagulability, and the new oral anticoagulants (NOACs) were not evaluated in patients with cancer.

Oral anticoagulation with warfarin is problematic in patients with cancer, typically requiring its suspension, due to wide fluctuations in international normalized ratio. Thus, low-molecular-weight heparin is frequently used by oncologists to treat or prevent thromboembolism in cancer.[115] The NOACs have been increasingly prescribed in patients with cancer, where thromboembolism incurs a poor prognosis,[116,117] but their limited experience in cancer and multiple drug interactions precludes firm recommendations.[118] For patients with cancer with HD, NOACs are limited at baseline, at 2 to 4 weeks, at 8 to 12 weeks, and every 3 months thereafter to thromboprophylaxis in nonvalvular AF.

The prolongation of the QTc interval greater than 460 milliseconds for women and 450 milliseconds for men or 60 milliseconds over baseline during chemotherapy should raise concern for the risk of torsades de pointes, and even SCD, even though QTc prolongation is present in up to one-third of patients with cancer. Risk factors for these malignant arrhythmias include female gender, older age, bradyarrhythmias, electrolyte abnormalities (hypokalemia, hypomagnesemia, and/or hypocalcemia, eg, due to diarrhea and/or vomiting), structural HDs (CAD, HF, LV hypertrophy), congenital long QT syndrome, and coadministration of QT-prolonging drugs (including 5-hydroxytryptamine receptor 3 antagonists, octreotide, tamoxifen, antipsychotics, antidepressants, antifungals, and quinolone antibiotics).[119,120] Renal and hepatic dysfunction furthermore increases the risk for QT prolongation, and in fact, some chemotherapy drugs can impair the clearance of QT-prolonging drugs by inhibiting hepatic metabolism (via cytochrome P450 3A4: imatinib) or renal clearance (cisplatin). In patients treated with QT-prolonging chemotherapeutics, ECG (at the very least at baseline, at 2–4 weeks, at 8–12 weeks, and every 3 months thereafter, but up to 1–2 times per week or even more often in those at higher risk or as needed), serum electrolyte, and other risk factors should be closely monitored and corrected, and coadministration of other QT-prolonging agents should be avoided before and during the treatment. In addition, patients should be informed of the risk of arrhythmias and asked to report any cardiac symptoms such as palpitations. Typical QTc cutoffs for therapy are 450 ms/460 ms at baseline, and a 60-millisecond increase

TABLE 18.2
National Cancer Institute's toxicity criteria for corrected QT interval prolongation and specific treatment according to the American College of Cardiology/American Heart Association Task Force and the European Society of Cardiology 2006 guidelines[120]

QTc Prolonging Grade	Definition	Recommendations
I	QTc (450 ms)	Removal of the offending agent is indicated (I, A)
II	QTc (470–500 ms or 60 ms above baseline)	
III	QTc (500 ms)	
IV	QTc (500 ms); life-threatening signs or symptoms (ie, arrhythmia, HF, hypotension, syncope), TdP	Intravenous magnesium sulfate is reasonable for patients who present with few episodes of TdP in which the QT remains long (IIa, B) Atrial or ventricular pacing or isoproterenol (IIa, B) Potassium ion repletion to 4.5–5 mmol/L (IIb, C)
V	Death	

Data in parentheses are recommendation, class.
Abbreviations: QTc, corrected QT interval; TdP, torsades de pointes.

or a value greater than 500 milliseconds. If these thresholds are surpassed, therapy is to be stopped and may be resumed at a reduced dose. Any grade 4 event, however, precludes any further therapy (Table 18.2).

REFERENCES

1. Balducci L, Extermann M. Cancer and aging. An evolving panorama. Hematol Oncol Clin North Am 2000;14(1):1–16.
2. Janssen-Heijnen ML, Szerencsi K, van de Schans SA, et al. Cancer patients with cardiovascular disease have survival rates comparable to cancer patients within the age-cohort of 10 years older without cardiovascular morbidity. Crit Rev Oncol Hematol 2010;76(3):196–207.
3. Davis MK, Rajala JL, Tyldesley S, et al. The prevalence of cardiac risk factors in men with localized prostate cancer undergoing androgen deprivation therapy in British Columbia, Canada. J Oncol 2015;2015:820403.
4. Popa MA, Wallace KJ, Brunello A, et al. Potential drug interactions and chemotoxicity in older patients with cancer receiving chemotherapy. J Geriatr Oncol 2014;5(3):307–14.
5. Krzych LJ, Bochenek A. Blood pressure variability: epidemiological and clinical issues. Cardiol J 2013;20(2):112–20.
6. Law MR, Morris JK, Wald NJ. Use of blood pressure lowering drugs in the prevention of cardiovascular disease: meta-analysis of 147 randomised trials in the context of expectations from prospective epidemiological studies. BMJ 2009;338:b1665.
7. Arai H, Saitoh S, Matsumoto T, et al. Hypertension as a paraneoplastic syndrome in hepatocellular carcinoma. J Gastroenterol 1999;34(4):530–4.
8. Rickman T, Garmany R, Doherty T, et al. Hypokalemia, metabolic alkalosis, and hypertension: Cushing's syndrome in a patient with metastatic prostate adenocarcinoma. Am J Kidney Dis 2001;37(4):838–46.
9. von Stempel C, Perks C, Corcoran J, et al. Cardiorespiratory failure secondary to ectopic Cushing's syndrome as the index presentation of small-cell lung cancer. BMJ Case Rep 2013;2013. pii: bcr2013009974.
10. Verges B, Walter T, Cariou B. Endocrine side effects of anti-cancer drugs: effects of anti-cancer targeted therapies on lipid and glucose metabolism. Eur J Endocrinol 2014;170(2):R43–55.
11. Zhong S, Zhang X, Chen L, et al. Statin use and mortality in cancer patients: systematic review and meta-analysis of observational studies. Cancer Treat Rev 2015;41(6):554–67.
12. Kutner JS, Blatchford PJ, Taylor DH Jr, et al. Safety and benefit of discontinuing statin therapy in the setting of advanced, life-limiting illness: a randomized clinical trial. JAMA Intern Med 2015;175(5):691–700.
13. Fleisher LA, Fleischmann KE, Auerbach AD, et al. 2014 ACC/AHA guideline on perioperative cardiovascular evaluation and management of patients undergoing noncardiac surgery: a report of the

American College of Cardiology/American Heart Association Task Force on practice guidelines. J Am Coll Cardiol 2014;64(22):e77–137.
14. Devereaux PJ, Mrkobrada M, Sessler DI, et al. Aspirin in patients undergoing noncardiac surgery. N Engl J Med 2014;370(16):1494–503.
15. Ahmed A. DEFEAT—Heart Failure: a guide to management of geriatric heart failure by generalist physicians. Minerva Med 2009;100(1):39–50.
16. Luciani A, Jacobsen PB, Extermann M, et al. Fatigue and functional dependence in older cancer patients. Am J Clin Oncol 2008;31(5):424–30.
17. Templin C, Ghadri JR, Diekmann J, et al. Clinical Features and Outcomes of Takotsubo (Stress) Cardiomyopathy. N Engl J Med 2015;373(10): 929–38.
18. Goel S, Sharma A, Garg A, et al. Chemotherapy induced Takotsubo cardiomyopathy. World J Clin Cases 2014;2(10):565–8.
19. Gangadhar TC, Von der Lohe E, Sawada SG, et al. Takotsubo cardiomyopathy in a patient with esophageal cancer: a case report. J Med Case Rep 2008;2:379.
20. Franco TH, Khan A, Joshi V, et al. Takotsubo cardiomyopathy in two men receiving bevacizumab for metastatic cancer. Ther Clin Risk Management 2008;4(6):1367–70.
21. Kepez A, Yesildag O, Erdogan O, et al. Takotsubo cardiomyopathy in a patient with lung adenocarcinoma. Heart Views 2012;13(3):107–10.
22. Geisler BP, Raad RA, Esaian D, et al. Apical ballooning and cardiomyopathy in a melanoma patient treated with ipilimumab: a case of takotsubo-like syndrome. J Immunother Cancer 2015;3:4.
23. Hope E, Smith M, Zeligs K, et al. Takotsubo cardiomyopathy following laparoscopic port placement in a patient with ovarian cancer. Gynecol Oncol Case Rep 2012;3:16–7.
24. Kasirye Y, Abdalrahman IB. Tako-tsubo cardiomyopathy in a patient with advanced colorectal adenocarcinoma. Case Rep Med 2010;2010: 487579.
25. Riber LP, Larsen TB, Christensen TD. Postoperative atrial fibrillation prophylaxis after lung surgery: systematic review and meta-analysis. Ann Thorac Surg 2014;98(6):1989–97.
26. Plana JC, Galderisi M, Barac A, et al. Expert Consensus for Multimodality Imaging Evaluation of Adult Patients during and after Cancer Therapy: A Report from the American Society of Echocardiography and the European Association of Cardiovascular Imaging. J Am Soc Echocardiogr 2014;27: 911–39.
27. Hensley ML, Hagerty KL, Kewalramani T, et al. American Society of Clinical Oncology 2008 clinical practice guideline update: use of chemotherapy and radiation therapy protectants. J Clin Oncol 2009;27:127–45.
28. Yancy CW, Jessup M, Bozkurt B, et al. 2013 ACCF/AHA guideline for the management of heart failure: a report of the American College of Cardiology Foundation/American Heart Association Task Force on Practice Guidelines. J Am Coll Cardiol 2013;62:e147–239.
29. National Comprehensive Cancer Network. NCCN Clinical Practice Guidelines in Survivorship. Version 2. 2015. Available at: www.nccn.org. Accessed September 23, 2016.
30. Romond EH, Perez EA, Bryant J, et al. Trastuzumab plus adjuvant chemotherapy for operable HER2-positive breast cancer. N Engl J Med 2005; 353:1673–84.
31. Slamon D, Eiermann W, Robert N, et al. Adjuvant trastuzumab in HER2-positive breast cancer. N Engl J Med 2011;365:1273–83.
32. Seidman A, Hudis C, Pierri MK, et al. Cardiac dysfunction in the trastuzumab clinical trials experience. J Clin Oncol 2002;20:1215–21.
33. Piccart-Gebhart MJ, Procter M, Leyland-Jones B, et al. Trastuzumab after adjuvant chemotherapy in HER2-positive breast cancer. N Engl J Med 2005;353:1659–72.
34. Cote GM, Sawyer DB, Chabner BA. ERBB2 inhibition and heart failure. N Engl J Med 2012;367:2150–3.
35. Thavendiranathan P, Grant AD, Negishi T, et al. Reproducibility of echocardiographic techniques for sequential assessment of left ventricular ejection fraction and volumes: application to patients undergoing cancer chemotherapy. J Am Coll Cardiol 2013;61:77–84.
36. Herceptin Prescribing Information. Genentech, Inc. October 29, 2010.
37. National Comprehensive Cancer Network. NCCN Clinical Practice Guidelines in Oncology. Breast Cancer. Version 1. 2012. Available at: www.nccn.org. Accessed June 30, 2015.
38. Swain SM, Baselga J, Kim SB, et al. Pertuzumab, trastuzumab, and docetaxel in HER2-positive metastatic breast cancer. N Engl J Med 2015; 372:724–34.
39. Ewer MS, Vooletich MT, Durand JB, et al. Reversibility of trastuzumab-related cardiotoxicity: new insights based on clinical course and response to medical treatment. J Clin Oncol 2005;23:7820–6.
40. Burstein HJ, Piccart-Gebhart MJ, Perez EA, et al. Choosing the best trastuzumab-based adjuvant chemotherapy regimen: should we abandon anthracyclines? J Clin Oncol 2012;30: 2179–82.
41. Cardinale D, Colombo A, Torrisi R, et al. Trastuzumab-induced cardiotoxicity: clinical and prognostic implications of troponin I evaluation. J Clin Oncol 2010;28:3910–6.

42. Sawaya H, Sebag IA, Plana JC, et al. Assessment of echocardiography and biomarkers for the extended prediction of cardiotoxicity in patients treated with anthracyclines, taxanes, and trastuzumab. Circ Cardiovasc Imaging 2012;5:596–603.
43. Folkman J. Tumor angiogenesis: therapeutic implications. N Engl J Med 1971;285(21):1182–6.
44. Li W, Croce K, Steensma DP, et al. Vascular and Metabolic Implications of Novel Targeted Cancer Therapies: Focus on Kinase Inhibitors. J Am Coll Cardiol 2015;66(10):1160–78.
45. Dy GK, Adjei AA. Understanding, recognizing, and managing toxicities of targeted anticancer therapies. CA Cancer J Clin 2013;63(4):249–79.
46. de Jesus-Gonzalez N, Robinson E, Moslehi J, et al. Management of antiangiogenic therapy-induced hypertension. Hypertension 2012;60(3):607–15.
47. Steeghs N, Gelderblom H, Roodt JO, et al. Hypertension and rarefaction during treatment with telatinib, a small molecule angiogenesis inhibitor. Clin Cancer Res 2008;14(11):3470–6.
48. Facemire CS, Nixon AB, Griffiths R, et al. Vascular endothelial growth factor receptor 2 controls blood pressure by regulating nitric oxide synthase expression. Hypertension 2009;54(3):652–8.
49. Eremina V, Jefferson JA, Kowalewska J, et al. VEGF inhibition and renal thrombotic microangiopathy. N Engl J Med 2008;358(11):1129–36.
50. Granger JP. Vascular endothelial growth factor inhibitors and hypertension: a central role for the kidney and endothelial factors? Hypertension 2009;54(3):465–7.
51. Vigneau C, Lorcy N, Dolley-Hitze T, et al. All anti-vascular endothelial growth factor drugs can induce 'pre-eclampsia-like syndrome': a RARe study. Nephrol Dial Transplant 2014;29(2):325–32.
52. Steingart RM, Bakris GL, Chen HX, et al. Management of cardiac toxicity in patients receiving vascular endothelial growth factor signaling pathway inhibitors. Am Heart J 2012;163(2):156–63.
53. Cardinale D, Sandri MT, Colombo A, et al. Prognostic value of troponin I in cardiac risk stratification of cancer patients undergoing high-dose chemotherapy. Circulation 2004;109(22):2749–54.
54. Groarke JD, Choueiri TK, Slosky D, et al. Recognizing and managing left ventricular dysfunction associated with therapeutic inhibition of the vascular endothelial growth factor signaling pathway. Curr Treat Options Cardiovasc Med 2014;16(9):335.
55. Yancy CW, Jessup M, Bozkurt B, et al. 2013 ACCF/AHA guideline for the management of heart failure: a report of the American College of Cardiology Foundation/American Heart Association Task Force on practice guidelines. Circulation 2013;128(16):e240–327.
56. Kusumoto S, Kawano H, Hayashi T, et al. Cyclophosphamide-induced Cardiotoxicity with a Prolonged Clinical Course Diagnosed on an Endomyocardial Biopsy Intern Med 2013;52:2311–5.
57. Zver S, Zadnik V, Bunc M, et al. Cardiac toxicity of high-dose cyclophosphamide in patients with multiple myeloma undergoing autologous hematopoietic stem cell transplantation. Int J Hematol 2007;85(5):408–14.
58. Morandi P, Ruffini PA, Benvenuto GM, et al. Cardiac toxicity of high-dose chemotherapy. Bone Marrow Transplantation 2005;35:323–34.
59. Cortes J, Mauro M, Steegmann JL, et al. Cardiovascular and pulmonary adverse events in patients treated with BCR-ABL inhibitors: Data from the FDA Adverse Event Reporting System. Am J Hematol 2015;90(4):E66–72.
60. Breccia M, Alimena G. Pleural/pericardic effusions during dasatinib treatment: incidence, management and risk factors associated to their development. Expert Opin Drug Saf 2010;9(5):713–21.
61. Kelly K, Swords R, Mahalingam D, et al. Serosal inflammation (pleural and pericardial effusions) related to tyrosine kinase inhibitors. Target Oncol 2009;4(2):99–105.
62. Stewart T, Pavlakis N, Ward M. Cardiotoxicity with 5-fluorouracil and capecitabine: more than just vasospastic angina. Intern Med J 2010;40(4):303–7.
63. Heidelberger C, Chaudhuri NK, Danneberg P, et al. Fluorinated pyrimidines, a new class of tumour-inhibitory compounds. Nature 1957;179(4561):663–6.
64. Talapatra K, Rajesh I, Rajesh B, et al. Transient asymptomatic bradycardia in patients on infusional 5-fluorouracil. J Cancer Res Ther 2007;3(3):169–71.
65. Wacker A, Lersch C, Scherpinski U, et al. High incidence of angina pectoris in patients treated with 5-fluorouracil. A planned surveillance study with 102 patients. Oncology 2003;65(2):108–12.
66. Labianca R, Beretta G, Clerici M, et al. Cardiac toxicity of 5-fluorouracil: a study on 1083 patients. Tumori 1982;68(6):505–10.
67. Schober C, Papageorgiou E, Harstrick A, et al. Cardiotoxicity of 5-fluorouracil in combination with folinic acid in patients with gastrointestinal cancer. Cancer 1993;72(7):2242–7.
68. Rezkalla S, Kloner RA, Ensley J, et al. Continuous ambulatory ECG monitoring during fluorouracil therapy: a prospective study. J Clin Oncol 1989;7(4):509–14.
69. Grunwald MR, Howie L, Diaz LA Jr. Takotsubo cardiomyopathy and Fluorouracil: case report and review of the literature. J Clin Oncol 2012;30(2):e11–14.
70. Kobayashi N, Hata N, Yokoyama S, et al. A case of Takotsubo cardiomyopathy during 5-fluorouracil

treatment for rectal adenocarcinoma. J Nippon Med Sch 2009;76(1):27–33.
71. Basselin C, Fontanges T, Descotes J, et al. 5-Fluorouracil-induced Tako-Tsubo-like syndrome. Pharmacotherapy 2011;31(2):226.
72. Radhakrishnan V, Bakhshi S. 5-Fluorouracil-induced acute dilated cardiomyopathy in a pediatric patient. J Pediatr Hematol Oncol 2011; 33(4):323.
73. Akhtar SS, Wani BA, Bano ZA, et al. 5-Fluorouracil-induced severe but reversible cardiogenic shock: a case report. Tumori 1996;82(5):505–7.
74. Kim L, Karas M, Wong SC. Chemotherapy-induced takotsubo cardiomyopathy. J Invasive Cardiol 2008;20(12):E338–40.
75. Ozturk MA, Ozveren O, Cinar V, et al. Takotsubo syndrome: an underdiagnosed complication of 5-fluorouracil mimicking acute myocardial infarction. Blood Coagul Fibrinolysis 2013;24(1):90–4.
76. Y-Hassan S, Tornvall P, Tornerud M, et al. Capecitabine caused cardiogenic shock through induction of global Takotsubo syndrome. Cardiovasc Revasc Med 2013;14(1):57–61.
77. Lim SH, Wilson SM, Hunter A, et al. Takotsubo cardiomyopathy and 5-Fluorouracil: getting to the heart of the matter. Case Rep Oncological Med 2013;2013:206765.
78. Polk A, Vaage-Nilsen M, Vistisen K, et al. Cardiotoxicity in cancer patients treated with 5-fluorouracil or capecitabine: a systematic review of incidence, manifestations and predisposing factors. Cancer Treat Rev 2013;39(8):974–84.
79. Kelly C, Bhuva N, Harrison M, et al. Use of raltitrexed as an alternative to 5-fluorouracil and capecitabine in cancer patients with cardiac history. Eur J Cancer 2013;49(10):2303–10.
80. Meyer CC, Calis KA, Burke LB, et al. Symptomatic cardiotoxicity associated with 5-fluorouracil. Pharmacotherapy 1997;17(4):729–36.
81. Meydan N, Kundak I, Yavuzsen T, et al. Cardiotoxicity of de Gramont's regimen: incidence, clinical characteristics and long-term follow-up. Jpn J Clin Oncol 2005;35(5):265–70.
82. Ng M, Cunningham D, Norman AR. The frequency and pattern of cardiotoxicity observed with capecitabine used in conjunction with oxaliplatin in patients treated for advanced colorectal cancer (CRC). Eur J Cancer 2005;41(11):1542–6.
83. Akhtar SS, Salim KP, Bano ZA. Symptomatic cardiotoxicity with high-dose 5-fluorouracil infusion: a prospective study. Oncology 1993;50(6):441–4.
84. Jensen SA, Sorensen JB. Risk factors and prevention of cardiotoxicity induced by 5-fluorouracil or capecitabine. Cancer Chemother Pharmacol 2006;58(4):487–93.
85. Kosmas C, Kallistratos MS, Kopterides P, et al. Cardiotoxicity of fluoropyrimidines in different schedules of administration: a prospective study. J Cancer Res Clin Oncol 2008;134(1):75–82.
86. Tsavaris N, Kosmas C, Vadiaka M, et al. 5-fluorouracil cardiotoxicity is a rare, dose and schedule-dependent adverse event: a prospective study. J BUON 2005;10(2):205–11.
87. Van Cutsem E, Hoff PM, Blum JL, et al. Incidence of cardiotoxicity with the oral fluoropyrimidine capecitabine is typical of that reported with 5-fluorouracil. Ann Oncol 2002;13(3):484–5.
88. Cianci G, Morelli MF, Cannita K, et al. Prophylactic options in patients with 5-fluorouracil-associated cardiotoxicity. Br J Cancer 2003;88(10): 1507–9.
89. Kim TD, le Coutre P, Schwarz M, et al. Clinical cardiac safety profile of nilotinib. Haematologica 2012;97:883–9.
90. Scappaticci FA, Skillings JR, Holden SN, et al. Arterial thromboembolic events in patients with metastatic carcinoma treated with chemotherapy and bevacizumab. J Natl Cancer Inst 2007;99(16): 1232–9.
91. Leighl NB, Bennouna J, Yi J, et al. Bleeding events in bevacizumab-treated cancer patients who received full-dose anticoagulation and remained on study. Br J Cancer 2011;104(3):413–8.
92. Tebbutt NC, Murphy F, Zannino D, et al. Risk of arterial thromboembolic events in patients with advanced colorectal cancer receiving bevacizumab. Ann Oncol 2011;22(8):1834–8.
93. Thygesen K, Alpert JS, Jaffe AS, et al. Third universal definition of myocardial infarction. Circulation 2012;126(16):2020–35.
94. Sarkiss MG, Yusuf SW, Warneke CL, et al. Impact of aspirin therapy in cancer patients with thrombocytopenia and acute coronary syndromes. Cancer 2007;109(3):621–7.
95. Shah KB, Kleinman BS, Rao TL, et al. Angina and other risk factors in patients with cardiac diseases undergoing noncardiac operations. Anesth Analg 1990;70:240–7.
96. Livhits M, Ko CY, Leonardi MJ, et al. Risk of surgery following recent myocardial infarction. Ann Surg 2011;253:857–64.
97. Livhits M, Gibbons MM, de VC, et al. Coronary revascularization after myocardial infarction can reduce risks of noncardiac surgery. J Am Coll Surg 2011;212:1018–26.
98. Maitland ML, Kasza KE, Karrison T, et al. Ambulatory monitoring detects sorafenib-induced blood pressure elevations on the first day of treatment. Clin Cancer Res 2009;15(19):6250–7.
99. Maitland ML, Bakris GL, Black HR, et al. Initial assessment, surveillance, and management of blood pressure in patients receiving vascular endothelial growth factor signaling pathway inhibitors. J Natl Cancer Inst 2010;102(9):596–604.

100. Rini BI, Quinn DI, Baum M, et al. Hypertension among patients with renal cell carcinoma receiving axitinib or sorafenib: analysis from the randomized phase III AXIS trial. Targeted Oncol 2015;10(1):45–53.
101. McKay RR, Rodriguez GE, Lin X, et al. Angiotensin system inhibitors and survival outcomes in patients with metastatic renal cell carcinoma. Clin Cancer Res 2015;21(11):2471–9.
102. Khakoo AY, Sidman RL, Pasqualini R, et al. Does the renin-angiotensin system participate in regulation of human vasculogenesis and angiogenesis? Cancer Res 2008;68(22):9112–5.
103. Rini BI, Cohen DP, Lu DR, et al. Hypertension as a biomarker of efficacy in patients with metastatic renal cell carcinoma treated with sunitinib. J Natl Cancer Inst 2011;103(9):763–73.
104. Estfan B, Byrne M, Kim R. Sorafenib in advanced hepatocellular carcinoma: hypertension as a potential surrogate marker for efficacy. Am J Clin Oncol 2013;36(4):319–24.
105. Jubb AM, Harris AL. Biomarkers to predict the clinical efficacy of bevacizumab in cancer. Lancet Oncol 2010;11(12):1172–83.
106. Langenberg MH, van Herpen CM, De Bono J, et al. Effective strategies for management of hypertension after vascular endothelial growth factor signaling inhibition therapy: results from a phase II randomized, factorial, double-blind study of Cediranib in patients with advanced solid tumors. J Clin Oncol 2009; 27(36):6152–9.
107. Porta C, Gore ME, Rini BI, et al. Long-term safety of sunitinib in metastatic renal cell carcinoma. Eur Urol 2016;69(2):345–51.
108. Chintalgattu V, Rees ML, Culver JC, et al. Coronary microvascular pericytes are the cellular target of sunitinib malate-induced cardiotoxicity. Sci Translational Med 2013;5(187):187ra169.
109. Chu TF, Rupnick MA, Kerkela R, et al. Cardiotoxicity associated with tyrosine kinase inhibitor sunitinib. Lancet (London, England) 2007;370(9604): 2011–9.
110. Pun SCP, Gupta D, Lakhman Y et al. Tissue Characteristics and Anatomic Distribution of Cardiac Metastases among Patients with Advanced Systemic Cancer Assessed by Cardiac Magnetic Resonance (CMR). Abstracts of the 19th Annual SCMR Scientific Sessions, 2016.
111. Neragi-Miandoab S, Kim J, Vlahakes GJ. Malignant tumours of the heart: a review of tumour type, diagnosis and therapy. Clin Oncol (R Coll Radiol) 2007;19(10):748–56.
112. Fahdi IE, Gaddam V, Saucedo JF, et al. Bradycardia during therapy for multiple myeloma with thalidomide. Am J Cardiol 2004;93:1052–5.
113. Farmakis D, Parissis J, Filippatos G. Insights into onco-cardiology: atrial fibrillation in cancer. J Am Coll Cardiol 2014;63(10):945–53.
114. Hu YF, Liu CJ, Chang PM, et al. Incident thromboembolism and heart failure associated with new-onset atrial fibrillation in cancer patients. Int J Cardiol 2013;165(2):355–7.
115. Lyman GH, Bohlke K, Khorana AA, et al. Venous thromboembolism prophylaxis and treatment in patients with cancer: american society of clinical oncology clinical practice guideline update 2014. J Clin Oncol 2015;33(6):654–6.
116. den Exter PL, van der Hulle T, Klok FA, et al. The newer anticoagulants in thrombosis control in cancer patients. Semin Oncol 2014;41(3):339–45.
117. Short NJ, Connors JM. New oral anticoagulants and the cancer patient. Oncologist 2014;19(1): 82–93.
118. Sanford D, Naidu A, Alizadeh N, et al. The effect of low molecular weight heparin on survival in cancer patients: an updated systematic review and meta-analysis of randomized trials. J Thromb Haemost 2014;12(7):1076–85.
119. Becker TK, Yeung SCJ. Drug-induced QT interval prolongation in cancer patients. Oncol Rev 2010; 4(4):223–32.
120. Zipes DP, Camm AJ, Borggrefe M, et al. ACC/AHA/ESC 2006 guidelines for management of patients with ventricular arrhythmias and the prevention of sudden cardiac death-executive summary: a report of the American College of Cardiology/American Heart Association Task Force and the European Society of Cardiology Committee for Practice Guidelines (Writing Committee to Develop Guidelines for Management of Patients with Ventricular Arrhythmias and the Prevention of Sudden Cardiac Death). Eur Heart J 2006;27: 2099–140.

CHAPTER 19

Cardiovascular Effects of Anthracycline Chemotherapy and Radiation Therapy in Children with Cancer

Shahnawaz M. Amdani, MBBS, MD[a], Neha Bansal, MD[a], Vivian I. Franco, MPH[b], Michael Jacob Adams, MD, MPH[c], Steven E. Lipshultz, MD[b,*]

INTRODUCTION

In the United States, cancer is diagnosed in more than 12,000 children every year.[1] Improvement in 5-year survival rates, from less than 58% in the 1970s to 83% today,[2] has increased the number of long-term survivors of childhood cancer to an estimated 420,000.[3] This improvement is partly the result of new chemotherapy and radiation treatments. However, improved survival also means that these patients are vulnerable to the late effects of these treatments.

Cardiovascular-related disease is the leading cause of non-cancer-related morbidity and mortality in long-term survivors of childhood cancer.[4] The risk of heart failure (HF), myocardial infarction (MI), pericardial disease, and valvular abnormalities is significantly greater in survivors than in their siblings.[5] Furthermore, survivors are 8 times as likely to die from cardiovascular-related disease as are people in the general population.[6]

Childhood cancer survivors receiving anthracycline chemotherapy are at a significantly increased risk of cardiotoxicity. This risk increases as the cumulative anthracycline dose increases[7] and persists for at least 45 years after treatment.[4] More than half of anthracycline-exposed childhood cancer survivors have subclinical cardiac abnormalities, including decreased left ventricular (LV) mass and wall thickness, increased LV afterload, and decreased LV contractility.[8] Clinicians are increasingly recognizing the importance of continuously monitoring these patients long after they have completed cancer treatment.[9]

Late cardiotoxicity is seen in survivors of adult cancers treated with the same agents, although the late effects in long-term survivors are just beginning to be understood. The overall scope of cardiovascular late effects is quite broad and not confined to cardiac function abnormalities even though these have remained the focus. The emergence of cardiovascular toxicities by the therapies that induced and consolidated cancer survival might differ in adults than in children, likely related to the comorbid conditions and a reduction in repair/regeneration capacity. The principles remain the same; however, there are likely to be some very important differences between childhood and adult cancer survivors, including the pathophysiology (Fig. 19.1).

PATHOPHYSIOLOGY OF CARDIOVASCULAR TOXICITY

Chemotherapeutic medications are designed to interfere with rapidly dividing neoplastic cells. However, in the process, they can adversely affect normal cell division, especially in tissues with rapid turnover. The cardiovascular system has limited regenerative capacity, so potential adverse events from these chemotherapeutic agents may be irreversible. Cardiotoxic effects have been

[a] Division of Pediatric Cardiology, Children's Hospital of Michigan, 3901 Beaubien Street, Detroit, MI 48201, USA; [b] Department of Pediatrics, Wayne State University School of Medicine, Children's Hospital of Michigan, 3901 Beaubien Boulevard, Suite 1K40, Detroit, MI 48201, USA; [c] Department of Public Health Sciences, University of Rochester School of Medicine and Dentistry, 601 Elmwood Avenue, Box 644, Rochester, NY 14619, USA
* Corresponding author.
E-mail address: slipshultz@med.wayne.edu

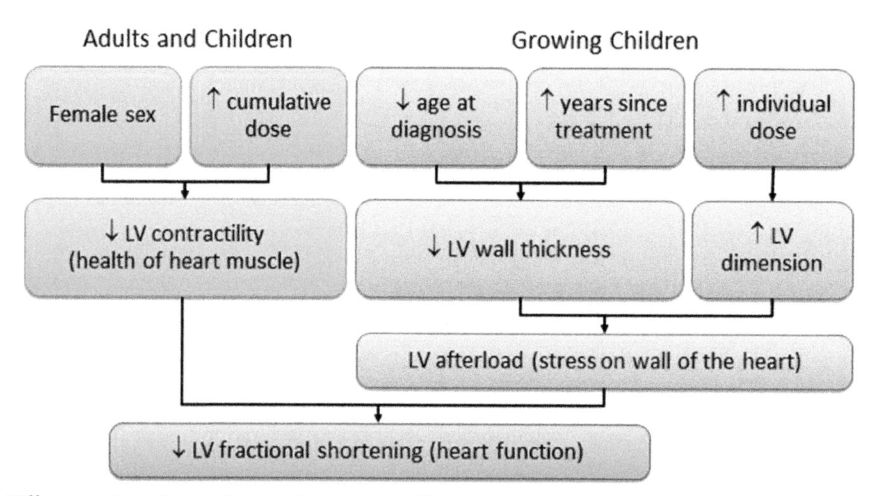

Fig. 19.1 Differences in anthracycline cardiotoxic late effects experienced between adults and children attributable to common risk factors. (*From* Lipshultz SE, Cochran TR, Franco VI, et al. Treatment-related cardiotoxicity in survivors of childhood cancer. Nat Rev Clin Oncol 2013;10:697; with permission).

documented for several classes of cancer treatments, including anthracyclines (eg, doxorubicin and epirubicin), alkylating agents (eg, busulfan and cyclophosphamide), antimetabolites (including 5-fluorouracil and cytarabine), antimicrotubule agents (eg, vinca alkaloids), targeted agents (eg, bevacizumab and trastuzumab), and radiation (Table 19.1).[10,11] Of these, anthracycline-related cardiotoxicity is particularly well known. Newer antineoplastic compounds, such as tyrosine kinase inhibitors, which have been reported to cause cardiotoxicity in adults, are now being used to treat children.[12]

Anthracyclines enter the cell through passive diffusion. In cardiomyocytes, anthracycline concentrations can be much higher in intracellular compartments, given the presence of high concentrations of cardiolipin and its high affinity for anthracycline.[13,14] The high intracellular concentration of anthracycline leads to membrane instability and damages mitochondrial DNA (mtDNA). This damage may inhibit the cell's ability to produce energy or to adjust to the increased demands of oxidative stress generated by free radicals, or reactive oxygen species (ROS).[15–18] In addition, glutathione peroxidase, one of the heart's crucial antioxidants, is depleted in the presence of anthracyclines.[19]

Once anthracycline enters the cell (Fig. 19.2), it forms complexes with iron and reduces the quinone moiety to subquinone. This reduction leads to a cascade production of ROS, which are the root cause for some of the deleterious effects on the cell and its components, and that ultimately causes cell death. Oxidative stress also induces nitric oxide synthase and produces nitric oxide and peroxynitrite, which inactivate myofibrillar creatine kinase and other important cardiac enzymes.[20,21] This damage, and that cardiomyocytes divide too slowly or too many are mitotically quiescent to replace these damaged cells, leads to organ damage.

Several other mechanisms for anthracycline-related cardiotoxicity have been postulated, including the induction of apoptosis, the production of vasoactive amines, the formation of toxic metabolites, the upregulation of nitric oxide synthase, and the inhibition of transcription and translation.[22–24] Anthracyclines cause the electron transport chain to uncouple, which creates highly ROS and impairs phosphorylation and ATP synthesis.[14] They also disturb mitochondrial calcium homeostasis, destabilize the mitochondrial membrane, and ultimately kill the cell. Cardiomyocytes exposed to anthracyclines show other changes, which may or may not depend on the oxidative pathway. These changes include depleted cardiac stem cells,[25] impaired DNA synthesis,[26] impaired cell signaling that triggers cell death,[27] altered gene expression,[28] inhibited calcium release from the sarcoplasmic reticulum,[29] impaired formation of the protein titin in sarcomeres,[30] and impaired mitochondrial creatine kinase activity and function.[31] These subcellular processes often continue for weeks after anthracycline exposure, which may provide insight into the mechanism of chronic cardiomyopathy.[32]

Anthracyclines can prolong QTc intervals, which indicates an increased risk of ventricular tachycardia.[33,34] In 10% to 30% of patients, anthracyclines have also been associated with premature ventricular contractions, sinus node dysfunction, ventricular late potentials, and decreased QRS voltage.[33,35,36] The mechanism

TABLE 19.1
Cardiotoxic effects of selected cytotoxic agents

Treatment	Cardiotoxic Effect
Anthracyclines: Daunorubicin, doxorubicin, epirubicin, idarubicin, mitoxantrone	Arrhythmias, pericarditis, myocarditis, HF, LV dysfunction
Liposomal anthracyclines: Pegylated liposomal doxorubicin hydrochloride (Doxil, Caelyx)	HF, LV dysfunction, arrhythmias
Antimetabolites: Capecitabine, carmustine, clofarabine, cytarabine, 5-fluorouracil, methotrexate	Ischemia, chest pain, MI, HF, arrhythmias, pericardial effusions, pericarditis, hemodynamic abnormalities
Anti-microtubule agents: Paclitaxel, vinca alkaloids	Hypotension or hypertension, ischemia, angina, MI, bradycardia, arrhythmias, conduction abnormalities, HF
Alkylating agents: Busulfan, chlormethine, cisplatin, cyclophosphamide, ifosfamide, mitomycin	Endomyocardial fibrosis, pericarditis, tamponade, ischemia, MI, hypertension, myocarditis, HF, arrhythmias
Small-molecule tyrosine kinase inhibitors: Dasatinib, gefitinib, imatinib mesylate, lapatinib, erlotinib, sorafenib, sunitinib	HF, edema, pericardial effusion, pericarditis, hypertension, arrhythmias, prolonged QT interval, ischemia, chest pain
Monoclonal antibodies: Alemtuzumab, bevacizumab, cetuximab, rituximab, trastuzumab	Hemodynamic abnormalities, LV dysfunction, HF, thromboembolism, angioedema, arrhythmias
Interleukins: Denileukin, IL-2	Hypotension, capillary leak syndrome, arrhythmias, coronary artery thrombosis, ischemia, LV dysfunction
Miscellaneous agents: All-trans-retinoic acid, arsenic trioxide, asparaginase, etoposide, interferon-α, lenalidomide, 6-mercaptopurine, pentostatin, teniposide, thalidomide	Electrocardiographic changes, QT prolongation, torsades de pointes, other arrhythmias, ischemia, angina, MI, HF, edema, hypotension, bradycardia, thromboembolism, and retinoid acid syndrome that includes fever, hypotension, respiratory distress, weight gain, peripheral edema, pleural-pericardial effusions

From Zerra P, Cochran TR, Franco VI, et al. An expert opinion on pharmacologic approaches to reducing the cardiotoxicity of childhood acute lymphoblastic leukemia therapies. Expert Opin Pharmacother 2013;14(11):1499; with permission.

for this electrophysiological toxicity is unknown, but could be related to free radical generation, as mentioned above. Often, these changes are transient and do not require interventions, but pacemakers have been placed in patients receiving doxorubicin, as well as epirubicin, which is less cardiotoxic.[36,37]

Over the last several years, there has been an increase in research about topoisomerase-II β (Top2β) alterations being the mechanism of doxorubicin-mediated cardiotoxicity.[38,39] The Top2β-doxorubicin-DNA ternary cleavage complex induces DNA double-strand breaks, causing cell death.[40] Zhang and colleagues[38] showed that cardiomyocyte-specific deletion of Top2β protects cardiomyocytes from doxorubicin-induced DNA double-strand breaks and transcriptome changes in mice, resulting in defective mitochondria. Furthermore, peripheral blood leukocyte Top2β levels were higher in anthracycline-sensitive patients (decreased LV ejection fraction [LVEF] ≥10% from baseline and LVEF <50%, despite receiving a cumulative doxorubicin dose ≤250 mg/m^2) than in anthracycline-resistant patients (received a cumulative doxorubicin dose ≥450 mg/m^2 with LVEF ≥50%), which suggests the potential use of Top2β as a surrogate marker for susceptibility of anthracycline-induced cardiotoxicity.[41]

RADIOTHERAPY

All components of the heart are susceptible to radiation damage. The pathophysiology of this damage has been studied extensively.[42] A hallmark of myocardial injury is nonspecific, diffuse, interstitial fibrosis.[43] Microscopically, not only does the total amount of collagen increase, but also the proportion of type I collagenase increases more than does type III. These changes

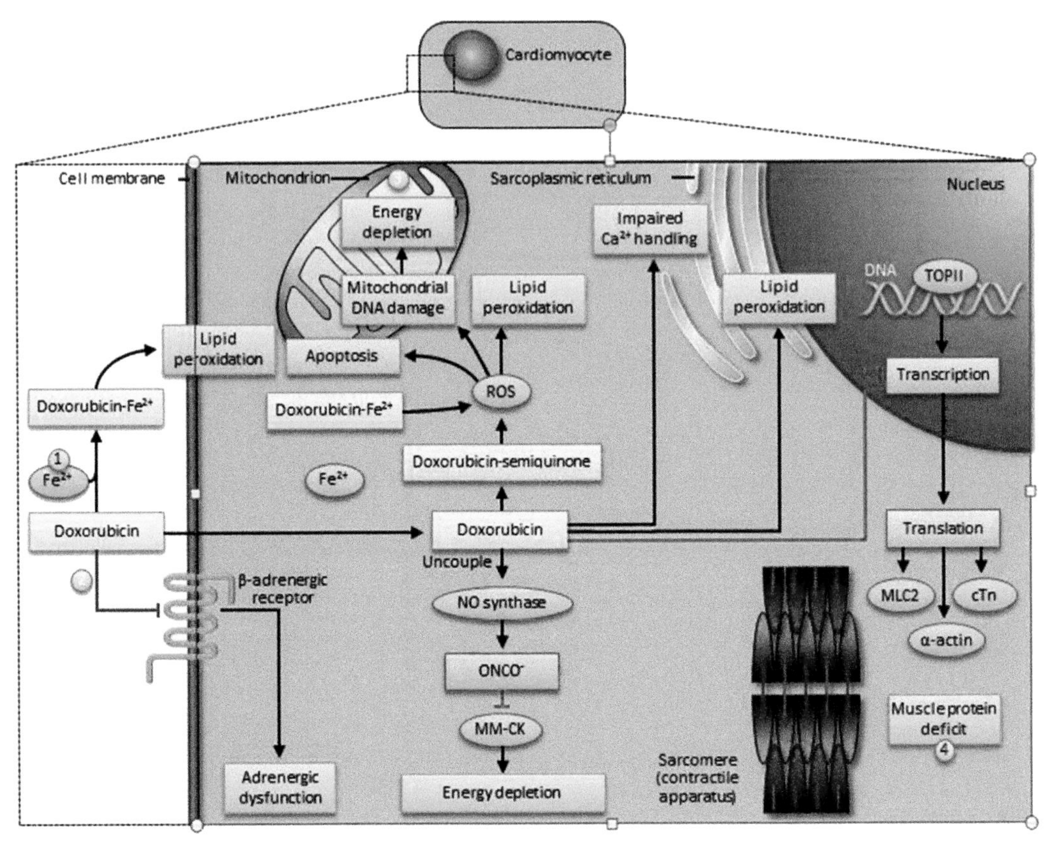

Fig. 19.2 Potential opportunities for cardioprotection in cardiomyocytes. MM-CK, myofibrillar isoform of the CK enzyme; NO, nitric oxide; ONCO, oncomodulin. (*From* Lipshultz SE, Cochran TR, Franco VI, et al. Treatment-related cardiotoxicity in survivors of childhood cancer. Nat Rev Clin Oncol 2013;10:697–710; with permission).

in collagen alter the compliance of the myocardium and contributes to diastolic dysfunction.[44] Even the conduction system is sensitive to this radiation-induced fibrosis, as indicated by several reports of arrhythmias and intracardiac conduction system abnormalities.[45–47]

Using a rabbit animal model of radiation damage, Stewart and colleagues[48,49] found that the myocardium was damaged in 3 phases. In the first, the small and medium-sized arteries were damaged after 6 hours of exposure to radiation, but the microvessels were not directly affected. A neutrophilic infiltrate also appeared, involving all layers of the heart. The second or latent phase began 2 days after radiation, characterized by progressive fibrosis. The healthy endothelial cells responded by replicating, but the rate was inadequate to avoid ischemia, and eventually more extensive fibrosis and myocardial death occurred. The third or late phase started 70 days after radiation and was characterized by extensive fibrosis.

Radiation also activates the inflammatory pathways.[50] ROS production increases, which creates an environment in which oxidative damage to proteins and lipids exacerbates other types of injuries.[51] This environment can lead to chronic inflammation, which may increase the risk of clinically important plaque development and rupture.[52] Extensive fibrous thickening of the pericardium, including pericardial adhesions and excessive pericardial fluid, is now rare with the radiotherapy (RT) doses and techniques used in children.[53] When the pericardium is damaged, small blood vessels proliferate, which are abnormal with increased permeability, causing ischemia and eventually fibrosis.

Irradiated valves become fibrotic, with or without calcification.[53,54] Because valves are basically avascular, this fibrosis is mysterious but might be explained as a late consequence of injury of the surrounding myocardial endothelium.[54] Because damage to the left-sided valves are often more severe and observed more commonly than the right-sided valves, the high systemic pressures may play an important role in the pathogenesis.[54,55]

The left anterior descending and the right coronary arteries are frequently affected after

RT.[56–58] Within the vessel, the narrowing may occur proximally and often involves the coronary ostia.[53,54,56,57] Some have found that the media and the intima are more densely thickened with fibrous tissue in radiation-induced atherosclerotic plaque. However, even in the general population, intimal plaques are largely composed of fibrous tissue.[53] Therefore, discriminating between radiation-induced atherosclerotic plaque and a typical nonradiation coronary artery disease plaque remains difficult.

In the brain, endothelial cell disruption starts an inflammatory response in the cerebral microvasculature, which causes endothelial perforation and increases platelet adherence and thrombus formation.[59,60] The loss of tight junctions and increased vascular permeability lead to histopathological changes that also result in luminal narrowing and thrombus formation.[59,61] Weakening of the vessel wall can result in abnormal dilation and tortuosity.[62] Neck irradiation increases the thickness of the intima and the media layer of the carotid wall.[63,64] These changes are associated with an increased risk of stroke, with preexisting atherosclerosis as an exacerbating factor.[64,65] In summary, the effects of radiation on cardiovascular tissue can be classified by the size of the vessel and time since exposure (Table 19.2).

PROGRESSION OF CARDIOVASCULAR TOXICITY

Anthracycline cardiotoxicity can present within a week or decades after initial treatment.[66] In fact, whether any time limit exists is uncertain. Early toxicity is not a prerequisite for toxicity presenting decades later, but the presence of measurable

TABLE 19.2
Vascular response to radiation

Time Phase	Small Arteries/ Arterioles (<1000 μm)	Medium Arteries (100–500 μm)	Large Arteries (>500 μm)
Acute/early delayed (<6 mo)	Detachment of endothelium from basement membrane; increased BBB permeability through loss of tight junction or increased vesicular activity; cell pyknosis; cytoplasmic vacuolation; nuclear swelling; perivascular edema; acute oxidative stress response		
Late delayed (>6 mo)	Progressive loss/ abnormal proliferation of endothelia; fibrinoid necrosis; adventitial fibrosis; media hyalinization; intimal thickening; chronic oxidative stress response; thrombus formation	Intimal fibrosis; myointimal formation; subintimal foam cell plaque formation; thrombosis	Intimal fibrosis; myointimal formation; subintimal foam cell plaque formation; thrombosis
Clinical sequelae	Mineralizing microangiopathy; impaired vasa vasorum; possible brain necrosis	Stenosis; aneurysm; vascular malformation	Stenosis; aneurysm; vascular malformation

Abbreviation: BBB, blood-brain barrier.

From Lipshultz SE, Adams MJ, Colan SD, et al. Long-term cardiovascular toxicity in children, adolescents, and young adults who receive cancer therapy: pathophysiology, course, monitoring, management, prevention, and research directions: a scientific statement from the American Heart Association. Circulation 2013;128(17):1936; with permission.

early cardiotoxicity probably indicates that late cardiotoxicity in long-term survivors is more likely to occur.[67] Cardiotoxicity is often classified by when the signs and symptoms appear. Cardiotoxicity within a week of treatment is referred to as acute onset. Cardiotoxicity between 1 week and 1 year is referred to as early-onset chronic progressive, and late-onset cardiotoxicity occurs 1 year after treatment (Table 19.3).

In each category, HF may occur because of LV dysfunction and decreased exercise capacity.[68] Acute-onset toxicity presents during treatment in less than 1% of patients[13,69,70] and often manifests as arrhythmias, electrocardiographic abnormalities, HF, or a myocarditis-pericarditis syndrome.[13,69–71] Early-onset chronic progressive cardiotoxicity has the same range of manifestations.[13,68,70,72,73] Although some patients may present with potentially fatal HF, especially with higher cumulative doses of anthracyclines, the condition is often transient and frequently resolves when treatment is discontinued.[13,71] However, cardiac abnormalities in survivors can be persistent and progressive, and even patients with lower cumulative doses may eventually experience effects of cardiotoxicity.[74]

In late-onset cardiotoxicity, LV function deteriorates, and cardiomyocytes are often decreased.[9,74,75] This cardiomyocyte loss results in LV dilation that progresses to a restrictive LV, LV wall thinning, and decreased LV contractility.[76] Echocardiographic findings include decreases in LV fractional shortening (FS), decreased LV mass, LV contractility, and LV end-diastolic posterior wall thickness.[13] With marked LV dysfunction, the heart may be unable to compensate for increased metabolic demands, such as acute viral illness, growth-hormone-induced growth spurts, weight-lifting, pregnancy-induced hypervolemia, and vaginal birth.[77–80]

Kremer and colleagues[81] reported a cumulative incidence of HF of 2.8% after a mean follow-up of 6.3 years and a mean cumulative dose of 301 mg/m^2 of doxorubicin, daunorubicin, idarubicin, or epirubicin. The progression of dilated cardiomyopathy was toward a restrictive-like pattern with extended follow-up (Fig. 19.3).[74] Serial echocardiograms obtained in 115 survivors treated with anthracyclines showed significantly reduced LV FS after doxorubicin therapy, which was inversely related to the cumulative dosing, with significantly depressed LV function in patients receiving more than 300 mg/m^2 of doxorubicin with this degree of intermediate follow-up. The authors observed a progressive and persistent decrease in the contractility with progressively increasing LV afterload with deficient LV mass for body surface area and a possibly reduced cardiac output. These changes were the worst with highest cumulative doses; however, changes were observed even with lower doses.[74] Long-term follow-up of this cohort showed a decrease in the LV dimension for body surface area with a subsequent increase in LV wall

TABLE 19.3
Characteristics of different types of anthracycline cardiotoxicity

Characteristic	Acute Cardiotoxicity	Early-Onset Progressive Cardiotoxicity	Late-Onset Progressive Cardiotoxicity
Onset	Within the first week of anthracycline treatment	<1 y after completion of anthracycline treatment	≥1 y after completion of anthracycline treatment
Risk factor dependence	Unknown	Yes[a]	Yes[a]
Clinical features in adults	Transient depression of myocardial contractility	Dilated cardiomyopathy	Dilated cardiomyopathy
Clinical features in children	Transient depression of myocardial contractility	Restrictive cardiomyopathy and/or dilated cardiomyopathy	Restrictive cardiomyopathy and/or dilated cardiomyopathy
Course	Usually reversible on discontinuation of anthracycline	Can be progressive	Can be progressive

[a] See Table 19.4 for risk factors.

From Lipshultz SE, Adams MJ, Colan SD et al. Long-term cardiovascular toxicity in children, adolescents, and young adults who receive cancer therapy: pathophysiology, course, monitoring, management, prevention, and research directions: a scientific statement from the American Heart Association. Circulation 2013;128(17):1951; with permission.

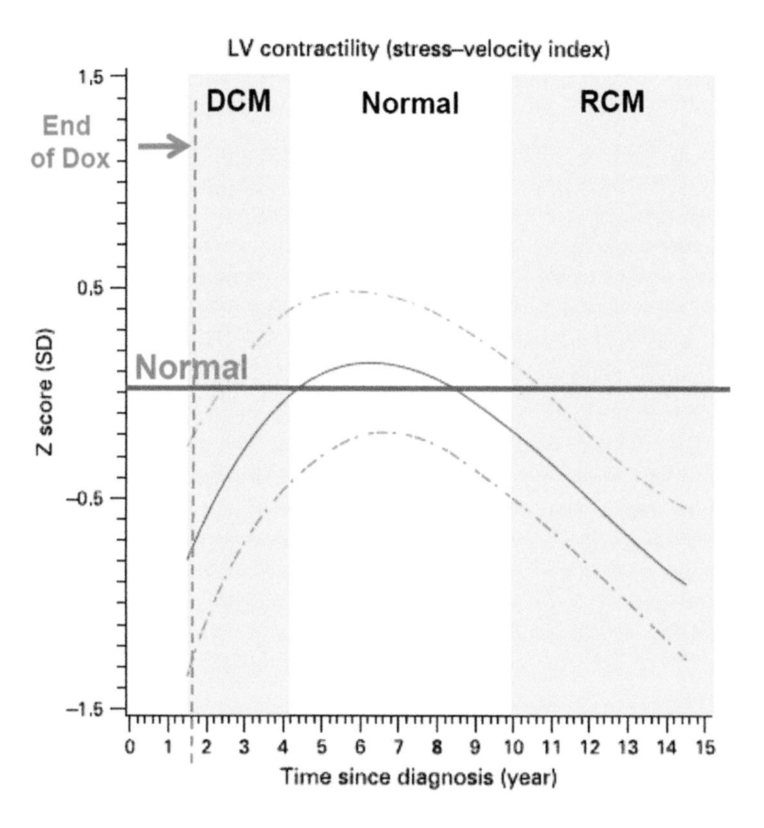

Fig. 19.3 Cardiac measurements from 115 long-term survivors of ALL treated with doxorubicin, by years since diagnosis showing how the dilated cardiomyopathy evolves into restrictive cardiomyopathy about 10 years after treatment. Solid line, mean Z-score; dashed lines, 95% confidence band. DCM, dilated cardiomyopathy; DOX, doxorubicin; RCM, restricted cardiomyopathy. (*Adapted from* Lipshultz SE, Lipsitz SR, Sallan SE, et al. Chronic progressive cardiac dysfunction years after doxorubicin therapy for childhood acute lymphoblastic leukemia. J Clin Oncol 2005;23:2629–36.)

thickness for body surface area resulting in a normal LV thickness-to-dimension ratio. This shrinking myocardial cavity size for body surface area ("Grinch syndrome") may result in HF, heart transplantation, or death in long-term survivors.[82] The various stages of ventricular dysfunction are depicted in Fig. 19.4.

Radiation-induced cardiotoxicity seems to be insidious, usually manifesting more than a decade after exposure. Because of changes in dosage and technique, radiation-associated pericarditis is now exceedingly rare. The most important consequence of clinical importance is diastolic dysfunction. Adams and colleagues[83] comprehensively studied 48 survivors of Hodgkin lymphoma treated with mediastinal RT; they observed that the cardiovascular abnormalities were often unsuspected because patients were asymptomatic. However, 37% showed evidence of a restrictive cardiomyopathy with diastolic dysfunction (reduced end-diastolic LV dimension and mass without changes in LV thickness) and a remarkably

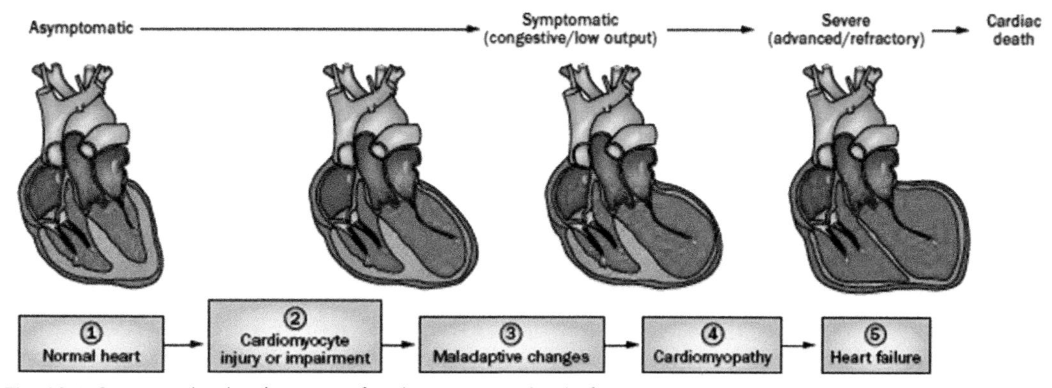

Fig. 19.4 Stages in the development of pediatric ventricular dysfunction. (*From* Lipshultz SE, Cochran TR, Franco VI, et al. Treatment-related cardiotoxicity in survivors of childhood cancer. Nat Rev Clin Oncol 2013;10:697–710; with permission).

lower average maximum oxygen consumption (Vo_{2max}) with exercise testing. Forty-two percent of the patients showed valvular defects, and 75% showed conduction defects. A significantly reduced Vo_{2max} was recognized in 30% of survivors, whereby blunting of the cardiac index increase with exercise is a nearly universal phenomenon in cancer survivors. Exercise capacity predicts mortality in HF patients, and thus, comprehensive cardiac screening was recommended for Hodgkin disease survivors.[82] A follow-up study on a cohort of 21 of these patients recently concluded that Vo_{2max} appeared to be associated with future reduced quality of life ($P = .021$).[84] The authors suggested cardiopulmonary exercise assessment, especially Vo_{2max}, should be considered in the assessment of fatigue in these survivors, and LV systolic function should not be the sole criteria for cardiotoxicity. The authors concluded that cardiopulmonary function correlated with physical functioning–related quality-of-life assessment years later in these survivors of Hodgkin lymphoma.

In adult patients diagnosed with Hodgkin lymphoma and treated with a mediastinal radiation dose of 35 Gy, 14% (40/282 patients) were found to have mild-to-moderate diastolic dysfunction. Furthermore, LV diastolic dysfunction was associated with stress-induced ischemia and a worse prognosis.[85] Survivors with LV dysfunction tend to have poor cardiac event-free survival and a worse quality of life than what is observed in LV dysfunction-free survivors.[83,85,86] Frequently associated with LV dysfunction is valvular dysfunction, which is often progressive and might lead to HF.[68] In the study by Adams and colleagues,[83] valvular abnormalities were noted in 47% of Hodgkin lymphoma survivors at levels higher than what would be expected in the age-matched healthy population. Valve disease appears to be a common clinically evident cardiovascular dysfunction within the first 20 years after mediastinal RT for Hodgkin lymphoma, along with coronary artery disease, cardiomyopathy, conduction disorders, and pericardial disease. Evidence-based guidelines for surveillance for these cardiovascular morbidities are lacking and need further research.[87]

RISK FACTORS FOR CARDIOTOXICITY

Cardiovascular effects do not manifest equally among all patients exposed to anthracyclines. For example, despite receiving the same cumulative dose, some children and adults may experience severe LV dysfunction, whereas others may experience no effects at all. Therefore, identifying factors that increase susceptibility to the cardiotoxic effects of anthracyclines is important.

TREATMENT-RELATED RISK FACTORS

Cumulative doses of anthracycline, chest-directed RT, and cranial irradiation increase risks for adverse cardiac effects. A higher cumulative anthracycline dose is associated with an increased risk of late cardiac dysfunction.[8,88] In a sample of long-term survivors of childhood acute lymphoblastic leukemia (ALL), LV end-diastolic dimension increased, indicating LV dilation, and LV FS declined with an increasing cumulative anthracycline dose years from therapy. Furthermore, compared with normal, the LV became dilated at a cumulative anthracycline dose greater than 320 mg/m^2, and LV FS was significantly reduced at cumulative anthracycline doses of 280 mg/m^2 or greater with intermediate follow-up of anthracycline-treated survivors of pediatric cancer.[88] However, cardiac damage has been found even in patients who received doses less than 240 mg/m^2, suggesting that there is no true "safe" dose of anthracycline, especially with longer follow-up.[89]

The association between chest-directed RT and long-term cardiac morbidity is well established. The average radiation dose was linearly related to the risk of cardiac mortality (60% estimated relative risk [RR] at 1 Gy) in a multicenter study of 4122 French and British childhood cancer survivors.[7,90] Other studies have shown an additive increased risk of cardiac mortality when high cumulative anthracycline doses were combined with RT.[91,92]

Cranial irradiation is a standard of treatment for childhood leukemia, for brain cancers, and to prevent brain metastases. Compared with patients who were unexposed to cranial irradiation, those who were exposed had decreased LV mass and LV dimensions over a 10-year follow-up.[91] These changes in LV structure were associated with a decrease in insulin-like growth factor 1 concentrations, which were possibly related to growth hormone (GH) deficiency, suggesting that cranial irradiation could be an additional risk factor for cardiotoxicity. This aspect, however, is unique to the growing heart and has not been seen in adults.

OTHER RISK FACTORS FOR ANTHRACYCLINE CARDIOTOXICITY

Other risk factors for anthracycline-related cardiotoxicity include female sex, younger age at treatment, longer follow-up after treatment, trisomy 21, certain genetic mutations, and preexisting cardiovascular disease and comorbidities (Table 19.4).[75,92]

Doxorubicin is poorly absorbed by the body fat, which comprises part of the calculated body surface area.[75] Therefore, intracellular cardiomyocyte doxorubicin concentrations may be increased during treatment for childhood cancer in patients with a larger percentage of body fat because dosage is often calculated based on body surface area. Girls tend to have a higher percentage of body fat than do boys, which may explain why girls are more susceptible to anthracycline-induced cardiotoxicity than boys are.[93] Young girls may also have less developed mechanisms to prevent or repair from free radical injury than boys. Follow-up studies have shown that survivors diagnosed before 1 year of age are more likely to experience LV wall thinning relative to body surface area,[75] and those with longer follow-up have a higher prevalence of LV dysfunction.[5]

Interest in potential genetic risk factors is increasing (Fig. 19.5). Hereditary hemochromatosis is a genetic disorder that can lead to iron overload. Among 184 high-risk ALL survivors screened for the frequency of HFE gene mutations, 10% had a mutation in the HFE C282Y allele, and their risk of doxorubicin-related myocardial injury was 9 times as high as that of noncarriers.[94] Preliminary studies have also found that patients exposed to low-to-moderate doses of anthracyclines who express homozygosity for the G allele of the CBR3 gene, which encodes carbonyl reductase 3, have an increased risk for cardiomyopathy (Fig. 19.6).[95,96] Associations between cardiotoxicity and 2 other polymorphisms, the ABCC5 A-1629T variant and NOS3 G894T variant, have also been shown in children diagnosed with high-risk ALL.[97] The ABCC5 gene is involved in the doxorubicin functional pathway and encodes for efflux transporters. Children with a polymorphism in the ABCC5 gene, the TT genotype of ABCC5 A-1629T, were shown to have decreased LVEF and LVFS. Furthermore, they were also more likely to have lower LVEF and LVFS values at the time of cancer diagnosis, which places them at higher risk of decreased LVEF and LVFS during and after cancer treatment. The NOS3 gene modulates reactive oxygen or nitrogen species in the metabolic pathway of doxorubicin. In contrast to the ABCC5 variant, polymorphism in the homozygous T allele of NOS3 G894T showed a cardioprotective effect in high-risk patients who received a higher dose of doxorubicin without dexrazoxane; LVEF in TT allele was 64% compared with 57% in AA and AT alleles, indicating a clinically significant difference in cardiac function. Furthermore, receipts of dexrazoxane abrogated this effect in patients with any of the 3 alleles, 64.4% for TT and 66.5% for the others, further supporting the use of dexrazoxane in this high-risk group. Identifying these potential genetic risk factors may assist in assessing the prognosis and guiding postchemotherapy monitoring and treatment (Fig. 19.7). Gene profiling cannot be recommended for routine clinical care at present because prospective studies comparing this with the conventional approach have not been

TABLE 19.4
Risk factors for anthracycline-induced cardiotoxicity

Risk Factors	Features
Total cumulative dose	Most important predictor of abnormal cardiac function
Age	For similar cumulative doses, younger age predisposes to greater cardiotoxicity (especially <5 y of age)
Length of follow-up	Longer follow-up reveals higher prevalence of myocardial impairment
Sex	Girls more vulnerable than boys for similar doses
Concomitant mantle irradiation	Evidence of enhanced cardiotoxicity; not clear whether additive or synergistic
Others	Concomitant exposure to cyclophosphamide, bleomycin, vincristine, amsacrine, or mitoxantrone may predispose to cardiotoxicity; trisomy 21 and black race have been associated with a higher risk of early clinical cardiotoxicity
Rate of anthracycline administration	Higher rate was thought to predispose to greater toxicity, but current trials in children do not support this finding

From Simbre VC, Duffy SA, Dadlani GH, et al. Cardiotoxicity of cancer chemotherapy: implications for children. Paediatr Drugs 2005;7(3):190; with permission.

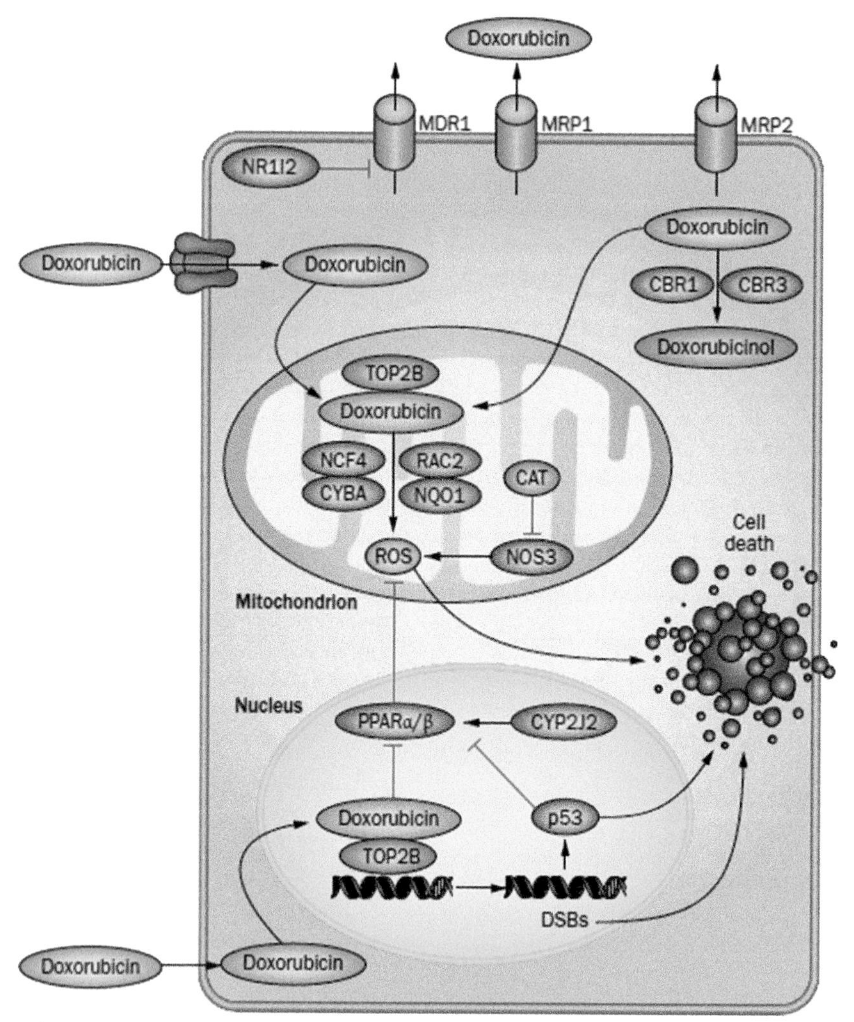

Fig. 19.5 Candidate genes implicated in doxorubicin-induced cardiotoxicity. Genomic variants have been identified in several proteins involved in the cardiotoxicity signaling cascade triggered by doxorubicin. Genes encoding cell membrane proteins, such as doxorubicin transporters and efflux pumps, include ABCB1, ABCC1, ABCC2, and SLC22A16, and can cause toxicity if mutations affect transporter function. Candidate genes encoding gene transcription regulators include PPARα, PPARβ, and TP53. Both TP53 and the doxorubicin–TOP2B complex inhibit expression of PPARα and PPARβ by binding to their gene promoters.[23,48] PPARα and PPARβ are nuclear receptors and transcriptional coactivators and are key regulators of oxidative phosphorylation and mitochondrial biogenesis involved in doxorubicin-induced cardiotoxicity.[23,47,49,50] Genes encoding mitochondrial proteins are critical for oxidative phosphorylation and generation of ATP and include CAT, NOS3, NQO1, CYBA, NCF4, and RAC2, which form the NAD(P)H oxidase complex. Genomic variants in these proteins contribute to mitochondrial dysfunction, thereby increasing ROS generation, which (along with apoptotic factors) ultimately culminates in cardiomyocyte death.[23] Proteins often found in the cytosol include CBR1 and CBR3 that metabolize doxorubicin to doxorubicinol, and NR1I2 that inhibits MDR1. ABCB1, ATP-binding cassette, subfamily B (MDR/TAP), member 1; ABCC1, ATP-binding cassette, subfamily C (CFTR/MRP), member 1; ABCC2, ATP-binding cassette, subfamily C (CFTR/MRP), member 2; CAT, catalase; CBR1, carbonyl reductase 1; CBR3, carbonyl reductase 3; CYBA, cytochrome B558 α subunit; CYP2J2, cytochrome P450 2J2; DSB, DNA double-stranded breaks; GRIN1, glutamate receptor, inotropic, N-methyl-D-aspartate 1; GRIN2D, glutamate receptor, inotropic, N-methyl-D-aspartate 2D; MDR1, multidrug resistance protein 1; MRP1, multidrug resistance-associated protein 1; MRP2, multidrug resistance-associated protein 2; NADPH, nicotinamide adenine dinucleotide phosphate oxidase; NCF4, neutrophil cytosolic factor 4, 40 kDa; NOS3, nitric oxide synthase 3; NQO1, NAD(P)H dehydrogenase, quinone 1; NR1I2, nuclear receptor subfamily 1 group I member 2; PPARα/β, peroxisome proliferator-activated receptor γ coactivator 1-α/β; RAC2, ras-related C3 botulinum toxin substrate 2 (rho family, small guanosine triphosphate–binding protein Rac2); SLC22A16, solute carrier family 22 (organic cation/carnitine transporter) member 16; TP53, tumor protein p53. (*From* Brown SA, Sandhu N, Herrmann J. Systems biology approaches to adverse drug effects: the example of cardio-oncology. Nat Rev Clin Oncol 2015;12:718–31; with permission).

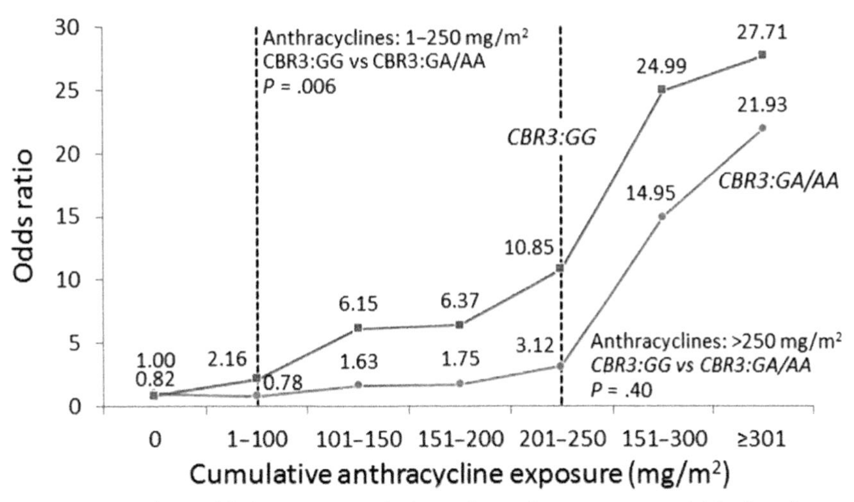

Fig. 19.6 Dose-response relationship between cumulative anthracycline exposure and risk of cardiomyopathy stratified by patients' CBR3 genotype status (CBR3:GG and CBR3:GA/AA). Patients with no exposure to anthracyclines and carrying CBR3:GA/AA genotype served as the referent group. Magnitude of risk is expressed as odds ratio, which was obtained using conditional logistic regression adjusting for age at diagnosis, sex, and chest radiation. (*From* Blanco JG, Sun CL, Landier W, et al. Anthracycline-related cardiomyopathy after childhood cancer: role of polymorphisms in carbonyl reductase genes–a report from the Children's Oncology Group. J Clin Oncol 2012;30:1415.)

performed using an endpoint of overall quality of life for a patient and their family that takes into account both oncologic efficacy and toxicity with late effects. Furthermore, the cost-effectiveness of gene profiling remains to be determined, especially as very simple clinical models already risk stratify very well (Fig. 19.8).

As in the general population, long-term childhood cancer survivors can also have one or more of the traditional risk factors for atherosclerosis, which could further increase the risk of future cardiovascular complications beyond that directly related to cancer therapies. Physical inactivity, obesity, tobacco use, and diabetes mellitus are some of the most commonly explored traditional modifiable atherosclerotic risk factors.[98] However, it is important to keep in mind that survivors might also have a lower threshold for cardiac problems than healthy individuals who have never had cancer.[7] An improved

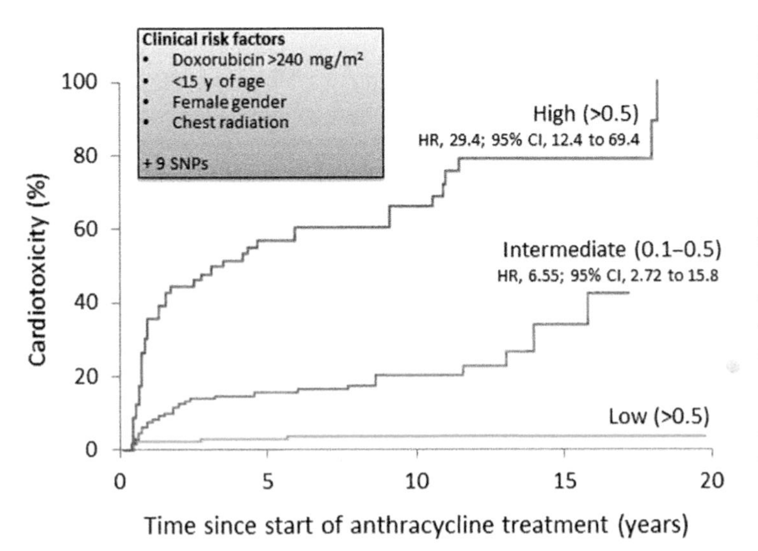

Fig. 19.7 Anthracycline-induced risk of cardiotoxicity FS ≤26%) in children. Kaplan-Meier graph of anthracycline-induced cardiotoxicity in 3 different risk groups (see Table 19.3) shows that in high-risk group, incidence of cardiotoxicity is highest in the first year but continues to increase over time. Similarly, cardiotoxicity continues to increase in the intermediate-risk group, although at a lower level. In contrast, few patients in the low-risk group developed cardiotoxicity over time (Ptrend = 6.7 × 10–25). HR, hazard ratio compared with low-risk group; SNPs, single-nucleotide polymorphisms. (*From* Visscher H, Ross CJ, Rassekh SR, et al. Pharmacogenomic prediction of anthracycline-induced cardiotoxicity in children. J Clin Oncol 2012;30:1422–8.)

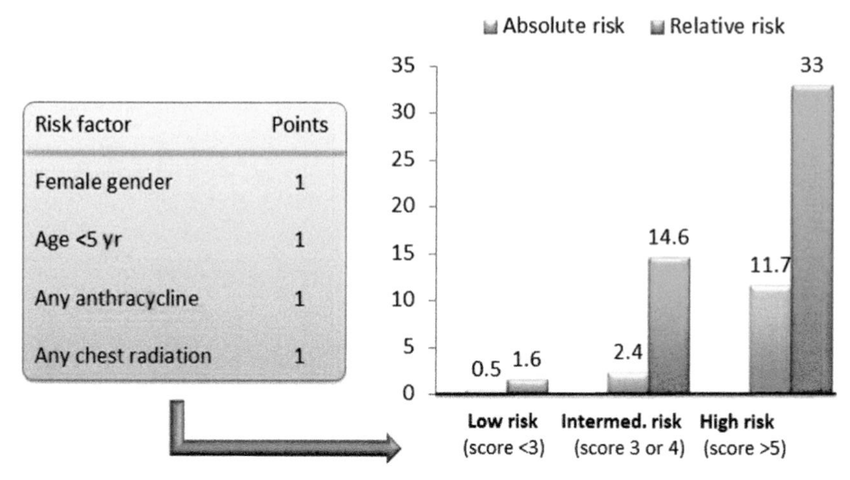

Fig. 19.8 Anthracycline-induced cardiotoxicity risk childhood cancer survivor study. (*Data from* Chow EJ, Asselin BL, Schwartz CL, et al. Late mortality after dexrazoxane treatment: a report from the Children's Oncology Group. J Clin Oncol 2015;33:2639–45; with permission).

understanding of the lifetime cardiovascular risk associated with these factors in long-term childhood cancer survivors may help guide treatment and predict any potential additional cardiovascular risk of specific cancer therapies, such as anthracyclines.[99]

MONITORING CARDIOTOXICITY

Serum cardiac biomarkers, such as cardiac troponin T (cTnT) and cardiac troponin I and N-terminal pro-brain natriuretic peptide (NT-proBNP), have been studied as methods for monitoring cardiotoxicity. In fact, cTnT and NT-proBNP have been validated as surrogate endpoints for late cardiotoxicity in long-term survivors.[100] Cardiac troponins are specific for myocardial damage, and increased concentrations indicate irreversible cardiomyocyte cell death in patients treated with anthracyclines.[101,102] Initial animal studies found that dose-dependent elevations in cTnT were related to the damage of cardiac tissue.[103] In a study of 134 children receiving moderate-dose anthracyclines for high-risk ALL, elevations in serum cTnT concentrations during the first 90 days of anthracycline treatment were significantly associated with reduced LV end-diastolic posterior wall thickness and LV mass and increased pathologic LV remodeling 4 years later.[100] In addition, elevations in serum concentrations of NT-proBNP, indicative of cardiomyopathy, during the first 90 days of treatment were correlated with abnormal LV thickness-to-dimension ratios 4 years after therapy (Fig. 19.9). Furthermore, during and after treatment, a higher percentage of patients had elevated concentrations of NT-proBNP than of cTnT.[100] Thus, as validated surrogate markers of late cardiotoxicity, serum biomarkers of cardiomyopathy (NT-proBNP) and cardiomyocyte injury or death (cTnT) might allow studies to determine whether these markers can be used to tailor anticancer therapy and to determine whether overall outcomes are improved. Future research should focus on developing a comprehensive panel of biomarkers, including patient characteristics and genetic markers, that have been validated as surrogate outcomes of late cardiotoxicity to assess for cardiac damage in survivors. Furthermore, monitoring NT-proBNP concentrations during therapy might predict which children are at higher risk of cardiotoxicity, allowing treatment to be modified before cardiomyocyte damage is irreversible.[89]

Numerous groups have recommended echocardiographic surveillance of the cardiovascular changes during and after cancer treatment in children, but currently no evidence-based monitoring guidelines exist. In 2006, van Dalen and colleagues[104] conducted a literature search of guidelines for monitoring cardiotoxicity in children during anthracycline treatment. Their search revealed only one published guideline during that time, and that was the 1992 guidelines published by Steinherz and colleagues.[105] However, these guidelines included recommendations to alter cancer treatment based on abnormal cardiac findings in the absence of clinical evidence during treatment. The authors took exception to those recommendations and stated that they were based on previously published literature that did not provide sufficient evidence to support dose

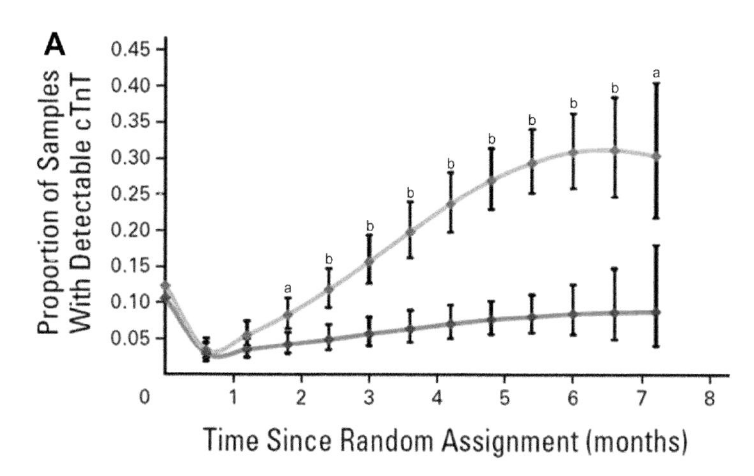

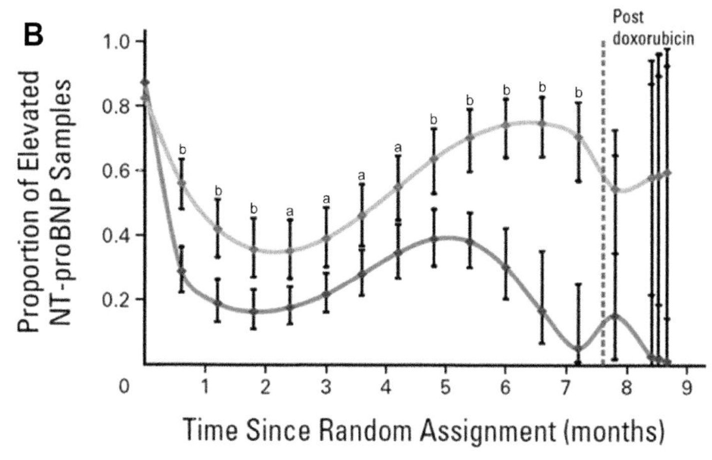

Fig. 19.9 (*A*) Model-based estimated probability of having an increased cTnT concentration over time in patients treated with doxorubicin, with or without dexrazoxane. The doxorubicin-dexrazoxane group is indicated by the blue line; the doxorubicin group is indicated by the gold line. Vertical bars show 95% confidence intervals. Increased cTnT is defined as a value >0.01 ng/mL. [a] *P* versus dexrazoxane group ≤.05; [b] *P* versus dexrazoxane group ≤.001. An overall test for dexrazoxane effect during treatment was significant (*P*<.001). (*B*) Model-based estimated probability of having an elevated NT-proBNP concentration over time in patients treated with doxorubicin, with or without dexrazoxane. The doxorubicin-dexrazoxane group is indicated by the blue line; the doxorubicin group is indicated by the gold line. Vertical bars show 95% confidence intervals. Increased NT-proBNP is defined as a value ≥150 pg/mL for children less than 1 year old and ≥100 pg/mL for children aged ≥1 year. [a] *P* versus dexrazoxane group ≤.05; [b] *P* versus dexrazoxane group ≤.001. An overall test for dexrazoxane effect during treatment was significant (*P*<.001) and after treatment was not significant (*P* = .24). (*From* Lipshultz SE, Miller TL, Scully RE, et al. Changes in cardiac biomarkers during doxorubicin treatment of pediatric patients with high-risk acute lymphoblastic leukemia: associations with long-term echocardiographic outcomes. J Clin Oncol 2012;30:1042–9; with permission).

modifications.[106] The overall outcome of the quality of life for a child with cancer and their family balanced by clinical efficacy and toxicity/late effects was not demonstrated to be improved by this recommendation. Thus, using such guidelines to modify cancer treatment could potentially cause more harm than good. When the main goal is to cure cancer, withholding potentially life-saving treatment because of cardiac abnormalities in the absence of clinical evidence of cardiac dysfunction, which may or may not be transient, may not achieve an overall improvement in curing cancer or in improving overall quality of life during a survivor's lifespan.

There is a difference between monitoring for cardiotoxicity during cancer therapy and in long-term survivors off therapy. There are also differences between children and adults. The American Society of Clinical Oncology Survivorship Expert Panel identified the need for optimal screening strategies and subsequent evidence-based treatment options for long-term cardiac and pulmonary toxicity secondary to chemotherapy or RT in symptomatic and asymptomatic adult cancer survivors in 2007.[107] In the current era, there are several guidelines available for this purpose with varying degrees of evidence to support recommendations. The American Heart Association (AHA) recommends close monitoring of cardiac function, but is not specific about the modality of choice or the frequency of the same.[108] The Children's Oncology Group released risk-based guidelines for monitoring for cardiotoxicity in survivors of pediatric cancer for late cardiac morbidity.[109] The optimal timing and frequency of cardiovascular monitoring in cancer survivors still remain controversial because the available guidelines are not consistent in their recommendations and are based on limited evidence. Long-term survivors treated with anthracyclines for childhood cancer appear to benefit by following Children's Oncology Group monitoring recommendations with less morbidity and mortality related to cardiotoxicity. A cost-effectiveness study of these guidelines showed that, compared with no screening, they could reduce the risk for HF in survivors at less than $100,000 per quality-adjusted life-years (QALYs), extend life expectancy by 6 months and QALYs by 1.6 months, and reduce the cumulative incidence of HF by 18% at 30 years after cancer diagnosis. However, less frequent screenings are more cost-effective than the guidelines and maintain 80% of the health benefits.[9] Finally, the International Late Effects of Childhood Cancer Guideline Harmonization Group just published the most recent set of recommendations.

Established traditional methods of cardiac function assessment often detect changes after damage had occurred, at which point the cardiotoxicity may be irreversible. It is important to annually monitor patients with a thorough history and physical examination with careful screening for signs of cardiac dysfunction. Electrocardiography is a universally available, inexpensive tool and may help in identifying at-risk patients.[110] However, it has a high interrater variability[111] and lacks the specificity and sensitivity to be a reliable tool.

When cardiac biomarkers are validated as predictors or surrogate endpoints for subsequent symptomatic cardiotoxicity, they take on added importance if their use to monitor patients and perform biomarker-guided therapy results in improved outcomes compared with conventional management. Echocardiography was suggested in one set of guidelines as the modality of choice for assessing cardiac structure and function after exposure to chemotherapy and RT.[112] The characteristics most often measured are LV systolic function in M-mode via LVFS or LVEF.[105] These characteristics are load-dependent and may have variable results: reports of anthracycline-related subclinical cardiotoxicity range from 0% to 57%.[113] The authors have not found this to be a validated predictor of outcome in children where it is assessed during anthracycline therapy but have observed it to be useful following anthracycline therapy.

M-mode echocardiographic measurements of the stress-velocity relationship are not load dependent.[114] Myocardial strain and strain rates have limited specificity in measuring myocardial injury. These are load-dependent variables whose role in patients with cardiotoxicity due to chemotherapy remains under active investigation.[115] This angle-independent, speckle-tracking type of echocardiography has been studied in both adults[116] and children[117] and shows promise in detecting subclinical cardiac dysfunction when compared with normal conventional measures of cardiac function.[118] However, the results of these imaging modalities vary with imaging system as well as quality, and more research is needed to determine the clinical utility of these newer techniques.[119]

Ultrasonic tissue characterization by integrated backscatter is a noninvasive means to measure changes in the myocardium. Its magnitude decreases in both ischemic and nonischemic myocardial diseases, making it highly sensitive but nonspecific for detecting subclinical changes.[120–122] Values from LV septal and posterior walls have been decreased in asymptomatic patients without systolic dysfunction after treatment with 5-fluorouracil.[123] However, results can vary with the angle of the ultrasound and the motion of the heart, and thus, the usefulness of this modality in long-term monitoring remains to be determined.

Cardiac MRI can detect perfusion abnormalities and subendocardial damage, which cannot be detected by other conventional methods. This modality does not use ionizing radiation, unlike radionuclide angiography, and it provides high resolution and numerous windows. Some small studies have evaluated its use in monitoring cardiotoxicity.[124–126] The modality is time-consuming, with limited availability, and often requires sedating younger children.

OTHER CARDIOVASCULAR SCREENING RECOMMENDATIONS FOR LATE CARDIOVASCULAR TOXICITY IN LONG-TERM CHILDHOOD CANCER SURVIVORS

Cerebrovascular: Stroke Prevention

The RR for cerebrovascular accidents (CVA) among cancer survivors is almost 10-fold as high as that of sibling controls.[127] Risks are highest among adult survivors of childhood ALL, patients with brain tumors, and patients with Hodgkin lymphoma—individuals most likely to have received cranial or neck irradiation.[128,129]

In a Dutch study of 2201 five-year survivors of Hodgkin lymphoma, cerebrovascular disease developed in 96 (55 with CVAs, 31 with transient ischemic attacks [TIAs], 10 with both CVAs and TIAs). The median time to first stroke or TIA was 17.4 years. Irradiation to the neck and mediastinum (the most important risk factor), treatment before age 21 years, and hypertension were significant risk factors for the occurrence of ischemic stroke.[130] One study by the Childhood Cancer Survivor Study cohort of 1926 five-year survivors of Hodgkin disease and 3846 matched siblings found that the RR of late-occurring stroke was 4.32 among survivors and 5.62 among survivors treated with mantle radiation.[129] In another study, the RR of stroke was 6.4 for leukemia survivors compared with their siblings and 29 for brain tumor survivors compared with their siblings. A mean cranial radiation therapy dose of 30 Gy or higher was associated with a dose-dependent increased risk in both leukemia and brain tumor survivors, with the highest risk after doses of 50 Gy or higher.[128]

Among 4227 five-year survivors of childhood cancer followed for a median of 29 years, each gray delivered to the prepontine cistern area of the brain increased the risk of death from cerebrovascular disease by 22%. Thus, the relationship between cerebrovascular mortality and radiation to the prepontine cistern appears to be dose dependent. Indeed, the prepontine cistern is close to the circle of Willis, a vascular network that provides all the terminal cerebral vasculature of the brain. Thus, radiation-induced damage to the arteries of this network could be the cause of stroke in the vascular territory of each of these arteries near to, or remote from, the site of the initial damage.[131]

Evidence supporting any routine surveillance strategies for carotid artery or cerebrovascular disease is currently lacking, although consideration can be given to the performance of carotid artery ultrasound in high-risk populations (eg, patients with hypertension, obesity, or diabetes mellitus who were treated with >40 Gy to the neck). However, definitions and implications of abnormal tests are not clear.[132,133]

Dedicated vascular imaging, such as magnetic resonance angiography, can be used to evaluate patients considered at high risk for stroke or who are symptomatic, but a specific screening recommendation cannot be identified.

Cardiovascular: Arrhythmias and Intracardiac Conduction Abnormalities

Patients with cancer appear to be at increased risk of sudden death from severe cardiac arrhythmias or intracardiac conduction abnormalities because of the high prevalence of predisposing risk factors, such as electrolyte abnormalities secondary to anorexia and concomitant medications, in conjunction with cardiotoxicity from cancer and its therapies. Different arrhythmias and conduction abnormalities have been reported during chemotherapy, including supraventricular and ventricular premature beats or tachycardias.[134–138] Interaction with cardiac ion channels has been considered to be important in the genesis of these arrhythmias as well as in changes detected by electrocardiogram (ECG), such as QT-interval prolongation and nonspecific T-wave changes.[137–140] Prolongation of QTc interval by antineoplastics may be dose dependent.[33,141,142]

Only scattered reports address the issue of late arrhythmias and conduction abnormalities after chemotherapy. A review of 11 leukemia patients reported that anthracycline treatment may be a risk factor for torsades de pointes weeks or years after therapy for leukemia, and such cases are generally related to QT-prolonging agents or to hypokalemia.[143] Another study on long-term survivors of childhood cancers treated with anthracyclines found that the incidence of abnormally prolonged QT dispersion intervals was greater than 38% and that the combination of a corrected QT interval dispersion greater than 110 milliseconds and an LVFS diminished to less than 29% was associated with sudden death.[144] In another study, patients who received a cumulative anthracycline dose greater than 200 mg/m^2 had abnormal standard and 24-hour ambulatory ECGs that were mostly limited to single supraventricular or ventricular premature complexes.[145] However, potentially serious ventricular ectopy, including ventricular tachycardia, was also noted.

Whether the risk of arrhythmia or conduction abnormalities exceeds that found in other causes of ventricular dysfunction is unknown. There are no formal evidence-based recommendations for rate and rhythm screening and evaluation in long-term survivors of cancer. The general recommendations in the American College of Cardiology/AHA HF guidelines include that Holter monitoring might be considered in patients presenting with HF who have a history of MI and who are being considered for an electrophysiological study to document ventricular tachycardia inducibility (class IIb: benefit ≥ risk – procedure/treatment may be considered; level of evidence C: very limited populations evaluated). The routine use of signal-averaged electrocardiography is not recommended for evaluating patients presenting with HF (class III: risk ≥ benefit – procedure/treatment should not be performed/administered because it is not helpful and can be harmful; level of evidence C: very limited populations evaluated).[146]

Prevention of Late Cardiotoxicity in Long-Term Survivors of Childhood Cancer

Antineoplastic drugs not only cause early morbidity and mortality but also can lead to persistent subclinical damage that can manifest later in life. Thus, minimizing or preventing this initial damage as early as possible is important (see Fig. 19.2).[7,11,13,66,67,72,78,97,100,147–157]

ANTHRACYCLINE-INDUCED CARDIOTOXICITY

Anthracycline Use

Over the years, treatment protocols have been tested to reduce the cardiac complications associated with anthracyclines. In the 1970s, before the association between cumulative dose and cardiotoxicity was recognized, children with ALL in clinical trials would receive cumulative doxorubicin doses greater than 400 mg/m^2. Cardiac abnormalities were persistent and progressive after anthracycline therapy. Inadequate LV mass for body surface area with chronic LV afterload excess was associated with a progressive LV contractile deficit and possibly reduced cardiac output with a restrictive cardiomyopathy. These abnormalities of LV structure and function were worst after the highest cumulative doses of doxorubicin, but they appeared even after low doses.[8,74,75] In response, cumulative doxorubicin doses in this population were initially reduced to between 45 and 60 mg/m^2 for children with standard-risk ALL and between 345 and 360 mg/m^2 for children with high-risk ALL, doses associated with a much lower risk of delayed cardiotoxicity.[158] The authors' study revealed that depressed LVFS and LV dilation relative to body surface area were uncommon with intermediate follow-up years after treatment of childhood leukemia when cumulative anthracycline doses were further reduced to none higher than 300 mg/m^2.[88] As a result, later protocols in childhood ALL lowered the cumulative doxorubicin dose even further for high-risk ALL patients, to 300 mg/m^2, to prevent these adverse effects.[158] Lowering the cumulative anthracycline doses may be cardioprotective, but they may also reduce treatment efficacy.[74,105,148] In addition, even the smallest doses of anthracyclines may still cause cardiac complications in this vulnerable group of children, suggesting that there is no safe dose of anthracyclines.[67]

Liposomal Anthracyclines

Another cardioprotective strategy is to modify the structure of the anthracycline compound. Encapsulation of doxorubicin inside a liposome alters its bioavailability and biodistribution and thus markedly changes its biological activity.[159] This formulation causes more of the doxorubicin to accumulate in the tumor and reduces the plasma concentrations of free doxorubicin, which is thought to reduce cardiotoxicity.[160]

Currently, Doxil is a pegylated liposomal doxorubicin (PLD) that is approved by the US Food and Drug Administration.[160] In a large, randomized, phase III trial of 509 women with metastatic breast cancer, the efficacy of PLD was similar to that of conventional doxorubicin, but PLD significantly reduced cardiac toxicity.[161] Although further research is required to fully understand the effect of liposomal-encapsulated anthracyclines in children, biopsy samples have shown that this structural modification lowers the chance of early cardiotoxicity without compromising the antineoplastic activity of conventional anthracyclines.[162–166]

Anthracycline Analogues

Anthracycline analogues with therapeutic indices better than daunorubicin and doxorubicin have been widely sought. Since the early 1970s, epirubicin, an epimer of doxorubicin, has been investigated.[167,168] In one randomized study of 172 patients with soft tissue sarcoma, the incidence of clinically manifest cardiomyopathy was 0% in 60 patients treated with epirubicin and 0.9% in 108 patients treated with doxorubicin.[168] Epirubicin was less toxic to cardiomyocytes than was doxorubicin at equimolar doses, but it increased cardiotoxicity slightly when administered at equally myelotoxic doses.[160,168,169]

Idarubicin appears to be a less cardiotoxic structural analogue of daunorubicin.[170] A phase 3 study of 230 patients at least 14 years old with acute myeloblastic leukemia treated with either idarubicin or daunorubicin found no significant difference in the frequency of HF.[171]

Mitoxantrone is an intravenous anthracenedione structurally related to anthracyclines. Some clinical trials that compared mitoxantrone with daunorubicin in previously untreated adults found no difference in cardiotoxicity.[172] Further randomized studies are required to determine whether other anthracycline structural analogues can prevent cardiac damage during therapy.

Continuous Anthracycline Infusion

Whether lowering the peak serum concentrations of doxorubicin by continuous infusion as opposed to bolus administration effectively reduces the associated cardiotoxic effects has been debated.[173] Continuous doxorubicin infusions over 48 or 96 hours appear less cardiotoxic in adults, when effects are assessed during or shortly after therapy. Such infusions allow the anthracycline cumulative dose to be increased in some patients by a factor of at least 2 and do not attenuate the oncologic effect of the drug.[147] However, in children diagnosed with high-risk ALL, continuous infusion provided no long-term cardioprotection over bolus infusion after a median of 8 years of cardiac follow-up.[174] Despite this lack of evidence, continuous infusion has been incorporated into pediatric protocols on the basis of the findings in adults. A randomized controlled trial of 121 children with high-risk ALL found that continuous doxorubicin infusion over 48 hours for childhood leukemia did not offer a cardioprotective advantage over bolus infusion. Both regimens were associated with progressive subclinical cardiotoxicity.[149] After a median follow-up of 8 years in this same cohort, both groups had similar echocardiographic changes (depressed LV systolic function, LV systolic dilation, reduced LV wall thickness, and reduced LV mass) at 3, 6, and 8 years; there were no statistically significant differences between groups.[174] Furthermore, children who received continuous infusion had higher charges and longer admissions, no improvement in oncologic efficacy, and increased mucositis and thromboembolic events. Other studies looking at bolus versus continuous infusions of anthracyclines have likewise not found any statistically significant differences in the degree of cardiotoxicity between the 2 types of administration.[173,175]

Dexrazoxane

Doxorubicin forms a complex with iron that is thought to facilitate the formation of toxic oxygen radicals in tissues. The attenuating effect of dexrazoxane on doxorubicin-induced cardiotoxicity may be attributable to its intracellular conversion to its active metal ion-binding form (ADR-925), which either removes iron from the doxorubicin-iron complex or binds free iron, thus preventing the formation of oxygen radicals.[40,158,176,177] Other methods independent of oxidative stress, such as DNA mutation mitigation, may mediate the cardiac protection involved with iron chelation. In fact, mitochondrial DNA (mtDNA) and oxidative phosphorylation activity were examined in a sample of childhood cancer survivors.[178] The authors' study showed that survivors who received doxorubicin alone had higher mtDNA copy numbers per cell than those who received concomitant doses of dexrazoxane, whereas no differences were seen in oxidative phosphorylation activity. These findings suggest a potential compensatory increase in mtDNA copies per cell to maintain mitochondrial function in the setting of mitochondrial dysfunction.[178]

Concern had arisen over whether dexrazoxane might increase the risk of second malignancies by reducing the antineoplastic effect of doxorubicin. Several studies have not found an association,[158,179–183] but one did,[184] although its findings have been questioned.[185,186] Furthermore, a recent study examined long-term overall and cause-specific mortality and disease relapse rates from 3 randomized clinical trials (Children's Oncology Group trials P9404 [T-cell ALL and non-Hodgkin lymphoma; n = 537], P9425 [intermediate-/high-risk Hodgkin lymphoma; n = 216], and P9426 [low-risk Hodgkin lymphoma; n = 255]), which were conducted between 1996 and 2001.[181] In the 1008 patients (507 received dexrazoxane) with a median follow-up of 12.6 years (range, 0–15.5 years), overall mortality did not vary by dexrazoxane status (12.8% with dexrazoxane at 10 years vs 12.2% without; hazard ratio, 1.03; 95% confidence interval, 0.73–1.45).[181] Hence, in pediatric patients with leukemia or lymphoma, after extended follow-up, dexrazoxane use did not seem to compromise long-term survival.

A randomized trial of children with high-risk ALL who received doxorubicin with or without dexrazoxane revealed that concentrations of the cardiac biomarkers cTnT and NT-proBNP were significantly higher in the doxorubicin-alone group, suggesting that dexrazoxane reduced myocardial injury and cardiomyopathy (Fig. 19.10).[99] Furthermore, the 8-year, event-free survival rate was 77% for the doxorubicin-alone group and 76% for the dexrazoxane plus doxorubicin group,[176] which indicates that dexrazoxane provides long-term cardioprotection without compromising oncologic efficacy in children with high-risk ALL (Fig. 19.11). Also, dexrazoxane exerted greater cardioprotection in girls than in boys in one study.[176]

In addition, a study by Asselin and colleagues,[182] which was part of the overarching study by Chow and colleagues,[181] found that dexrazoxane was cardioprotective, did not compromise oncologic efficacy, and was not associated with an increased risk of second malignancies. In fact, the cardiac results were similar to that of the study by Lipshultz and colleagues,[176] in that LV wall thickness and thickness-to-dimension ratio were worse than normal in those who received doxorubicin alone, but were within the normal range in those who received dexrazoxane with doxorubicin, at 3 to 5 years after ALL diagnosis.

Dexrazoxane has also shown benefits in children with osteosarcoma.[183,187] Schwartz and colleagues[183] examined the effect of dexrazoxane as a cardioprotectant to support doxorubicin dose escalation, if it affects tumor response, and if it increases the risk of second malignancies. As the authors had hypothesized, dexrazoxane safely

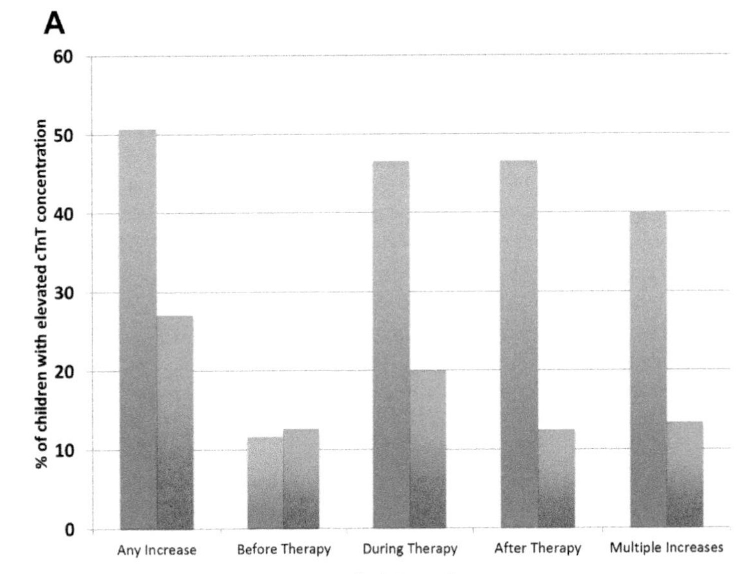

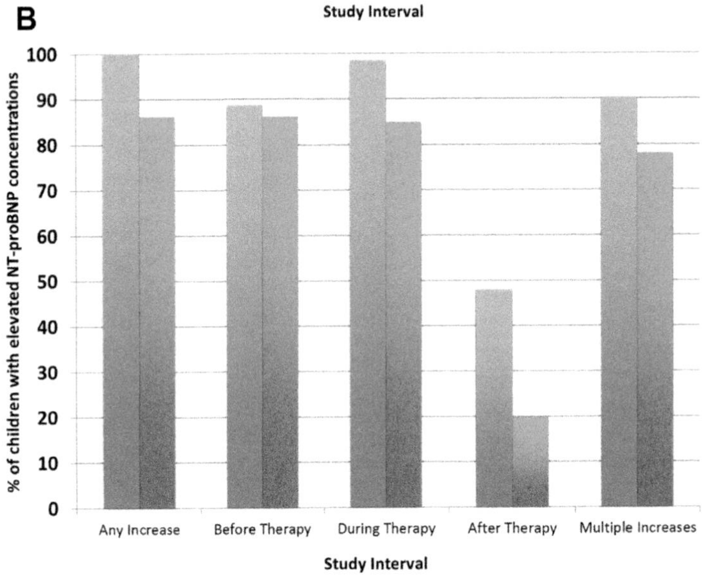

Fig. 19.10 Frequency of biomarker elevations in 156 children with high-risk ALL, by study interval. Blue bar, doxorubicin; red bar, doxorubicin plus dexrazoxane. (*A*) cTnT; (*B*) NT-proBNP. (*Data from* Lipshultz SE, Miller TL, Scully RE, et al. Changes in cardiac biomarkers during doxorubicin treatment of pediatric patients with high-risk acute lymphoblastic leukemia: associations with long-term echocardiographic outcomes. J Clin Oncol 2012;30:1042–9.)

allowed dose escalation of doxorubicin to more than 450 mg/m^2, did not interfere with tumor response, and did not increase the risk of second malignancies.

The safety and feasibility of delivering trastuzumab, a targeted biologic therapy known to be cardiotoxic especially in combination with doxorubicin, were tested in children with metastatic osteosarcoma and HER2 overexpression.[187] The authors purposely added dexrazoxane to the treatment protocol to protect patients from the combined cardiotoxic effects of doxorubicin and trastuzumab. They concluded that although oncologic outcomes were poor in children who received trastuzumab, they were able to safely deliver it in an anthracycline-based regimen using dexrazoxane, because there was no measurable acute myocardial injury using additive cardiotoxic chemotherapeutic agents indicating dexrazoxane cardioprotection.[187]

Together, these studies support the use of dexrazoxane as a primary cardioprotectant in children and adolescents who are diagnosed with malignancies and treated with cardiotoxic agents, such as anthracyclines.[176,181–183,187]

Angiotensin-Converting Enzyme Inhibitors and β-Adrenergic Antagonists

A common late effect of doxorubicin therapy for childhood cancer is reduced LV wall

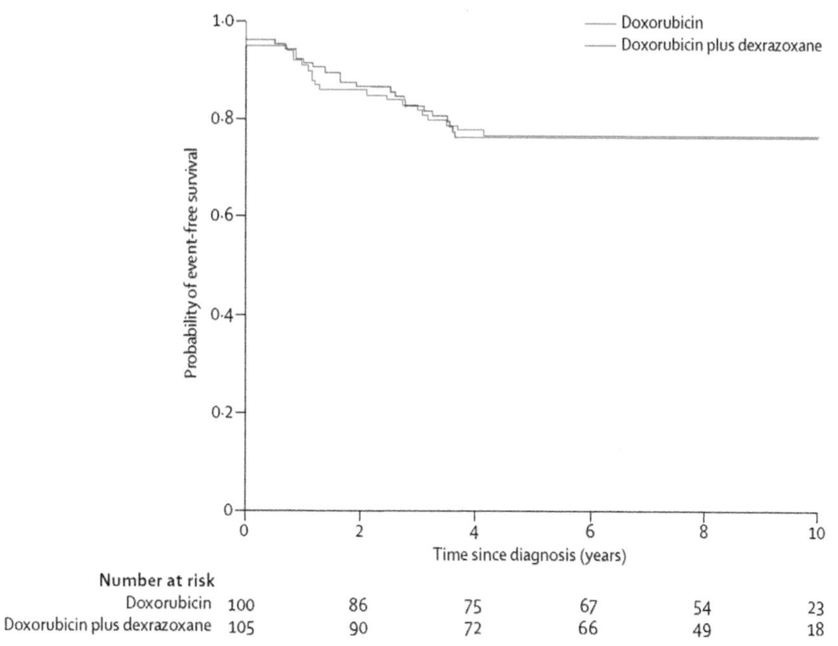

Fig. 19.11 Event-free survival for 205 children treated with doxorubicin alone or with dexrazoxane, indicating that dexrazoxane does not reduce the efficacy of doxorubicin. (*From* Lipshultz SE, Scully RE, Lipsitz SR, et al. Assessment of dexrazoxane as a cardioprotectant in doxorubicin-treated children with high-risk acute lymphoblastic leukaemia: long-term follow-up of a prospective, randomised, multicentre trial. Lancet Oncol 2010;11:950–61; with permission).

thickness for body surface area resulting in elevated LV afterload and depressed LV function. Because anthracycline-related structural changes often progress from a dilated cardiomyopathy to a restrictive-like cardiomyopathy during late follow-up of long-term survivors of childhood cancer, it is critically important to understand the type of cardiomyopathy causing HF in these patients. Many treatments appropriate for HF caused by dilated cardiomyopathy are inappropriate for HF caused by restrictive cardiomyopathy.[89] Two studies have assessed these effects in children who had received anthracyclines.[149,188] In adults without cancer, adding enalapril to conventional therapy significantly reduced mortality and hospitalizations for HF in patients with chronic HF with reduced LVEFs.[189,190] Afterload reduction therapy with enalapril with these drugs in long-term survivors of childhood cancer were associated with an early improvement in LV dimension, afterload, mass, and FS[149]; however, these improvements were lost after 6 to 10 years. Children with HF who had started treatment had either died or undergone cardiac transplantation by 6 years of enalapril therapy. Thus, treatment with angiotensin-converting enzyme inhibitors improves structure and function in the short term in this population, but does not prevent LV wall thinning for body surface area and exacerbates the long-term consequences of inadequate cardiac hypertrophy.[147]

β-Blockade reduces all-cause mortality in non-oncology patients with HF.[191,192] Although the mechanism of β-blockade is not fully understood, it is thought to prevent the reversal of adrenergically mediated intrinsic myocardial dysfunction and remodeling.[193] In one study, metoprolol improved ventricular function in some children with dilated cardiomyopathy and HF.[194] In another study in children with HF, carvedilol was associated with an improved modified New York Heart Association functional class in 67% of patients after 3 months, and an improved mean LVFS from 16.2% to 19.0%. Side effects, mainly dizziness, hypotension, and headache, occurred in 54% of patients, but were well tolerated. Adverse outcomes (death, cardiac transplantation, and ventricular-assist device placement) occurred in 30% of patients.[195] Hence, further investigation is required to determine whether β-blocker therapy is beneficial to children with HF.

Radiation-Induced Cardiotoxicity: Strategies to Reduce Radiation-Associated Cardiovascular Toxicity

Determining the risk for cardiotoxicity is confounded by several variables, including the technique, dosage, patient's age, time since irradiation, other cancer therapies received, and other traditional cardiovascular disease risk factors. Moreover, the spectrum of radiation-induced cardiac injury is broad and includes direct and indirect cardiovascular effects. Reducing or eliminating the risk of radiation-induced cardiotoxicity relies primarily on minimizing both the radiation dose and the exposed cardiac volume while maintaining therapeutic effectiveness. As a general guideline, radiation fields must be carefully defined to achieve this objective. Field definition for any malignancy depends on the anatomy of the region, including the lymph node distribution and the patterns of disease extension. Similarly, a succession of clinical trials in children has determined the lowest radiation doses that maintain treatment effectiveness with long-term safety.[196,197]

A prime example of this decrease in radiation dosage is that of pediatric Hodgkin lymphoma, for which radiation dosages have been reduced from historic levels between 35 and 45 Gy to currently between 15 and 25 Gy in most clinical trials. All the while, radiation volumes have been decreased from territorial RT (ie, mantle radiation), to involved-field RT, to involved-node RT. The significance of this reduction is represented by information from patients treated for Hodgkin lymphoma, in whom cardiovascular (subcarinal) blocking lessened the RR of death from cardiovascular reasons (other than MI) from 5.3 to 1.4. The rate of pericarditis diminished when the LV and subcarinal locales were shielded.[196] In a study comparing the doses to normal tissue, the mean heart dose from involved-node RT was an average of 50% lower than that from involved-field RT.[197]

Computed tomographic–based planning and anterior-posterior opposed parallel pair beam radiation remain common treatments of childhood malignancies; however 3-dimensional conformal RT using nonopposed beams, intensity-modulated RT (IMRT), or proton therapy can reduce the dose to cardiac structures adjacent (in any direction) to the target tumor volume. Proton treatment may further reduce the mean dosage to typical neighboring or encompassing ordinary tissues below that of IMRT or of 3-dimensional conformal RT without expanding the volume of ordinary tissue that receives less radiation. Despite the fact that the viability of these more conformal methods has been accounted for in organs other than the heart, the advantages of a lower dose to critical organs are unlikely to be fully appreciated/confirmed for decades.

Finally, targeted radiation fields are appropriate in some situations, such as in treating pulmonary metastases adjacent to cardiac structures. In this situation, stereotactic RT can target the involved tumor while largely eliminating potentially harmful radiation exposure to adjacent tissues. With stereotactic RT, high doses of radiation are administered in a small number of fractions.

MANAGEMENT OF CARDIAC MORBIDITY IN CANCER SURVIVORS

Chemotherapy-Induced Heart Failure

HF encompasses a variety of clinical, neurohormonal, and structural abnormalities.[198] The incidence of HF increases over time, which highlights the ongoing risk of cardiovascular events these patients incur as they grow older. The American College of Cardiology/AHA "Guidelines for the Diagnosis and Management of Heart Failure in Adults" use a classification system that divides the spectrum of HF into 4 stages, which range from patients at risk for ventricular dysfunction (stage A) to patients with intractable HF not responsive to medical therapy (stage D).[146] The classification has also been applied to HF in children,[199] but without evidence of its application in survivors of childhood cancer; caution must be used when applying it in this vulnerable patient population. In a recent review, Colan[200] points out there are specific areas of rapid change in the evaluation and management of HF in the pediatric population that are undoubtedly worthy of updating. These areas include use of serum and imaging biomarkers, wearable and implantable monitoring devices, acute HF management, and mechanical support.[200]

Cardiotoxic chemotherapeutic agents place survivors at risk for HF (stage A), and as subsequent manifestations of HF appear, survivors may progress to stage D. Unlike children with idiopathic cardiomyopathy, who often present in stages C and D, the asymptomatic survivor of childhood cancer in whom regular cardiac follow-up identifies stage B disease may be treated before symptoms appear. This concept is supported in adult patients with cancer in whom early identification of stage B HF was key for restoration of cardiac function, which was the prognostically determining factor. In adults with HF, the critical drop in survival occurs with the transition from stage B to stage C HF, further supporting the early recognition and treatment of cardiac dysfunction.

Most of the existing literature for managing children comes from clinical trials in adults; hence, data from children are sparse. Therefore, the cause and pathophysiology of HF must be extrapolated cautiously because these characteristics in adults differ widely from those in children. HF in adults is most commonly caused by ischemic heart disease or idiopathic cardiomyopathy, whereas the causes in children are multifactorial. In particular, the mechanisms of cardiac injury after chemotherapy or radiation differ greatly from those involved in ischemic or genetic cardiomyopathies. Hence, treatment without understanding the differences in pathophysiology may lead to treatment with less benefit and more adverse effects.[148]

Therapeutic approaches to pediatric HF can be classified into 3 categories: pharmacologic interventions directed to reversal of remodeling, pharmacologic therapies directed to the relief of symptoms, and surgical interventions, such as mechanical assist device support, cardiac replacement, or cardiac regeneration. An overview of the integrated approach to childhood cancer survivors at risk of HF is outlined in Fig. 19.12.

Heart Failure Stage A: Patients at High Risk for Heart Failure

The same behavior changes for adults at risk for HF are recommended for children: Management should follow contemporary guidelines for treating systolic and diastolic hypertension, lipid disorders, diabetes mellitus, and behaviors that may increase the risk of HF (eg, smoking, excessive alcohol consumption, and illicit drug use). Health care providers should periodically evaluate children for signs and symptoms of HF in those at high risk for HF and, in patients with known atherosclerotic vascular disease, should follow current guidelines for secondary prevention and perform a noninvasive evaluation of LV function (ie, LVEF) and validate cardiac biomarkers predictive of outcome in patients with a strong family history of cardiomyopathy or in those receiving cardiotoxic interventions. Lifestyle interventions should be tailored to personalize interventions based on survivor needs and capabilities in a closely supervised program for

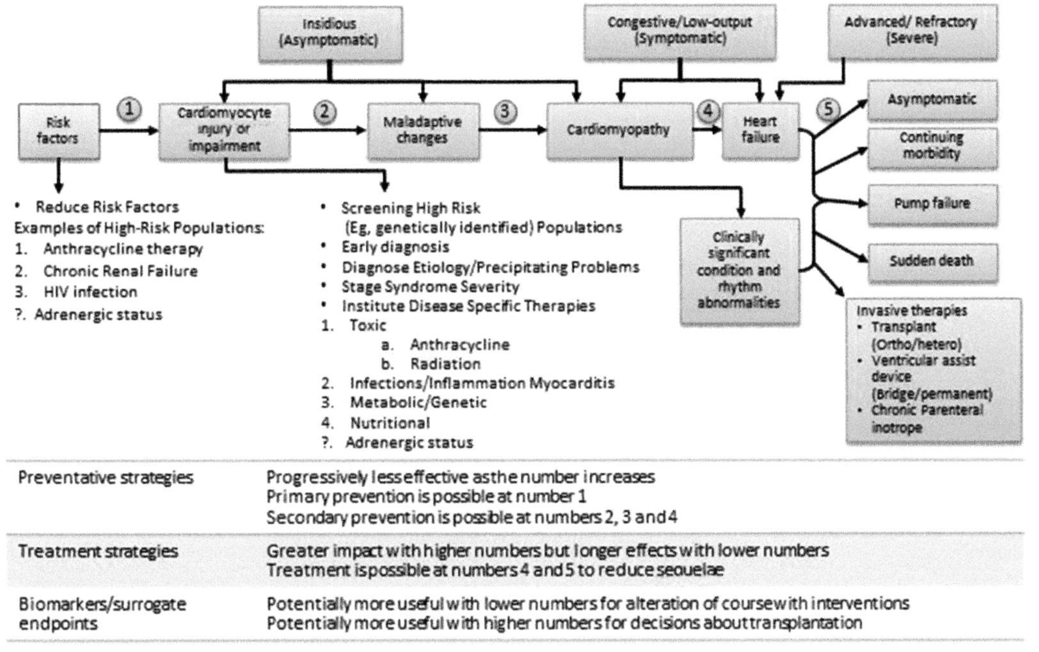

Fig. 19.12 Stages in the course of pediatric ventricular dysfunction. A review of the stages in the course of pediatric ventricular dysfunction that can be followed by echocardiographic measurements of LV structure and function in conjunction with cardiac biomarkers that have been validated as surrogates for clinically significant cardiac endpoints. The identification of risk factors and high-risk populations for ventricular dysfunction are highlighted where their use may lead to preventive or early therapeutic strategies, whereas the determination of etiology may lead to cause-specific therapies. The numbers 1 to 5 indicate stage-related points of intervention for preventive and therapeutic strategies and where biomarkers and surrogate markers may be used. (*Modified from* Lipshultz SE. Ventricular dysfunction clinical research in infants, children and adolescents. Prog Pediatr Cardiol 2000;12:1–28; with permission from Elsevier; and *From* Lipshultz SE, Wilkinson JD. Beta-adrenergic adaptation in idiopathic dilated cardiomyopathy: differences between children and adults. Eur Heart J 2014;35:10.)

this population at higher risk for cardiovascular disease than the generally noncancer survivor population.

Heart Failure Stage B: Patients with Evidence of Ventricular Dysfunction Without Signs or Symptoms of Heart Failure

Angiotensin-converting enzyme inhibitors or angiotensin receptor blockers and β-blockers can improve LVEF and decrease LV dilation in adults with LV dysfunction. These agents have been recommended for treating some survivors at risk for LV dysfunction.[146] In a retrospective study of 18 patients, Lipshultz and colleagues[149] found that in doxorubicin-treated long-term survivors of childhood cancer, over the first 6 years of enalapril therapy, there was progressive improvement toward normal values in LV dimension, afterload, FS, and mass, but all these parameters deteriorated between 6 and 10 years. LV wall thickness deteriorated throughout the study period, as did LV contractility and systolic blood pressure. Diastolic blood pressure also decreased slightly. By 6 years on enalapril, all 6 patients who had had HF at the start of enalapril therapy had either died or undergone cardiac transplantation, compared with 3 of the 12 patients with asymptomatic LV dysfunction. Hence, the short-term benefit in enalapril-induced improvement in LV structure and function is transient and mostly related to lowering diastolic blood pressure.

However, a multicenter, randomized, placebo-controlled trial of 135 long-term survivors of pediatric cancer with LV dysfunction after anthracycline therapy found no difference in the rate of change in maximal cardiac index per year between enalapril and placebo groups.[201] Hence, there are no randomized controlled clinical trial data to support the use of enalapril to prevent progression of LV dysfunction in anthracycline-treated survivors of childhood cancer. However, there are theoretic model–based studies suggesting that enalapril may be effective for this purpose.[9] β-Blockade has also not been studied in a randomized controlled study in asymptomatic anthracycline-treated survivors with ventricular dysfunction.

Heart Failure Stage C: Patients with Ventricular Dysfunction and Prior or Current Symptoms of Heart Failure

The most common manifestations of HF in children include gastrointestinal symptoms and dyspnea. Diuretic therapy and salt restriction are indicated in patients who have evidence of fluid retention. Angiotensin-converting enzyme inhibitors should be considered for all patients with current or prior symptoms of HF and reduced LVEF, unless contraindicated.[146,199] In a multicenter, placebo-controlled, randomized trial of carvedilol in children and adolescents with symptomatic systolic HF but not cancer, carvedilol did not significantly improve clinical HF outcomes.[202] However, given the lower-than-expected event rates, the trial may have been underpowered. Despite these limitations, clinicians continue to use β-blockers in children with acquired or idiopathic cardiomyopathy.

Heart Failure Stage D: Patients in Heart Failure Refractory to Medical Management

As alluded to, childhood cancer survivors may experience improvement in their cardiac function with medical therapy, but ultimately these may fail, hence calling for ongoing cardiac surveillance even if the patient is doing relatively well. Those who developed stage C HF will remain at higher risk for deterioration. As outlined in adults with anthracycline-induced HF, those with a low LV mass are at the highest risk of further deterioration.

Many childhood cancer survivors in clinical HF who progress to marked functional impairment refractory to medical therapy may have no specific contraindication for extracorporeal membrane oxygenation or implantable pulsatile or continuous-flow ventricular assist devices to provide short- and mid-term cardiac support. For those eligible patients, these devices have been used to rescue cancer survivors from acute decompensated HF or as a bridge to transplantation.[203–205]

There is no literature about the optimal timing of implanting mechanical assist devices in childhood cancer survivors in HF. The risk of adverse events with mechanical assist devices, including infection, thrombosis, bleeding, and neurologic impairment, can be as high as 40%.[206] Hence, the risks should be balanced against the benefits in this decision because of the high risk of serious device-related morbidity and mortality.

Heart transplantation is highly effective in children with cardiomyopathy.[207] Survival 10 years after transplant in children with dilated cardiomyopathy and HF is 72%.[208] Heart transplantation has been performed in patients with doxorubicin-induced cardiomyopathy since the earliest days of transplantation.[209–211] Survival of children with doxorubicin-induced cardiomyopathy appears to be similar to that of children with cardiomyopathy from other causes.[208,212] Cancer survivors are at higher risk of malignancy after heart transplantation because the degree of immune suppression is higher. Hence, a multidisciplinary team of cardiologists, oncologists, and infectious disease specialists should evaluate candidates to assess the risk for posttransplantation malignancy. Excellent cancer-free survival has been reported after heart transplantation in pediatric cancer survivors.[213]

Growth Hormone Deficiency

Treatment of adults with GH deficiency was not possible until recombinant human GH was introduced in the late 1980s.[214] Patients with GH deficiency are more likely to have dyslipidemia and metabolic syndrome, but those with chronic HF are also generally resistant to GH. A study revealed that as many as 40% of adults with HF are GH deficient. GH replacement therapy improves exercise capacity, vascular reactivity, LV function, and quality of life.[215] In a case-control study of 34 anthracycline-treated childhood cancer survivors compared with 86 similar cancer survivors without GH therapy evaluated by serial echocardiography while undergoing GH replacement therapy, Lipshultz and colleagues[78] found that LV wall thickness increased during GH therapy (from −1.38 SD to −1.09 SD after 3 years of GH therapy), but the effect was lost shortly after GH therapy ended and the LV wall thickness diminished over time (−1.50 SD at 1 year after therapy and −1.96 SD at 4 years). During GH therapy, the LV wall thickness for the GH-treated group was greater than that for the control group; however, by 4 years after stopping GH therapy, there was no difference between the GH-treated group and the control group. Moreover, GH therapy did not affect the progressive LV dysfunction.[78]

Concern over the use of GH in childhood cancer survivors has been raised, however. First, GH replacement might increase the risk of recurrence or second cancers. These concerns stem from the biological mechanisms of GH; specifically, that it has mitogenic and proliferating properties, as evidenced by some early case reports of cancer in patients receiving GH,[216,217] including one of a second cancer in a childhood cancer survivor.[218] In a cohort of 6284 patients, Fradkin and colleagues[219] found that patients treated with GH had a significantly higher rate of leukemia than that of age-, race-, and sex-matched controls from the general population. However, in their study, 5 of the 6 patients in whom leukemia developed had antecedent cranial tumors (4 craniopharyngioma, 1 astrocytoma) as the cause of GH deficiency, and 4 had received RT. Thus, the increased risk of leukemia in cancer survivors could have resulted more likely from the toxic effects of therapy and not GH replacement. The comparison group was the general US population, so adjustment for cancer therapies that increase the risk of second cancers, and of leukemia in particular, was not possible.

Among a cohort of 1848 patients in the United Kingdom treated during childhood and early adulthood with human pituitary GH between 1959 and 1985, GH was significantly associated with an increased the risk of mortality from cancer overall (standardized mortality ratio, 2.8), colorectal cancer (10.8), and Hodgkin lymphoma (11.4).[220] However, 2 large studies of childhood cancer survivors[221,222] suggested that GH replacement does not increase the risk of recurrence, the risk of a second cancer, or the risk of mortality in survivors of most types of childhood cancer. However, for survivors of childhood brain cancers and of ALL, these studies cannot eliminate the possibility that GH replacement increases the incidence of second tumors. Thus, these risks need to be considered in the decision to start GH therapy in these survivors. These results also highlight the need for studies on survivors of these 2 diagnoses, especially because cranial irradiation is now used much less frequently in survivors of ALL compared with the ALL survivors in these 2 studies, who were diagnosed before 1986.

A third major issue is that GH therapy may exacerbate insulin resistance.[223–231] This finding is especially concerning in childhood cancer survivors who have received large doses of cranial irradiation and are therefore already at risk for insulin resistance and diabetes mellitus, although this has not yet been explored in this patient population. A retrospective study comparing 1411 adults with hypopituitarism and GH deficiency with the normal population and then a prospective comparison with 289 patients with hypopituitarism on long-term GH replacement revealed that overall mortality and the rate of MIs were higher in patients not receiving GH replacement. The rate of malignancies was higher in the adults with hypopituitarism not receiving GH therapy, with a predominance of colorectal cancer. GH replacement appeared to protect against MIs.[232] These results suggest that any perturbation in glucose control caused by GH replacement is not clinically important enough to increase the risk of coronary heart disease, which is the leading cause of death in those with diabetes mellitus, and that GH replacement improves survival among adults with GH deficiency.

Not many trials have evaluated GH replacement in adult survivors of childhood cancer. An open-label, nonrandomized trial compared 16 GH-deficient survivors after 5 years of GH replacement with 13 untreated GH-deficient survivors. All participants had been treated for childhood ALL, with therapy that included 18 to 24 Gy of cranial irradiation, and were between 19 and 32 years old at the end of the study. GH therapy significantly improved concentrations of plasma glucose, apolipoprotein B/apolipoprotein A1, and high-density lipoprotein-cholesterol and significantly reduced the prevalence of metabolic syndrome. Hence, GH therapy was associated with reduced cardiovascular risk in these young ALL patients.[233] In a study by Landy and colleagues,[91] childhood cancer survivors exposed to cranial irradiation had an additional 12% decrease in LV mass compared with unexposed survivors (*P*<.01), and an additional 3.6% decrease in LV dimension (*P* = .03). Survivors exposed to cranial irradiation also had a 30.8% decrease in insulin growth factor-1 relative to normal, which was greater than the 10.5% decrease in unexposed survivors (*P*<.01). Because these abnormalities in LV mass and dimension appear to be associated with decreased GH functioning, they may be treatable using GH replacement therapy.

In summary, evidence mostly from the general population with some from childhood cancer survivors indicates that GH replacement has many positive effects on metabolism and cardiovascular disease risk factors and so has the potential to increase both the quantity and the quality of life in GH-deficient survivors. Concerns about GH replacement increasing the risk of diabetes mellitus and metabolic syndrome were based on shorter-term studies and have mostly been eliminated because longer studies have found opposite results, at least for the general population. The one remaining concern is that in childhood cancer survivors, GH replacement may increase the risk of second cancers, but this possibility is not clear, and even if true, the risk is minimal and does not appear to affect overall mortality. This concern should be considered and suggests the need for further research, particularly in survivors of childhood ALL and childhood brain tumors treated since 1986 who received only recombinant human GH.

Metabolic Syndrome and Insulin Resistance

In addition to the general risk factors for metabolic syndrome and type 2 diabetes mellitus, such as obesity, race, and age, cancer survivors have additional characteristics that put them at a higher risk than the general population. Examples are cranial radiation dose and increasing time since treatment. Many treatment risk factors act not only through increasing overall body mass index but also by decreasing lean body mass. Indeed, even cancer survivors who are not overweight or obese may experience fatty liver and metabolic abnormalities.[234] This paradox was recently shown in a cross-sectional study comparing 319 childhood cancer survivors at least 5 years after diagnosis with 208 siblings.[235]

Unfortunately, the efficacy of treating diabetes mellitus or metabolic syndrome in childhood cancer survivors in the absence of GH deficiency has not been studied. A recent scientific statement from the AHA and other committees on reducing cardiovascular risk in high-risk children indicates that treating diabetes mellitus or insulin resistance is likely to be as effective in childhood cancer survivors as in the general population, unless there are underlying causes for glucose metabolism dysfunction, such as hypothalamus-pituitary axis abnormalities.[236]

In cancer survivors, as in the general population, lifestyle and behavior changes are as important to therapy as are medications. However, considering that many of the medications used to treat diabetes mellitus and metabolic syndrome are not as well studied in children as in adults and that they have unknown or harmful effects on the unborn child, it might be more beneficial to encourage lifestyle or behavior changes until there is more evidence available.[92]

The 2006 and 2010 AHA scientific statements describe the most effective strategies for improving physical activity among people of all ages.[237,238] An intriguing strategy that could help not only survivors during childhood but also their siblings and parents as well is to engage the parents as "agents of change" to improve the lifestyle habits of the entire family. Unfortunately, a recent AHA review of randomized trials studying this approach to treat childhood obesity in the general population did not conclusively show that greater parental involvement was associated with better outcomes in children, although some studies showed better outcomes 2 to 5 years after an intervention that included parents.[239] Miller and colleagues[240] compared measures of physical fitness—peak oxygen consumption, time to anaerobic threshold, and time to peak exercise—from 72 survivors with those of 32 siblings without cancer at a mean of 13.4 years after cancer diagnosis (range, 4.5–31.6 years). Survivors were similar in age at diagnosis, time since diagnosis, and chemotherapeutic agents received. Importantly, they had a mix of cancer diagnoses, which would improve the generalizability of the results. The use of sibling controls also strengthens the validity of the results. The study provided compelling evidence that survivors had significantly lower exercise capacity, less endurance, and lower anaerobic thresholds than did their siblings. The study also confirmed other reports that physical fitness is lower in young adult survivors than in their siblings, even years after treatment, and that it is lower in women.[148,241] This paper showed that certain characteristics, such as restrictive cardiomyopathy, may justify or require supervised exercise because patients with restrictive cardiomyopathy may worsen with strenuous exercise. As a result, Miller and colleagues[240] suggest that these patients be closely monitored during exercise.

Restrictive Cardiomyopathy

Another important cardiac complication from chemotherapy-induced or radiation-induced cardiac injury is the subsequent development in some survivors of a restrictive cardiomyopathy. Treatment of this condition is similar to that for idiopathic restrictive cardiomyopathy; however, treatment options must be considered in the context of the patient's overall health and comorbidities. Treatment of restrictive cardiomyopathy consists of appropriate fluid management to minimize cardiovascular symptoms and includes limiting dietary sodium and fluid intake and the use of diuretics. Because the ventricles are less compliant, the goal of treatment is to reduce intravascular filling pressures, which are the source of early symptoms of HF. Unfortunately, this treatment does not alter the progression of the underlying myopathic process. Ultimately, many of these patients eventually require cardiac transplantation. Cardiac transplantation is constrained by donor availability, and the applicability of transplantation must be carefully evaluated in terms of the underlying prognosis and the relevant comorbidities using the principles established in all heart transplantation evaluations. Of particular concern are the recurrence rates of the primary cancer, the occurrence rates of new malignancies, and the health of the kidneys. In addition, the optimal timing of transplantation in patients with restrictive cardiomyopathy is controversial, with some groups advocating for transplantation at the time of diagnosis and others advocating a less aggressive approach.[242,243] The natural history of restrictive cardiomyopathy is described only in several small series, so this issue cannot be definitively addressed and remains an area of individual decision making. Notwithstanding these difficulties, heart transplantation can be lifesaving in carefully selected candidates with restrictive cardiomyopathy.

SUMMARY

Advances in treatment have increased survival in children with cancer, but their cardiovascular-related health burden will increase as they age. As cardio-oncology evolves, it is beginning to provide clinicians with a better understanding to identify adverse cardiac effects of antineoplastic therapy. Even then, definitive data supporting evidence-based guidelines for cardiovascular monitoring during cancer therapy are lacking. It is critical to base an optimal monitoring regimen on clinical evidence.

As clinicians continue to learn about the cardiovascular effects of cancer treatment, the importance of primary prevention becomes abundantly clear. The aim of vigilant monitoring is to identify signs of cardiac disease early enough to potentially prevent, slow, or reverse the deterioration of the structure and function of the heart. More research is needed to identify tailored therapies to decrease the risk of cardiotoxicity while maintaining the efficacy of the cancer therapy.

Further long-term, prospective studies are needed to better understand the risks of cardiac events in this population and to improve treatment strategies. The cardiovascular effects may appear decades after treatment and are often progressive and irreversible. Thus, screening, preventing, or reducing treatment-related cardiovascular damage with agents such as dexrazoxane, screening for risk factors, and implementing serial cardiac monitoring are important measures for survivors of childhood cancer. Furthermore, the importance of a stable multidisciplinary medical home for childhood cancer survivors throughout their lifespan will facilitate the optimization of functional status and quality of life as well as improve the understanding of the course, risk factors, and most appropriate evidence-based monitoring and treatment of this first generation of survivors.

REFERENCES

1. Li J, Thompson TD, Miller JW, et al. Cancer incidence among children and adolescents in the United States, 2001-2003. Pediatrics 2008;121(6):e1470–1477.
2. Siegel RL, Miller KD, Jemal A. Cancer statistics, 2015. CA Cancer J Clin 2015;65(1):5–29.
3. Armstrong GT, Ross JD. Late cardiotoxicity in aging adult survivors of childhood cancer. Prog Pediatr Cardiol 2014;36(1):19–26.

4. Armstrong GT, Kawashima T, Leisenring W, et al. Aging and risk of severe, disabling, life-threatening, and fatal events in the childhood cancer survivor study. J Clin Oncol 2014;32(12):1218–27.
5. Mulrooney DA, Yeazel MW, Kawashima T, et al. Cardiac outcomes in a cohort of adult survivors of childhood and adolescent cancer: retrospective analysis of the Childhood Cancer Survivor Study cohort. BMJ 2009;339:b4606.
6. Mertens AC, Liu Q, Neglia JP, et al. Cause-specific late mortality among 5-year survivors of childhood cancer: the Childhood Cancer Survivor Study. J Natl Cancer Inst 2008;100(19):1368–79.
7. Lipshultz SE, Adams MJ. Cardiotoxicity after childhood cancer: beginning with the end in mind. J Clin Oncol 2010;28(8):1276–81.
8. Lipshultz SE, Colan SD, Gelber RD, et al. Late cardiac effects of doxorubicin therapy for acute lymphoblastic leukemia in childhood. N Engl J Med 1991;324(12):808–15.
9. Wong FL, Bhatia S, Landier W, et al. Cost-effectiveness of the Children's Oncology Group long-term follow-up screening guidelines for childhood cancer survivors at risk for treatment-related heart failure. Ann Intern Med 2014;160(10):672–83.
10. Fulbright JM. Review of cardiotoxicity in pediatric cancer patients: during and after therapy. Cardiol Res Pract 2011;2011:942090.
11. Simbre VC, Duffy SA, Dadlani GH, et al. Cardiotoxicity of cancer chemotherapy: implications for children. Paediatr Drugs 2005;7(3):187–202.
12. Kerkela R, Grazette L, Yacobi R, et al. Cardiotoxicity of the cancer therapeutic agent imatinib mesylate. Nat Med 2006;12(8):908–16.
13. Lipshultz SE, Alvarez JA, Scully RE. Anthracycline associated cardiotoxicity in survivors of childhood cancer. Heart 2008;94(4):525–33.
14. Simunek T, Sterba M, Popelova O, et al. Anthracycline-induced cardiotoxicity: overview of studies examining the roles of oxidative stress and free cellular iron. Pharmacol Rep 2009;61(1):154–71.
15. Ashley N, Poulton J. Mitochondrial DNA is a direct target of anti-cancer anthracycline drugs. Biochem Biophys Res Commun 2009;378(3):450–5.
16. Lebrecht D, Setzer B, Ketelsen UP, et al. Time-dependent and tissue-specific accumulation of mtDNA and respiratory chain defects in chronic doxorubicin cardiomyopathy. Circulation 2003;108(19):2423–9.
17. Thompson KL, Rosenzweig BA, Zhang J, et al. Early alterations in heart gene expression profiles associated with doxorubicin cardiotoxicity in rats. Cancer Chemother Pharmacol 2010;66(2):303–14.
18. Wallace KB. Doxorubicin-induced cardiac mitochondrionopathy. Pharmacol Toxicol 2003;93(3):105–15.
19. Doroshow JH, Locker GY, Myers CE. Enzymatic defenses of the mouse heart against reactive oxygen metabolites: alterations produced by doxorubicin. J Clin Invest 1980;65(1):128–35.
20. Fogli S, Nieri P, Breschi MC. The role of nitric oxide in anthracycline toxicity and prospects for pharmacologic prevention of cardiac damage. FASEB J 2004;18(6):664–75.
21. Mihm MJ, Bauer JA. Peroxynitrite-induced inhibition and nitration of cardiac myofibrillar creatine kinase. Biochimie 2002;84(10):1013–9.
22. Chen B, Peng X, Pentassuglia L, et al. Molecular and cellular mechanisms of anthracycline cardiotoxicity. Cardiovasc Toxicol 2007;7(2):114–21.
23. Ito H, Miller SC, Billingham ME, et al. Doxorubicin selectively inhibits muscle gene expression in cardiac muscle cells in vivo and in vitro. Proc Natl Acad Sci U S A 1990;87(11):4275–9.
24. Peng X, Chen B, Lim CC, et al. The cardiotoxicology of anthracycline chemotherapeutics: translating molecular mechanism into preventative medicine. Mol Interv 2005;5(3):163–71.
25. De Angelis A, Piegari E, Cappetta D, et al. Anthracycline cardiomyopathy is mediated by depletion of the cardiac stem cell pool and is rescued by restoration of progenitor cell function. Circulation 2010;121(2):276–92.
26. Kalyanaraman B, Joseph J, Kalivendi S, et al. Doxorubicin-induced apoptosis: implications in cardiotoxicity. Mol Cell Biochem 2002;234-235(1–2):119–24.
27. Jurcut R, Wildiers H, Ganame J, et al. Detection and monitoring of cardiotoxicity-what does modern cardiology offer? Support Care Cancer 2008;16(5):437–45.
28. Rusconi P, Gomez-Marin O, Rossique-Gonzalez M, et al. Carvedilol in children with cardiomyopathy: 3-year experience at a single institution. J Heart Lung Transplant 2004;23(7):832–8.
29. Lowis S, Lewis I, Elsworth A, et al. A phase I study of intravenous liposomal daunorubicin (DaunoXome) in paediatric patients with relapsed or resistant solid tumours. Br J Cancer 2006;95(5):571–80.
30. Lebrecht D, Kokkori A, Ketelsen UP, et al. Tissue-specific mtDNA lesions and radical-associated mitochondrial dysfunction in human hearts exposed to doxorubicin. J Pathol 2005;207(4):436–44.
31. Ryberg M, Nielsen D, Cortese G, et al. New insight into epirubicin cardiac toxicity: competing risks analysis of 1097 breast cancer patients. J Natl Cancer Inst 2008;100(15):1058–67.
32. Tokarska-Schlattner M, Zaugg M, Zuppinger C, et al. New insights into doxorubicin-induced cardiotoxicity: the critical role of cellular energetics. J Mol Cell Cardiol 2006;41(3):389–405.

33. Bagnes C, Panchuk PN, Recondo G. Antineoplastic chemotherapy induced QTc prolongation. Curr Drug Saf 2010;5(1):93–6.
34. Albini A, Pennesi G, Donatelli F, et al. Cardiotoxicity of anticancer drugs: the need for cardio-oncology and cardio-oncological prevention. J Natl Cancer Inst 2010;102(1):14–25.
35. Pratila MG, Steinherz LJ, Pratilas V. Sick sinus syndrome in a teenager treated with idarubicin. J Cardiothorac Vasc Anesth 1993;7(1):125–6.
36. Kilickap S, Akgul E, Aksoy S, et al. Doxorubicin-induced second degree and complete atrioventricular block. Europace 2005;7(3):227–30.
37. Okamoto T, Ogata J, Minami K. Sino-atrial block during anesthesia in a patient with breast cancer being treated with the anticancer drug epirubicin. Anesth Analg 2003;97(1):19–20.
38. Zhang S, Liu X, Bawa-Khalfe T, et al. Identification of the molecular basis of doxorubicin-induced cardiotoxicity. Nat Med 2012;18(11):1639–42.
39. Khiati S, Dalla Rosa I, Sourbier C, et al. Mitochondrial topoisomerase I (TOP1mt) is a novel limiting factor of doxorubicin cardiotoxicity. Clin Cancer Res 2014;20(18):4873–81.
40. Lyu YL, Kerrigan JE, Lin CP, et al. Topoisomerase IIbeta mediated DNA double-strand breaks: implications in doxorubicin cardiotoxicity and prevention by dexrazoxane. Cancer Res 2007;67(18):8839–46.
41. Vejpongsa P, Yeh ET. Prevention of anthracycline-induced cardiotoxicity: challenges and opportunities. J Am Coll Cardiol 2014;64(9):938–45.
42. Adams MJ, Hardenbergh PH, Constine LS, et al. Radiation-associated cardiovascular disease. Crit Rev Oncol Hematol 2003;45(1):55–75.
43. Fajardo LF, Stewart JR, Cohn KE. Morphology of radiation-induced heart disease. Arch Pathol 1968;86(5):512–9.
44. Chello M, Mastroroberto P, Romano R, et al. Changes in the proportion of types I and III collagen in the left ventricular wall of patients with post-irradiative pericarditis. Cardiovasc Surg 1996;4(2):222–6.
45. Orzan F, Brusca A, Gaita F, et al. Associated cardiac lesions in patients with radiation-induced complete heart block. Int J Cardiol 1993;39(2):151–6.
46. Cohen SI, Bharati S, Glass J, et al. Radiotherapy as a cause of complete atrioventricular block in Hodgkin's disease. An electrophysiological-pathological correlation. Arch Intern Med 1981;141(5):676–9.
47. La Vecchia L. Physiologic dual chamber pacing in radiation-induced atrioventricular block. Chest 1996;110(2):580–1.
48. Stewart JR, Fajardo LF, Gillette SM, et al. Radiation injury to the heart. Int J Radiat Oncol Biol Phys 1995;31(5):1205–11.
49. Stewart JR, Fajardo LF. Radiation-induced heart disease. Clinical and experimental aspects. Radiol Clin North Am 1971;9(3):511–31.
50. Schultz-Hector S, Trott KR. Radiation-induced cardiovascular diseases: is the epidemiologic evidence compatible with the radiobiologic data? Int J Radiat Oncol Biol Phys 2007;67(1):10–8.
51. Robbins ME, Zhao W. Chronic oxidative stress and radiation-induced late normal tissue injury: a review. Int J Radiat Biol 2004;80(4):251–9.
52. Little MP, Tawn EJ, Tzoulaki I, et al. A systematic review of epidemiological associations between low and moderate doses of ionizing radiation and late cardiovascular effects, and their possible mechanisms. Radiat Res 2008;169(1):99–109.
53. Brosius FC 3rd, Waller BF, Roberts WC. Radiation heart disease. Analysis of 16 young (aged 15 to 33 years) necropsy patients who received over 3,500 rads to the heart. Am J Med 1981;70(3):519–30.
54. Veinot JP, Edwards WD. Pathology of radiation-induced heart disease: a surgical and autopsy study of 27 cases. Hum Pathol 1996;27(8):766–73.
55. Carlson RG, Mayfield WR, Normann S, et al. Radiation-associated valvular disease. Chest 1991;99(3):538–45.
56. McEniery PT, Dorosti K, Schiavone WA, et al. Clinical and angiographic features of coronary artery disease after chest irradiation. Am J Cardiol 1987;60(13):1020–4.
57. King V, Constine LS, Clark D, et al. Symptomatic coronary artery disease after mantle irradiation for Hodgkin's disease. Int J Radiat Oncol Biol Phys 1996;36(4):881–9.
58. Annest LS, Anderson RP, Li W, et al. Coronary artery disease following mediastinal radiation therapy. J Thorac Cardiovasc Surg 1983;85(2):257–63.
59. Yuan H, Gaber MW, Boyd K, et al. Effects of fractionated radiation on the brain vasculature in a murine model: blood-brain barrier permeability, astrocyte proliferation, and ultrastructural changes. Int J Radiat Oncol Biol Phys 2006;66(3):860–6.
60. Verheij M, Dewit LG, Boomgaard MN, et al. Ionizing radiation enhances platelet adhesion to the extracellular matrix of human endothelial cells by an increase in the release of von Willebrand factor. Radiat Res 1994;137(2):202–7.
61. Li YQ, Chen P, Haimovitz-Friedman A, et al. Endothelial apoptosis initiates acute blood-brain barrier disruption after ionizing radiation. Cancer Res 2003;63(18):5950–6.
62. Fajardo LF. The pathology of ionizing radiation as defined by morphologic patterns. Acta Oncol 2005;44(1):13–22.
63. Muzaffar K, Collins SL, Labropoulos N, et al. A prospective study of the effects of irradiation on the carotid artery. Laryngoscope 2000;110(11):1811–4.

64. O'Leary DH, Polak JF, Kronmal RA, et al. Carotid-artery intima and media thickness as a risk factor for myocardial infarction and stroke in older adults. Cardiovascular Health Study Collaborative Research Group. N Engl J Med 1999;340(1):14–22.
65. Smith GL, Smith BD, Buchholz TA, et al. Cerebrovascular disease risk in older head and neck cancer patients after radiotherapy. J Clin Oncol 2008; 26(31):5119–25.
66. Goorin AM, Chauvenet AR, Perez-Atayde AR, et al. Initial congestive heart failure, six to ten years after doxorubicin chemotherapy for childhood cancer. J Pediatr 1990;116(1):144–7.
67. Trachtenberg BH, Landy DC, Franco VI, et al. Anthracycline-associated cardiotoxicity in survivors of childhood cancer. Pediatr Cardiol 2011; 32(3):342–53.
68. Adams MJ, Lipshultz SE. Pathophysiology of anthracycline- and radiation-associated cardiomyopathies: implications for screening and prevention. Pediatr Blood Cancer 2005;44(7):600–6.
69. Giantris A, Abdurrahman L, Hinkle A, et al. Anthracycline-induced cardiotoxicity in children and young adults. Crit Rev Oncol Hematol 1998;27(1):53–68.
70. Krischer JP, Epstein S, Cuthbertson DD, et al. Clinical cardiotoxicity following anthracycline treatment for childhood cancer: the Pediatric Oncology Group experience. J Clin Oncol 1997; 15(4):1544–52.
71. Bristow MR, Mason JW, Billingham ME, et al. Doxorubicin cardiomyopathy: evaluation by phonocardiography, endomyocardial biopsy, and cardiac catheterization. Ann Intern Med 1978; 88(2):168–75.
72. Barry E, Alvarez JA, Scully RE, et al. Anthracycline-induced cardiotoxicity: course, pathophysiology, prevention and management. Expert Opin Pharmacother 2007;8(8):1039–58.
73. Grenier MA, Lipshultz SE. Epidemiology of anthracycline cardiotoxicity in children and adults. Semin Oncol 1998;25(4 Suppl 10):72–85.
74. Lipshultz SE, Lipsitz SR, Sallan SE, et al. Chronic progressive cardiac dysfunction years after doxorubicin therapy for childhood acute lymphoblastic leukemia. J Clin Oncol 2005;23(12):2629–36.
75. Lipshultz SE, Lipsitz SR, Mone SM, et al. Female sex and drug dose as risk factors for late cardiotoxic effects of doxorubicin therapy for childhood cancer. N Engl J Med 1995;332(26):1738–43.
76. Kim DH, Landry AB 3rd, Lee YS, et al. Doxorubicin-induced calcium release from cardiac sarcoplasmic reticulum vesicles. J Mol Cell Cardiol 1989;21(5):433–6.
77. Ali MK, Ewer MS, Gibbs HR, et al. Late doxorubicin-associated cardiotoxicity in children. The possible role of intercurrent viral infection. Cancer 1994;74(1):182–8.
78. Lipshultz SE, Vlach SA, Lipsitz SR, et al. Cardiac changes associated with growth hormone therapy among children treated with anthracyclines. Pediatrics 2005;115(6):1613–22.
79. Steinherz LJ, Steinherz PG, Tan C. Cardiac failure and dysrhythmias 6-19 years after anthracycline therapy: a series of 15 patients. Med Pediatr Oncol 1995;24(6):352–61.
80. Steinherz LJ, Steinherz PG, Tan CT, et al. Cardiac toxicity 4 to 20 years after completing anthracycline therapy. JAMA 1991;266(12):1672–7.
81. Kremer LC, van Dalen EC, Offringa M, et al. Anthracycline-induced clinical heart failure in a cohort of 607 children: long-term follow-up study. J Clin Oncol 2001;19(1):191–6.
82. Lipshultz SE, Scully RE, Stevenson KE, et al. Hearts too small for body size after doxorubicin for childhood leukemia: Grinch syndrome [abstract]. J Clin Oncol 2014;32:10021.
83. Adams MJ, Lipsitz SR, Colan SD, et al. Cardiovascular status in long-term survivors of Hodgkin's disease treated with chest radiotherapy. J Clin Oncol 2004;22(15):3139–48.
84. Adams MJ, Ng AK, Mauch P, et al. Peak oxygen consumption in Hodgkin's lymphoma survivors treated with mediastinal radiotherapy as a predictor of quality of life 5 years later. Prog Pediatr Cardiol 2015;39(2, Part A):93–8.
85. Heidenreich PA, Hancock SL, Vagelos RH, et al. Diastolic dysfunction after mediastinal irradiation. Am Heart J 2005;150(5):977–82.
86. Heidenreich PA, Schnittger I, Strauss HW, et al. Screening for coronary artery disease after mediastinal irradiation for Hodgkin's disease. J Clin Oncol 2007;25(1):43–9.
87. Xie Y, Collins WJ, Audeh MW, et al. Breast cancer survivorship and cardiovascular disease: emerging approaches in cardio-oncology. Curr Treat Options Cardiovasc Med 2015;17(12):60.
88. Nysom K, Holm K, Lipsitz SR, et al. Relationship between cumulative anthracycline dose and late cardiotoxicity in childhood acute lymphoblastic leukemia. J Clin Oncol 1998; 16(2):545–50.
89. Lipshultz SE, Franco VI, Miller TL, et al. Cardiovascular disease in adult survivors of childhood cancer. Annu Rev Med 2015;66:161–76.
90. Tukenova M, Guibout C, Oberlin O, et al. Role of cancer treatment in long-term overall and cardiovascular mortality after childhood cancer. J Clin Oncol 2010;28(8):1308–15.
91. Landy DC, Miller TL, Lipsitz SR, et al. Cranial irradiation as an additional risk factor for anthracycline cardiotoxicity in childhood cancer survivors: an analysis from the cardiac risk factors in childhood cancer survivors study. Pediatr Cardiol 2013;34(4): 826–34.

92. Lipshultz SE, Adams MJ, Colan SD, et al. Long-term cardiovascular toxicity in children, adolescents, and young adults who receive cancer therapy: pathophysiology, course, monitoring, management, prevention, and research directions: a scientific statement from the American Heart Association. Circulation 2013;128(17):1927–95.
93. Rodvold KA, Rushing DA, Tewksbury DA. Doxorubicin clearance in the obese. J Clin Oncol 1988; 6(8):1321–7.
94. Lipshultz SE, Lipsitz SR, Kutok JL, et al. Impact of hemochromatosis gene mutations on cardiac status in doxorubicin-treated survivors of childhood high-risk leukemia. Cancer 2013;119(19):3555–62.
95. Blanco JG, Leisenring WM, Gonzalez-Covarrubias VM, et al. Genetic polymorphisms in the carbonyl reductase 3 gene CBR3 and the NAD(P)H:quinone oxidoreductase 1 gene NQO1 in patients who developed anthracycline-related congestive heart failure after childhood cancer. Cancer 2008;112(12):2789–95.
96. Blanco JG, Sun CL, Landier W, et al. Anthracycline-related cardiomyopathy after childhood cancer: role of polymorphisms in carbonyl reductase genes–a report from the Children's Oncology Group. J Clin Oncol 2012;30(13):1415–21.
97. Krajinovic M, Elbared J, Drouin S, et al. Polymorphisms of ABCC5 and NOS3 genes influence doxorubicin cardiotoxicity in survivors of childhood acute lymphoblastic leukemia. Pharmacogenomics J 2015. http://dx.doi.org/10.1038/tpj.2015.63.
98. Franco VI, Henkel JM, Miller TL, et al. Cardiovascular effects in childhood cancer survivors treated with anthracyclines. Cardiol Res Pract 2011;2011: 134679.
99. LeClerc JM, Billett AL, Gelber RD, et al. Treatment of childhood acute lymphoblastic leukemia: results of Dana-Farber ALL Consortium Protocol 87-01. J Clin Oncol 2002;20(1):237–46.
100. Lipshultz SE, Miller TL, Scully RE, et al. Changes in cardiac biomarkers during doxorubicin treatment of pediatric patients with high-risk acute lymphoblastic leukemia: associations with long-term echocardiographic outcomes. J Clin Oncol 2012; 30(10):1042–9.
101. Lipshultz SE, Rifai N, Sallan SE, et al. Predictive value of cardiac troponin T in pediatric patients at risk for myocardial injury. Circulation 1997; 96(8):2641–8.
102. Cardinale D, Sandri MT, Colombo A, et al. Prognostic value of troponin I in cardiac risk stratification of cancer patients undergoing high-dose chemotherapy. Circulation 2004;109(22):2749–54.
103. Herman EH, Zhang J, Lipshultz SE, et al. Correlation between serum levels of cardiac troponin-T and the severity of the chronic cardiomyopathy induced by doxorubicin. J Clin Oncol 1999;17(7): 2237–43.
104. van Dalen EC, van den Brug M, Caron HN, et al. Anthracycline-induced cardiotoxicity: comparison of recommendations for monitoring cardiac function during therapy in paediatric oncology trials. Eur J Cancer 2006;42(18):3199–205.
105. Steinherz LJ, Graham T, Hurwitz R, et al. Guidelines for cardiac monitoring of children during and after anthracycline therapy: report of the Cardiology Committee of the Childrens Cancer Study Group. Pediatrics 1992;89(5 Pt 1):942–9.
106. Lipshultz SE, Sanders SP, Goorin AM, et al. Monitoring for anthracycline cardiotoxicity. Pediatrics 1994;93(3):433–7.
107. Carver JR, Shapiro CL, Ng A, et al. American Society of Clinical Oncology clinical evidence review on the ongoing care of adult cancer survivors: cardiac and pulmonary late effects. J Clin Oncol 2007; 25(25):3991–4008.
108. Hunt SA, Abraham WT, Chin MH, et al. ACC/AHA 2005 guideline update for the diagnosis and management of chronic heart failure in the adult: a report of the American College of Cardiology/American Heart Association task force on practice guidelines (writing committee to update the 2001 guidelines for the evaluation and management of heart failure): developed in collaboration with the American College of Chest Physicians and the International Society for Heart and Lung Transplantation: endorsed by the heart rhythm society. Circulation 2005;112(12):e154–235.
109. Landier W, Bhatia S, Eshelman DA, et al. Development of risk-based guidelines for pediatric cancer survivors: the Children's Oncology Group long-term follow-up guidelines from the children's oncology group late effects committee and nursing discipline. J Clin Oncol 2004;22(24):4979–90.
110. Nakamae H, Tsumura K, Akahori M, et al. QT dispersion correlates with systolic rather than diastolic parameters in patients receiving anthracycline treatment. Intern Med 2004;43(5):379–87.
111. Altena R, Perik PJ, van Veldhuisen DJ, et al. Cardiovascular toxicity caused by cancer treatment: strategies for early detection. Lancet Oncol 2009; 10(4):391–9.
112. Cheitlin MD, Armstrong WF, Aurigemma GP, et al. ACC/AHA/ASE 2003 guideline update for the clinical application of echocardiography: summary article. A report of the American College of Cardiology/American Heart Association task force on practice guidelines (ACC/AHA/ASE committee to update the 1997 guidelines for the clinical application of echocardiography). J Am Soc Echocardiogr 2003;16(10):1091–110.
113. Kremer LC, van der Pal HJ, Offringa M, et al. Frequency and risk factors of subclinical cardiotoxicity

after anthracycline therapy in children: a systematic review. Ann Oncol 2002;13(6):819–29.
114. Colan SD, Borow KM, Neumann A. Left ventricular end-systolic wall stress-velocity of fiber shortening relation: a load-independent index of myocardial contractility. J Am Coll Cardiol 1984;4(4):715–24.
115. Colan SD, Lipshultz SE, Sallan SE. Balancing the oncologic effectiveness versus the cardiotoxicity of anthracycline chemotherapy in childhood cancer. Prog Pediatr Cardiol 2014;36(1):7–10.
116. Amundsen BH, Helle-Valle T, Edvardsen T, et al. Noninvasive myocardial strain measurement by speckle tracking echocardiography: validation against sonomicrometry and tagged magnetic resonance imaging. J Am Coll Cardiol 2006;47(4):789–93.
117. Singh GK, Cupps B, Pasque M, et al. Accuracy and reproducibility of strain by speckle tracking in pediatric subjects with normal heart and single ventricular physiology: a two-dimensional speckle-tracking echocardiography and magnetic resonance imaging correlative study. J Am Soc Echocardiogr 2010;23(11):1143–52.
118. Ganame J, Claus P, Uyttebroeck A, et al. Myocardial dysfunction late after low-dose anthracycline treatment in asymptomatic pediatric patients. J Am Soc Echocardiogr 2007;20(12):1351–8.
119. Kaul S, Miller JG, Grayburn PA, et al. A suggested roadmap for cardiovascular ultrasound research for the future. J Am Soc Echocardiogr 2011;24(4):455–64.
120. Colonna P, Montisci R, Galiuto L, et al. Effects of acute myocardial ischemia on intramyocardial contraction heterogeneity: a study performed with ultrasound integrated backscatter during transesophageal atrial pacing. Circulation 1999;100(17):1770–6.
121. Vered Z, Mohr GA, Barzilai B, et al. Ultrasound integrated backscatter tissue characterization of remote myocardial infarction in human subjects. J Am Coll Cardiol 1989;13(1):84–91.
122. Perez JE, McGill JB, Santiago JV, et al. Abnormal myocardial acoustic properties in diabetic patients and their correlation with the severity of disease. J Am Coll Cardiol 1992;19(6):1154–62.
123. Ceyhan C, Meydan N, Barutca S, et al. Ultrasound tissue characterization by integrated backscatter for analyzing Fluorouracil induced myocardial damage. Echocardiography 2005;22(3):233–8.
124. Oberholzer K, Kunz RP, Dittrich M, et al. Anthracycline-induced cardiotoxicity: cardiac MRI after treatment for childhood cancer. Rofo 2004;176(9):1245–50 [in German].
125. Basar EZ, Corapcioglu F, Babaoglu K, et al. Are cardiac magnetic resonance imaging and radionuclide ventriculography good options against echocardiography for evaluation of anthracycline induced chronic cardiotoxicity in childhood cancer survivors? Pediatr Hematol Oncol 2014;31(3):237–52.
126. Lunning MA, Kutty S, Rome ET, et al. Cardiac magnetic resonance imaging for the assessment of the myocardium after doxorubicin-based chemotherapy. Am J Clin Oncol 2015;38(4):377–81.
127. Oeffinger KC, Mertens AC, Sklar CA, et al. Chronic health conditions in adult survivors of childhood cancer. N Engl J Med 2006;355(15):1572–82.
128. Bowers DC, Liu Y, Leisenring W, et al. Late-occurring stroke among long-term survivors of childhood leukemia and brain tumors: a report from the Childhood Cancer Survivor Study. J Clin Oncol 2006;24(33):5277–82.
129. Bowers DC, McNeil DE, Liu Y, et al. Stroke as a late treatment effect of Hodgkin's Disease: a report from the Childhood Cancer Survivor Study. J Clin Oncol 2005;23(27):6508–15.
130. De Bruin ML, Dorresteijn LD, van't Veer MB, et al. Increased risk of stroke and transient ischemic attack in 5-year survivors of Hodgkin lymphoma. J Natl Cancer Inst 2009;101(13):928–37.
131. Haddy N, Mousannif A, Tukenova M, et al. Relationship between the brain radiation dose for the treatment of childhood cancer and the risk of long-term cerebrovascular mortality. Brain 2011;134(Pt 5):1362–72.
132. Qureshi AI, Alexandrov AV, Tegeler CH, et al. Guidelines for screening of extracranial carotid artery disease: a statement for healthcare professionals from the multidisciplinary practice guidelines committee of the American Society of Neuroimaging; cosponsored by the Society of Vascular and Interventional Neurology. J Neuroimaging 2007;17(1):19–47.
133. Lorenz MW, Polak JF, Kavousi M, et al. Carotid intima-media thickness progression to predict cardiovascular events in the general population (the PROG-IMT collaborative project): a meta-analysis of individual participant data. Lancet 2012;379(9831):2053–62.
134. Shan K, Lincoff AM, Young JB. Anthracycline-induced cardiotoxicity. Ann Intern Med 1996;125(1):47–58.
135. Singal PK, Iliskovic N. Doxorubicin-induced cardiomyopathy. N Engl J Med 1998;339(13):900–5.
136. Wojnowski L, Kulle B, Schirmer M, et al. NAD(P)H oxidase and multidrug resistance protein genetic polymorphisms are associated with doxorubicin-induced cardiotoxicity. Circulation 2005;112(24):3754–62.
137. Doroshow JH. Doxorubicin-induced cardiac toxicity. N Engl J Med 1991;324(12):843–5.
138. Lipshultz SE, Grenier MA, Colan SD. Doxorubicin-induced cardiomyopathy. N Engl J Med 1999;340(8):653–4 [author reply: 655].

139. Wang YX, Korth M. Effects of doxorubicin on excitation-contraction coupling in guinea pig ventricular myocardium. Circ Res 1995;76(4):645–53.
140. Arai M, Yoguchi A, Takizawa T, et al. Mechanism of doxorubicin-induced inhibition of sarcoplasmic reticulum Ca(2+)-ATPase gene transcription. Circ Res 2000;86(1):8–14.
141. Ferrari S, Figus E, Cagnano R, et al. The role of corrected QT interval in the cardiologic follow-up of young patients treated with Adriamycin. J Chemother 1996;8(3):232–6.
142. Arbel Y, Swartzon M, Justo D. QT prolongation and Torsades de Pointes in patients previously treated with anthracyclines. Anticancer Drugs 2007;18(4):493–8.
143. Chen C, Heusch A, Donner B, et al. Present risk of anthracycline or radiation-induced cardiac sequelae following therapy of malignancies in children and adolescents. Klin Padiatr 2009;221(3):162–6.
144. Gupta M, Thaler HT, Friedman D, et al. Presence of prolonged dispersion of QT intervals in late survivors of childhood anthracycline therapy. Pediatr Hematol Oncol 2002;19(8):533–42.
145. Larsen RL, Jakacki RI, Vetter VL, et al. Electrocardiographic changes and arrhythmias after cancer therapy in children and young adults. Am J Cardiol 1992;70(1):73–7.
146. Hunt SA, Abraham WT, Chin MH, et al. 2009 focused update incorporated into the ACC/AHA 2005 guidelines for the diagnosis and management of heart failure in adults a report of the American College of Cardiology Foundation/American Heart Association Task force on practice guidelines developed in collaboration with the International Society for Heart and Lung Transplantation. J Am Coll Cardiol 2009;53(15):e1–90.
147. Wouters KA, Kremer LC, Miller TL, et al. Protecting against anthracycline-induced myocardial damage: a review of the most promising strategies. Br J Haematol 2005;131(5):561–78.
148. Lipshultz SE, Colan SD. Cardiovascular trials in long-term survivors of childhood cancer. J Clin Oncol 2004;22(5):769–73.
149. Lipshultz SE, Lipsitz SR, Sallan SE, et al. Long-term enalapril therapy for left ventricular dysfunction in doxorubicin-treated survivors of childhood cancer. J Clin Oncol 2002;20(23):4517–22.
150. Alvarez JA, Scully RE, Miller TL, et al. Long-term effects of treatments for childhood cancers. Curr Opin Pediatr 2007;19(1):23–31.
151. van Dalen EC, Caron HN, Dickinson HO, et al. Cardioprotective interventions for cancer patients receiving anthracyclines. Cochrane Database Syst Rev 2005;(1):CD003917.
152. Scully RE, Lipshultz SE. Anthracycline cardiotoxicity in long-term survivors of childhood cancer. Cardiovasc Toxicol 2007;7(2):122–8.
153. Lipshultz SE, Sallan SE. Cardiovascular abnormalities in long-term survivors of childhood malignancy. J Clin Oncol 1993;11(7):1199–203.
154. Lipshultz SE. Exposure to anthracyclines during childhood causes cardiac injury. Semin Oncol 2006;33(3 Suppl 8):S8–14.
155. Lipshultz SE. Heart failure in childhood cancer survivors. Nat Clin Pract Oncol 2007;4(6):334–5.
156. Simbre IV, Adams MJ, Deshpande SS, et al. Cardiomyopathy caused by antineoplastic therapies. Curr Treat Options Cardiovasc Med 2001;3(6): 493–505.
157. Zerra P, Cochran TR, Franco VI, et al. An expert opinion on pharmacologic approaches to reducing the cardiotoxicity of childhood acute lymphoblastic leukemia therapies. Expert Opin Pharmacother 2013;14(11):1497–513.
158. Lipshultz SE, Rifai N, Dalton VM, et al. The effect of dexrazoxane on myocardial injury in doxorubicin-treated children with acute lymphoblastic leukemia. N Engl J Med 2004;351(2):145–53.
159. Tardi PG, Boman NL, Cullis PR. Liposomal doxorubicin. J Drug Target 1996;4(3):129–40.
160. Fulbright JM, Huh W, Anderson P, et al. Can anthracycline therapy for pediatric malignancies be less cardiotoxic? Curr Oncol Rep 2010;12(6): 411–9.
161. O'Brien ME, Wigler N, Inbar M, et al. Reduced cardiotoxicity and comparable efficacy in a phase III trial of pegylated liposomal doxorubicin HCl (CAELYX/Doxil) versus conventional doxorubicin for first-line treatment of metastatic breast cancer. Ann Oncol 2004;15(3):440–9.
162. Safra T. Cardiac safety of liposomal anthracyclines. Oncologist 2003;8(Suppl 2):17–24.
163. Marina NM, Cochrane D, Harney E, et al. Dose escalation and pharmacokinetics of pegylated liposomal doxorubicin (Doxil) in children with solid tumors: a pediatric oncology group study. Clin Cancer Res 2002;8(2):413–8.
164. Batist G, Ramakrishnan G, Rao CS, et al. Reduced cardiotoxicity and preserved antitumor efficacy of liposome-encapsulated doxorubicin and cyclophosphamide compared with conventional doxorubicin and cyclophosphamide in a randomized, multicenter trial of metastatic breast cancer. J Clin Oncol 2001;19(5):1444–54.
165. Harris L, Batist G, Belt R, et al. Liposome-encapsulated doxorubicin compared with conventional doxorubicin in a randomized multicenter trial as first-line therapy of metastatic breast carcinoma. Cancer 2002;94(1):25–36.
166. Gabizon AA, Lyass O, Berry GJ, et al. Cardiac safety of pegylated liposomal doxorubicin (Doxil/Caelyx) demonstrated by endomyocardial biopsy in patients with advanced malignancies. Cancer Invest 2004;22(5):663–9.

167. Bonadonna G, Gianni L, Santoro A, et al. Drugs ten years later: epirubicin. Ann Oncol 1993;4(5):359–69.
168. Stohr W, Paulides M, Brecht I, et al. Comparison of epirubicin and doxorubicin cardiotoxicity in children and adolescents treated within the German Cooperative Soft Tissue Sarcoma Study (CWS). J Cancer Res Clin Oncol 2006;132(1):35–40.
169. Feijen EA, Leisenring WM, Stratton KL, et al. Equivalence ratio for daunorubicin to doxorubicin in relation to late heart failure in survivors of childhood cancer. J Clin Oncol 2015;33(32):3774–80.
170. Buckley MM, Lamb HM. Oral idarubicin. A review of its pharmacological properties and clinical efficacy in the treatment of haematological malignancies and advanced breast cancer. Drugs Aging 1997;11(1):61–86.
171. Vogler WR, Velez-Garcia E, Weiner RS, et al. A phase III trial comparing idarubicin and daunorubicin in combination with cytarabine in acute myelogenous leukemia: a Southeastern Cancer Study Group Study. J Clin Oncol 1992;10(7):1103–11.
172. Thomas X, Archimbaud E. Mitoxantrone in the treatment of acute myelogenous leukemia: a review. Hematol Cell Ther 1997;39(4):63–74.
173. Levitt GA, Dorup I, Sorensen K, et al. Does anthracycline administration by infusion in children affect late cardiotoxicity? Br J Haematol 2004;124(4):463–8.
174. Lipshultz SE, Miller TL, Lipsitz SR, et al. Continuous versus bolus infusion of doxorubicin in children with ALL: long-term cardiac outcomes. Pediatrics 2012;130(6):1003–11.
175. Gupta M, Steinherz PG, Cheung NK, et al. Late cardiotoxicity after bolus versus infusion anthracycline therapy for childhood cancers. Med Pediatr Oncol 2003;40(6):343–7.
176. Lipshultz SE, Scully RE, Lipsitz SR, et al. Assessment of dexrazoxane as a cardioprotectant in doxorubicin-treated children with high-risk acute lymphoblastic leukaemia: long-term follow-up of a prospective, randomised, multicentre trial. Lancet Oncol 2010;11(10):950–61.
177. Lipshultz SE. Dexrazoxane for protection against cardiotoxic effects of anthracyclines in children. J Clin Oncol 1996;14(2):328–31.
178. Lipshultz SE, Anderson LM, Miller TL, et al. Impaired mitochondrial function is abrogated by dexrazoxane in doxorubicin-treated childhood acute lymphoblastic leukemia survivors. Cancer 2016;122(6):946–53.
179. Barry EV, Vrooman LM, Dahlberg SE, et al. Absence of secondary malignant neoplasms in children with high-risk acute lymphoblastic leukemia treated with dexrazoxane. J Clin Oncol 2008; 26(7):1106–11.
180. Vrooman LM, Neuberg DS, Stevenson KE, et al. The low incidence of secondary acute myelogenous leukaemia in children and adolescents treated with dexrazoxane for acute lymphoblastic leukaemia: a report from the Dana-Farber Cancer Institute ALL Consortium. Eur J Cancer 2011;47(9): 1373–9.
181. Chow EJ, Asselin BL, Schwartz CL, et al. Late mortality after dexrazoxane treatment: a report from the Children's Oncology Group. J Clin Oncol 2015;33(24):2639–45.
182. Asselin BL, Devidas M, Chen L, et al. Cardioprotection and safety of dexrazoxane in patients treated for newly diagnosed T-cell acute lymphoblastic leukemia or advanced-stage lymphoblastic non-Hodgkin lymphoma: a report of the Children's Oncology Group randomized trial Pediatric Oncology Group 9404. J Clin Oncol 2016;34(8): 854–962.
183. Schwartz CL, Wexler LH, Krailo MD, et al. Intensified chemotherapy with dexrazoxane cardioprotection in newly diagnosed nonmetastatic osteosarcoma: a report from the Children's Oncology Group. Pediatr Blood Cancer 2016;63(1):54–61.
184. Tebbi CK, London WB, Friedman D, et al. Dexrazoxane-associated risk for acute myeloid leukemia/myelodysplastic syndrome and other secondary malignancies in pediatric Hodgkin's disease. J Clin Oncol 2007;25(5):493–500.
185. Lipshultz SE, Lipsitz SR, Orav EJ. Dexrazoxane-associated risk for secondary malignancies in pediatric Hodgkin's disease: a claim without compelling evidence. J Clin Oncol 2007;25(21): 3179 [author reply: 3180].
186. Hellmann K. Dexrazoxane-associated risk for secondary malignancies in pediatric Hodgkin's disease: a claim without evidence. J Clin Oncol 2007;25(29):4689–90 [author reply: 4690–1].
187. Ebb D, Meyers P, Grier H, et al. Phase II trial of trastuzumab in combination with cytotoxic chemotherapy for treatment of metastatic osteosarcoma with human epidermal growth factor receptor 2 overexpression: a report from the children's oncology group. J Clin Oncol 2012;30(20): 2545–51.
188. van Dalen EC, van der Pal HJ, van den Bos C, et al. Treatment for asymptomatic anthracycline-induced cardiac dysfunction in childhood cancer survivors: the need for evidence. J Clin Oncol 2003;21(17):3377 [author reply: 3377–8].
189. Effect of enalapril on survival in patients with reduced left ventricular ejection fractions and congestive heart failure. The SOLVD Investigators. N Engl J Med 1991;325(5):293–302.
190. Pouleur H, Rousseau MF, van Eyll C, et al. Effects of long-term enalapril therapy on left ventricular diastolic properties in patients with depressed ejection fraction. SOLVD Investigators. Circulation 1993;88(2):481–91.

191. Heidenreich PA, Lee TT, Massie BM. Effect of beta-blockade on mortality in patients with heart failure: a meta-analysis of randomized clinical trials. J Am Coll Cardiol 1997;30(1):27–34.
192. Lechat P, Packer M, Chalon S, et al. Clinical effects of beta-adrenergic blockade in chronic heart failure: a meta-analysis of double-blind, placebo-controlled, randomized trials. Circulation 1998; 98(12):1184–91.
193. Bristow MR. Mechanism of action of beta-blocking agents in heart failure. Am J Cardiol 1997;80(11A): 26L–40L.
194. Shaddy RE, Tani LY, Gidding SS, et al. Beta-blocker treatment of dilated cardiomyopathy with congestive heart failure in children: a multi-institutional experience. J Heart Lung Transplant 1999;18(3):269–74.
195. Bruns LA, Chrisant MK, Lamour JM, et al. Carvedilol as therapy in pediatric heart failure: an initial multicenter experience. J Pediatr 2001;138(4): 505–11.
196. Weber DC, Peguret N, Dipasquale G, et al. Involved-node and involved-field volumetric modulated arc vs. fixed beam intensity-modulated radiotherapy for female patients with early-stage supra-diaphragmatic Hodgkin lymphoma: a comparative planning study. Int J Radiat Oncol Biol Phys 2009;75(5):1578–86.
197. Maraldo MV, Brodin NP, Vogelius IR, et al. Risk of developing cardiovascular disease after involved node radiotherapy versus mantle field for Hodgkin lymphoma. Int J Radiat Oncol Biol Phys 2012;83(4): 1232–7.
198. Auerbach SR, Richmond ME, Lamour JM, et al. BNP levels predict outcome in pediatric heart failure patients: post hoc analysis of the Pediatric Carvedilol Trial. Circ Heart Fail 2010;3(5):606–11.
199. Rosenthal D, Chrisant MR, Edens E, et al. International Society for Heart and Lung Transplantation: Practice guidelines for management of heart failure in children. J Heart Lung Transplant 2004; 23(12):1313–33.
200. Colan SD. Review of the International Society for Heart and Lung Transplantation Practice guidelines for management of heart failure in children. Cardiol Young 2015;25(Suppl 2):154–9.
201. Silber JH, Cnaan A, Clark BJ, et al. Enalapril to prevent cardiac function decline in long-term survivors of pediatric cancer exposed to anthracyclines. J Clin Oncol 2004;22(5):820–8.
202. Shaddy RE, Boucek MM, Hsu DT, et al. Carvedilol for children and adolescents with heart failure: a randomized controlled trial. JAMA 2007;298(10): 1171–9.
203. Castells E, Roca J, Miralles A, et al. Recovery of ventricular function with a left ventricular axial pump in a patient with end-stage toxic cardiomyopathy not a candidate for heart transplantation: first experience in Spain. Transplant Proc 2009;41(6):2237–9.
204. Kanter KR, McBride LR, Pennington DG, et al. Bridging to cardiac transplantation with pulsatile ventricular assist devices. Ann Thorac Surg 1988; 46(2):134–40.
205. Simsir SA, Lin SS, Blue LJ, et al. Left ventricular assist device as destination therapy in doxorubicin-induced cardiomyopathy. Ann Thorac Surg 2005;80(2):717–9.
206. Blume ED, Naftel DC, Bastardi HJ, et al. Outcomes of children bridged to heart transplantation with ventricular assist devices: a multi-institutional study. Circulation 2006;113(19):2313–9.
207. Dipchand AI, Naftel DC, Feingold B, et al. Outcomes of children with cardiomyopathy listed for transplant: a multi-institutional study. J Heart Lung Transplant 2009;28(12):1312–21.
208. Kirk R, Naftel D, Hoffman TM, et al. Outcome of pediatric patients with dilated cardiomyopathy listed for transplant: a multi-institutional study. J Heart Lung Transplant 2009;28(12):1322–8.
209. Arico M, Nespoli L, Pedroni E, et al. Heart transplantation in a child with doxorubicin-induced cardiomyopathy. N Engl J Med 1988;319(20): 1353.
210. Goenen M, Baele P, Lintermans J, et al. Orthotopic heart transplantation eleven years after left pneumonectomy. J Heart Transplant 1988;7(4):309–11.
211. Aldouri MA, Lopes ME, Yacoub M, et al. Cardiac transplantation for doxorubicin-induced cardiomyopathy in acute myeloid leukaemia. Br J Haematol 1990;74(4):541.
212. Armitage JM, Kormos RL, Griffith BP, et al. Heart transplantation in patients with malignant disease. J Heart Transplant 1990;9(6):627–9 [discussion: 630].
213. Ward KM, Binns H, Chin C, et al. Pediatric heart transplantation for anthracycline cardiomyopathy: cancer recurrence is rare. J Heart Lung Transplant 2004;23(9):1040–5.
214. Svensson J, Bengtsson BA. Safety aspects of GH replacement. Eur J Endocrinol 2009;161(Suppl 1): S65–74.
215. Cittadini A, Saldamarco L, Marra AM, et al. Growth hormone deficiency in patients with chronic heart failure and beneficial effects of its correction. J Clin Endocrinol Metab 2009;94(9):3329–36.
216. Ogawa M, Mori O, Kamijo T, et al. The occurrence of acute lymphoblastic leukemia shortly after the cessation of human growth hormone therapy. Jpn J Clin Oncol 1988;18(3):255–60.
217. Endo M, Kaneko Y, Shikano T, et al. Possible association of human growth hormone treatment with an occurrence of acute myeloblastic leukemia with an inversion of chromosome 3 in a child of

pituitary dwarfism. Med Pediatr Oncol 1988;16(1): 45–7.

218. Sasaki U, Hara M, Watanabe S. Occurrence of acute lymphoblastic leukemia in a boy treated with growth hormone for growth retardation after irradiation to the brain tumor. Jpn J Clin Oncol 1988;18(1):81–4.
219. Fradkin JE, Mills JL, Schonberger LB, et al. Risk of leukemia after treatment with pituitary growth hormone. JAMA 1993;270(23):2829–32.
220. Swerdlow AJ, Higgins CD, Adlard P, et al. Risk of cancer in patients treated with human pituitary growth hormone in the UK, 1959-85: a cohort study. Lancet 2002;360(9329):273–7.
221. Sklar CA, Mertens AC, Mitby P, et al. Risk of disease recurrence and second neoplasms in survivors of childhood cancer treated with growth hormone: a report from the Childhood Cancer Survivor Study. J Clin Endocrinol Metab 2002;87(7): 3136–41.
222. Ergun-Longmire B, Mertens AC, Mitby P, et al. Growth hormone treatment and risk of second neoplasms in the childhood cancer survivor. J Clin Endocrinol Metab 2006;91(9):3494–8.
223. Gotherstrom G, Svensson J, Koranyi J, et al. A prospective study of 5 years of GH replacement therapy in GH-deficient adults: sustained effects on body composition, bone mass, and metabolic indices. J Clin Endocrinol Metab 2001;86(10): 4657–65.
224. O'Neal DN, Kalfas A, Dunning PL, et al. The effect of 3 months of recombinant human growth hormone (GH) therapy on insulin and glucose-mediated glucose disposal and insulin secretion in GH-deficient adults: a minimal model analysis. J Clin Endocrinol Metab 1994;79(4):975–83.
225. Fowelin J, Attvall S, Lager I, et al. Effects of treatment with recombinant human growth hormone on insulin sensitivity and glucose metabolism in adults with growth hormone deficiency. Metabolism 1993;42(11):1443–7.
226. Bramnert M, Segerlantz M, Laurila E, et al. Growth hormone replacement therapy induces insulin resistance by activating the glucose-fatty acid cycle. J Clin Endocrinol Metab 2003;88(4):1455–63.
227. Maison P, Griffin S, Nicoue-Beglah M, et al. Impact of growth hormone (GH) treatment on cardiovascular risk factors in GH-deficient adults: a metaanalysis of Blinded, Randomized, Placebo-Controlled Trials. J Clin Endocrinol Metab 2004; 89(5):2192–9.
228. Weaver JU, Monson JP, Noonan K, et al. The effect of low dose recombinant human growth hormone replacement on regional fat distribution, insulin sensitivity, and cardiovascular risk factors in hypopituitary adults. J Clin Endocrinol Metab 1995; 80(1):153–9.
229. Rosenfalck AM, Maghsoudi S, Fisker S, et al. The effect of 30 months of low-dose replacement therapy with recombinant human growth hormone (rhGH) on insulin and C-peptide kinetics, insulin secretion, insulin sensitivity, glucose effectiveness, and body composition in GH-deficient adults. J Clin Endocrinol Metab 2000;85(11):4173–81.
230. Hoffman AR, Kuntze JE, Baptista J, et al. Growth hormone (GH) replacement therapy in adult-onset GH deficiency: effects on body composition in men and women in a double-blind, randomized, placebo-controlled trial. J Clin Endocrinol Metab 2004;89(5):2048–56.
231. al-Shoumer KA, Gray R, Anyaoku V, et al. Effects of four years' treatment with biosynthetic human growth hormone (GH) on glucose homeostasis, insulin secretion and lipid metabolism in GH-deficient adults. Clin Endocrinol (Oxf) 1998;48(6): 795–802.
232. Svensson J, Bengtsson BA, Rosen T, et al. Malignant disease and cardiovascular morbidity in hypopituitary adults with or without growth hormone replacement therapy. J Clin Endocrinol Metab 2004;89(7):3306–12.
233. Follin C, Thilen U, Osterberg K, et al. Cardiovascular risk, cardiac function, physical activity, and quality of life with and without long-term growth hormone therapy in adult survivors of childhood acute lymphoblastic leukemia. J Clin Endocrinol Metab 2010;95(8):3726–35.
234. Tomita Y, Ishiguro H, Yasuda Y, et al. High incidence of fatty liver and insulin resistance in long-term adult survivors of childhood SCT. Bone Marrow Transplant 2011;46(3):416–25.
235. Steinberger J, Sinaiko AR, Kelly AS, et al. Cardiovascular risk and insulin resistance in childhood cancer survivors. J Pediatr 2012;160(3):494–9.
236. Kavey RE, Allada V, Daniels SR, et al. Cardiovascular risk reduction in high-risk pediatric patients: a scientific statement from the American Heart Association expert panel on population and prevention science; the councils on cardiovascular disease in the young, epidemiology and prevention, nutrition, physical activity and metabolism, high blood pressure research, cardiovascular nursing, and the kidney in heart disease; and the interdisciplinary working group on quality of care and outcomes research: endorsed by the American Academy of Pediatrics. Circulation 2006; 114(24):2710–38.
237. Marcus BH, Williams DM, Dubbert PM, et al. Physical activity intervention studies: what we know and what we need to know: a scientific statement from the American Heart Association Council on Nutrition, Physical Activity, and Metabolism (Subcommittee on Physical Activity); Council on Cardiovascular Disease in the Young; and the

Interdisciplinary Working Group on Quality of Care and Outcomes Research. Circulation 2006; 114(24):2739–52.

238. Artinian NT, Fletcher GF, Mozaffarian D, et al. Interventions to promote physical activity and dietary lifestyle changes for cardiovascular risk factor reduction in adults: a scientific statement from the American Heart Association. Circulation 2010; 122(4):406–41.
239. Faith MS, Van Horn L, Appel LJ, et al. Evaluating parents and adult caregivers as "agents of change" for treating obese children: evidence for parent behavior change strategies and research gaps: a scientific statement from the American Heart Association. Circulation 2012; 125(9):1186–207.
240. Miller AM, Lopez-Mitnik G, Somarriba G, et al. Exercise capacity in long-term survivors of pediatric cancer: an analysis from the cardiac risk factors in childhood cancer survivors study. Pediatr Blood Cancer 2013;60(4):663–8.
241. Steiner R. Increasing exercise in long-term survivors of pediatric cancer and their siblings: should treatment be a family affair? Pediatr Blood Cancer 2013;60(4):529–30.
242. Chen SC, Balfour IC, Jureidini S. Clinical spectrum of restrictive cardiomyopathy in children. J Heart Lung Transplant 2001;20(1):90–2.
243. Zangwill SD, Naftel D, L'Ecuyer T, et al. Outcomes of children with restrictive cardiomyopathy listed for heart transplant: a multi-institutional study. J Heart Lung Transplant 2009;28(12):1335–40.

CHAPTER 20

Supportive and Palliative Care and Issues in Cardio-oncology

Sara E. Wordingham, MD[a,*], Keith M. Swetz, MD, MA[b]

WHAT ARE THE ISSUES AND WHAT IS PALLIATIVE CARE: AN INTRODUCTION

Patients who endure treatment for life-threatening situations with cancer often are left facing challenges with subsequent cardiac disease resulting from the life-prolonging treatment that was previously received. In this setting of uncertainty and symptom burden, palliative care has been increasingly used to treat both advanced cardiac and serious cancer-associated illness. The goal of palliative care, by definition, is to improve comfort and quality of life for patients facing illnesses that are not fully responsive to curative therapy.[1–3] Although previously considered only for patients with cancer, palliative care has been increasingly accepted for patients with advanced heart disease and has been promoted as an integral part of shared decision-making and holistic, patient-centered care by the American Heart Association, American College of Cardiology, and other organizations.[4–6]

Palliative care is a growing interdisciplinary field focusing on quality of life for patients with advanced illness. Such care focuses on the physical, social, psychological, existential, and spiritual needs of a patient and their loved ones and is provided by an interdisciplinary team that is typically made up of physicians, advanced practitioners, social workers, and chaplains to name a few (Box 20.1). Palliative care can be provided alongside any disease-directed interventions, and no treatments are excluded while a patient is receiving concurrent palliative care.

Palliative care should not be thought of a distinct transition point in a patient's care, rather, as supportive care along the continuum of a patient's advanced illness (Fig. 20.1). Palliative care should be contrasted from hospice care, which is a specific program of care associated with an anticipated life expectancy of six months or less if the disease follows its anticipated course. Hospice care in the United States has been associated with a specific benefit of Medicare that replaces Part A (hospital-based coverage), and this allows for a plan of care that focuses primarily on comfort to be undertaken in the home setting or other locations when appropriate. Since the benefit's inception in 1982, hospice care is offered by other insurance providers and in some cases to the uninsured via charity care or state-funded programs. Palliative care consultation could be considered for any patient with an advanced, life-limiting illness whose disease-associated burdens require subspecialty management and programs have introduced triggers for cardiac conditions[7,8] (Box 20.2).

Patients with advanced cardiac disease often have unmet needs regarding quality of life, as evident, for instance, in an estimated two-thirds of patients with advanced heart failure who experience suboptimal symptom relief.[9] It is fair to assume that there are palliative care, quality-of-life, or symptom-burden issues in the cardio-oncology populations as well with multiple factors, facets, and overlap phenomena. However, given limited palliative care evidence specifically in this emerging field, many of the concepts and data are extrapolated from advanced heart failure populations, where symptom burden and quality-of-life issues are often analogous.

For patients in a cardio-oncology practice, special consideration is required to meet the needs of patients and their loved ones who have faced a

[a] Department of Medicine, Division of Hematology-Oncology, Palliative Medicine, Mayo Clinic, 5777 East Mayo Boulevard, Phoenix, AZ 85253, USA; [b] Birmingham Veteran Affairs Medical Center and UAB Center for Palliative and Supportive Care, 1720 2nd Avenue South, BDB 650, Birmingham, AL 35294-0012, USA
* Corresponding author.
E-mail address: Wordingham.Sara@mayo.edu

BOX 20.1
Common members of the palliative care team

The patient

The patient's loved ones

Palliative medicine subspecialty physician

Other subspecialist physicians

Advanced care practitioners (nurse practitioners, physician assistants, clinical nurse specialists)

Nurses

Social workers

Pharmacists

Chaplains

Dieticians

Other specialized providers (bereavement/grief; music therapy, art therapy, pet therapy)

Volunteers

From Wordingham SE, Swetz KM. Overview of palliative care and hospice services. Clin Liver Dis (Hoboken) 2015;5(7):30–32; with permission.

"double hit" in terms of serious diagnoses. Various clinical scenarios involving advanced heart failure and malignancy can be encountered in a sequential and/or synchronous fashion. Patients who are treated and cured of their malignancy may later be facing end-of-life challenges with cardiovascular diseases. Conversely, patients with advanced heart failure who faced the uncertainty of awaiting orthotopic heart transplantation and finally received their organ may later develop immunosuppression-associated malignancy. Patients and families who have placed tremendous hope in the possibility of transcatheter aortic valve replacement or a ventricular assist device may be found to have a concurrent malignancy, which not only takes their hopes for advanced cardiac therapies but also places them in the cross-fire of two potentially lethal processes. Last, a patient who has been faithfully served by a permanent pacemaker or implantable cardioverter-defibrillator over the years may find the device rendered superfluous by the diagnosis of a progressive metastatic malignancy.

Although the examples are endless and heartbreaking, clinicians in the cardio-oncology field are charged with important tasks in each of these situations—eliciting and focusing on the goals, preferences, and values of the patient, presenting anticipatory guidance, and engaging in a process of shared decision-making that prioritizes the patient's goal (Fig. 20.2). Such care can be done in a fashion that maintains hope, because hope is a dynamic and flexible construct that can evolve and grow stronger in the setting of uncertainty.

As access to palliative care varies regionally, it has be posited that all providers should have skills in basic symptom management and aligning treatment plans with patients' goals, preferences, and values.[2] Although it is contended that such patients as described may benefit from early palliative care referral to address the multifaceted supportive care needs of this population, the supply of subspecialty trained palliative care providers would not be able to meet such a demand.[10,11] The authors present situations wherein palliative care consultation may be considered (see Box 20.2); however, specific symptom management and advanced care planning (ACP) strategies are also reviewed in later discussion.

SYMPTOM MANAGEMENT CHALLENGES AND PROMOTING QUALITY OF LIFE

Patients with advanced cardiac disease can experience a complex interplay of symptoms that can include dyspnea, fatigue, nausea, anorexia, altered mentation, anxiety, depression, and pain. With diverse pathophysiologic changes in

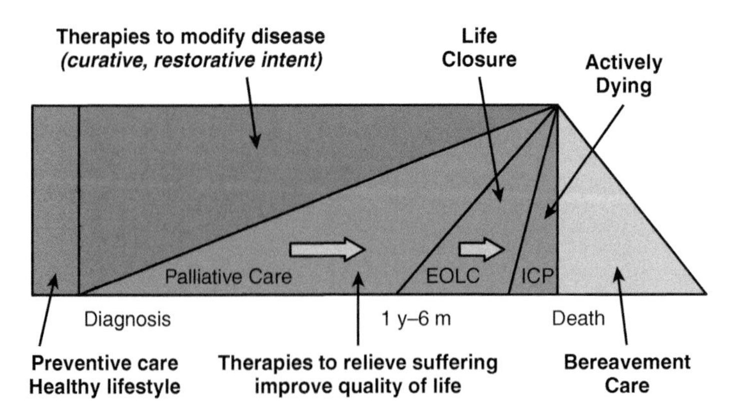

Fig. 20.1 The role of palliative care in consort with disease-modifying therapy. Note that while progression of these events appears linear, for many patients the move from a predominantly disease-modifying trajectory to a predominantly palliative plan of care occurs episodically. EOLC, end-of-life care; ICP, integrated care pathway. (*From* Macaden SC. Moving toward a national policy on palliative and end of life care. Indian J Palliat Care 2011;17(Suppl):S43).

BOX 20.2
Reasons to consider a palliative care consult

Assistance with complex symptom management

- Managing escalating or refractory symptoms (eg, pain, dyspnea, and nausea)
- Complex pharmacologic management in patients facing a life-limiting illness (eg, opioid infusions, opioid rotations, patient-controlled analgesia, methadone initiation, and ketamine initiation)
- Addressing complex depression, anxiety, grief and existential, spiritual, or psychosocial distress
- Respite and/or palliative sedation for intractable symptoms

Care of complex, severely ill patients over time

- New diagnosis with metastatic cancer and/or malignancy with high symptom burden
- Frequent hospital admissions for the same diagnosis of a serious illness
- Intensive care unit admission with metastatic cancer
- Intensive care unit admission with poor prognosis
- Prolonged intensive care unit stay

Assistance with medical decision-making and determining goals of care

- Discussing transitions in care
- Discussing complex and/or evolving goals of care
- Assisting with conflict resolution regarding goals or methods of treatment, whether that conflict is within the family, between the family and the medical teams, or between treatment teams
- Redefining hope in the setting of complex illness
- Discussing complex code status
- Managing patient and/or family conflict or complex social issues
- Discussing ethical dilemmas

Questions regarding future planning needs

- Determining and discussing prognosis where desired
- Care and planning in the setting of advanced illness (Consider referral when one would answer "yes" to the question: Would I be surprised if my patient died within 12 months?)
- Discussing issues pertaining to artificial feeding or hydration
- Determining present and future care needs
- Help with determining hospice eligibility and providing hospice education

From Strand JJ, Mansel JK, Swetz KM. The growth of palliative care. Minn Med 2014;97(6):41. Reprinted with permission, Minnesota Medical Association.

advanced heart disease, leading to increased release of catecholamines and proinflammatory cytokines, activation of the renin-angiotensin system, pulmonary congestion, and sleep-disordered breathing, it can be difficult to delineate and manage the exact cause of a particular symptom. Thus, approaching symptom management in the broader context of a patient's goals of care and focus on promoting quality of life can be most helpful as patients near end of life (see Fig. 20.2). Notably, aggressive symptom management and supportive care for patients with cancer and heart disease can occur concurrently with any advanced or disease-directed therapies.[12–14]

CLINICAL CORRELATION

Ms R. is a 63-year-old woman who has a diagnosis of metastatic breast cancer (negative estrogen and progesterone receptor status, positive for HER2/neu amplification). At the time of diagnosis, she has multiple osseous spinal metastases that are treated surgically with stabilization of the spine with improvement in pain. After completion of adjuvant radiation to the spine and whole brain radiation for some 2 small cerebral metastases, her cancer is managed with maintenance pertuzumab and trastuzumab for 18 months.

During that time, Ms R. is doing fairly well, but struggles with some mild cognitive impairment

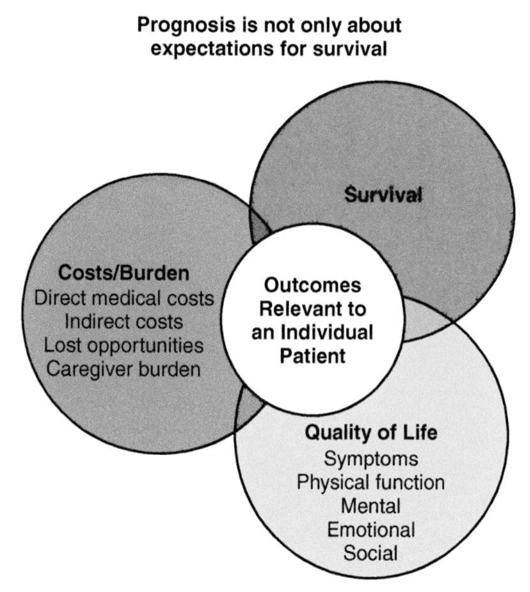

Fig. 20.2 In promoting patient-centered outcomes, survival is not the only issue to consider, but all outcomes relevant to the patient must be considered. (*From* Allen LA, Stevenson LW, Grady KL, et al. Decision making in advanced heart failure: a scientific statement from the American Heart Association. Circulation 2012;125(15):1928–52; with permission.)

and associated clinical depression. She continues have chronic axial back pain, which is predominantly myofascial in nature, but responds well to oxycodone 5 mg twice daily, and she has never requested early refill or shown signs of medication misuse. During routine follow-up, the patient notes some worsening fatigue, mild dyspnea on exertion, and new onset pedal edema, and she reports occasional palpitations. Laboratories reveal a stable CA27.29 level, normal calcium levels and thyroid function, and no anemia. Her Patient Health Questionnaire (PHQ)-9 depression assessment suggests "mild-moderate depression." A transthoracic echocardiogram reveals "longitudinal strain changes" with preserved left ventricular ejection fraction (LVEF), but some mildly increased filling pressures. In addition to cardiac medical managements, how can burdensome symptoms be optimized for Ms R.?

Chronic Pain

Although not commonly considered as a symptom directly attributable to advanced cardiac disease, moderate to severe pain is reported in nearly 70% of patients with advanced heart failure and can be associated with low cardiac output and myocardial/muscle ischemia, peripheral neuropathy, osteoarthritis and degenerative joint disease, and other causes.[15,16] When possible, the underlying cause of pain should be assessed and addressed. Surgical intervention for advanced degenerative conditions can still be considered for patients with heart disease and malignancy if the risks and goals of the intervention and subsequent expectations are discussed. Specifically, procedures to improve quality of life should not be excluded simply because of the diagnosis of cardiac or oncologic issues, but must be couched in the context of expected survival and overall goals of care.

Notably, opioids can be among the safest medications used to treat pain in the population of advanced cardiac disease and malignancy, as long as patients are dosed and monitored appropriately. Nonsteroidal anti-inflammatory drugs are usually contraindicated because of the risks of kidney injury, hypertension, sodium retention, and gastrointestinal bleed. Medications such as tramadol are often tried in this population, but there are significant risks of drug-drug interaction in this population, for example, with selective serotonin reuptake inhibitors, and tramadol can be associated with a higher rate of adverse reactions in this population.[17] Thus, some have proposed that opioids may be the most appropriate analgesic in advanced heart failure, because opioids may have more predictable efficacy and less risk of side effects.[18]

Although concern about safe and appropriate use of opioids sometimes limits their use, low-dose opioids can be titrated to provide adequate symptom relief[19] (further discussed later in the Dyspnea section), and as discussed in this case, many patients can use low-dose opioids safely and reliably without any aberrant behavior or issues with addiction. Notably, the prevalence of pain symptoms has been shown to increase as functional class worsens, and quality of life is negatively affected by the experience of pain, highlighting the importance of its assessment and management in this population.[20]

Fatigue

Fatigue and effort intolerance are among the most common and disabling symptoms of heart disease. Fatigue has also been associated with higher rates of depression in heart failure[21,22] and is frequently a troubling chronic symptom for cancer survivors, even long after chemotherapy has been completed.[23] The cause of fatigue is typically multifactorial and can be related to both clinical and psychological characteristics—including worsening heart failure, nonrestorative sleep, mood, and medication side effects.[24] Enrollment in an exercise program has been shown to increase functional capacity, improve quality of life, and decrease in all-cause mortality in heart failure.[25,26] However, given that treatment of fatigue is often less successful than treatment of other symptoms of advanced cardiac disease, patient and family education can be of significant value in terms of setting realistic expectations. Loved ones may interpret tiredness, subjective weakness, and subjective decrement in mental capacity as "giving up" or that the patient is not trying hard enough, even though symptoms may be beyond the patient's control. Providers can encourage patients to remain active, but also give patients "permission to rest," which may serve to decrease pressure on the patient and family. In addition, medications that may exacerbate fatigue (statins, antihypertensive agents) can be mindfully discontinued as a patient nears end of life.[27,28]

Nausea, Anorexia, and Cachexia

Nausea in advanced heart disease and malignancy can be related to multiple factors, such as decreased intestinal perfusion, medication side effects, and constipation. Nausea can exacerbate anorexia and weight loss in the catabolic state precipitated by advanced cardiac and oncologic diseases. Pharmacologic interventions can include ongoing optimization of heart failure–directed therapies, withdrawal of nonessential medication that may cause or exacerbate nausea, and trials of antiemetics. For patients with malignancy, the benefit of chemotherapy must be balanced with the side effects and burdens to the patient, including gastrointestinal upset. Education should be provided for patients and families identifying the catabolic state seen in advanced cardiac disease and advanced malignancy, so that anorexia and cachexia can be recognized as part of the natural history of the illness, as opposed to a lack of dietary will or suboptimal nutritional effort by the patient. Although corticosteroids can be useful in stimulating appetite and improving energy in patients with cancer,[29] such benefits may be offset by worsening sodium and fluid retention amplified in patients with reduced cardiac function. Although megestrol has been shown to have some utility in cancer populations,[30] unfortunately pharmacologic interventions tend to be less beneficial for patients with heart failure, and nutritional recommendations for patients with cardiac cachexia remain notional.[31]

Cognitive Impairment and Delirium

The association between heart failure and cognitive impairment has been linked to decreased cerebral perfusion, the ongoing risk of delirium, and the multifactorial precipitants of heart disease, including atherosclerosis.[32] Patients who have previously received chemotherapy may already struggle with fatigue and "chemobrain" (memory loss and cognitive changes related to previous chemotherapy) and related challenges on a day-to-day basis.[33] In heart failure, the severity of cognitive dysfunction has been related to the severity of heart failure symptoms and left ventricular systolic function.[32] For patients with underlying cardiac disease, care should focus on prevention of delirium and careful attention to potentially reversible causes when delirium arises, recognizing that patients with pre-existing cognitive impairment are at a higher risk of delirium when they become acutely unwell. Patients with advanced heart disease and malignancy have many reasons to become delirious, including frequent hospitalizations, age, medications (often including opioids), high overall symptom burden, and physiologic derangements due to renal impairment and low-flow state. In the setting of agitated delirium, low doses of antidopaminergic agents can be helpful, all the while ensuring that nonpharmacologic interventions are maximized. For patients whose goals of care focus more squarely on comfort and quality of life, there is a limited to absent role for QT interval monitoring with use of haloperidol.[34]

Depression and Anxiety

Similar to other serious and life-limiting illnesses, depression and anxiety are common symptoms in advanced heart disease[35,36] and cancer survivors.[23] Approximately 18% of patients with advanced serious illness meet the clinical criteria for major or minor depression,[37] and approximately 1 in 5 patients with heart failure meet criteria for major depression, a rate 2 to 3 times that of the general population.[35,36] The American Heart Association recommends screening all cardiac patients with the PHQ-2,[38] and previous work in terminally ill patients with cancer has shown that even the question, "Are you depressed?," can provide meaningful insight into a patient's needs.[39] Higher rates of depression have been seen among patients assessed with questionnaires or those with more advanced heart failure.[36] Rates of mortality, rehospitalization, and general health care use are higher in heart failure patients with more severe depression,[36] which is important because depression increases mortality risk in patients with pre-existing cardiovascular disease.[40]

Patients with advance heart failure may be undertreated for their depression, as illustrated in reports that 90% of depressed patients with heart failure did not receive treatment for their depression.[41] Options for treatment include pharmacologic and nonpharmacologic interventions. Depending on prognosis and goals of care, antidepressants must be used judiciously given the increased risk of deleterious side effects in the advance cardiac disease population, including fluid retention, electrolyte disturbances, and QT interval prolongation.

Anxiety is less well studied in the advanced heart disease population; however, a dyspnea-anxiety cycle[42] has been explored in the chronic obstructive pulmonary disease literature, the concepts of which are relevant to patients cardiac and oncologic bases for their symptoms (further discussed later in the Dyspnea section).

CLINICAL CORRELATION

Ms L. is a 48-year-old woman with a history of Hodgkin lymphoma from age 24. She was successfully treated with high-dose mantle radiation and chemotherapy and later developed mild-moderate dyspnea around the age of 42. Cardiac evaluation was suggestive of mild pericardial restriction and a mildly reduced LVEF at 50% as well as changes consistent with early mitral and pulmonic valvular heart disease. Ms L. is managed medically for the next 5 years, but then develops a "secondary" breast cancer at age 47. She undergoes radical mastectomy and selective lymphadenectomy. The diagnosis of grade III adenocarcinoma of the breast is made, and although lymph nodes were negative for malignancy, her estrogen receptor, progesterone receptor, and Her2/neu status were all negative.

Given "triple-negative" disease status, tumor size, and high tumor grade, Ms L. receives adjuvant doxorubicin and cyclophosphamide, with the anthracycline dose adjusted for prior radiation exposure and LVEF of 45%, which is followed by dose-dense paclitaxel.

Ms L. tolerated surgery and chemotherapy well and remains in clinical remission for several months at her 3-, 6-, and 9-month surveillance visits. Between her 9-month and 1-year recheck regarding her breast cancer, she develops worsening class IV dyspnea, moderate lower extremity edema, and moderate bilateral pleural effusions, which are drained and found to be a transudate, with negative cytology and no evidence of malignancy. Echocardiogram now shows a markedly reduced LVEF at 18% with mild-moderate restrictive changes. Attempts at palliating Ms L.'s symptoms with low-dose opioids, optimal medical management with lisinopril, carvedilol, and furosemide are not helpful. Spironolactone was not tolerated due to hyperkalemia.

The patient experiences frequent hospitalizations and marked impairment of quality of life. As the patient remained symptomatic and with a depressed LVEF, the patient undergoes implantation with cardiac resynchronization therapy and defibrillator. Despite adjustments made over next 3 months, the patient's symptoms remain profound. Ms L. has a 16-year-old son who has been learning to drive, and she would really like to see him graduate from high school 18 months from now. Given this, the patient is considered for a left ventricular assist device as destination therapy. At this time, Ms L. does not appear to have recurrent malignant disease, but all are concerned about her limited prognosis, and transplantation is not considered given the short time since cancer diagnosis and concerns about recurrence in the future.

Dyspnea

Dyspnea is a common symptom of advanced heart disease and one by which the disease is classified, although symptoms of shortness of breath and edema are frequently seen in cancer and other chronic disease states. Breathlessness may persist despite optimal medical management of cancer or heart disease, and data are emerging on pharmacologic and nonpharmacologic interventions for the management of dyspnea.[43,44] Dyspnea has been referred to as an important "patient-driven agenda," in an effort to highlight symptom burden as well as survival in advanced heart disease.[45] Although the primary treatment of dyspnea is to address its underlying cause, one must be mindful of the concept of "total dyspnea" in which a patient's previous experiences, physical sensations, comorbidities, social situation, and functional impairment are all considered as playing a role in the sensation of shortness of breath.[46] Caregivers of patients with heart failure who suffer with breathlessness report high levels of unmet needs and caregiver burden as well as less positive caregiving experiences, similar to caregivers of patients with lung cancer.[47,48]

As mentioned earlier, low-dose opioids have been shown to be safe and effective to improve subjective dyspnea, and several studies and systematic reviews have demonstrated that opioids can be used in proportionate doses with excellent efficacy and minimal side effects,[49–51] even in patients with chronic obstructive pulmonary disease.[52,53] Opioid receptors are found throughout the cardiorespiratory system, and although providers may be hesitant to prescribe opioids, it has been argued that opioids can be used safely in patients for treatment of dyspnea without hastening death.[54]

Although opioids have been shown to improve quality of life and relieve refractory breathlessness, providers have cited both a lack of experience in the use of opioids for dyspnea and concerns about the physiologic and legal consequences of prescribing these medications.[55] Thus, referral to or collaboration with palliative care experts may help to mollify these concerns. In addition, short-acting benzodiazepines can be effective in alleviating anxiety associated with breathlessness that is not relieved by other interventions; however, there appears to be a dose response whereby higher doses of benzodiazepines for the treatment of dyspnea can be associated with an increased risk of mortality.[52]

Last, supplemental oxygen is often prescribed for treatment of dyspnea and hypoxia, but its use in the home in the United States is often limited by Medicare criteria. Although a nasal cannula is viewed by many patients and families as "essential" for the treatment of breathlessness, the evidence to support this is less robust for some patient populations. A double-blinded randomized controlled trial of palliative oxygen therapy versus room air for relief of breathlessness in patients with refractory dyspnea did not show a difference between either treatment modality in terms of efficacy of symptom relief.[56] Further systematic analyses have suggested that continuous (not only as needed) oxygen therapy during exertion may reduce for patients with chronic obstructive pulmonary disease who were either mildly hypoxic or normoxic, and who would not have qualified for home oxygen therapy otherwise.[57] Given the ongoing evolution of the literature in this regard, the authors encourage clinicians to treat dyspnea as an entity that is distinct from hypoxic or tachypnea and affects patients' quality of life. Often, symptom palliation seems to be better accomplished with low-dose opioids and circulating fans over supplemental oxygen therapy.

Advanced Care Planning

ACP plays an important role in the care of all patients with advanced illness, but becomes even more important in patients who may have multiple advanced illnesses. A new diagnosis of heart failure, for example, represents an important transition in someone's care and an important opportunity to readdress patients' goals of care and their ACP documentation.[4] Standard advance directives documents often fail to address the most common scenarios that precipitate end of life for a particular illness. For example, the advanced illness trajectory of heart failure is very different from that of advanced dementia. Providers can use the time of a new diagnosis to assist patients in their understanding of their condition and help to understand their goals and values and accept the significant uncertainty that lies ahead. Yearly discussions regarding advanced care preferences are recommended for patients with heart failure[4]; the importance of such discussions is only compounded for patients with concurrent oncologic diagnoses. Palliative care consultation (see Box 20.2) to facilitate the honing of advanced directives into a personalized preparedness plan may be beneficial for patients like the ones described in the vignettes, as competing goals of care and prioritization of quality and quantity of life are sometimes challenging to discern.[14] Further research is warranted to see if similar planning can be of benefit to cardio-oncology populations before considering high-risk procedures such as transarterial valve replacement, mechanical circulatory support device implantation, or treatment of secondarily developed hematological malignancy with allogenic stem cell transplantation.

SUMMARY

Patients with a history of cancer who subsequently develop cardiac disease, or those with cardiac disease who are facing challenging decisions regarding antineoplastic therapy, represent vulnerable groups who may be at a higher risk of physical and psychological comorbidity. Herein, the authors have presented guidance for clinicians to address these complex situations, which has been aimed at empowering clinicians to explore these issues and to stimulate further reflection and discussion, versus presenting an authoritative collection of absolutes that must be followed. As this field continues to develop, so too must the art and science of communication and efforts at improving quality of life develop for this multidimensional population.

REFERENCES

1. World Palliative Care Alliance, World Health Organization. Global atlas of palliative care at the end of life. 2014. Available at: http://www.who.int/cancer/publications/palliative-care-atlas/en/.
2. Quill TE, Abernethy AP. Generalist plus specialist palliative care—creating a more sustainable model. N Engl J Med 2013;368(13):1173–5.
3. Strand JJ, Mansel JK, Swetz KM. The growth of palliative care. Minn Med 2014;97(6):39–43.
4. Allen LA, Stevenson LW, Grady KL, et al. Decision making in advanced heart failure: a scientific statement from the American Heart Association. Circulation 2012;125(15):1928–52.

5. Feldman D, Pamboukian SV, Teuteberg JJ, et al. The 2013 International Society for Heart and Lung Transplantation Guidelines for mechanical circulatory support: executive summary. J Heart Lung Transplant 2013;32(2):157–87.
6. Fang JC, Ewald GA, Allen LA, et al. Advanced (stage D) heart failure: a statement from the Heart Failure Society of America Guidelines Committee. J Card Fail 2015;21(6):519–34.
7. Bakitas M, Macmartin M, Trzepkowski K, et al. Palliative care consultations for heart failure patients: how many, when, and why? J Card Fail 2013;19(3): 193–201.
8. Bekelman DB, Nowels CT, Allen LA, et al. Outpatient palliative care for chronic heart failure: a case series. J Palliat Med 2011;14(7):815–21.
9. McCarthy M, Lay M, Addington-Hall J. Dying from heart disease. J R Coll Physicians Lond 1996;30(4): 325–8.
10. Kamal AH, Maguire JM, Meier DE. Evolving the palliative care workforce to provide responsive, serious illness care. Ann Intern Med 2015;163(8): 637–8.
11. Lupu D, American Academy of Hospice and Palliative Medicine Workforce Task Force. Estimate of current hospice and palliative medicine physician workforce shortage. J Pain Symptom Manage 2010;40(6):899–911.
12. Temel JS, Greer JA, Muzikansky A, et al. Early palliative care for patients with metastatic non-small-cell lung cancer. N Engl J Med 2010;363(8):733–42.
13. Goodlin SJ. Palliative care in congestive heart failure. J Am Coll Cardiol 2009;54(5):386–96.
14. Swetz KM, Freeman MR, Abouezzeddine OF, et al. Palliative medicine consultation for preparedness planning in patients receiving left ventricular assist devices as destination therapy. Mayo Clin Proc 2011;86(6):493–500.
15. Godfrey CM, Harrison MB, Friedberg E, et al. The symptom of pain in individuals recently hospitalized for heart failure. J Cardiovasc Nurs 2007;22(5):368–74 [discussion: 366–7].
16. Goebel JR, Doering LV, Evangelista LS, et al. A comparative study of pain in heart failure and non-heart failure veterans. J Card Fail 2009;15(1): 24–30.
17. Swetz KM, Carey EC, Bundrick JB. Clinical pearls in palliative medicine 2012. Mayo Clin Proc 2012; 87(11):1118–23.
18. Goodlin SJ, Wingate S, Albert NM, et al. Investigating pain in heart failure patients: the pain assessment, incidence, and nature in heart failure (PAIN-HF) study. J Card Fail 2012;18(10):776–83.
19. Pergolizzi J, Boger RH, Budd K, et al. Opioids and the management of chronic severe pain in the elderly: consensus statement of an International Expert Panel with focus on the six clinically most often used World Health Organization Step III opioids (buprenorphine, fentanyl, hydromorphone, methadone, morphine, oxycodone). Pain Pract 2008;8(4):287–313.
20. Evangelista LS, Sackett E, Dracup K. Pain and heart failure: unrecognized and untreated. Eur J Cardiovasc Nurs 2009;8(3):169–73.
21. Sullivan M, Levy WC, Russo JE, et al. Depression and health status in patients with advanced heart failure: a prospective study in tertiary care. J Card Fail 2004;10(5):390–6.
22. Yu DS, Lee DT, Woo J, et al. Correlates of psychological distress in elderly patients with congestive heart failure. J Psychosom Res 2004;57(6):573–81.
23. Pachman DR, Barton DL, Swetz KM, et al. Troublesome symptoms in cancer survivors: fatigue, insomnia, neuropathy, and pain. J Clin Oncol 2012;30(30):3687–96.
24. Smith OR, Michielsen HJ, Pelle AJ, et al. Symptoms of fatigue in chronic heart failure patients: clinical and psychological predictors. Eur J Heart Fail 2007;9(9):922–7.
25. Belardinelli R, Georgiou D, Cianci G, et al. Randomized, controlled trial of long-term moderate exercise training in chronic heart failure: effects on functional capacity, quality of life, and clinical outcome. Circulation 1999;99(9):1173–82.
26. O'Connor CM, Whellan DJ, Lee KL, et al. Efficacy and safety of exercise training in patients with chronic heart failure: HF-ACTION randomized controlled trial. JAMA 2009;301(14):1439–50.
27. Kutner JS, Blatchford PJ, Taylor DH Jr, et al. Safety and benefit of discontinuing statin therapy in the setting of advanced, life-limiting illness: a randomized clinical trial. JAMA Intern Med 2015;175(5): 691–700.
28. LeBlanc TW, McNeil MJ, Kamal AH, et al. Polypharmacy in patients with advanced cancer and the role of medication discontinuation. Lancet Oncol 2015; 16(7):e333–41.
29. Yennurajalingam S, Bruera E. Role of corticosteroids for fatigue in advanced incurable cancer: is it a 'wonder drug' or 'deal with the devil'. Curr Opin Support Palliat Care 2014;8(4):346–51.
30. Mateen F, Jatoi A. Megestrol acetate for the palliation of anorexia in advanced, incurable cancer patients. Clin Nutr 2006;25(5):711–5.
31. von Haehling S, Lainscak M, Springer J, et al. Cardiac cachexia: A systematic overview. Pharmacol Ther 2009;121(3):227–52.
32. Heckman GA, Patterson CJ, Demers C, et al. Heart failure and cognitive impairment: challenges and opportunities. Clin Interv Aging 2007; 2(2):209–18.
33. Moore HC. An overview of chemotherapy-related cognitive dysfunction, or 'chemobrain'. Oncology 2014;28(9):797–804.

34. Vella-Brincat J, Macleod AD. Haloperidol in palliative care. Palliat Med 2004;18(3):195–201.
35. Evans DL, Charney DS, Lewis L, et al. Mood disorders in the medically ill: scientific review and recommendations. Biol Psychiatry 2005;58(3):175–89.
36. Rutledge T, Reis VA, Linke SE, et al. Depression in heart failure a meta-analytic review of prevalence, intervention effects, and associations with clinical outcomes. J Am Coll Cardiol 2006;48(8):1527–37.
37. Block SD. Diagnosis and treatment of depression in patients with advanced illness. Epidemiol Psichiatr Soc 2010;19(2):103–9.
38. Lichtman JH, Bigger JT Jr, Blumenthal JA, et al. Depression and coronary heart disease: recommendations for screening, referral, and treatment: a science advisory from the American Heart Association Prevention Committee of the Council on Cardiovascular Nursing, Council on Clinical Cardiology, Council on Epidemiology and Prevention, and Interdisciplinary Council on Quality of Care and Outcomes Research: endorsed by the American Psychiatric Association. Circulation 2008;118(17):1768–75.
39. Chochinov HM, Wilson KG, Enns M, et al. "Are you depressed?" Screening for depression in the terminally ill. Am J Psychiatry 1997;154(5):674–6.
40. Chamberlain AM, Vickers KS, Colligan RC, et al. Associations of preexisting depression and anxiety with hospitalization in patients with cardiovascular disease. Mayo Clin Proc 2011;86(11):1056–62.
41. Koenig HG. Depression in hospitalized older patients with congestive heart failure. Gen Hosp Psychiatry 1998;20(1):29–43.
42. Carrieri-Kohlman V, Douglas MK, Gormley JM, et al. Desensitization and guided mastery: treatment approaches for the management of dyspnea. Heart Lung 1993;22(3):226–34.
43. Ekstrom MP, Abernethy AP, Currow DC. The management of chronic breathlessness in patients with advanced and terminal illness. BMJ 2015;349:g7617.
44. Kamal AH, Maguire JM, Wheeler JL, et al. Dyspnea review for the palliative care professional: treatment goals and therapeutic options. J Palliat Med 2012;15(1):106–14.
45. Johnson MJ, Oxberry SG. The management of dyspnoea in chronic heart failure. Curr Opin Support Palliat Care 2010;4(2):63–8.
46. Kamal AH, Maguire JM, Wheeler JL, et al. Dyspnea review for the palliative care professional: assessment, burdens, and etiologies. J Palliat Med 2011;14(10):1167–72.
47. Malik FA, Gysels M, Higginson IJ. Living with breathlessness: a survey of caregivers of breathless patients with lung cancer or heart failure. Palliat Med 2013;27(7):647–56.
48. Abernethy AP, Wheeler JL. Total dyspnoea. Curr Opin Support Palliat Care 2008;2(2):110–3.
49. Abernethy AP, Currow DC, Frith P, et al. Randomised, double blind, placebo controlled crossover trial of sustained release morphine for the management of refractory dyspnoea. BMJ 2003;327(7414):523–8.
50. Currow DC, McDonald C, Oaten S, et al. Once-daily opioids for chronic dyspnea: a dose increment and pharmacovigilance study. J Pain Symptom Manage 2011;42(3):388–99.
51. Ben-Aharon I, Gafter-Gvili A, Leibovici L, et al. Interventions for alleviating cancer-related dyspnea: a systematic review and meta-analysis. Acta Oncol 2012;51(8):996–1008.
52. Ekstrom MP, Bornefalk-Hermansson A, Abernethy AP, et al. Safety of benzodiazepines and opioids in very severe respiratory disease: national prospective study. BMJ 2014;348:g445.
53. Ekstrom M, Bornefalk-Hermansson A, Abernethy A, et al. Low-dose opioids should be considered for symptom relief also in advanced chronic obstructive pulmonary disease (COPD). Evid Based Med 2015;20(1):39.
54. Hallenbeck J. Pathophysiologies of dyspnea explained: why might opioids relieve dyspnea and not hasten death? J Palliat Med 2012;15(8):848–53.
55. Rocker G, Young J, Donahue M, et al. Perspectives of patients, family caregivers and physicians about the use of opioids for refractory dyspnea in advanced chronic obstructive pulmonary disease. Can Med Assoc J 2012;184(9):E497–504.
56. Abernethy AP, McDonald CF, Frith PA, et al. Effect of palliative oxygen versus room air in relief of breathlessness in patients with refractory dyspnoea: a double-blind, randomised controlled trial. Lancet 2010;376(9743):784–93.
57. Uronis HE, Ekstrom MP, Currow DC, et al. Oxygen for relief of dyspnoea in people with chronic obstructive pulmonary disease who would not qualify for home oxygen: a systematic review and meta-analysis. Thorax 2015;70(5):492–4.

CHAPTER 21

Cardio-oncology in Practice: Goals and Principles

Daniel J. Lenihan, MD

Throughout our health care system, there are major opportunities for improvement in the delivery of effective medical care. In so many ways, we as health care providers must look to avoid polypharmacy, attempt to manage health care costs, improve the administration and application of guideline-directed therapy, learn to be mindful of overtesting and defensive medicine as well as carefully assess the existing barriers to optimal cardiac care. Furthermore, we should be compelled to share our knowledge gained from our direct experience to improve our colleagues' practice characteristics in a progressive and collaborative manner. In fact, these ideas are spelled out in the Hippocratic Oath we are sworn to uphold. These goals are all laudable goals that each of us can strive for, and it is hoped at least some aspects of this can be accomplished in our daily practices (Box 21.1). As it turns out, the emerging discipline of Cardio-oncology is a microcosm of the larger health care challenges and is an example of what we can collectively achieve if we are committed to improving all aspects of the cardiac care of patients with cancer.

There are several overarching principles that can guide practitioners in the development of an effective cardio-oncology practice (Box 21.2). These principles are intended to form a basis for the cardio-oncology interaction, but exactly how specific interactions occur is completely dependent on the local environment. In addition, these suggestions are from the perspective of a cardiologist, and it is acknowledged that other important perspectives, such as those from the hematologist/oncologist, primary care provider, or patient/family, may be substantially different. It is necessary to keep in mind that cardiologists, as an example, cannot be afraid to propose a sound cardiology-based observation to the diagnosis and treatment of a patient with cancer because this may have a major impact.[1,2] Practitioners also need to understand that the patient with cancer is vulnerable and is asked to do a lot already when one considers all the testing and treatments that are prescribed for long periods of time. As a cardiologist, you can provide your best cardiac care, and if that is delivered, this will prevent or minimize cardiac limitation.[3] A quality cardiovascular consultation will have a huge impact on the cancer care provided. Furthermore, a vibrant collaboration with other colleagues outside of your primary practice area is always very rewarding and can be one of the most satisfactory components in your practice.[4,5] A critical component of cardio-oncology is to have disciplined reporting of clinical events, and it is imperative that we collectively share our experiences with others. One must also keep an open mind to new observations because we do not have a long history and comfort with many of the new therapies for cancer.[6,7]

BOX 21.1
Goals for the development of cardio-oncology as a discipline

Manage health care costs

Avoid polypharmacy

Improve the application of guideline based diagnosis and treatment

Be mindful of overtesting and defensive medicine

Carefully assess barriers to effective clinical care

Commit to collective research in the field

Share our experiences with other colleagues

1215 21st Avenue South, Suite 5209, Nashville, TN 37232, USA
E-mail address: daniel.lenihan@vanderbilt.edu

BOX 21.2
Principles for the practice of cardio-oncology

Understand the patient is vulnerable and is asked to do a lot already

You can provide your best cardiac care and that will prevent or minimize cardiac limitation

A quality cardiovascular consultation will have a huge impact on the cancer care provided

A vibrant collaboration with other colleagues outside of your primary area is very rewarding

Disciplined reporting of clinical observations is imperative for patient safety

Keep your mind open to new observations because we do not have a long history and comfort with new medications and treatments

Patients and families are universally appreciative of an effective health care team that communicates well

Therefore, exactly how is cardio-oncology as a discipline actually done at a particular location? The "how-to" is outlined in specific areas in subsequent chapters. In my experience of setting up a cardio-oncology practice personally in 2 different locations and institutions as well as directly observing many other situations firsthand, I would suggest the goals and principles discussed form the blueprint, and the actual building of a "cardio-oncology house" requires the following: (1) a true interest in assisting and supporting a patient with cancer through their complex journey; (2) a recognition that sound cardiac-based treatment, including prevention strategies, will have a major positive impact on the overall outcome; and (3) truly understanding that being part of good team is always fun.[8]

SUPPLEMENTARY MATERIAL

Go to ExpertConsult.com to listen to an interview with the author.

REFERENCES

1. Yoon GJ, Telli ML, Kao DP, et al. Left ventricular dysfunction in patients receiving cardiotoxic cancer therapies are clinicians responding optimally? J Am Coll Cardiol 2010;56:1644–50.
2. Sarkiss MG, Yusuf SW, Warneke CL, et al. Impact of aspirin therapy in cancer patients with thrombocytopenia and acute coronary syndromes. Cancer 2007; 109:621–7.
3. Ewer MS, Vooletich MT, Durand JB, et al. Reversibility of trastuzumab-related cardiotoxicity: new insights based on clinical course and response to medical treatment. J Clin Oncol 2005;23: 7820–6.
4. O'Gara PT, Ness DL, Harold JG. Medical professionalism and the American College of Cardiology: a renewed commitment. J Am Coll Cardiol 2015;65: 503–6.
5. O'Gara PT, Oetgen WJ. Innovation and implementation in cardiovascular medicine: challenges in the face of opportunity. JAMA 2015;313:1007–8.
6. Hall PS, Harshman LC, Srinivas S, et al. The frequency and severity of cardiovascular toxicity from targeted therapy in advanced renal cell carcinoma patients. JACC Heart Fail 2013;1:72–8.
7. Khakoo AY, Kassiotis CM, Tannir N, et al. Heart failure associated with sunitinib malate: a multitargeted receptor tyrosine kinase inhibitor. Cancer 2008;112: 2500–8.
8. Lenihan DJ. Tyrosine kinase inhibitors: can promising new therapy associated with cardiac toxicity strengthen the concept of teamwork? J Clin Oncol 2008;26:5154–5.

CHAPTER 22

Structure and Implementation of Cardio-oncology Care

Joerg Herrmann, MD[a,*], Maria Chiara Todaro, MD[b], Bijoy K. Khandheria, MD[c]

CARDIO-ONCOLOGY AT NON-PRIMARY CANCER CENTERS

Cardiology services at major primary cancer centers such as MD Anderson and Sloan Kettering and other institutions have a distinctly different history. At non-primary cancer centers, the different service lines grew independently, and cardiology services were not started and integrated to fulfill the special needs of 1 patient population such as those with cancer. Accordingly, the initiation, development, and establishment of a cardio-oncology clinic or service line at those centers are met with various challenges.[1]

In distinction from primary cancer centers with a defined scenario, the initial challenged is the vision and the mission at other institutions. At nonprimary cancer centers, awareness might not be a given, and once raised, there is the need to outline, and sometimes even prove, the need and demand for this line of service. An example in the published literature is the Cardiac Oncology Clinic at the Ottawa Hospital Cancer Center, where more than 400 patients were seen in the first 50 months, more than 50% being patients with breast cancer (but also gastrointestinal, genitourinary, and hematological malignancies).[2] These numbers the initial experience at the Mayo Clinic Rochester with a notable increase in demand over time (100% increase to 15 patients per months from 2014 to 2015) and changing referral patterns. However, even if there is demand, a common next question is if oncologists and hematologists would not be able to look after these patients. In fact, oncologists and hematologists have done so for numerous years, and it therefore sometimes also becomes a matter of mindset and openness to practice changes. From an administration perspective, any additional service requires additional resources, which includes far more than physician interest in this field, namely appointment coordinators, desk staff, and possibly even nurses, nurse practitioners, and pharmacists. These conceptual, logistical, and financial aspects are not minute, and institutional support is paramount.

Secondly, it is a key necessity that those who provide cardio-oncology service not only have an interest but also a commitment and availability as well as in-depth expertise in this area. With these traits, the cardio-oncologist can take some of the demands in an ever more complex practice environment and add to the care of the patient in a very practical and meaningful way. In order to provide expert consultations, physicians as well as paramedicals involved in cardio-oncology need to receive, expand, and maintain specialized education in this field. Although symptomatic or asymptomatic cardiac dysfunction is often the most common referral reason, arrhythmias, pericardial, valvular, and coronary artery disease are not uncommon referral reasons as are hypertension and prechemotherapy assessment. Indeed, the cardio-oncology clinic can play a crucial part in patients completing their chemotherapy (>80% during or after cardiac therapy in the Ottawa experience).[2] For this reason, the scope of practice and knowledge required for the clinic is quite broad and yet very specific and detailed at the same time to meet the demand of a range of different cancer groups with a range of very

[a] 200 First Street Southwest, Rochester, MN 55905, USA; [b] Via sacro cuore di Gesù 7, Messina 98122, Italy; [c] University of Wisconsin School of Medicine, The Karen Yontz Center for Cardio Oncology at Aurora Health Care, 2801 West Kinnickinnic River Parkway, #840, Milwaukee, WI 53215, USA
* Corresponding author.
E-mail address: herrmann.joerg@mayo.edu

different referral questions. Understandably, very often, a vacuum is present in this area even if the infrastructure could otherwise be built. Accordingly, there is the need for leadership and mentorship. The novelty aspects in this area, lack of evidence-based clinical standards, and relative limited opportunities for education and training pose true barriers. Valuable experience and expertise from primary cancer centers is an invaluable asset for this demand.

A third key element for a successful cardio-oncology clinic, in addition to buy-in and expertise, is collaboration. In distinction from primary cancer centers, which integrate cardiology services naturally into the care of patients with cancer, collaboration becomes a much more active effort at nonprimary cancer centers. Depending on the initiating department, there are different levels of and responses to collaboration efforts. For instance, if the initiative stems from the oncology or hematology group, cardiology departments are likely willing to meet these needs and invest in these endeavors of a large referral population, that is, the focus will be on training cardiologists in cardio-oncology. On the contrary, if a cardio-oncology service line is initiated by cardiologists, then the main need will be to reach out to the oncologists and hematologists and to define the level and extent of interaction for the establishment of a referral practice. Accordingly, the cardiologists need to get to know the oncologists and hematologists and vice versa. No matter where a cardio-oncology clinic gets started, the long-term success depends on the communication and interaction between the disciplines. Approaches to facilitate a cardio-oncology program are highlighted in Table 22.1.

Historically, the decision on the location of a cardio-oncology clinic was made by the existing infrastructures and initiating departments. Ideally, there should be sound thought to this decision whether the cardio-oncology clinic will be in a cancer or cardiovascular (CV) center, because it can greatly influence the success of the clinic. Arguments in favor of one or the other are listed in Table 22.2. The main factors to consider are those that resonate with the 3 essential keys to a successful cardio-oncology clinic outlined above: institutional support (including hospital administration, funding, staffing, and workflow), practice expertise, accessibility, and availability, and collaboration and communication between faculty members. Accordingly, the physical location can have a tremendous impact to further proximity or distance of CV and oncology/hematology clinics and services and opportunities for joint practice and education. Survivorship programs are a prime example for natural integration of CV aspects into the care of patients with cancer. At the end, three main practice models of a cardio-oncology clinic can be envisioned, based on the primary ownership and interaction infrastructure, as illustrated in Fig. 22.1.

In addition to these considerations, which pertain to the outpatient practice, there also is a need for review of demands, scope, and format of inpatient consultation services. Very likely, a deciding factor is the extent of the cancer practice relative to other services offered at an institution. A dedicated cardio-oncology in-patient service would be well placed at a primary cancer center and can be justified at institutions with large cancer care facilities. On the other hand, when a broad spectrum of care is provided in a hospital, it might be more advisable to provide general cardiology consultation services with input from cardio-oncologists as needed and arrangement for cardio-oncology outpatient follow-up.

At the Mayo Clinic Rochester, for instance, the second care model was chosen even though all in-patient cancer service is provided at Rochester Methodist Hospital. However, numerous other patient populations are seen at this hospital as well, including orthopedic patients, gynecologic patients, urology patients, and intensive care patients, which favors a general cardiology consultation service. Also, the staffing needs are too demanding that only those with interest in cardio-oncology could cover completely throughout the year and still staff the outpatient practice. For any emerging cardio-oncology practice, it might be more efficient and effective to invest in an outpatient clinic that can not only cover patient visits but also provide expert advice to in-patient teams, answer curbside questions, and provide consultations that do not require fact-to-face consultation, so-called e-consults. Depending on the initial demand, it might be advisable to start with a half-day clinic and to have at least 1 slot available every day as well as 1 provider available for calls and e-consults. An example of a triage model is outlined in Fig. 22.2.

In summary, the key steps in establishing a Cardio-oncology clinic may be summarized as follows:

- Step 1: Interaction between oncologists, hematologists, and cardiologists
- Step 2: Defining the need for a cardio-oncology service line
- Step 3: Outlining the scope of cardio-oncology practice at the individual institution
- Step 4: Organizing a comprehensive program that meets the specific institutional needs

TABLE 22.1
Approaches to facilitate a cardio-oncology service line

Process Measures	Methods
Creating awareness	• Educating and establishing cognizance of the necessity for cardio-oncology within the entire hospital, including other physicians, physician extenders, nurses, and administrative staff including the hospital leaders and decision-makers • May involve multiple presentations on the necessity for and embodiment of cardio-oncology at different forums, including hospital grand rounds, various administrative committees, hospital symposia, and so on • The onco-cardiologist should be prepared to attend (and even seek) meetings with leadership and be prepared with relevant highlights on what necessitates this field
Patient education	• Seminars, community events, symposia, and so on • Informs patients to be attentive to the downstream effects of their cancer therapy • Patients are generally interested in learning how to care for their health and may seek out the onco-cardiologist especially for this reason
Hospital staff education	• Includes teaching and providing educational materials on cardio-oncology; CV risks of cancer therapeutic agents; diagnoses, management, and treatment; when to refer to cardio-oncology; as well as updates in the published data • Lectures on various cardio-oncology topics should be provided to medical trainees and house staff
Organizing a comprehensive program	• Should involve exchange of patient information with discussions and updates on change in clinical status
Input at oncology forums	• Includes tumor board conferences and oncology grand rounds • Makes for more comprehensive decision making on cancer therapies and overall patient care; oncologists value this sort of input
Providing evidence of growth	• Eventually necessary to convince administration of the need for cardio-oncology • Alerts administration to the need for resources and/or the fact that already provided resources are being applied in a constructive manner
Providing outcome data	Providing data on better patient outcomes as a result of the establishment of a cardio-oncology clinic would provide the ultimate driving force for establishment and growth of the program

From Okwuosa TM, Barac A. Burgeoning cardio-oncology programs: challenges and opportunities for early career cardiologists/faculty directors. J Am Coll Cardiol 2015;66(10):1193–7; with permission.

Step 5: Seeking institutional support
Step 6: Developing an infrastructure for clinical practice
Step 7: Educating the clinic staff
Step 8: Commitment to practice and continuous education
Step 9: Planning of joint conferences and meetings

STRUCTURE AND IMPLEMENTATION OF CARDIO-ONCOLOGY CARE IN GROUP PRACTICES

The survival rate of patients with cancer, as well as those with CV disease, has greatly increased over the past 3 decades; moreover, most of the common CV risk factors, such as obesity, alcohol abuse, and smoking, are also predisposing conditions to cancer and, as consequence, it is increasingly probable that a patient may have both cancer and CV disease. The increase in survival is partially explained by early diagnosis, improvements in anticancer pharmacologic treatment, and more tailored therapeutic approaches.

The use of chemotherapeutic agents, radiation therapy, and molecular-targeted therapies is an approach that can injure the CV system, both at a central level by deteriorating the heart function and in the periphery by inducing hypertension and/or thrombotic events, often present in oncology patients.[1]

TABLE 22.2
Pros and cons of cardio-oncology clinic locations

	Cardio-oncology Clinic in Cardiovascular Center	Cardio-oncology Clinic in Cancer Center
Pros	• Support staff that are familiar with the spectrum of CV disease • Patient and provider proximity to CV services such as ECG and echocardiography services	• Easy patient access to cardio-oncology • Capacity for more comprehensive patient care • Improved contact with the oncologists for immediate questions, consultations, and tumor board opinions, and a generally more inclusive care of the patient with cancer
Cons	• Loss of exclusivity to the special needs of the patient with cancer • Lack of awareness by the oncologists about a special cardiology service dedicated to serving their patients • Less spontaneous consultations and interactions between oncologists and serving cardiologist(s), which may hamper the evolution of a comprehensive service	• Limited access to CV studies such as ECG, echocardiography, and stress tests (depending on size and funding in institution) • Less availability of staff trained in performing ECGs/other cardiac studies, and can answer cardiac questions/educate patients on cardiac care
Circumvent the cons	• The cardiologist should be proactive in fostering relationships with the oncologist and the oncology team • Attendance—and contribution to—tumor board conferences and oncology grand rounds with the goal of integrating the cardio-oncologist into the day-to-day practices of the oncology team • Additional training of the cardiology clinic staff, including knowledge of common chemotherapies with relevance to CV health, need for more frequent monitoring, psychosocial needs of the patient with cancer, and so on	• ECG, and possibly, echocardiography machine(s)/services in the cancer center to effect more efficient CV diagnosis and care of these patients • Institute effective transportation between the cardiac imaging center and oncology clinic • Train oncology staff in CV care and assistance (including performing ECGs)

Abbreviation: ECG, electrocardiogram.
From Okwuosa TM, Barac A. Burgeoning cardio-oncology programs: challenges and opportunities for early career cardiologists/faculty directors. J Am Coll Cardiol 2015;66(10):1193–7; with permission.

For this reason, cardiology and oncology in the past few years have developed a tight connection, and specialists now collaborate in order to achieve the global health of the patient. This multi-disciplinary interaction is evolving not only at major medical centers but also in group practices. The focus has been on cardiotoxicity as one of the most common and feared complications with direct impact on the quality of life, life expectancy, and option of further cancer therapy.

CARDIOTOXICITY PREVENTION

Drug-associated cardiotoxicity is defined as 1 or more of the following: (1) cardiomyopathy, in terms of a reduction in left ventricular ejection fraction (LVEF), either global or more severe in the septum; (2) symptoms associated with heart failure (HF); (3) signs associated with HF, such as S3 gallop, tachycardia, or both; (4) reduction in LVEF from baseline that is in the range of less than or equal to 5% to less than 55% with accompanying signs or symptoms of HF, or a reduction in LVEF in the range of equal to or greater than 10% to less than 55%, without accompanying signs or symptoms.

This definition does not include subclinical CV damage that may occur early in response to some chemotherapeutic agents.[2] However, identification of early myocardial damage before its

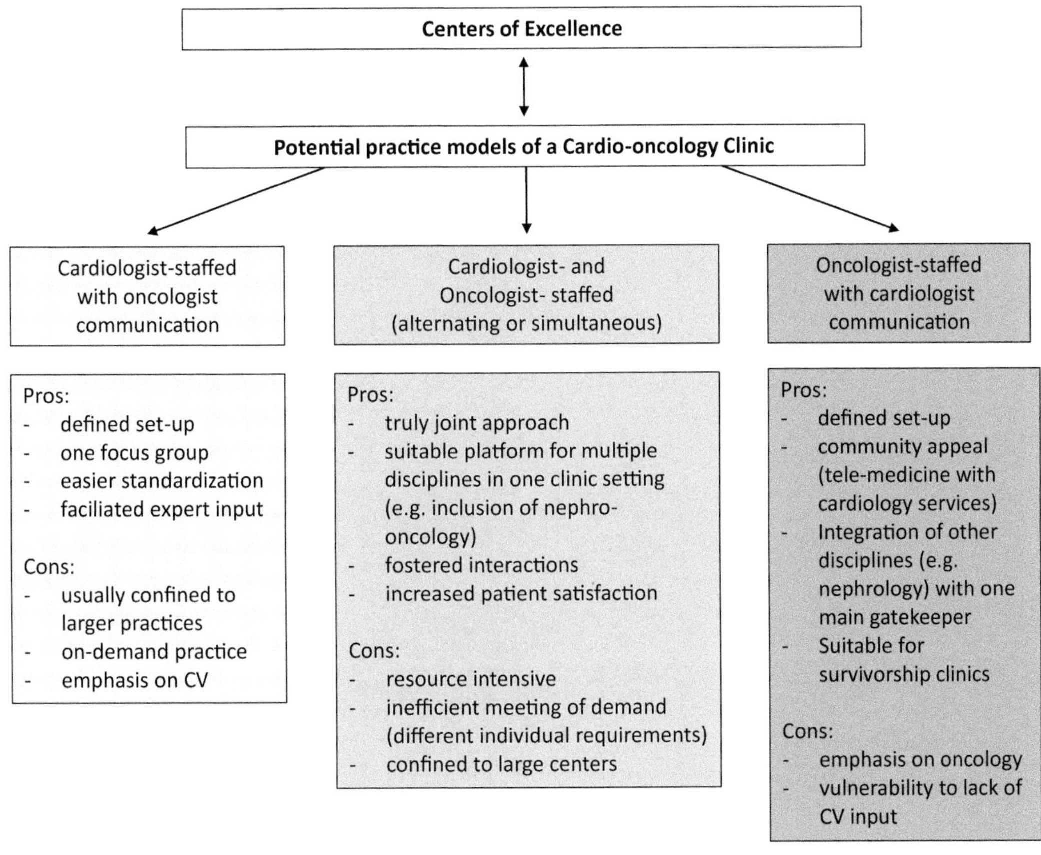

Fig. 22.1 Number of cardio-oncology consultations at the Mayo Clinic Rochester in 2014 and 2015 and the growth in demand over time.

phenotypic expression is key and can be accomplished through accurate selection of patient candidates receiving potentially cardiotoxic treatments and the prompt initiation of appropriate clinical, and when needed, instrumental follow-up.

Clinical and instrumental surveillance should be carried out before, during, and after treatment and should be tailored to the most common toxic effect caused by the specific chemotherapeutic agent used. For example, anthracyclines are generally associated with irreversible type I cardiac dysfunction and require a closer follow-up that necessarily will include periodic evaluation of ejection fraction and left ventricular (LV) longitudinal function by echocardiography.

An increasing role in the early identification of patients at risk of developing myocardial damage is attributed to biomarkers. Cardinale and colleagues[3] demonstrated that the systematic use of troponin I obtains both qualitative (identification of patients at risk) and quantitative information (the higher the troponin level, the higher the functional cardiac damage). Moreover, thanks to the high negative predictive value of troponin I (99%), it is possible to identify patients at low risk of developing cardiac events, limiting close cardiologic surveillance to "troponin-positive patients."

Brain natriuretic peptide (BNP) and its amino-terminal peptide (NT-proBNP) are also widely used and validated in clinical practice for diagnostic and prognostic purposes in HF and have been identified as possible predictors of LV dysfunction during chemotherapy. However, although higher levels of both BNP and NT-proBNP were observed during chemotherapy (doxorubuicin, trastuzumab, epirubicin treatment) and radiotherapy, contrasting evidence on their role in both adult and pediatric populations has limited their routine use in clinical practice.[4]

In private practice, the accomplishment of this ambitious target might be hampered by reimbursement issues and cost-effectiveness problems related to echocardiographic surveillance and measurement of troponin levels at baseline as well as during and after treatment. On the

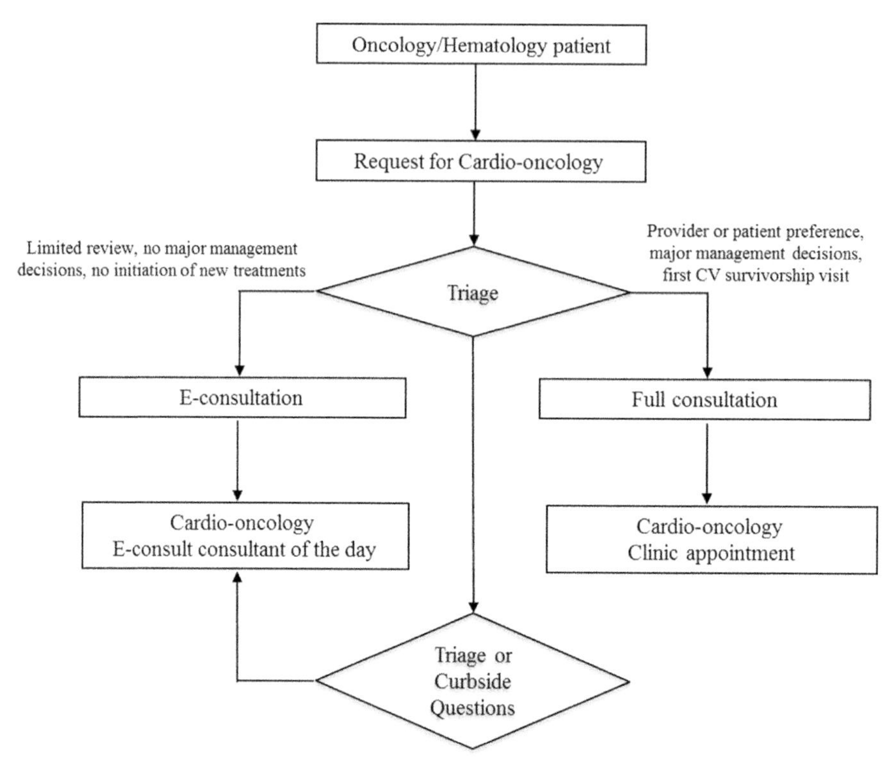

Fig. 22.2 Cardio-oncology triage model used at the Mayo Clinic Rochester.

other hand, general practitioners and physicians in private practices should be aware of the clinical relevance of cardio-oncology and encouraged to implement cardio-oncology prevention programs. Informative seminars and meetings between specialists working in referral cen ters and private practice physicians could play a key role.

CARDIO-ONCOLOGY COOPERATION IN PRACTICE

The impelling need of cooperation between cardiologists and oncologists led to the formation of the International CardiOncology Society (ICOS) in 2010, whose aim is to facilitate communication among specialists and develop best practice models.[5] The goals of ICOS can be summarized as follows:

1. Eliminate cardiac disease as a barrier to effective cancer therapy;
2. Prevent the development of HF wherever possible;
3. Establish a multi-institutional and international database;
4. Promote the development of clinical decisions with optimal patient outcomes as the focal point;
5. Develop Web-based educational tools and interactive case study questions;
6. Develop the Common Terminology Criteria, to include sophisticated cardiac-based diagnostic tools and ultimately extend these common reporting criteria to CV clinical research;
7. Disseminate practical multidisciplinary guidelines, which are lacking at the moment, for cardiac monitoring of cancer treatments.

It is important to emphasize that this network is not only for those in referral centers but also for physicians in private and group practices. For obvious reasons, it is important to have at least 1 physician in this group taking the lead and providing organization; this could be in the form of units or clinics.

FROM A DISEASE-CENTERED TO A PATIENT-CENTERED ORGANIZATION: THE CREATION OF "CARDIO-ONCOLOGY" INTERDISCIPLINARY CLINICAL UNITS

In private practice, the cardio-oncology consultation focuses almost exclusively on patients who will receive potentially cardiotoxic drugs, ideally tailored to the patient and type of chemotherapy that he or she will receive. For this purpose, it

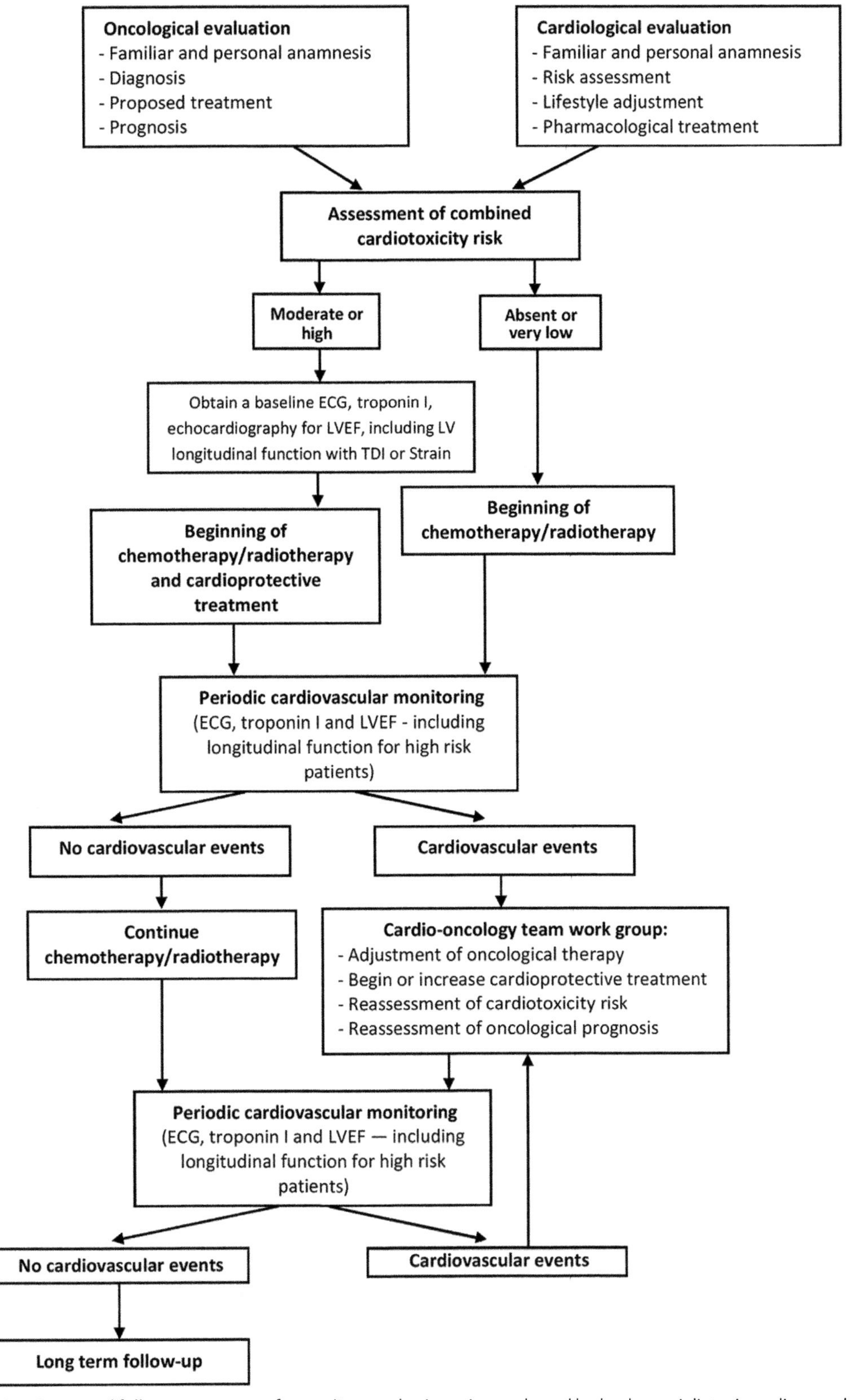

Fig. 22.3 Proposed follow-up program for cardio-oncologic patients, shared by both specialists. A cardio-oncologic unit with a dedicated multidisciplinary team would promote the centrality of the patients, encouraging the best clinical care especially for those at high risk.

could be opportune to produce a source document for each patient showing personal CV risk factors (family history for coronary artery disease, age, obesity, cigarette smoking, hypertension, diabetes, and so forth), previous history of coronary artery disease (previous percutaneous or surgical myocardial revascularization), and functional capacity through patient's exercise tolerance assessment and administration of questionnaires for angina score evaluation. On the same document, the site of primitive tumor, the eventual involvement of organs, and finally, the oncologic prognosis of the patient should be clearly indicated. An ideal organization of interdisciplinary cardio-oncology units should contemplate dedicated periodic meetings where each patient is discussed, individual CV risk profile is defined by cardiologists, a chemotherapeutic and/or radiotherapeutic approach is proposed by oncologists, an integrated cardiotoxicity risk score is derived from interdisciplinary evaluation, and, finally, a patient-tailored follow-up program is arranged by both specialists (Fig. 22.3). This system will lead to a targeted follow-up based on the cocktail of drugs the patient will receive and the most common side effect produced on the CV system. In this way, a patient-centered attitude will be promoted over a pathology-centered attitude, reducing the chance of patients surviving cancer, being defeated by irreversible HF.

A suitable cardio-oncology care model in private practice thus consists of expert medical doctors on staff that periodically check the clinical status of patients with a high level of suspicion for oncologic disease and CV risk stratification. Practical steps toward establishing such a model in private practice include accurate medical history, physical examination, laboratory tests, and clinical questionnaires. Patients with suspected oncologic disease and high CV risk burden should be referred to a cardio-oncology prevention protocol as the one proposed in Fig. 22.3.

The main challenges are related to the need of a strong link between private practices and main reference hospitals for cardio-oncology care. However, the patient will be the first to benefit from this widespread organization model, because most of the care for these patients is ambulatory, thus justifying the possibility and need for the expansion to group practices whose care model is not hospital based.

This system will lead to a targeted follow-up based on the cocktail of drugs the patient will receive and the most common side effect produced on the CV system. In this way, a patient-centered attitude will be promoted over a pathology-centered attitude, reducing the chance of patients surviving cancer being defeated by irreversible HF.

REFERENCES

1. Okwuosa TM, Barac A. Burgeoning cardio-oncology programs: challenges and opportunities for early career cardiologists/faculty directors. J Am Coll Cardiol 2015;66(10):1193–7.
2. Sulpher J, Mathur S, Graham N, et al. Clinical experience of patients referred to a multidisciplinary cardiac oncology clinic: an observational study. J Oncol 2015;2015:671232.
3. Cardinale D, Sandri MT, Martinoni A, et al. Left ventricular dysfunction predicted by early troponin I release after high-dose chemotherapy. J Am Coll Cardiol 2000;36:517–22.
4. Tian S, Hirshfield KM, Jabbour SK, et al. Serum biomarkers for the detection of cardiac toxicity after chemotherapy and radiation therapy in breast cancer patients. Front Oncol 2014;4:277.
5. Lenihan DJ, Cardinale D, Cipolla CM. The compelling need for a cardiology and oncology partnership and the birth of the International CardiOncology Society. Prog Cardiovasc Dis 2010;53(2):88–93.

CHAPTER 23

Cardio-oncology Fellowship Programs

Ana Barac, MD, PhD[a,*], Rupal O'Quinn, MD[b], Susan Dent, MD[c], Olexie Aseyev, MD, PhD[d], Joseph R. Carver, MD[e]

EDUCATIONAL NEEDS AND GOALS

Educational needs in cardio-oncology are broad and rapidly growing, in reflection of the dynamic nature of this multidisciplinary field. Although resources and tools are needed to advance the education of a spectrum of health care providers that participate in the cardiovascular care of patients with active cancer and cancer survivors,[1] here the focus is on the educational gaps and opportunities within fellowship programs that provide training and education for cardiovascular disease specialists.

The national cardio-oncology survey of adult and pediatric cardiology program directors conducted in May 2014 identified the lack of educational resources as an important barrier for the development of cardio-oncology programs, together with the lack of guidelines, lack of funding, and limited infrastructure.[1] In the same report, participating program directors, 76% of whom came from the academic centers, noted that they would be likely to use educational and training materials if they were available. Professional societies have a long-standing legacy of supporting their members through creation and dissemination of knowledge and development and implementation of professional standards of training. An excellent example is the recommendations for training in adult cardiovascular disease that evolved with the growth of cardiovascular specialty: a consensus statement of the Core Cardiology Training Symposium held at the American College of Cardiology (ACC) Heart House in June 2014 represented the basis for what is known as the Core Cardiology Training Statement, under the commonly used acronym "COCATS,"[2] that provides guidelines for training of cardiovascular specialists. Both the original and subsequently the updated COCATS documents follow the recommendations of the Accreditation Council for Graduate Medical Education (ACGME) that regulates training in internal medicine and subspecialties and establishes infrastructure and program content requirements for program accreditation. With the growth of the cardiovascular field and increasing needs for further subspecialty training, updated COCATS documents have continued to add content components, such as multimodality imaging, critical care cardiology, and vascular medicine in the most recent COCATS4.[3] These areas also demonstrate how standardization of training requirements and delineation of competencies not only meets the needs for trained workforce but importantly also advances the field by providing a path for faculty and facility development, the incorporation of technologies, and the dissemination of knowledge.[4]

The overarching educational goal of the cardio-oncology fellowship program is to improve care of patients with cancer and cancer survivors by increasing the understanding and ability to modify the interactions between cancer, cancer treatment, and cardiovascular health. For cardiovascular specialists, this includes understanding of the basic principles and types of cancer therapies, their cardiovascular complications, optimization of cardiovascular risk factors, monitoring

[a] MedStar Heart and Vascular Institute, Georgetown University, Washington, DC, USA; [b] Penn Heart and Vascular Center, Perelman Center for Advanced Medicine, Philadelphia, PA 19104, USA; [c] The Ottawa Hospital Cancer Centre, Division of Medical Oncology, Ottawa, Ontario, Canada; [d] The Ottawa Hospital Cancer Center, Department of Medicine, University of Ottawa, Ottawa, Ontario, Canada; [e] Abramson Family Cancer Research Institute, Abramson Cancer Center of the University of Pennsylvania, Philadelphia, PA, USA
* Corresponding author. MedStar Heart and Vascular Institute, Georgetown University, 110 Irving street, NW, 1F1218, Washington DC, 20010, USA
E-mail address: ana.barac@medstar.net

and early detection of toxicities during active cancer treatment, management of toxicities, as well as extended surveillance during cancer survivorship. The importance of training in cardiovascular research and scholarly activity has been recognized as an integral component of COCATS 4,[5] and it is an essential area of training in cardio-oncology. Understanding of basic and translational research is particularly relevant in this field, wherein interactions of novel molecular therapies with cardiovascular systems continue to provide unique insights into cardiovascular (patho)physiology, thus opening new horizons for cardiovascular disease treatments.[6] Similarly, understanding of and participation in clinical and epidemiology research, charged with broad aims of developing cancer treatment–related evidence-based guidelines for cardiovascular risk prevention and treatment, development of care coordination, and implementation of standards and evaluation measures[7] will form an important part of training in cardio-oncology. In addition to recognizing growing professional needs, the national cardio-oncology survey identified several ongoing educational and training activities,[1] primarily in tertiary academic centers, that are forming a fertile ground for coordination of efforts and creation of professional standards for practice and training. A conceptual framework for cardio-oncology training development using the overarching ACGME 6 domain structure is provided in Box 23.1.

Collaboration among active tertiary cardio-oncology centers and professional groups, such

BOX 23.1
A conceptual framework of cardio-oncology training within Accreditation Council for Graduate Medical Education core competencies

1. Patient care
   - To deliver compassionate, appropriate, and effective cardiovascular care to patients undergoing cancer therapies and cancer survivors
2. Medical knowledge
   - Knowledge of cardiovascular effects of agents used in cancer treatment
   - Understanding of cardiovascular complications of diverse cancer therapies in the acute setting and long- term cardiovascular risks in cancer survivorship
   - Knowledge of cardiovascular monitoring, including cardiovascular imaging and use of biomarkers
   - Knowledge of cardiovascular intervention and treatment strategies specific to patients undergoing cancer treatment
3. Practice-based learning and improvement
   - Participation in cardio-oncology studies, including basic, translational, and clinical research with the following aims: (a) to improve the understanding of the mechanisms of cardiovascular effects of cancer therapies, (b) to advance monitoring techniques, and (c) to develop and implement early prevention and treatment strategies
   - Presentation of clinical cases and development of practice improvement initiatives
4. Interpersonal and communication skills
   - Active participation in multidisciplinary forums, such as tumor board and understanding of the critical role of a multidisciplinary approach to patient care
   - Promotion of interdisciplinary communication and collaborative decision making with other health care professionals involved in the care of patients with cancer and cancer survivors
5. Professionalism
   - Adherence to ethical principles and sensitivity to complex psychological, medical, and social issues of patients with cancer
   - Professional commitment to contribute to dialogue and facilitate decision making in complex and life-threatening situations
6. Systems-based practice
   - Integration of care through interdisciplinary platforms, such as incorporating cardiovascular monitoring and intervention strategies in observational and therapeutic oncology trials as well as cancer survivorship programs

as International CardiOncology Society and Canadian Cardiac Oncology Network Cardio-oncology and ACC's Cardio-oncology Section, will be important in setting milestones for different levels of training and delineation of cardio-oncology–specific professional activities in different domains, such as cardiovascular consultation, acute care, cardiovascular testing, disease prevention, and lifelong learning.

In summary, the cardio-oncology field has seen an impressive growth of research and clinical activities over the last decade[1] that provide a rich platform for creation of educational and training curriculum and, in turn, lead to further synchronized advancement of the field.

CURRICULUM ORGANIZATION

The recognition of the important interrelationship between cardiology and oncology has been recognized as well as the impact on the patient with cancer from diagnosis, through treatment and survivorship.[8] The increased understanding of cancer biology, advances in cancer therapy, and improved survivorship strategies over the past 2 decades has increased the number of both adult and pediatric cancer survivors, with almost 19 million predicted by 2024, up from 3 million in 1971.[9] Although cardiotoxicity can develop during the acute management of cancer, most patients remain at risk for cardiovascular complications for the rest of their lifetime.[8,10–19] In adult survivors of pediatric malignancies, treatment-related cardiac death remains the top noncancer cause of mortality.[20–22] Despite the growing realization of the importance of long-term follow-up care for cancer survivors, as well as the many evidence-based clinical guidelines for the diagnosis and treatment of cancer, there is a paucity of evidence-based clinical care guidelines giving recommendations about survivorship.[23] There are even fewer guidelines/position statements addressing surveillance for cardiovascular issues, such as cardiomyopathy,[24] ischemic heart disease,[25,26] and so forth. As a result, cancer survivors who are at risk of cardiovascular effects from their cancer treatment may present years later after a prolonged asymptomatic latency period with advanced cancer-induced cardiac damage. A multidisciplinary and comprehensive team focused on a collaborative effort that includes the expertise of individuals with expertise in cardio-oncology is critical in optimizing patient outcomes, even after the malignancy has been treated.

The aforementioned survey, through the ACC, showed that 2 of 3 hospital centers across the United States added cardio-oncology services in response to this growing patient need.[27] This is reflected in the burgeoning number of new cardio-oncology programs.[28,29] In addition, the survey highlighted that 43% of the centers did not offer formal training to fellows or house-staff in the growing discipline of cardio-oncology. There is clearly a need to establish a formal structure to train the future generation of cardio-oncologists.

When we speak of cardio-oncologists, who are we talking about? Cardio-oncologists are medical providers who are focused on the cardiovascular health of patients who have, or had, cancer. They help ensure that optimal cancer treatment is administered by preventing, or at least mitigating, treatment-related cardiotoxicity whenever possible. They shoulder the responsibility of managing any resulting cardiovascular complications to avoid limiting effective cancer therapy. They also play a role in the management and treatment of any cardiovascular effects that either exist before treatment or occur as a result of the cancer therapy, or cancer itself. Cardio-oncologists also endeavor to improve clinical cardiovascular care, enhance education, and promote research for patients who have an active or prior history of malignancy.

Despite the known complex interaction between cancer, its treatment, underlying cardiovascular disease, and the cardiovascular effects of the cancer and its treatment, most cardiologists and oncologists are not trained in, or are unaware of, the multifaceted relationship between these parameters, and how to navigate them to ensure that patient management is optimized.[26] There is thus a growing need to add formal cardio-oncology modules to basic/traditional training curriculum as well as postfellowship advanced training to those individuals who have already received formal instruction in the fields of cardiovascular diseases or hematology/oncology.

The Goals of a Cardio-oncology Training Program

The goals of cardio-oncology training are listed in Box 23.2 and focus on knowledge, patient care, and research with an overarching goal of delivering optimal cost-effective care to patients with cancer from diagnosis through long-term survivorship.

The cardiovascular trainee

Starting with a basic cardiovascular knowledge base, training should increase the awareness of the natural history and treatment options for common cancers along with an understanding of evolving cancer treatments that include surgery,

BOX 23.2
Goals of cardio-oncology training

To acquire basic knowledge in a "nondominant" discipline (pathophysiology, treatment complications, "jargon")
To receive leveled intensity training in cardio-oncology based on trainee's career path
To be involved in a facility with a comprehensive cardiology-oncology infrastructure
To recognize and address/triage common cancer treatment complications
To improve cardiology and oncology care

chemotherapy, targeted agents, and radiotherapy. A basic understanding of the mechanism of action of anticancer therapies with special emphasis on the types, pathophysiology, and prevalence of known cardiac side effects are fundamental and critical skills to becoming a cardio-oncologist. Because cancer treatment has become a rapidly evolving and dynamic process with new drug approvals and the use of new combinations of old drugs, so too does the landscape of cardiotoxicity evolve. It is essential that training also stress the availability and use of oncology data sources to maintain and enhance expertise during and following formal training.

Training should also provide an advanced understanding of systemic effects of cancer and potential oncologic emergencies affecting the cardiovascular system (eg, tumor lysis syndrome, disseminated intravascular coagulation), as well as their management, and oncologic pharmacology that specifically affects the cardiovascular system.

After providing a strong fundamental oncology knowledge base ("Oncology 101"), the next goal is to focus on early detection of cancer treatment-related cardiac injury at every stage of cancer care starting with basic risk assessment and risk factor modification at diagnosis to follow-up evaluation coupled with the use of biomarkers and imaging.[30–42]

Trainees should learn which treatments effectively prevent, reduce, or treat the cardiac consequences of cancer therapy. They should also share this education with relevant health care providers in order to maximize the benefits of cancer treatment for patients while minimizing the potential toxicity to the cardiovascular system.

The trainee should be able to use his/her knowledge to not only understand the complicated relationships between cancer and the cardiovascular system but also be able to use this new awareness to modify the interactions between cancer treatment and cardiovascular disease.

Given that cardio-oncology is a relatively new discipline, the importance of research touching upon all aspects of this field cannot be overemphasized. Basic science research and translational research are necessary to further the understanding of the myriad ways in which different cancer therapies impact the cellular level of the cardiovascular system, causing widespread effects that are clinically relevant at the time of therapy as well as years later. Basic science research can help the development of effective cardioprotective strategies (finally answer the question of the value/risks of dexrazoxane as a treatment to mitigate cardiac toxicity in adults undergoing therapy with anthracyclines[43,44]) and ultimately will unlock the genetic keys to susceptibility and cardiac protection that currently are not understood.

Advanced imaging training and imaging research are also important components to nurture. Cost-effective screening tools and reproducible and valid imaging parameters must be developed based on the pathophysiology of cardiotoxicity that can reliably predict early, preclinical disease and enable the discovery of prevention and treatment strategies. Research in different imaging modalities, including echocardiography and cardiac magnetic resonance, continue to broaden the ways of detecting cardiotoxicity[30–41] as well as providing tools that potentially can determine prognosis. Prospective clinical trials will continue to help validate these strategies, and fine-tune them to offer maximum benefit to patients. Further work in outcomes research and epidemiology is necessary to guide in identifying cancer survivors most at risk in developing cardiotoxicity both during and after treatment of their cancer. Trainees should participate in one of the many burgeoning areas of research in cardio-oncology.

The oncology trainee

Training for oncologists in cardio-oncology takes on a slightly different focus. Existing training programs already stress the cancer aspect of this specialty—from natural history to treatment pharmacokinetics and a strong foundation of oncology is a given.

These trainees need a refresher in "Cardiology 101" to refresh and review an understanding of the pathophysiology of the cardiovascular system with a focus on the common cellular pathways shared by the cardiovascular system and cancer's effect on involved organs. In addition, these trainees should acquire a basic understanding of how to use and interpret cardiac imaging modalities (such as electrocardiography, echocardiography, and stress tests) and biomarkers to diagnose as well as monitor the cardiac effects of cancer therapy.

The goals of training are therefore related to enhancing bedside diagnostic and examination skills, reinforcement of the natural history of myocardial, coronary, pericardial, and electrophysiological disease and how best to use the existing biomarker and imaging modalities in cost-effective patient care.

Those with a background in hematology/oncology should have a general familiarity with the presentation, evaluation, and treatment of the common cardiac comorbidities and common cardiovascular side effects of cancer therapy that include hypertension, heart failure and cardiomyopathy, arrhythmias (especially supraventricular), coronary ischemia, pericardial disease, and vascular complications. They, too, should have a comfortable familiarity with the cardiovascular effects of common cancer treatments.

Participation in research as described for the cardiovascular trainee is similarly relevant and a critical component of training.

Common components

For both the cardiology and the oncology trainee and their programs, there must be a formal didactic curriculum and ability to care for both inpatients and outpatients. The differences between basic training (a rotation or block of time) and advanced training (cardio-oncology specialization) are basically differences in time of exposure, volume of patient experiences, and time dedicated to research that will be described subsequently.

In the community

Family practice and internal medicine practitioners represent the "army" of caregivers for most cancer survivors. They are on the frontlines to detect subclinical cardiotoxicity and cancer-treatment–induced cardiac problems. They should have continuing medical education (CME) opportunities to better understand and recognize the more common cardiovascular complications that can occur after cancer treatment and when to refer to cardio-oncology and to be updated on the cardiovascular effects of emerging therapies as well as the ever-changing recommendations for cardiac risk factor modification.

The institutional requirements for training in cardio-oncology are listed in Box 23.3 and require an existing cardio-oncology program. The definition of the latter is broad but minimally requires either or both a cardiologist and medical oncologist with expertise through dedicated patient care experience, time spent shadowing recognized cardio-oncologists, a clinical research focus that includes cardio-oncology publications, and/or participation in past and ongoing national and international cardio-oncology conferences. Having a dedicated professional, cardiologist or an oncologist, with expertise in cardio-oncology field is a starting point for didactic teaching and basic trainee exposure and to transmit the basic principles that can be taught and included in fellowship curriculum.

BOX 23.3
Institutional requirements for cardio-oncology training

Institutional commitment (financial, promotion, support personnel)

People (cardiologists and/or oncologists with dedicated practice time for specialty)

"Comprehensive services" (cancer center) for patient disease diversity and volume

Full range of cardiovascular services (diagnostic and interventional)

For more advanced training, at least one clinician with a dedicated practice in cardio-oncology with dedicated practice time to see patients with cancer with cardiac issues or cardiac patients with cancer is a minimal requirement. There is no preset amount of dedicated practice time—for a rotation, a small percentage of time may be sufficient, that is, 1 or 2 outpatient clinics per week. For a posttraining completion fellowship, it has to be a larger percentage of time with potential exposure to multiple outpatient clinics and inpatient consultation. For example, at the Abramson Cancer Center in Philadelphia, 2 cardiologists spend 100% of their time practicing cardio-oncology and 1 cardiologist spends 80% of their time focused on cardio-oncology research and 20% of the time taking care of cardio-oncology patients.

As a start, there has to be a program. Then, there has to be a full spectrum of solid and hematological malignancy patients who have the potential for cardiac toxicity. Exposure to broad oncology pathology requires the equivalence of a comprehensive cancer program with a full cadre of medical oncologists, surgical oncologists, and radiation oncologists complemented by, but not required, a clinical research infrastructure.

Comprehensive cancer program has to coexist with a comprehensive cardiovascular program that offers state-of-the-art cardiac imaging, interventional cardiology and electrophysiology, and cardiothoracic surgery.

Ideally, because collaboration and communication between cardiologists and oncologists are the fundamental precepts, in addition to comprehensive programs and a defined cardio-oncologist or oncocardiologist, the onus for patient referral and program success lies with oncology. Fundamental to a program is the recognition by medical and radiation oncologists that cardiovascular disease—either as pretreatment comorbidity or treatment-related cardiac complications—are prevalent and that comanagement with cardio-oncology is beneficial for everyone so that there is patient flow.

Training requirements

As previously discussed, recognition, evaluation, and treatment of patients with cancer with coexisting cardiac comorbidity or those with complications of cardiotoxic chemotherapy or radiation therapy are important skills for those practicing cardiology and oncology. Recognition of a problem and knowledge about when to refer to a specialist are important skills for family medicine practitioners and internists. All of these practitioners take care of patients with cancer or cancer survivors and should have some exposure to cardio-oncology through educational opportunities, such as cardio-oncology sessions/conferences/presentations, grand rounds, core lectures, CME-based learning, and review articles of relevant topics. Going forward, the authors propose that all cardiology and medical oncology fellowship trainees be exposed to the fundamental concepts of cardio-oncology described above. In order to achieve competency beyond a simple exposure to this area, 3 distinct training levels are defined, as listed in following discussion.

Level 1 training: exposure and basic overview: basic core curriculum. All cardiology and oncology fellowship training programs will provide, at a minimum, a level 1 curriculum in cardio-oncology. The goal of Level 1 training is to provide exposure and appreciation for the nuances of the cardiovascular care in patients with cancer. The goal is not to train cardio-oncologists with this exposure.

Ideally, medical students, residents in internal or family medicine, or medical oncology fellows could take this rotation. The experience would be a combination of core didactic lectures, exposure to a "library" of key review articles, and clinical in-patient and outpatient patient care. More specifically, through these tools, level 1 training will provide a basic familiarity with the classes of cancer drugs and amount/location of radiation that may cause both short-term and long-term functional and/or anatomic changes. For medical oncology fellows, the drug portion would focus on common cardiac medications. Trainees will also develop understanding about the importance of preventing, diagnosing, and monitoring cardiovascular side effects to ensure that optimal cancer therapy can be given and to improve patient outcomes. They will learn about cardiovascular monitoring and treatment in general terms and begin to learn the nuances of the early detection via biomarkers and cardiac imaging modalities. Last, they will develop an understanding of when to refer their patients to more experienced cardio-oncologists if necessary. This rotation could be a minimum of 2 weeks and a maximum of 4 weeks during their training. The goals of level 1 training are listed in Box 23.4.

Level 2 training: advanced clinical experience and knowledge. It is assumed that all participants in level 2 have had a prior level 1 experience. If not, the first month of the rotation would mirror level 1 to assure an exposure to a "core curriculum."

This rotation is for those individuals who wish to broaden their experience with cardio-oncology patients and increase their knowledge about cardio-oncology practices for a minimum of 2 months. This rotation is for trainees who expect more than casual interaction with cardio-oncology patients and allows more primary patient contact and a wider range of clinical experience and the ability to start and/or complete a clinical cardio-oncology research project.

This training should enrich their understanding of the different categories of cancer therapies and their individual potential for cardiac injury. It should acquaint them with the most pertinent

BOX 23.4
Level 1 training goals

- To become familiar with cancer treatments and cardiovascular risk
- To manage cardiac comorbidity in a patient with cancer
- To learn the mode of optimal detection of subclinical cardiac disease
- To understand when to refer a patient to a cardio-oncologist

cardio-oncology trials and research that have shaped the field thus far. After a 2-month exposure, trainees should appreciate the importance of cardiovascular risk assessment and be comfortable with risk factor modification in light of the patient's cancer treatment regimen before starting and during cancer therapy because the basic substrate of pre-existing cardiac risk factors contribute to subsequent complications. Trainees will also understand the need and method to monitor patients for immediate cardiovascular consequences from both a cardiology and an oncologic standpoint.

Because the population of cancer survivors continues to rapidly increase and because survivors may have decades of cancer-free life after treatment completion, a distinct element of the curriculum will be to train clinicians to recognize the potential of late cardiac damage in patients with and especially without the traditional cardiovascular risk factors. This experience should allow the development of a working algorithm for long-term care with regard to surveillance strategies that include the use of biomarkers and cardiac imaging and a familiarity with the pitfalls of these modalities. For the medical oncology fellow, there should be enough exposure to cardiac imaging to provide the opportunity to learn basic cardiac echocardiogram patterns for diagnosis so that they are not just report readers and a basic exposure to cardiac MRI to understand its benefits, indications, and limitations.

The knowledge obtained during this time should enable them to play a role in the multidisciplinary approach to patient care and management, with an understanding about the importance of communication and collaboration among all the members of the team, and the need to continue this relationship with the patient and team members into survivorship. This knowledge base will also allow trainees to understand the complexity of the physical, logistical, and psychosocial issues that patients face not only at the time of diagnosis and during active treatment but also for the rest of their lives as well. After completing level 2 training, individuals should also be able to treat basic problems, feel comfortable in following long-term asymptomatic survivors of potentially cardiotoxic cancer treatment, and recognize which situations call for the need for a referral to providers with greater cardio-oncology experience.

The outpatient clinical experience should include specific cardio-oncology clinics, survivorship clinics, and oncology clinics with exposure tailored to individual trainee preference among all disease-specific cancer clinics. Exposure to the inpatient setting can be accomplished by participating in cardio-oncology consults and/or by rounding with an inpatient hematology/oncology team. The latter has multiple benefits that include a real-time patient-oriented opportunity to learn about different malignancies, their treatment, and complications; to provide the trainee with an opportunity to offer insight into the cardiovascular health and management; and to reinforce the collaborative nature of the subspecialty. In addition to clinical patient exposure, the level 2 trainee in cardio-oncology should also contribute to weekly clinical case conferences and/or multidisciplinary tumor boards and journal clubs. The goals of level 2 training are listed in Box 23.5.

Level 3 training. This level of training is for those who anticipate focusing most of their subsequent clinical or research activities within cardio-oncology to obtain advanced knowledge on prevention, management, and follow-up strategies for patients who experience cardiovascular complications during or following their cancer therapy. Level 3 training is a commitment for an additional 12 months of fellowship training beyond that required for cardiology or medical oncology boards by the American Board of Internal Medicine, that is, a dedicated year to become a cardio-oncologist. At the present time, it is unclear whether this year can be short-tracked in time equal to prior cardio-oncology rotations during prior training. In addition, it is still also unclear whether a trainee can spend the entire third year of fellowship specializing in cardio-oncology similar to spending the third year of a cardiology fellowship in the catheterization laboratory, imaging, electrophysiology, or heart failure or the third year of oncology fellowship in this format. The latter concept is tricky because cardio-oncology is not an approved ACGME rotation at this time.

A fellowship in cardio-oncology should be offered at a center with the characteristics described under Institutional Requirements above. A formal year-long curriculum should take place in a setting that has comprehensive cardiac and

BOX 23.5
Level 2 training goals

- All components of level 1
- To be exposed to a wider range of cardio-oncology patients, including survivorship
- To follow individual patients through their cancer treatment
- To participate in a clinical research project

cancer care for adequate patient volume and complexity of care.

During this year-long exposure, there should be dedicated time for enhancement of basic primary fellowship skills: cardiologists should have regular "reading" time for cardiac studies, and oncology-based trainees should have an equal amount of time to maintain and upgrade the skills basic to their specialty. Both should have a dedicated block in radiation oncology to thoroughly understand the nuances of treatment planning, execution, and its "jargon."

A major benefit of a year-long program is the ability to participate in longitudinal care beyond a one-time consultation. The authors have encouraged and supported the development of a "practice" during the year with the fellow accumulating a cohort of patients that he/she follows. With supervision, they make primary-care decisions and participate on the front-line with day-to-day care recognizing the complexity of long-term care of a cardio-oncology patient and understanding changing cancer and cardiology environments for individual patients and applying that understanding more universally. They should also have the opportunity to care for patients after completion of their active cancer treatment into survivorship.

Level 3 trainees should be expected to participate in the advancement of the discipline through basic science/translational research, participation as coinvestigators in clinical trials and in academic pursuits: writing reviews, book chapters, abstract submissions, or other publications. The authors have also encouraged fellows to give local presentations at their training site, participate in national and international cardio-oncology meetings, and require the completion of an original research project.

Opportunities should exist to obtain increased exposure or training in other areas relevant to cardio-oncology, such as cardiac magnetic resonance, advanced echocardiography techniques such as myocardial strain and 3D image acquisition/interpretation, radiation oncology, PET-computed tomography, and exercise physiology. Finally, individuals who undergo level 3 training should be able to provide instruction in cardio-oncology to other health care providers interested in expanding their own fund of knowledge of this growing discipline.

Implementation of a cardio-oncology training program

The establishment of cardio-oncology training programs across North America and Europe has been hampered by the lack of formal structure and guidance needed to establish and implement a successful cardio-oncology training program. In this article, the authors have described the core elements required for a cardio-oncology program; however, there is little in the literature to guide program directors on how to implement such a program. A solid infrastructure represents only one key element of a successful program. Although centers may have the necessary tools, including staff, diagnostic equipment, patients, and so forth, for trainees, the implementation of such a training program may be more difficult. Educational institutions face the challenge of balancing clinical workloads of trainees, with established education and research objectives. A successful training program requires support and engagement from the host institution at ALL levels, including the University, hospital administration, senior management, Department of Medicine, and the respective divisions (hematology/oncology and cardiology). Coordination of the cardio-oncology fellowship training program (level 3) should be conducted through the postgraduate training office at the University affiliated with the host institution. In centers/institutions where there is no postgraduate office, linkages need to be established with other centers to facilitate coordination of the planned training program year. Cardio-oncology trainees should have a clear educational plan established at the beginning of their program, including objectives to be achieved, and timelines to follow. A multidisciplinary team, including health care providers with expertise in cardio-oncology, must be an integral part of the trainee's educational program. Ideally, the cardio-oncology team should be in close physical proximity to each other in order to facilitate a multidisciplinary approach. Research projects should be encouraged for all trainees, thus necessitating the need for a listing of potential projects and research supervisors at the beginning of the training program. Evaluations of the trainee should occur on a regular basis. Although regular feedback is appropriate, formal evaluations should take place periodically (every 3 months) to provide the trainee with the greatest opportunity for a successful year. Training requirements for those individuals (eg, family physicians, internists) taking part in level I or II cardio-oncology training are more flexible and thus could be coordinated through the postgraduate education office or respective department/division. In addition, the success of a cardio-oncology curriculum will depend on on-going evaluation and adaptation based on feedback from both the trainees and the multidisciplinary team involved in the program.

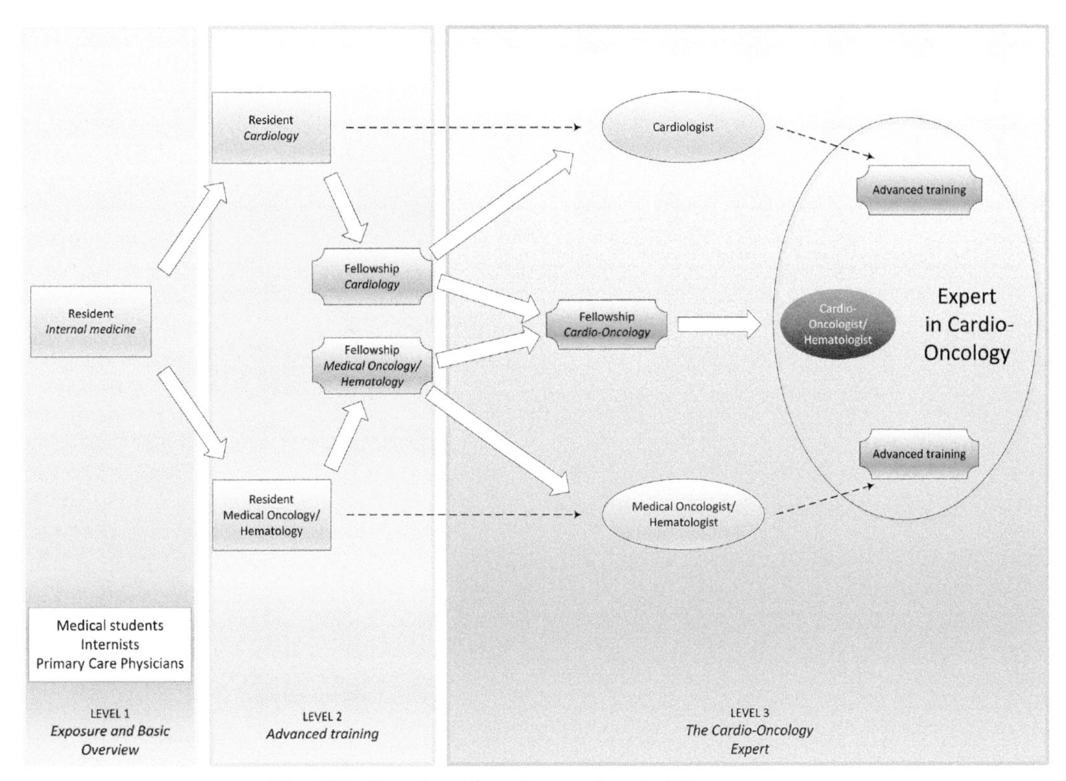

Fig. 23.1 Overview of cardio-oncology training program.

SUMMARY

Cardio-oncology has become a recognized subspecialty over the past decade. The complexity of medical care of patients with cancer with cardiac issues has mandated the existence of a trained multidisciplinary team as an integral component of cancer care from diagnosis to survivorship. An overview of a Cardio-oncology Training Format is illustrated in Fig. 23.1. The most essential element of this is the training of a work force for the future. This chapter discussed the beginning of that process and presented training principles to enable future success.

SUPPLEMENTARY MATERIAL

Go to ExpertConsult.com to listen to an interview with the author.

REFERENCES

1. Barac A, Murtagh G, Carver JR, et al. Cardiovascular health of patients with cancer and cancer survivors: a roadmap to the next level. J Am Coll Cardiol 2015; 65(25):2739–46.
2. COCATS Guidelines. Guidelines for Training in Adult Cardiovascular Medicine, Core Cardiology Training Symposium. June 27-28, 1994. American College of Cardiology. J Am Coll Cardiol 1995; 25(1):1–34.
3. Halperin JL, Williams ES, Fuster V. COCATS 4 Introduction. J Am Coll Cardiol 2015;65(17): 1724–33.
4. Okwuosa TM, Barac A. Burgeoning cardio-oncology programs: challenges and opportunities for early career cardiologists/faculty directors. J Am Coll Cardiol 2015;66(10):1193–7.
5. Harrington RA, Barac A, Brush JE Jr, et al. COCATS 4 task force 15: training in cardiovascular research and scholarly activity. J Am Coll Cardiol 2015; 65(17):1899–906.
6. Li W, Croce K, Steensma DP, et al. Vascular and metabolic implications of novel targeted cancer therapies: focus on kinase inhibitors. J Am Coll Cardiol 2015;66(10):1160–78.
7. Shelburne N, Adhikari B, Brell J, et al. Cancer treatment-related cardiotoxicity: current state of knowledge and future research priorities. J Natl Cancer Inst 2014;106(9). http://dx.doi.org/10.1093/jnci/dju232.
8. Albini A, Pennesi G, Donatelli F, et al. Cardiotoxicity of anticancer drugs: the need for cardio-oncology and cardio-oncological prevention. J Natl Cancer Inst 2010;102(1):14–25.
9. Available at: www.cdc.org. Accessed September 8, 2016.

10. Oeffinger KC, Mertens AC, Sklar CA, et al. Chronic health conditions in adult survivors of childhood cancer. N Engl J Med 2006;355:1572–8.
11. Chatterjee K, Zhang J, Honbo N, et al. Doxorubicin cardiomyopathy. Cardiology 2010;115:155–62.
12. Mertens AC, Liu Q, Neglia JP, et al. Cause-specific late mortality among 5-year survivors of childhood cancer: the Childhood Cancer Survivor Study. J Natl Cancer Inst 2008;100(19):1368–79.
13. Tukenova M, Guibout C, Oberlin O, et al. Role of cancer treatment in long-term overall and cardiovascular mortality after childhood cancer. J Clin Oncol 2010;28(8):1308–15.
14. Lipshultz SE, Alvarez JA, Scully RE. Anthracycline associated cardiotoxicity in survivors of childhood cancer. Heart 2008;94(4):525–33.
15. Lipshultz SE, Colan SD, Gelber RD, et al. Late cardiac effects of doxorubicin therapy for acute lymphoblastic leukemia in childhood. N Engl J Med 1991;324(12):808–15.
16. Jaworski C, Mariani JA, Wheeler G, et al. Cardiac complications of thoracic irradiation. J Am Coll Cardiol 2013;61:2319–28.
17. De Azambuja E, Ameya L, Diaz M, et al. Cardiac assessment of early breast cancer patients 18 years after treatment with cyclophosphamide-, methotrexate-, fluorouracil-, or epirubicin-based chemotherapy. Eur J Cancer 2015;51(17):2517–24.
18. Maraldo MV, Giusti F, Vogelius IR, et al. Cardiovascular disease after treatment for Hodgkin's lymphoma: an analysis of nine collaborative EORTC-LYSA trials. Lancet Haematol 2015;2(11):e492–502.
19. Gupta A, Long JB, Chen J, et al. Risk of vascular toxicity with platinum based chemotherapy in elderly patients with bladder cancer. J Urol 2016;195(1):33–40.
20. van der Pal HJ, van Dalen EC, van Delden E, et al. High risk of symptomatic cardiac events in childhood cancer survivors. J Clin Oncol 2012;30:1429–37.
21. Mertens AC, Liu Q, Neglia JP, et al. Cause-specific late mortality among 5-year survivors of childhood cancer: the Childhood Cancer Survivor Study. J Natl Cancer Inst 2008;100:1368–79.
22. Armstrong GT, Oeffinger KC, Chen Y, et al. Modifiable risk factors and major cardiac events among adult survivors of childhood cancer. J Clin Oncol 2013;31:3673–80.
23. Runowicz CD, Leach CR, Henry NL, et al. American Cancer Society/American Society of Clinical Oncology Breast Cancer Survivorship Care Guideline. CA Cancer J Clin 2016. http://dx.doi.org/10.3322/caac.21319.
24. Ammon M, Arenja N, Leibundgut G, et al. Cardiovascular management of cancer patients with chemotherapy-associated left ventricular systolic dysfunction in real-world clinical practice. J Card Fail 2013;19:629–34.
25. Darby SC, Ewertz M, McGale P, et al. Risk of ischemic heart disease in women after radiotherapy for breast cancer. N Engl J Med 2013;368:987–98.
26. Gyenes G, Rutqvist LE, Liedberg A, et al. Long-term cardiac morbidity and mortality in a randomized trial of pre- and postoperative radiation therapy versus surgery alone in primary breast cancer. Radiother Oncol 1998;48:185–90.
27. Barac A, Murtagh G, Carver JR, et al. Cardiovascular health of patients with cancer and cancer survivors: a roadmap to the next level. J Am Coll Cardiol 2015;65(25):2739–46.
28. Okwuosa TM, Barac A. Burgeoning cardio-oncology programs: challenges and opportunities for early career cardiologists/faculty directors. J Am Coll Cardiol 2015;66(10):1193–7.
29. Yu AF, Ky B. Roadmap for biomarkers of cancer therapy cardiotoxicity. Heart 2016. http://dx.doi.org/10.1136/heartjnl-2015-307894.
30. Calleja A, Poulin F, Khorolsky C, et al. Right ventricular dysfunction in patients experiencing cardiotoxicity during breast cancer therapy. J Oncol 2015;2015:609194.
31. Armstrong GT, Joshi VM, Zhu L, et al. Increased tricuspid regurgitant jet velocity by Doppler echocardiography in adult survivors of childhood cancer: a report from the St Jude Lifetime Cohort Study. J Clin Oncol 2013;31:774–81.
32. Armstrong GT, Joshi VM, Ness KK, et al. Comprehensive echocardiographic detection of treatment-related cardiac dysfunction in adult survivors of childhood cancer: results from the St. Jude Lifetime Cohort Study. J Am Coll Cardiol 2015;65:2511–22.
33. Negishi K, Negishi T, Hare JL, et al. Independent and incremental value of deformation indices for prediction of trastuzumab-induced cardiotoxicity. J Am Soc Echocardiogr 2013;26:493–8.
34. Negishi K, Negishi T, Haluska BA, et al. Use of speckle strain to assess left ventricular responses to cardiotoxic chemotherapy and cardioprotection. Eur Heart J Cardiovasc Imaging 2014;15:324–31.
35. Stanton T, Jenkins C, Haluska BA, et al. Association of outcome with left ventricular parameters measured by two-dimensional and three-dimensional echocardiography in patients at high cardiovascular risk. J Am Soc Echocardiography 2014;27:65–73.
36. Thavendiranathan P, Grant AD, Negishi T, et al. Reproducibility of echocardiographic techniques for sequential assessment of left ventricular ejection fraction and volumes: application to patients undergoing cancer chemotherapy. J Am Coll Cardiol 2013;61:77–84.

37. Thavendiranathan P, Wintersperger BJ, Flamm SD, et al. Cardiac MRI in the assessment of cardiac injury and toxicity from cancer chemotherapy: a systematic review. Circ Cardiovasc Imaging 2013;6:1080–91.
38. Kongbundansuk S, Hundley WG. Noninvasive imaging of cardiovascular injury related to the treatment of cancer. JACC Cardiovasc Imaging 2014;7:824–38.
39. Pizzino F, Vizzari G, Qamar R, et al. Multimodality imaging in cardiooncology. J Oncol 2015;2015:263950.
40. Thavendiranathan P, Poulin F, Lim K, et al. Use of myocardial strain imaging by echocardiography for the early detection of cardiotoxicity in patients during and after cancer chemotherapy: a systematic review. J Am Coll Cardiol 2014;63(25 Pt A):2751–68.
41. Villarraga HR, Herrmann J, Nkomo VT. Cardio-oncology: role of echocardiography. Prog Cardiovasc Dis 2014;57:10–8.
42. Grover S, Lou PW, Bradbrook C, et al. Early and late changes in markers of aortic stiffness with breast cancer therapy. Intern Med J 2015;45(2):140–7.
43. Myers C. The role of iron in doxorubicin-induced cardiomyopathy. Semin Oncol 1998;25(4 Suppl 10):10–4.
44. Xu X, Persson HL, Richardson DR. Molecular pharmacology of the interaction of anthracyclines with iron. Mol Pharmacol 2005;68(2):261–71.

Appendix: Drug Guide

CHEMOTHERAPEUTIC DRUG/TREATMENT GUIDE

The number of drugs used in cancer therapy is ever increasing. Still, several classes remain key elements in treatment regimens with a defined cardiovascular toxicity profile. One of the best examples are the anthracyclines, which also could be labeled as antitumor antibiotics based on their discovery, and topoisomerase inhibitors, based on their mechanism. Table 1 summarizes these classes of drugs. Alkylating agents are the next major historical class of chemotherapeutics with known cardiovascular side effects (Table 2), followed by the antimetabolites (Table 3) and the microtubule-targeting agents (Table 4). Monoclonal antibodies (Table 5) have taken an important role in modern-day cancer therapy as have tyrosine kinase inhibitors (Table 6). Biological response modifiers and differentiating agents (Table 7) as well as other miscellaneous drugs (Table 8) complete the list. For each of the agents within these classes of drugs, the main therapeutic indication (malignancy it is used for) is outlined followed by a listing of known mechanisms of cardiovascular toxicity, its risk factors and presentations, as well as prevention/risk reduction strategies. These tables are intended to serve as a reference to the main cardiovascular disease manifestations of chemotherapeutics. They might also prove useful as a quick guide at the bedside when reviewing and discussing the cardiovascular toxicity profile of any given or planned chemotherapy regimen.

TABLE 1
Anticancer treatment, mechanisms, risk factors, manifestations, and prevention of cardiotoxicity with anthracycline and nonanthracycline antibiotic and topoisomerase inhibitors

Treatments/Drugs	Max Limited Dose (mg/m^2)	Therapeutic Indication	Mechanisms of Cardiotoxicity	Risk Factors	Manifestations of Cardiotoxicity	Prevention & Risk Reduction Strategies
Anthracycline and analogues						
Doxorubicin Daunorubicin Epirubicin Idarubicin	450–500 400–550 800–900 60	Breast cancer Gastric tumor Leukemias Lymphomas Lung cancer Ovarian tumor Sarcomas	↑Toxic oxygen free radical production ↑Oxidative stress Lipid peroxidation of membrane ↓Endogenous antioxidant enzymes Intracellular iron accumulation DNA damage Topoisomerase IIb inhibition Cellular apoptosis Replacement fibrosis	• Concurrent chemotherapy • Prior/concurrent chest radiation • High dose per cycle (>50 mg/m^2) • High cumulative dose (≥300 mg/m^2 of doxorubicin, ≥600 mg/m^2 of epirubicin) • IV bolus • Extreme age (elderly >65, children <18) • Woman, pregnancy • Pre-existing CV disease (CAD, HT, LV dysfunction) • Hematopoietic stem cell transplantation	Acute (initial to several weeks after Tx) • Arrhythmia (AF, SVT, VT, CHB, Mobitz II) • ST-T wave abnormalities • Anginal pain • LV dysfunction/CHF • Pericarditis/ myocarditis • Myocardial ischemia/infarction Chronic (early within 1 y and late onset beyond 1 y after Tx) • Asymptomatic diastolic/systolic dysfunction, overt HF • Dilated cardiomyopathy • Stroke	• Limiting lifetime cumulative dose • Structural modification (liposomal encapsulated formulation) & prolonged infusion (>6 h) • CV risk assessment before start of chemotherapy • Intensive monitoring of cardiac function during & after Tx • F/U ECG if QRS in limb leads ↓≥30% as associated with cardiomyopathy (daunorubicin) • Adjunctive cardioprotective agent Dexrazoxane β-Blocker (carvedilol, nebivolol) ACE-I/ARB Spironolactone Statins

Mitoxantrone	140	Breast cancer NHL, AML Multiple sclerosis	↑Toxic oxygen free radical ↑Oxidative stress	• Concurrent chemotherapy • Prior/concurrent chest irradiation • High cumulative dose	Pericarditis-myocarditis syndrome CHF, arrhythmias Myocardial ischemia/infarction	• Limiting lifetime cumulative dose • CV risk assessment before start of chemotherapy • Intensive monitoring of cardiac function during and after treatment

Treatments/Drugs	Therapeutic Indication	Mechanisms of Cardiotoxicity	Risk Factors	Manifestations of Cardiotoxicity	Prevention & Risk Reduction Strategies
Non-Anthracycline Chemotherapy					
Antitumor Antibiotics		Unknown	• High cumulative dose >30 mg/m^2 [mytomycin C] • Concomitant with anthracycline or nonanthracycline based chemotherapy • Prior coronary artery disease	CHF Substernal chest pain Pericarditis (Bleomycin) Myocardial ischemia/infarction (Bleomycin) Interstitial pneumonitis/fibrosis/pulmonary hypertension (Bleomycin)	• Dose adjustment and limitation of other chemotherapies • Supportive care • Termination of treatment in case of pericarditis due to bleomycin
Mitomycin C Bleomycin	Gastric cancer Pancreatic cancer Bladder cancer Lung cancer Lymphomas Germ cell tumors Squamous cell CA				
Topoisomerase Inhibitors		Coronary artery vasospasm Direct injury to the myocardium Immune response induction	• Concurrent chemotherapy (esp. bleomycin, cisplatin, ifosfamide) • Pre-existing CV disease	Myocardial ischemia/infarction	Unknown
Etoposide	Testicular cancer SCLC Hematologic cancer				

Abbreviations: ACE-1, angiotensin-converting-enzyme inhibitor; AF, atrial fibrillation; AML, acute myeloid leukemia; ARB, angiotensin receptor blocker; CAD, coronary artery disease; CHB, complete heart block; CHF, congestive heart failure; CV, cardiovascular; ECG, electrocardiogram; HF, heart failure; HT, hormone therapy; IV, intravenous; LV, left ventricular; NHL, non-Hodgkin lymphoma; SVT, supraventricular tachycardia; VT, ventricular tachycardia.

Modified from Kongbundansuk S, Hundley WG. Noninvasive imaging of cardiovascular injury related to the treatment of cancer. JACC Cardiovasc Imaging 2014;7(8):824–38.

TABLE 2
Anticancer treatment, mechanisms, risk factors, manifestations, and prevention of cardiotoxicity with alkylating agents

Treatments/Drugs	Therapeutic Indication	Mechanisms of Cardiotoxicity	Risk Factors	Manifestations of Cardiotoxicity	Prevention & Risk Reduction Strategies
Cyclophosphamide	Leukemias Lymphomas Various solid tumors	Endothelial capillary damage	• High dose (not related to cumulative dose) • Elderly • Prior abnormal ejection fraction • Prior irradiation to chest wall • Prior anthracyclines	Hemorrhagic myocarditis/ pericarditis (common 1st week after cyclophosphamide) Pericardial effusion/ tamponade LV dysfunction/CHF LVH	• Corticosteroid & analgesic with termination of treatment • Dose adjustment
Ifosfamide	Lymphomas Various solid tumors	Myocardial fiber fragmentation	• High-dose regimen • Use for lymphoma	Arrhythmias, ST-T wave change CHF	• Dose adjustment • ECG monitoring
Busulfan	CML	Unknown	Unknown	Endocardial/pulmonary fibrosis HTN, arrhythmias Pericardial effusion	Unknown
Cisplatin	Germ cell tumors Ovarian cancer Lymphomas Head/neck tumors Lung cancer Sarcomas	Anaphylaxis and hypersensitivity reaction Endothelial injury/apoptosis Arterial thrombosis Vascular fibrosis E'lyte disturbance (hypokalemia, hypomagnesemia)	• Elderly • Prior mediastinal irradiation • Use for metastatic testicular cancer • Use with cyclophosphamide	Early manifestation • Myocardial ischemia/ infarction • CHF Late manifestation • Myocardial ischemia/ infarction • HTN, stroke, LVH • Arrhythmia (SVT, bradycardia, LBBB) • LV dysfunction/CHF • Ischemic cardiomyopathy • Vascular toxicity • Raynaud's phenomenon	• Adequate hydration and fluid balance • E'lyte check-up and correction • Avoid concomitant renally toxic drug • Continuous infusion with monitoring for hypersensitivity reaction

Abbreviations: CHF, congestive heart failure; CML, chronic myelogenous leukemia; ECG, electrocardiogram; HTN, hypertension; LBBB, left bundle branch block; LV, left ventricular; LVH, left ventricular hypertrophy; SVT, supraventricular tachycardia.

Modified from Kongbundansuk S, Hundley WG. Noninvasive imaging of cardiovascular injury related to the treatment of cancer. JACC Cardiovasc Imaging 2014;7(8):824–38.

TABLE 3
Anticancer treatment, mechanisms, risk factors, manifestations, and prevention of cardiotoxicity with antimetabolites

Treatments/Drugs	Therapeutic Indication	Mechanisms of Cardiotoxicity	Risk Factors	Manifestations of Cardiotoxicity	Prevention & Risk Reduction Strategies
Fluorouracil (5-FU) Capecitabine	Breast cancer Colorectal cancer Pancreatic cancer	Myocardial ischemia due to • Coronary vasoconstriction (alteration of PKC signaling in vascular smooth muscle cells and endothelial injury) • Increased cardiac metabolism • Oxidative stress • Diminished ability of RBCs to transfer oxygen • Exaggerated sympathetic drive	• Underlying CV disease • Infusion length and dose both long term & short term • Previous treatment with 5-FU (Capecitabine) • Concomitant chemotherapy	Chest pain/angina (5-FU) Myocardial ischemia/ infarction Myocarditis/pericarditis CHF Stress-induced cardiomyopathy (Takotsubo) (5-FU)	• Termination of treatment (reversible), retreatment after symptom improvement • IV bolus regimen, lower dose regimen • Antianginal treatment • Prophylactic coronary vasodilator therapy (limited efficacy)
Fludarabine Pentostatin Cladribine Cytarabine Methotrexate (MTX)	Leukemias Lymphomas Various solid tumors Autoimmune disease	Unknown	Unknown	Pericarditis (pericardial effusion/tamponade) (cytarabine) Arrhythmia (bradycardia, supra/ventricular arrhythmia) (MTX) Hypotension/chest pain (Fludarabine) Myocardial ischemia/ infarction CHF	• Termination of treatment (reversible), retreatment after symptom improvement • Steroid treatment in case of pericarditis from cytarabine • Antianginal treatment • Prophylactic coronary vasodilator therapy (limited efficacy)

Abbreviations: CHF, congestive heart failure; CV, cardiovascular; IV, intravenous; PKC, protein kinase C; RBC, red blood cells.
Modified from Kongbundansuk S, Hundley WG. Noninvasive imaging of cardiovascular injury related to the treatment of cancer. JACC Cardiovasc Imaging 2014;7(8):824–38.

TABLE 4
Anticancer treatment, mechanisms, risk factors, manifestations, and prevention of cardiotoxicity with microtubule-targeting agents

Treatments/Drugs	Therapeutic Indication	Mechanisms of Cardiotoxicity	Risk Factors	Manifestations of Cardiotoxicity	Prevention & Risk Reduction Strategies
Vinca alkaloids Vinblastine Vincristine Vinorelbine	Leukemias Lymphomas Nephroblastoma TTP/chronic ITP Breast cancer SCLC	Possible coronary vasospasm and thrombosis Endothelial injury/ apoptosis	Unknown	Hypertension Myocardial ischemia/ infarction Vaso-occlusive complication Raynaud phenomenon	Unknown
Taxane derivative Paclitaxel Docetaxel Eribulin Ixabepilone	Breast cancer Ovarian cancer NSCLC Kaposi sarcoma Prostate cancer Gastric adenocarcinoma	Possible coronary vasospasm Endothelial injury Anaphylaxis and hypersensitivity reaction	• Congenital long QT syndrome • Concomitant chemotherapy • Concomitant QTc prolonging drugs • Underlying CV disease	Conduction abnormalities (bradycardia, CHB) Arrhythmia (SVT), angina QTc prolongation (Eribulin) Myocardial ischemia/ infarction Ventricular dysfunction Hypotension	• Pretreatment with corticosteroid, H1 and H2 blocker • Dose adjustment and limitation of anthracycline • ECG monitoring (Paclitaxel, Eribulin) • Continuous infusion with monitoring for hypersensitivity reaction

Abbreviations: CHB, complete heart block; CV, cardiovascular; ECG, electrocardiogram; ITP, idiopathic thrombocytopenic purpura; SCLC, small cell lung carcinoma; SVT, supraventricular tachycardia; TTP, thrombotic thrombocytopenic purpura.

Modified from Kongbundansuk S, Hundley WG. Noninvasive imaging of cardiovascular injury related to the treatment of cancer. JACC Cardiovasc Imaging 2014;7(8):824–38.

TABLE 5
Mechanisms, risk factors, manifestations, and prevention of cardiotoxicity with monoclonal antibodies

Treatments/ Drugs	Therapeutic Indication	Mechanisms of Cardiotoxicity	Risk Factors	Manifestations of Cardiotoxicity	Prevention & Risk Reduction Strategies
Trastuzumab Pertuzumab	Breast cancer Gastric cancer Esophageal cancer	Inhibition of the HER2 signaling stress adaptation pathway Hypersensitivity reaction Anaphylaxis	• Prior or concurrent anthracycline use (cumulative doxorubicin dose equivalent >300 mg/m^2) • Pre-existing poor LV function • Age >50 y • High BMI • Women with underlying DM • Antihypertensive treatment	Asymptomatic LV dysfunction Anaphylactic reaction CHF, nonischemic cardiomyopathy Arrhythmias Myocardial ischemia/ infarction	• Limiting prior dose of anthracyclines • Increasing time interval from anthracycline treatment • Avoidance of myocardial ischemia and severe systemic hypertension • Temporary hold or termination of treatment based on clinical scenario • Continuous infusion with monitoring for hypersensitivity reaction • Monitoring per consensus guidelines (baseline and every 3 months on therapy, and 6 months after if prior anthracycline) • cTn elevation may predict risk and prognosis (irreversibility)
Rituximab	Lymphomas Leukemias Autoimmune Ds	Unknown Anaphylaxis and hypersensitivity reaction	• Pre-existing CV disease • High number of circulating malignant cells (≥25,000/ mm^3) with or without evidence of high tumor burden	Angina Arrhythmia (ventricular fibrillation) Myocardial ischemia/ infarction Takotsubo/apical balloon syndrome Cardiogenic shock	• Termination of treatment (reversible) • Continuous infusion with infusion monitoring for hypersensitivity reaction

(continued on next page)

TABLE 5
(continued)

Treatments/ Drugs	Therapeutic Indication	Mechanisms of Cardiotoxicity	Risk Factors	Manifestations of Cardiotoxicity	Prevention & Risk Reduction Strategies
Bevacizumab	Colorectal cancer Glioblastoma Breast cancer NSCLC RCC	Unknown Possible exacerbation of pre-existing coronary and peripheral arterial disease Endothelial dysfunction Infusion hypersensitivity reaction	• Pre-existing CV disease • Prior or concurrent anthracyclines • Age >65 y • Previous arterial thrombo-embolic event	Angina, dyspnea Myocardial ischemia/ infarction Stroke, arterial thromboembolic event Severe hypertension CHF	• Monitoring BP during and after treatment • Infusion monitoring for hy-persensitivity reaction
Alemtuzumab	Lymphoma Leukemias Multiple Sclerosis GVHD	Unknown Anaphylaxis and hypersensitivity reaction	Unknown	Hypotension, cardiogenic shock Arrhythmia (AF, VT) CHF Myocardial ischemia/ infarction	• Termination of treatment (reversible) • Continuous infusion with monitoring for hypersensi-tivity reaction • Premedication with cortico-steroid and H1 and H2 blockers
Cetuximab	Colorectal cancer Head/neck tumors	Unknown Anaphylaxis and hypersensitivity reaction E'lyte imbalance (hypomagnesemia)	Pre-existing CV disease (previous CAD, HTN, LV dysfunction or arrhythmia)	Arrhythmia, QTc prolongation CHF Myocardial ischemia/ infarction Sudden cardiac arrest	• Termination of treatment (reversible) • Continuous infusion with monitoring for hypersensi-tivity reaction • Monitor and correction of serum e'lyte and magnesium • Dose modification

Abbreviations: AF, atrial fibrillation; BMI, body mass index; BP, blood pressure; CAD, coronary artery disease; CHF, congestive heart failure; cTn, cardiac troponin; CV, cardiovascular; DM, diabetes mellitus; GVHD, graft-versus-host disease; HTN, hypertension; ITP, idiopathic thrombocytopenic purpura; LV, left ventricular; NCLC, non–small-cell lung carcinoma; RCC, renal cell carcinoma; VT, ventricular tachycardia.

Modified from Kongbundansuk S, Hundley WG. Noninvasive imaging of cardiovascular injury related to the treatment of cancer. JACC Cardiovasc Imaging 2014;7(8):824–38.

TABLE 6
Mechanisms, risk factors, manifestations, and prevention of cardiotoxicity with multi-targeted tyrosine kinase inhibitors

Treatments/ Drugs	Therapeutic Indication	Mechanisms of Cardiotoxicity	Risk Factors	Manifestations of Cardiotoxicity	Prevention & Risk Reduction Strategies
Sorafenib Sunitinib Pazaponib Axitinib Lenvatinib	RCC/HCC/GIST Pancreatic neuroendocrine tumors Melanoma Thyroid cancer	Inhibition of ribosomal S6 kinase Inhibition of RAF1 kinase activity Activation of apoptotic pathways resulting in myocyte loss ATP depletion leading to LV dysfunction	History of HTN and CAD	Arrhythmias (bradycardia) Prolongation of QTc/ ST-T changes LV dysfunction/CHF Angina, ACS, and stroke DVT/PE HTN	• Termination of treatment (reversible) • Monitoring of EKG and LV function • Cardiac troponin (and BNP) monitoring
Regorafenib	Colorectal cancers GIST	Unknown	Pre-existing CV disease	Myocardial ischemia/ infarction (rare)	Unknown
Vandetanib	Medullary thyroid cancer Breast/lung cancers CML/CEL/ALL Mesothelioma	Unknown	• Congenital long QT syndrome • E'lyte imbalance, hypocalcemia, and hypomagnesemia • Concurrent use of drugs that prolong the QTc interval	Prolongation of QTc/ torsades de pointes/SCD LV dysfunction/CHF HTN	• Termination of treatment (reversible) • Monitoring of EKG and QTc interval prior and during treatment • Correction of serum e'lyte, Ca and Mg before and during treatment • Avoidance of concurrent use of drugs with properties to prolong QTc or strongly inhibit CYP3A4
Imatinib Dasatinib Bosutinib Nilotinib Ponatinib	GIST CML	Mitochondrial dysfunction Decline in ATP concentration Endothelial dysfunction	• Pre-existing CV disease • Congenital long QT syndrome • E'lyte imbalance, hypocalcemia, and hypomagnesemia • Concurrent use of drugs that prolong the QTc interval	Prolongation of QTc Systolic and diastolic dysfunction Chest pain, HT Pericardial effusion Fatal myocardial ischemia/infarction, critical limb ischemia, and stroke (nilotinib and ponatinib) LV dysfunction/CHF	• Dose reduction of termination • Monitoring EKG and LV function • Correction of serum e'lyte and Mg before and during treatment • Avoidance of concurrent use of drugs with properties to prolong QTc or strongly inhibit CYP3A4

(continued on next page)

TABLE 6
(*continued*)

Treatments/ Drugs	Therapeutic Indication	Mechanisms of Cardiotoxicity	Risk Factors	Manifestations of Cardiotoxicity	Prevention & Risk Reduction Strategies
Lapatinib	Breast cancer Brain cancer	Unknown (rare cardiotoxicity, usually occurs in combination with other cardiotoxic agents)	Concurrent use of systemic cardiotoxic agents	Prinzmetal angina LV dysfunction/CHF	• Termination of treatment (reversible) • Dose adjustment and limitation of other chemotherapies
Crizotinib Vemurafenib	NSCLC Melanoma	Unknown	• Congenital long QT syndrome • E'lyte imbalance and hypomagnesemia • Concurrent drugs that prolong QTc interval	Severe sinus bradycardia (≤45 bpm) (Crizotinib) Arrhythmia, QTc prolongation, torsades de pointes CHF, hypotension, syncope (Crizotinib)	• Termination of treatment (reversible) • QTc >500 ms during treatment advice for termination of Tx • Monitoring of EKG & correction of e'lyte and Mg before and during Tx • Avoidance of concurrent use of drugs with properties to prolong QTc or strongly inhibit CYP3A4

Abbreviations: ALL, acute lymphoblastic leukemia; CAD, coronary artery disease; CEL, chronic eosinophilic leukemia; CHF, congestive heart failure; CML, chronic myelogenous leukemia; CYP3A4, cytochrome p450 3a4; DVT, deep vein thrombosis; EKG, electrocardiogram; GIST, gastrointestinal stroma tumor; HCC, hepatocellular carcinoma; HTN, hypertension; LV, left ventricular; NCLC, non–small-cell lung carcinoma; PE, pulmonary embolism; RCC, renal cell carcinoma; SCD, sudden cardiac death.

Modified from Kongbundansuk S, Hundley WG. Noninvasive imaging of cardiovascular injury related to the treatment of cancer. JACC Cardiovasc Imaging 2014;7(8):824–38.

TABLE 7
Anticancer treatment, mechanisms, risk factors, manifestations, and prevention of cardiotoxicity with biological response modifiers and differentiation agents

Treatments/ Drugs	Therapeutic Indication	Mechanisms of Cardiotoxicity	Risk Factors	Manifestations of Cardiotoxicity	Prevention & Risk Reduction Strategies
Interferon-α	Leukemia Lymphomas Melanoma Various solid tumor	Unknown Complex of interferon and cardiac tissue stimulating an autoimmune or inflammatory reaction (unclear mechanism)	• Pre-existing CV disease • History of CAD disease	Early manifestation • Arrhythmias (supraventricular/ventricular) and heart block • Sudden cardiac death (case report) • Hypertension • Acute pericarditis (effusion/tamponade, high dose related case report) Late manifestation • LV dysfunction/CHF • Dilated cardiomyopathy	Termination of treatment (reversible)
Interleukin-2	Melanoma RCC	Capillary leakage syndrome with increased vascular permeability (high dose) Direct myocardial toxicity (unclear mechanism)	Unknown	Early manifestation • Hypotension (↓SVR, ↑HR)-peak at 4 h after Tx • Arrhythmias (SVT/VT) • Myocarditis • Thrombotic events Late manifestation • Dilated cardiomyopathy	• Termination of treatment (reversible) • Hydration/fluid replacement • Vasopressors as indicated
Denileukin difitox	Lymphomas Leukemias	Fatal capillary leakage syndrome Hypersensitivity reaction	Pre-existing CV disease	Hypotension, tachycardia Chest pain Myocardial ischemia/infarction Arrhythmias CHF	• Termination of treatment (reversible) • Continuous infusion with monitoring for hypersensitivity reaction
All-trans retinoic acid Arsenic trioxide (ATO)	Leukemias (AML esp. in acute promyeloblastic leukemia)	Direct myocyte injury and damage ↑Oxidative stress and DNA fragmentation ↑Apoptosis of myocardial cells Capillary leakage syndrome	• WBC $\geq$10,000/mm^3 • Rapidly increasing WBC count • Presence of CD13 expression on leukemic cells • Hypokalemia, Hypomagnesemia (ATO)	Differentiation syndrome (Both) • Hypotension • CHF/pulmonary edema • Pericardial effusion/tamponade • Myocardial ischemia/infarction QTc prolongation/torsades de pointes/SCD (ATO)	• Prompt IV corticosteroid • Continue chemotherapy (termination recommended only in case of severe differentiation syndrome) • General supportive care (oxygen, diuretic) • Monitoring of EKG and correction of serum e'lyte and magnesium (ATO) • Resveratrol treatment (ATO-case report)

Abbreviations: AML, acute myeloid leukemia; CAD, coronary artery disease; CHF, congestive heart failure; CV, cardiovascular; EKG, electrocardiogram; HR, heart rate; LV, left ventricular; SVR, stroke volume ratio; SVT, supraventricular tachycardia; VT, ventricular tachycardia; WBC, white blood cells.

Modified from Kongbundansuk S, Hundley WG. Noninvasive imaging of cardiovascular injury related to the treatment of cancer. JACC Cardiovasc Imaging 2014;7(8):824–38.

TABLE 8
Mechanisms, risk factors, manifestations, and prevention of cardiotoxicity with miscellaneous agents

Treatments/ Drugs	Therapeutic Indication	Mechanisms of Cardiotoxicity	Risk Factors	Manifestations of Cardiotoxicity	Prevention & Risk Reduction Strategies
Diethylstilbestrol Estramustine	Breast cancer Prostate cancer	Unknown Estrogen-related CV side effects	Pre-existing CV disease	Arterial thrombosis-myocardial ischemia/infarct/stroke Venous thrombosis-DVT, PE Hypertension ↑CV death	• Use with precaution in patient with CV risk factors • Diethylstilbestrol: no longer available in US due to teratogenic effect
Proteasome inhibitors • Bortezomib • Carfilzomib	Multiple myeloma Mantel cell lymphoma	Decreased ATP synthesis Decreased cardiac myocyte contractility Protein accumulation Relaxation impairment	• Pre-existing CV disease and cardiovascular risk factors • Concurrent systemic cardiotoxic chemotherapies • Concomitant with drug-associated hypotension	Orthostatic hypotension, syncope Arrhythmia (bradycardia, heart block, AF) New-onset/worsening pre-existing HF (diastolic and systolic) Myocardial ischemia/infarction Pulmonary arterial hypertension Cardiac arrest	• Optimization of CV risk factor and disease (eg, hypertension) • Dose modification or termination • Cautious use in patients with a history of syncope • Avoidance of dehydration
Histone deacetylase inhibitors (HDAC-I) • Vorinostat • Romidepsin	T-cell lymphoma NSCLC	Unknown	• Pre-existing CV disease • Congenital long QT syndrome • Concurrent drugs that prolong QTc interval or inhibit CYP3A4 • E'lyte disturbance or hypomagnesemia	Prolongation of QTc, ST-T changes [transient changes] Arrhythmias [supraventricular/ventricular] Hypotension, syncope DVT	• No routine EKG monitoring, only in high-risk individuals • Correction of e'lyte, including magnesium, levels before start of medication • Avoidance of concurrent use of drugs with QTc prolonging or CYP3A4 inhibition potential

Abbreviations: AF, atrial fibrillation; CV, cardiovascular; CYP3A4, cytochrome p450 3a4; DVT, deep vein thrombosis; EKG, electrocardiogram; HF, heart failure; NCLC, non–small-cell lung carcinoma; PE, pulmonary embolism.

Modified from Kongbundansuk S, Hundley WG. Noninvasive imaging of cardiovascular injury related to the treatment of cancer. JACC Cardiovasc Imaging 2014;7(8):824–38.

Index

Note: Page numbers of article titles are in **boldface** type.

Q

T